Molecular Pathways in Cancers

Molecular Pathways in Cancers

Editors

Ion Cristóbal
Marta Rodríguez

MDPI • Basel • Beijing • Wuhan • Barcelona • Belgrade • Manchester • Tokyo • Cluj • Tianjin

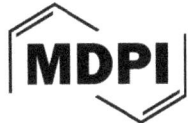

Editors
Ion Cristóbal
Translational Oncology Division
Health Research
Institute-Fundacion Jimenez
Diaz-UAM, Oncohealth Institute
Madrid
Spain

Marta Rodríguez
Pathology
Health Research
Institute-Fundacion Jimenez
Diaz-UAM
Madrid
Spain

Editorial Office
MDPI
St. Alban-Anlage 66
4052 Basel, Switzerland

This is a reprint of articles from the Special Issue published online in the open access journal *Cancers* (ISSN 2072-6694) (available at: www.mdpi.com/journal/cancers/special_issues/MP-Cancers).

For citation purposes, cite each article independently as indicated on the article page online and as indicated below:

LastName, A.A.; LastName, B.B.; LastName, C.C. Article Title. *Journal Name* **Year**, *Volume Number*, Page Range.

ISBN 978-3-0365-3682-8 (Hbk)
ISBN 978-3-0365-3681-1 (PDF)

© 2022 by the authors. Articles in this book are Open Access and distributed under the Creative Commons Attribution (CC BY) license, which allows users to download, copy and build upon published articles, as long as the author and publisher are properly credited, which ensures maximum dissemination and a wider impact of our publications.

The book as a whole is distributed by MDPI under the terms and conditions of the Creative Commons license CC BY-NC-ND.

Contents

Preface to "Molecular Pathways in Cancers" vii

Marta Rodríguez and Ion Cristóbal
Advances in the Knowledge of the Molecular Pathogenesis of High-Prevalence Tumors and Its Relevance for Their Future Clinical Management
Reprinted from: *Cancers* **2021**, *13*, 6053, doi:10.3390/cancers13236053 1

Javier Martinez-Useros, Mario Martin-Galan, Maria Florez-Cespedes and Jesus Garcia-Foncillas
Epigenetics of Most Aggressive Solid Tumors: Pathways, Targets and Treatments
Reprinted from: *Cancers* **2021**, *13*, 3209, doi:10.3390/cancers13133209 5

Rohit Gundamaraju, Wenying Lu and Rishya Manikam
Revisiting Mitochondria Scored Cancer Progression and Metastasis
Reprinted from: *Cancers* **2021**, *13*, 432, doi:10.3390/cancers13030432 33

Maria Isaguliants, Ekaterina Bayurova, Darya Avdoshina, Alla Kondrashova, Francesca Chiodi and Joel M. Palefsky
Oncogenic Effects of HIV-1 Proteins, Mechanisms Behind
Reprinted from: *Cancers* **2021**, *13*, 305, doi:10.3390/cancers13020305 47

Yaiza Senent, Daniel Ajona, Antonio González-Martín, Ruben Pio and Beatriz Tavira
The Complement System in Ovarian Cancer: An Underexplored Old Path
Reprinted from: *Cancers* **2021**, *13*, 3806, doi:10.3390/cancers13153806 71

Naoshi Nishida
Role of Oncogenic Pathways on the Cancer Immunosuppressive Microenvironment and Its Clinical Implications in Hepatocellular Carcinoma
Reprinted from: *Cancers* **2021**, *13*, 3666, doi:10.3390/cancers13153666 91

Ana Guijarro-Hernández and José Luis Vizmanos
A Broad Overview of Signaling in *Ph*-Negative Classic Myeloproliferative Neoplasms
Reprinted from: *Cancers* **2021**, *13*, 984, doi:10.3390/cancers13050984 107

Kyoung-Jin Lee, Yuri Kim, Min Seo Kim, Hyun-Mi Ju, Boyoung Choi and Hansoo Lee et al.
CD99–PTPN12 Axis Suppresses Actin Cytoskeleton-Mediated Dimerization of Epidermal Growth Factor Receptor
Reprinted from: *Cancers* **2020**, *12*, 2895, doi:10.3390/cancers12102895 131

María del Mar Noblejas-López, Igor López-Cade, Jesús Fuentes-Antrás, Gonzalo Fernández-Hinojal, Ada Esteban-Sánchez and Aránzazu Manzano et al.
Genomic Mapping of Splicing-Related Genes Identify Amplifications in *LSM1*, *CLNS1A*, and *ILF2* in Luminal Breast Cancer
Reprinted from: *Cancers* **2021**, *13*, 4118, doi:10.3390/cancers13164118 155

Marta Sanz-Álvarez, Ion Cristóbal, Melani Luque, Andrea Santos, Sandra Zazo and Juan Madoz-Gúrpide et al.
Expression of Phosphorylated BRD4 Is Markedly Associated with the Activation Status of the PP2A Pathway and Shows a Strong Prognostic Value in Triple Negative Breast Cancer Patients
Reprinted from: *Cancers* **2021**, *13*, 1246, doi:10.3390/cancers13061246 171

Marta Sanz-Álvarez, Ester Martín-Aparicio, Melani Luque, Sandra Zazo, Javier Martínez-Useros and Pilar Eroles et al.
The Novel Oral mTORC1/2 Inhibitor TAK-228 Reverses Trastuzumab Resistance in HER2-Positive Breast Cancer Models
Reprinted from: *Cancers* **2021**, *13*, 2778, doi:10.3390/cancers13112778 183

Desirée Martínez-Martínez, María-Val Toledo Lobo, Pablo Baquero, Santiago Ropero, Javier C. Angulo and Antonio Chiloeches et al.
Downregulation of Snail by DUSP1 Impairs Cell Migration and Invasion through the Inactivation of JNK and ERK and Is Useful as a Predictive Factor in the Prognosis of Prostate Cancer
Reprinted from: *Cancers* **2021**, *13*, 1158, doi:10.3390/cancers13051158 207

Md Imtiaz Khalil, Ishita Ghosh, Vibha Singh, Jing Chen, Haining Zhu and Arrigo De Benedetti
NEK1 Phosphorylation of YAP Promotes Its Stabilization and Transcriptional Output
Reprinted from: *Cancers* **2020**, *12*, 3666, doi:10.3390/cancers12123666 229

Vasiliki Papadaki, Ken Asada, Julie K. Watson, Toshiya Tamura, Alex Leung and Jack Hopkins et al.
Two Secreted Proteoglycans, Activators of Urothelial Cell–Cell Adhesion, Negatively Contribute to Bladder Cancer Initiation and Progression
Reprinted from: *Cancers* **2020**, *12*, 3362, doi:10.3390/cancers12113362 247

Preface to "Molecular Pathways in Cancers"

Despite continuous advances in anticancer therapies, the survival rates in most tumor types remain very poor, especially in those patients with advanced stages of the disease, due to a complex network of alterations that change and increase the oncogenic behaviour of tumor cells. Therefore, a better understanding of the main molecular mechanisms that govern the different human cancer types is and will be the best strategy to improve patient outcomes.

Ion Cristóbal and Marta Rodríguez
Editors

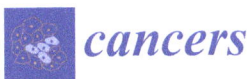

Editorial

Advances in the Knowledge of the Molecular Pathogenesis of High-Prevalence Tumors and Its Relevance for Their Future Clinical Management

Marta Rodríguez [1,2,*,†] and Ion Cristóbal [3,4,*,†]

1. Pathology Department, IIS-Fundación Jiménez Díaz-UAM, E-28040 Madrid, Spain
2. Center for the Biomedical Research Network in Oncology (CIBERONC), E-28040 Madrid, Spain
3. Cancer Unit for Research on Novel Therapeutic Targets, Oncohealth Institute, IIS-Fundación Jiménez Díaz-UAM, E-28040 Madrid, Spain
4. Translational Oncology Division, Oncohealth Institute, IIS-Fundación Jiménez Díaz-UAM, E-28040 Madrid, Spain
* Correspondence: marta.rodriguezm@quironsalud.es (M.R.); ion.cristobal@fjd.es (I.C.); Tel.: +34-91-550-4800 (ext. 2057) (M.R.); +34-91-550-4800 (ext. 2820) (I.C.)
† These authors have contributed equally to this work.

Citation: Rodríguez, M.; Cristóbal, I. Advances in the Knowledge of the Molecular Pathogenesis of High-Prevalence Tumors and Its Relevance for Their Future Clinical Management. *Cancers* **2021**, *13*, 6053. https://doi.org/10.3390/cancers13236053

Received: 22 November 2021
Accepted: 24 November 2021
Published: 1 December 2021

Publisher's Note: MDPI stays neutral with regard to jurisdictional claims in published maps and institutional affiliations.

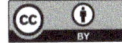

Copyright: © 2021 by the authors. Licensee MDPI, Basel, Switzerland. This article is an open access article distributed under the terms and conditions of the Creative Commons Attribution (CC BY) license (https://creativecommons.org/licenses/by/4.0/).

This Special Issue aims to include relevant works that increase our knowledge about the molecular pathways that govern the development and progression of high-prevalence human cancers, which are responsible for most cancer-related deaths worldwide. This is one of the ways to provide oncologists with novel therapeutic tools that can improve the clinical management and outcome of cancer patients. In addition to original articles providing relevant results that will be commented upon in more detail below, this Special Issue also contains several review articles that summarize the current state of the art in crucial aspects of human cancer. Thus, the work by Martinez-Useros et al. [1] reviewed epigenetic pathways and treatments (several under study in current clinical trials) that target epigenetic modifications in highly aggressive tumors. Gundamaraju et al. [2] focused in their manuscript on the molecular mechanisms by which the mitochondria influence cancer biology and their usefulness to develop therapeutic strategies. Another relevant challenge, reviewed by Isaguliants et al. [3], is the increased risk of developed cancer observed in people living with human immunodeficiency virus type 1 (HIV-1), despite a long-term successful implementation of antiretroviral therapy. The authors focused on the oncogenic properties of five viral proteins: envelope protein gp120, accessory protein negative factor Nef, matrix protein p17, transactivator of transcription Tat, and reverse transcriptase RT. All proteins either led to the proliferation of pre-existing malignant cells or induced the malignant transformation of normal cells, which is responsible for the carcinogenic effects of HIV-1. Moreover, Senent et al. [4] reported the importance of the complement system in ovarian cancer, highlighting how certain elements of this system play tumor-promoting roles that decrease the efficacy of distinct therapeutic approaches, and discussing the potential usefulness of the complement as a target of treatments for ovarian cancer. In addition, the work by Nishida [5] reviewed the role of oncogenic signaling pathways on the cancer immunosuppressive microenvironment in hepatocellular carcinoma. Interestingly, this manuscript summarizes the molecular factors that could be determining the efficacy of therapies based on immune checkpoint inhibition. Finally, Guijarro-Hernández and Vizmanos [6] carried out a systematic review summarizing the signaling pathways affected in Ph-negative mieloproliferative neoplasms (MPNs). MPNs are driven not only by a constitutive activation of the JAK2/STAT signaling and JAK2-related pathways, but a complex network of non-canonical pathways that affects key cellular functions such as epigenetic and transcriptional regulation, splicing and additional pathways that confer a highly complex and coordinated program in the tumor cells of these blood disorders.

Regarding the contribution of original articles, our Special Issue contains four pieces of work about breast cancer focused on the identification of molecular aberrations that can serve as novel molecular targets and prognostic markers. Thus, Lee et al. [7] reported that the use of a CD99-derived agonist ligand inhibited EGF-induced EGFR dimerization. This issue involved a PTPN12-dependent c-Src/FAK inactivation that impaired cytoskeletal reorganization and suppressed tumor growth in vivo of the triple negative breast cancer cell line MDA-MB-231. Furthermore, Noblejas-López et al. [8] carried out a genomic mapping that evaluated the presence of alterations in 304 splicing-related genes and their prognostic value in luminal breast cancer patients. They identified that amplifications in *CLNS1A*, *LSM1*, and *ILF2* determined poor outcome. At the functional level, they found that these alterations conferred enhanced proliferation in luminal cell lines that can be pharmacologically reversed by using BET inhibitors. In this line of thinking, an increasing number of publications have shown that the use of BET inhibitors could be a therapeutic approach in triple negative breast cancer (TNBC), and that PP2A is a tumor suppressor that directly targets the bromodomain-containing protein 4 (BRD4) regulating its stabilization and activation. The work of Sanz-Alvarez et al. [9] evaluated the clinical impact of BRD4 phosphorylation levels in TNBC patients. Notably, they observed BRD4 hyperphosphorylation in around 34% of cases, and strongly associated with PP2A inhibition status. Moreover, this alteration was markedly associated with patient recurrence and predicted unfavorable prognosis, suggesting the clinical relevance of the PP2A/BET axis as a potential novel marker in TNBC. Considering these results, and the fact that the PP2A pathway has also been previously reported to be affected in luminal breast cancer, it seems that the PP2A/BET interplay could represent a plausible druggable target to develop alternative therapeutic strategies in certain breast cancer patient subgroups from different molecular subtypes. The same research group also published another study in this Special Issue, in this case about HER2-positive breast cancer models. In their work, Sanz-Alvarez et al. [10] evaluated the efficacy of three different PI3K/AKT/mTOR inhibitors (BEZ235, everolimus, and TAK-228) in a panel of HER2-positive breast cancer cell lines with primary and acquired resistance to Trastuzumab. They found promising results combining TAK-228 with Trastuzumab in all resistant cell lines, observing decreased cell proliferation together with increased apoptosis and G0/G1 cell cycle arrest. Considering these results, the combination of Trastuzumab with PI3K/AKT/mTOR inhibitors emerges as a potential alternative strategy to overcome Trastuzumab resistance in HER2-positive breast cancer.

In the context of prostate cancer, the work by Martínez-Martínez et al. [11] provides novel findings about the role of dual specificity phosphatase 1 (DUSP1). The authors demonstrated that this tumor suppressor leads to Snail downregulation and decreased migration and invasion capabilities of prostate cancer cells through the inhibition of c-Jun N-terminal Kinase (JNK) and extracellular-signal-regulated kinase (ERK). Notably, they also found that the subgroup of prostate cancer patients with an expression pattern $DUSP_{high}$/activated JNK_{low}/activated ERK_{low}/$Snail_{low}$ showed better clinical outcome, suggesting its potential utility as molecular marker in this disease. Moreover, Khalil et al. [12] showed relevant results suggesting that the TLK1/NEK1/YAP1 signaling axis plays a key role during the process of androgen-sensitive to androgen-independent conversion, facilitating progression to metastatic castration-resistant prostate cancer. Finally, Papadaki et al. [13] published a comprehensive study in bladder cancer. They found that two secreted extracellular matrix proteins, osteomodulin (OMD), and proline/arginine-rich and leucine repeat protein (PRELP), were selectively expressed in bladder umbrella epithelial cells but markedly downregulated in bladder cancer cells. These two proteins act as tumor suppressors, regulating epithelial to mesenchymal transition (EMT), which was mediated by the inhibition of the TGF-β and EGF pathways.

Altogether, this Special Issue includes several reviews and unique articles with novel, interesting findings that allow the readers to improve their knowledge about the molecular mechanisms involved in high-prevalence tumors and the recent advances in targeted therapies for these diseases.

Funding: This research received no external funding.

Conflicts of Interest: The authors declare no conflict of interest.

References

1. Martinez-Useros, J.; Martin-Galan, M.; Florez-Cespedes, M.; Garcia-Foncillas, J. Epigenetics of Most Aggressive Solid Tumors: Pathways, Targets and Treatments. *Cancers* **2021**, *13*, 3209. [CrossRef] [PubMed]
2. Gundamaraju, R.; Lu, W.; Manikam, R. Revisiting Mitochondria Scored Cancer Progression and Metastasis. *Cancers* **2021**, *13*, 432. [CrossRef] [PubMed]
3. Isaguliants, M.; Bayurova, E.; Avdoshina, D.; Kondrashova, A.; Chiodi, F.; Palefsky, J.M. Oncogenic Effects of HIV-1 Proteins, Mechanisms Behind. *Cancers* **2021**, *13*, 305. [CrossRef] [PubMed]
4. Senent, Y.; Ajona, D.; González-Martín, A.; Pio, R.; Tavira, B. The Complement System in Ovarian Cancer: An Underexplored Old Path. *Cancers* **2021**, *13*, 3806. [CrossRef] [PubMed]
5. Nishida, N. Role of Oncogenic Pathways on the Cancer Immunosuppressive Microenvironment and Its Clinical Implications in Hepatocellular Carcinoma. *Cancers* **2021**, *13*, 3666. [CrossRef] [PubMed]
6. Guijarro-Hernández, A.; Vizmanos, J.L. A Broad Overview of Signaling in *Ph*-Negative Classic Myeloproliferative Neoplasms. *Cancers* **2021**, *13*, 984. [CrossRef] [PubMed]
7. Lee, K.-J.; Kim, Y.; Kim, M.S.; Ju, H.-M.; Choi, B.; Lee, H.; Jeoung, D.; Moon, K.-W.; Kang, D.; Choi, J.; et al. CD99–PTPN12 Axis Suppresses Actin Cytoskeleton-Mediated Dimerization of Epidermal Growth Factor Receptor. *Cancers* **2020**, *12*, 2895. [CrossRef]
8. Noblejas-López, M.M.; López-Cade, I.; Fuentes-Antrás, J.; Fernández-Hinojal, G.; Esteban-Sánchez, A.; Manzano, A.; García-Sáenz, J.Á.; Pérez-Segura, P.; La Hoya, M.D.; Pandiella, A.; et al. Genomic Mapping of Splicing-Related Genes Identify Amplifications in *LSM1*, *CLNS1A*, and *ILF2* in Luminal Breast Cancer. *Cancers* **2021**, *13*, 4118. [CrossRef]
9. Sanz-Álvarez, M.; Cristóbal, I.; Luque, M.; Santos, A.; Zazo, S.; Madoz-Gúrpide, J.; Caramés, C.; Chiang, C.-M.; García-Foncillas, J.; Eroles, P.; et al. Expression of Phosphorylated BRD4 Is Markedly Associated with the Activation Status of the PP2A Pathway and Shows a Strong Prognostic Value in Triple Negative Breast Cancer Patients. *Cancers* **2021**, *13*, 1246. [CrossRef] [PubMed]
10. Sanz-Álvarez, M.; Martín-Aparicio, E.; Luque, M.; Zazo, S.; Martínez-Useros, J.; Eroles, P.; Rovira, A.; Albanell, J.; Madoz-Gúrpide, J.; Rojo, F. The Novel Oral mTORC1/2 Inhibitor TAK-228 Reverses Trastuzumab Resistance in HER2-Positive Breast Cancer Models. *Cancers* **2021**, *13*, 2778. [CrossRef] [PubMed]
11. Martínez-Martínez, D.; Toledo Lobo, M.-V.; Baquero, P.; Ropero, S.; Angulo, J.C.; Chiloeches, A.; Lasa, M. Downregulation of Snail by DUSP1 Impairs Cell Migration and Invasion through the Inactivation of JNK and ERK and Is Useful as a Predictive Factor in the Prognosis of Prostate Cancer. *Cancers* **2021**, *13*, 1158. [CrossRef] [PubMed]
12. Khalil, M.I.; Ghosh, I.; Singh, V.; Chen, J.; Zhu, H.; De Benedetti, A. NEK1 Phosphorylation of YAP Promotes Its Stabilization and Transcriptional Output. *Cancers* **2020**, *12*, 3666. [CrossRef] [PubMed]
13. Papadaki, V.; Asada, K.; Watson, J.K.; Tamura, T.; Leung, A.; Hopkins, J.; Dellett, M.; Sasai, N.; Davaapil, H.; Nik-Zainal, S.; et al. Two Secreted Proteoglycans, Activators of Urothelial Cell–Cell Adhesion, Negatively Contribute to Bladder Cancer Initiation and Progression. *Cancers* **2020**, *12*, 3362. [CrossRef] [PubMed]

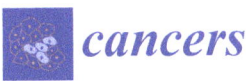

Review

Epigenetics of Most Aggressive Solid Tumors: Pathways, Targets and Treatments

Javier Martinez-Useros [1,*], Mario Martin-Galan [1], Maria Florez-Cespedes [2] and Jesus Garcia-Foncillas [1,*]

- [1] Translational Oncology Division, OncoHealth Institute, Fundacion Jimenez Diaz University Hospital, Avenida Reyes Catolicos 2, 28040 Madrid, Spain; mariomgtics@gmail.com
- [2] Imperial College London, Exhibition Road, South Kensington, London SW7 2BX, UK; maria.florez-cespedes17@imperial.ac.uk
- * Correspondence: javier.museros@oncohealth.eu (J.M.-U.); jesus.garciafoncillas@oncohealth.eu (J.G.-F.); Tel.: +34-91-550-48-00 (J.G.-F.)

Simple Summary: The large amount of knowledge regarding epigenetic pathways has opened a broad range of treatments that provide hope for adult patients with highly aggressive forms of solid tumors. The most commonly used treatments for epigenic modifications are based on the specific inhibitors of DNA methyltransferases, azacitidine and decitabine (5-AZA-dC), and on histone deacetylases inhibitors, such as trichostatin A (TSA) or vorinostat (SAHA). However, many other compounds are under investigation, and some are being evaluated in clinical trials. In this review, we have extracted relevant information about epigenetic pathways and treatments that target epigenetic modifications in highly aggressive tumors, as a new hope for these patients.

Abstract: Highly aggressive tumors are characterized by a highly invasive phenotype, and they display chemoresistance. Furthermore, some of the tumors lack expression of biomarkers for target therapies. This is the case of small-cell lung cancer, triple-negative breast cancer, pancreatic ductal adenocarcinoma, glioblastoma, metastatic melanoma, and advanced ovarian cancer. Unfortunately, these patients show a low survival rate and most of the available drugs are ineffective. In this context, epigenetic modifications have emerged to provide the causes and potential treatments for such types of tumors. Methylation and hydroxymethylation of DNA, and histone modifications, are the most common targets of epigenetic therapy, to influence gene expression without altering the DNA sequence. These modifications could impact both oncogenes and tumor suppressor factors, which influence several molecular pathways such as epithelial-to-mesenchymal transition, WNT/β–catenin, PI3K–mTOR, MAPK, or mismatch repair machinery. However, epigenetic changes are inducible and reversible events that could be influenced by some environmental conditions, such as UV exposure, smoking habit, or diet. Changes in DNA methylation status and/or histone modification, such as acetylation, methylation or phosphorylation, among others, are the most important targets for epigenetic cancer therapy. Therefore, the present review aims to compile the basic information of epigenetic modifications, pathways and factors, and provide a rationale for the research and treatment of highly aggressive tumors with epigenetic drugs.

Keywords: epigenetic; methylation; acetylation; non-coding RNA; small-cell lung cancer; triple-negative breast cancer; pancreatic ductal adenocarcinoma; glioblastoma; metastatic melanoma; advanced ovarian cancer

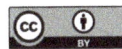

1. Introduction

DNA is organized inside the nucleus, in a very complex structure called chromatin. The negative charge of DNA is supported by basic proteins that are rich in arginine and lysine residues, called histones. There are five families of histones and according to their function they are called core histones (H2, H3, and H4) that form the nucleosome core, or linker histones (H1 and H5), which contribute to the condensation of the nucleosome.

The nucleosome core is composed by two H2A–H2B dimers and a H3–H4 tetramer. The electrostatic attraction between the positively charged histones and negatively charged DNA allows the complex structure of chromatin to form [1,2]. Chromatin is composed of nucleosomes wrapped by 146–147 bp DNA [3]. The H1 histone serves as a linker between the nucleosomes, in order to provide a highly stable chromatin structure [4]. Histones possess amino-terminal tails that allow gene regulation, by epigenetic modifications, due to their flexible shaping [4]. Deregulation in the deposition of histone modification is associated with several human diseases, such as cancer [5]. Moreover, some epigenetic modifications could be influenced by specific molecular pathways involved in cancer, such as epithelial-to-mesenchymal transition (EMT) [6], Wnt/β-catenin signaling [7], the MAPK signaling pathway [8], DNA repair [9], hypoxia [10], and the PI3K–mTOR pathway [11]. Interestingly, some environmental conditions, such as UV exposure or diet, are also able to induce epigenetic changes. For example, compounds such as folate, choline, betaine, and methionine act as cofactors or methyl donors for DNA methylation reactions. A diet rich in resveratrol, curcumin, genistein, epigallocatechin-3-gallate, sulforaphane, and quercetin is able to reactivate certain tumor suppressive genes by inducing DNA demethylation; however, fungi-contaminated agricultural foods contain mycotoxins that may also lead to cancer [12].

Clinical research has achieved several advances in cancer treatment that have led to a longer survival of patients. However, treatment strategies for highly aggressive tumors remains almost constant, without any significant improvements. In the new era of targeted therapy, epigenetic therapies appear as a potential approach for the treatment of highly aggressive tumors, offering new hope for these patients. Methylation and hydroxymethylation of DNA, and histone modifications, are the most common targets of epigenetic therapy, to influence gene expression without any DNA alteration. On the other hand, increasing reports support the use of non-coding RNA as epigenetic treatment to intercept translation, and negatively regulate the expression of oncogenes.

1.1. DNA Methylation

DNA methylation plays a crucial role in normal cell metabolism; therefore, changes in the methylation status of cells, by methyltransferases, can lead to cell transformation and represent the difference between normal and tumor cells [13] (Figure 1). Cytosine and adenine are the only bases susceptible to methylation. DNA methylation consists of the transfer of methyl groups (-CH$_3$) to the cytosine in position C5, which is followed by a guanine (G). These sites are termed CpG dinucleotides and result in 5-methylcytosine. These sites occur with high frequency in CpG genomic regions. Non-cytosine methylation, such as the methylation of adenine or thymine, appears in very low probability [14]. CpG islands are located in ~60% of human promoters, and methylation of these sites results in a transcriptional repression of the genes [5,15]. Furthermore, 60–80% of CpG islands of somatic cells genome are methylated [16]. The DNA methyltransferase (DNMT) (Figure 1) family regulates the process of DNA methylation [17]. This protein family is composed of the following five members: DNMT1, DNMT2, DNMT3a, DNMT3b and DNMT3L. Interestingly, mutations in some of these members are usually associated with some types of cancer [18]. For example, the DNMT3b subtype is significantly overexpressed in some tumors [19,20]. The methylation status of DNA can be read by MBD (methyl-CpG binding domain) proteins, which are divided into three families. The first family includes MeCP2, MBD1, MBD2, MBD3 and MBD4 [21]; although, MBD3 can only detect hydroxymethylated DNA [22]. The second family is characterized by a BTB domain (also called as the POZ domain) and comprises ZBTB33, ZBTB4 and ZBTB38 [23]. The third family includes the following two proteins: UHRF1 and UHRF2 [24]. Some drugs are able to modulate the expression levels of these proteins. Decitabine and 5-azacytidine trigger calcium-calmodulin kinase (CamK) activity, leading to MeCP2 nuclear export, which induces the epigenetic reactivation of some tumor suppressive genes in colorectal cancer [25]. Other drugs, such as 5-azacytidine, doxorubicin, vorinostat, paclitaxel, or cisplatin, regulate the expression of different MBD proteins. MBD1 was upregulated after treatment with all those drugs. Downregulation of MBD2 was observed after 5-azacytidine, doxorubicin, or vorinostat treatment, MBD3 downregulation after vorinostat, and the inhibition of MBD4 varied in a time- and drug-dependent manner [26]. Another study reported the decrease in ZBTB4 levels after roscovitine treatment [27]. Concerning UHRF1, its downregulation enables the demethylation, and the subsequent reactivation, of some epigenetically silenced tumor-suppressive genes [28]. Giovinazzo et al. reported the pharmacological inhibition of UHRF1 by the anthracycline derivatives, idarubicin and mitoxantrone [29]. Therefore, several drugs allow the negative modulation of these MBD proteins, implying a high potential to be used as target therapies.

Aberrant DNA methylation has been associated with drug resistance, and as predictive biomarker [30]. Also, inadequate methylation is associated to inflammatory diseases, premalignant lesions and cancer led by chromatin instability [31]. Hypermethylation and hypomethylation of DNA are usual phenomena in cancer; indeed, tumor-suppressive genes are hypermethylated in cancer cells, while they remain hypomethylated in normal cells [32]. Therefore, the demethylation of target genes could be a promising approach in clinical practice. Physiologically, demethylation of DNA sequences is carried out by the ten-eleven translocation (TET) proteins. The three mammalian TET proteins, called TET1, TET2 and TET3, enable the oxidation of 5-methylcytosine (5mC) of nucleic acids, to 5-hydroxymethylcytosine (5hmC), 5-formylcytosine (5fC) or 5-carboxylcytosine (5caC) [33]. The mutation or inhibition of TET proteins is associated with aging and tumorigenesis [34]. Indeed, mutation in *TET2* is frequently found in hematopoietic malignancies [35], and the downregulation of TET proteins has been observed in several solid tumors, such as breast cancer, gastric, glioblastoma, liver, lung, melanoma and prostate [34,36–38].

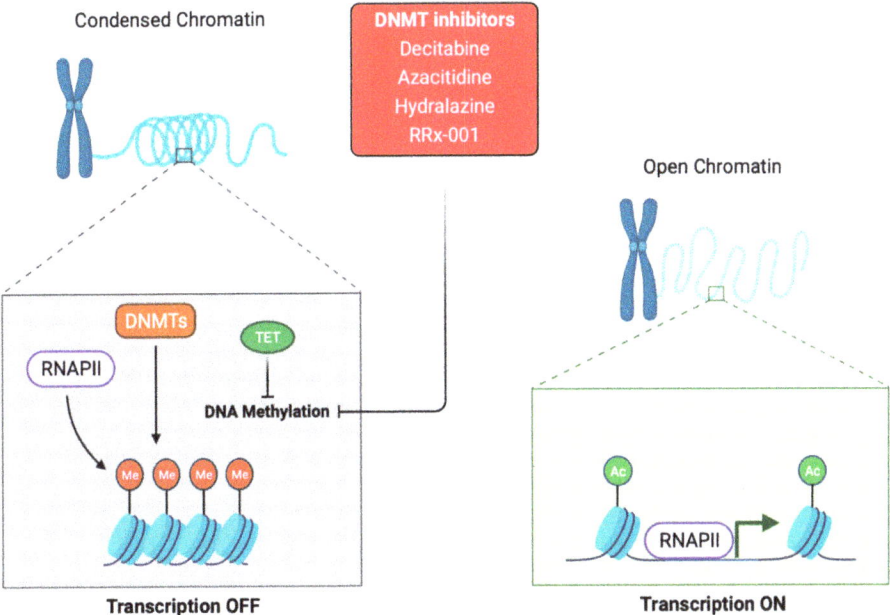

Figure 1. Schematic representation of the DNA methylation process. DNMTis inhibits DNA methylation by downregulation of DNMTs. The action of DNA methylation inhibitors (DNMTs inhibitors and TET proteins) triggers a chromatin-remodeling process and chromatin structure becomes transcriptionally accessible to RNA polymerase II, which will begin the transcription process. DNMTis: DNA methyltransferases inhibitors. DNMTs: DNA methyltransferases. TET: ten-eleven translocation proteins. RNAPII: RNA polymerase II. Me: methyl. Ac: acetyl.

1.2. Histone Modification

Histone modification can take place in the following two locations: the flexible tails of the nucleosomes and the internal sites in the core of the histone (Figure 2) [39]. The residues most susceptible for modification are lysine and arginine residues, and hydroxyl group-containing serine/threonine/tyrosine residues [40]. Histone modification includes several reactions, such as the methylation and acetylation of lysine and arginine residues, phosphorylation of threonine and serine residues, SUMOylation of lysine residues, isomerization of proline residues, ADP-ribosylation, ubiquitylation, citrullination, deamination, formylation, O-GlcNAcylation, propionylation, butyrylation and crotonylation [41]. Histone acetylation of lysine limits the interactions between the histones H3 and H4, and DNA; while deacetylation leads to gene inactivation [42]. Acetylation is associated with active transcription, and facilitates the recruitment of co-regulators and elements to promote transcription. Modifications of histones are driven by protein effectors and are crucial in the regulation of gene expression. HATs (histone acetyltransferases) are a group of effectors that transfer the acetyl groups to lysine residues of histones [43]. Notably, aberrations in the histone modification pattern may induce cancer [44]. For example, tumor cells present a loss of Lys16 acetylation and Lys20 trimethylation of histone H4 at the early phase of tumor initiation [45]. In contrast, histone deacetylases are another group of effectors that remove the acetyl groups from acetyl-lysine residues, which allows DNA to wrap tightly to histones [46]. Histone deacetylases (HDACs) have been recently reported as a target for cancer therapy (Figure 2) [46]. HDAC1-11 and other histone deacetylases, termed sirtuins, normally play a role as gene silencers [47]. Other effectors are histone demethylases that remove methyl groups from lysine residues. The lysine-specific demethylase 1 (LSD1) exhibits tumor-prone abilities in glioblastoma, and its inhibition sensitizes tumor cells to vorinostat, increasing apoptosis [48]. Other histone demethylases, such as KDM4, produce genome instability, while KDM6 is considered a tumor-suppressive factor [49].

On the other hand, readers of these modifications determine the functional outcome of specific epigenetic change. Some of the proteins involved in the recognition of histone modifications are BET (bromodomain and extraterminal domain-containing). This family is composed of four proteins (BRD2, BRD3, BRD4 and BRDT), and plays important roles in tumor development, since they also lead to transcriptional activity [50,51]. For this reason, BET inhibitors have been evaluated as anti-tumor therapies, showing encouraging results in several malignancies, without significant toxicities or adverse events (Figure 2) [51].

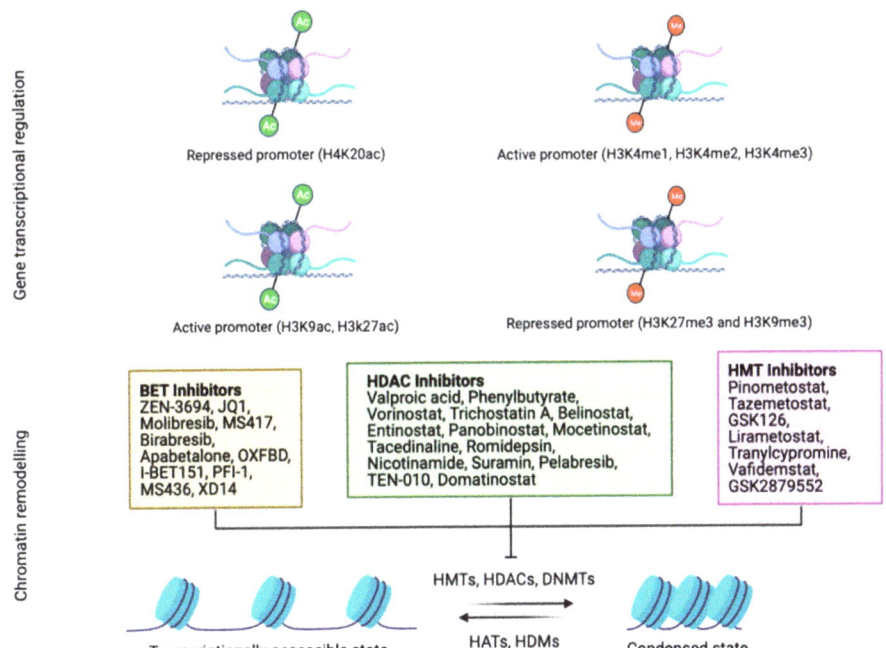

Figure 2. Schematic representation of the main histone modification processes. Both acetylation and methylation positively and negatively regulate gene transcription according to the methylated or acetylated residue (up). Several drugs have been designed to allow chromatin remodeling by the inhibition of BET, HDAC or HMT proteins that condense chromatin and hamper transcription (down). Histones acetylation and cytosines unmethylation will result in an open chromatin structure and gene transcription is active. BET: bromodomain and extra-terminal motif (BET) proteins. HDAC: histone deacetylases. HMT: histone methyltransferase. DNMTs: DNA methyltransferases. HAT: histone acetyltransferase. HDM: histone demethylase.

1.3. Non-Coding RNA

This family includes several factors, but the most notable, in regards to cancer, are small interfering RNA (siRNAs), microRNAs (miRNAs), PIWI-interacting RNA (piRNAs), and long non-coding RNAs (lncRNAs) (Figure 3) [5].

The small interfering RNA (siRNA) transcripts are double-stranded RNA fragments, about 21–25 base pairs long. The function of siRNA is thought to be related to erasing viral double-stranded sequences to avoid infection. SiRNA is cleaved by Dicer from long double-stranded RNA sequences [52]. The double-stranded siRNA is processed by the RNA-induced silencing complex (RISC), to produce single-stranded siRNA [53]. This strand is able to recognize the target mRNA. The perfect match induces mRNA degradation, and a partial match results in translational repression [54].

MiRNA are the most known non-coding RNA and they are involved in several cell functions. Several miRNAs are linked to cancer initiation and development. Furthermore, miRNAs can be tumor-prone or tumor-suppressive factors [55]. MiRNAs are very similar to siRNAs; however, miRNAs originate from double-stranded RNA hairpins, rather than long double-stranded RNA that need additional manipulation by DROSHA [56].

P-element-induced wimpy testis (PIWI) proteins belong to the Argonaute (AGO) family and were discovered in the germline [57]. They also bind a unique type of non-coding small RNAs, called piRNAs (PIWI-interacting RNAs). This tandem, composed of PIWI and piRNAs, constitute the piRNA-induced silencing complex (piRISC). PiRNAs are special mediators, because depending on the factors that modulate, some piRNAs are considered oncogenic, while others are considered tumor-suppressive factors [58].

Long non-coding RNAs (lncRNAs) constitute a huge subgroup of ncRNAs, defined as RNA transcripts, with more than 200 nucleotides [59]. LncRNAs play an important role in the development of various cancers [60]. The lncRNA, HOTAIR, is closely related to epigenetic modifications. The knockdown of HOTAIR activates transcription-reducing H3K27 trimethylation [61]. Moreover, HOTAIR is able to interact with lysine-specific histone demethylase 1A (LSD1) [62]. Aberrant HOTAIR expression has been observed in several tumors, and its positive expression has been associated with several hallmarks of cancer, such as high cell proliferation, angiogenesis or drug resistance, by the direct regulation of several downstream factors involving multiple signaling pathways [63–65]. Another crucial lncRNA is MALAT-1 (metastasis-associated lung adenocarcinoma transcript-1), which is aberrantly upregulated in multiple tumor types, and yields high proliferative and metastatic profiles [66]. High expression of MALAT-1 has been associated with high-grade and advanced-stage melanoma, glioma and lung cancers [67–69].

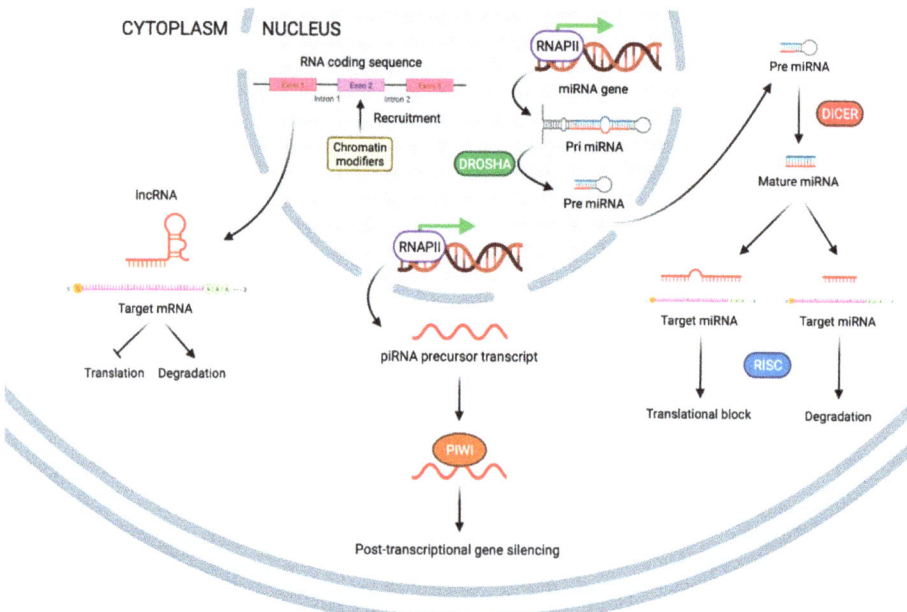

Figure 3. Schematic representation of non-coding RNA. LncRNA targets mRNA to inhibit translation or degrade mRNA (left). PIWI proteins stabilize piRNAs and lead to post-translational control (middle). MiRNA are originated from double-stranded RNA hairpins. The ribonuclease III enzyme, DROSHA, binds and cleaves hairpin structures in primary RNA transcripts into precursor miRNAs. Once transported to cytoplasm, precursor miRNAs are processed by DICER into mature miRNAs that regulate expression of mRNA (right). miRNA: microRNA. DICER: ribonuclease III enzyme. DROSHA: ribonuclease III enzyme. RISC: RNA-induced silencing complex. piRNA: PIWI-interacting RNA.

The large amount of knowledge regarding epigenetic modifications has opened a broad palette of treatment strategies for the most aggressive solid tumors in adulthood. Thus, the objective of this review is to compile basic knowledge about epigenetic pathways and treatments, and provide a rational for further clinical trials, based on the use of these treatments in highly aggressive solid tumors.

2. Epigenetic Modulation in Highly Aggressive Solid Tumors

The most commonly drugs used as hypomethylating agents are specific inhibitors of DNA methyltransferase (DNMT), for example, azacitidine and decitabine (5-AZA-dC) (Figure 1) [70]. These drugs lead to a reduction in whole DNA methylation status [71], and damage DNA by inducing genomic instability that hampers DNA synthesis [72]. Trichostatin A (TSA) and vorinostat (SAHA) are the most used inhibitors for the class I and II histone deacetylases (HDAC), demonstrating a broad spectrum of epigenetic activities [73]. Sodium phenylbutyrate is also a histone deacetylase inhibitor that is under investigation for its potential use in malignant brain tumors [74]. Although epigenetic drugs have a great potential to improve patient prognosis, there are also important considerations concerning global transcriptional effects. Epigenetic modifications by drugs may result in an aberrant gene expression pattern, leading to a global transcriptional alteration that will drive severe genome instability and cancer [75]. At the molecular level, several studies have reported the upregulation of P21 after epigenetic treatment [76]. On the other hand, since germ cells drive broad epigenetic reprogramming, these drugs could influence histone modifications and alterations in the non-coding RNAs of sperm and oocytes, which may influence progeny development [77]. Furthermore, these drugs have been demonstrated to impair normal hematopoiesis. Indeed, some of the adverse events in the clinical evaluation of epigenetic drugs are hematologic toxicity [76], as well as severe cardiac toxicity, as previously reported with the administration of the histone deacetylase inhibitor [78]. Nevertheless, these drugs exhibited promising results for cancer patients, and due to the growing interest and hope in epigenetic modulation in the clinical practice, we focus this review on different pathways and treatments for the most aggressive solid tumors, specifically small-cell lung cancer, triple-negative breast cancer, pancreatic ductal adenocarcinoma, glioblastoma, metastasic melanoma and ovarian cancer (Figure 4).

Melanoma
- UV radiation induce DNA methyltransferase and histone acetylation.
- Epigenetic upregulation of CCR7 and CXCR4.
- Hypermethylation of DAPK, MGMT, RASSF1A and RAR-β2.
- Downregulation of TET2.
- H3K4 acetylation.
- Epigenetic activation of BRAFV600E and epigenetic inhibition of PTEN.
- High expression of EZH2.
- Upregulation of miRNA-125b, and downregulation of mir-376a and mir-376c.

SCLC
- TRIM36 hypermethylation.
- Diagnostic biomarkers: methylation in P16, TERT, WT1 and RASSF1.
- Hypomethylation of TTF1.
- Hypermethylation of DCCK1 in liquid biopsies of SCLC.
- Hypermethylation signature of ITK, RUNX3, CTLA4, PLG, EMR3, SLC22A18, TRIP6IL10, PECAM1, S100A2, MMP9, ERCC1, CSF3R and CAV1.

PDAC
- Mutation in epigenetic regulators: ARID1B, PBRM1, SMARCA2, KDM6A, ARID1A, SMARCA4 and MLL2.
- H3K4me3 is present in low-grade tumors.
- H3K4me1 is present in high-grade tumors.
- High expression of EZH2 is associated with poorly-differentiation.
- Overexpression of DNMT1, DNMT3A and DNMT3B.
- Hypermethylation in APC, BRCA1, P16/INK4a, P15/INK4b, RARβ and P73.
- Hypermethylation of genes involved in TGF-β, WNT, Integrin or ROBO.
- Downregulation of P300 and upregulation of HDAC1, HDAC2 and HDAC7.
- Upregulation of miR-21, miR-196a-2, miR-203, miR-155, miR-210 and miR-222; and downregulation of miR-132.
- Upregulation of HOTAIR, HOTTIP, MALAT1 and PVT1.

AOC
- Overexpression of HDAC2 and HP1 hampers DNA damage responses induced by platinum.
- Inhibition of H4K16 acetylation.
- Patients with high expression levels of hMOF present better outcome.
- Expression of class I HDACs associate with progression disease.
- SIRT1 upregulation inactivates TP53 and confers chemoresistance to platinum compounds.
- Downregulation of SIRT3.
- Overexpression of EZH2 and LSD1.
- KDM3A expression regulates cancer undifferentiation and platinum resistance.

TNBC
- Hypermethylation of ER promoter.
- Histone modification activates NF-κB and NIK.
- BRCA1 hypermethylation.
- Hypermethylation of PRSS8, VAMP8 and CLDN4.
- Histone acetylation overexpress CD24.
- H3K9 acetylation of TGFβR2 promoter.
- High expression of EZH2.
- Hypermethylation of miR-31.
- Overexpression of MALAT-1 and HOTAIR.
- Downregulation of GAS5.

GBM
- Three groups:
  1) IDH-mutant, 1p/19q co-deletion status low-grade group.
  2) IDH-mutant-non-co-deletion status, G-CIMP-low group with low DNA methylation status.
  3) IDH-mutant-non-co-deletion status, G-CIMP-high group with high levels of DNA methylation status.
- Hypermethylation of MGMT predicts Carmustine and Temozolomide response.
- Patients with high expression of MBD3 protein may obtain benefit from Pyrvinium pamoate treatment.
- Upregulation of HOTAIR and MALAT1.

Figure 4. Summary of the most representative epigenetic modifications of most aggressive solid tumors observed in adulthood. UV: ultraviolet. SCLC: small-cell lung cancer. PDAC: pancreatic ductal adenocarcinoma. AOC: advanced ovarian cancer. TNBC: triple-negative breast cancer. GBM: glioblastoma.

2.1. Epigenetic Modulation in Small-Cell Lung Cancer

Small-cell lung cancer (SCLC) incidence over time has decreased, reducing by 10–11% in all the cases of lung cancer, which may reflect decreases in smoking habits and changes in the type of cigarettes [79]. One of the causes that leads to a malignant phenotype in lung cancer is the exposure to polycyclic aromatic hydrocarbons, such as benzo (a) pyrene. This induces *TRIM36* hypermethylation, and its subsequent inhibition is associated with the acquisition of an aggressive phenotype [80]. SCLC is the highest aggressive subtype of lung cancer, since tumor cells are highly proliferative, and they spread and metastasize quickly throughout the body [81].

The methylation status of bronchial washings from different types of lung cancers provided a signature, based on four DNA methylated factors (*P16*, *TERT*, *WT1*, and *RASSF1*), which could improve the efficiency of SCLC diagnosis when compared with cytologic evaluation [82]. Another study found that SCLC frequently express thyroid transcription factor 1 (TTF1) at high levels, due to hypomethylation of its promoter [83]. TTF1 overexpression has been reported to confer high tumor cell proliferation and survival [84]. Also, the hypermethylation status in *DCLK1*, which has been associated to colorectal cancer and cholangiocarcinoma, has been found in liquid biopsies in 75% of SCLC patients, and has been associated with poor survival; therefore, this could represent a promising biomarker for early diagnosis and disease prognostic for this cancer subtype [85]. Several other genes have also been found methylated in SCLC, for example *ITK*, *RUNX3*, *CTLA4*, *PLG*, *EMR3*, *SLC22A18*, *TRIP6IL10*, *PECAM1*, *S100A2*, *MMP9*, *ERCC1*, *CSF3R* and *CAV1* [86].

In the treatment scenario, one study reported that 5-AZA-dC and the HDAC inhibitors, LBH589 or MGCD0103, synergistically reduced proliferation in five out of nine SCLC cell lines in vitro [87]. Interestingly, the authors observed higher expression of IFN-stimulated genes in the resistant cell lines after treatment, which determine SCLC cell sensitivity to epigenetic modulators [87]. Another study describes that TSA is able to induce an increase in ABCB1, a protein that confers drug resistance to tumor cells [88]. In clinical trials, a new epigenetic treatment, called RRx-001, is under investigation (NCT02489903; Table 1; Figures 1 and 2). RRx-001 is an alkylating agent based on a dinitroazetidine derivative that inhibits DNA methyltransferase (DNMT) and induces DNA damage via ATM/γ-H2AX, and apoptosis by the activation of caspases [89]. This drug is being tested in platinum refractory or resistant SCLC patients, with 3.8% complete responses and 23.1% partial responses, which increased the overall survival OS [90].

The progress in the treatment of SCLC has been very limited in the last decade, especially when compared to the numerous results that arise for NSCLC. Although the FDA approved the use of immunotherapy anti-PD-L1 in combination with carboplatin and etoposide as an induction therapy in extensive-stage SCLC, much remains to be done to achieve a cure for SCLC patients. In fact, the combination of immunotherapy plus chemotherapy has only represented an improvement in the overall survival of two months [91]. Therefore, there is much left to be done, and, in this sense, drugs directed against epigenetic targets may represent potential treatment approaches.

2.2. Epigenetic Modulation in Triple-Negative Breast Cancer

Triple-negative breast cancers (TNBC) comprise 7–14% of all breast cancers [92]. TNBC is considered the most aggressive subtype due to the lack of expression of estrogen receptors (ER), progesterone (PR), and HER2 receptors that make the currently used drugs ineffective. One study reported a highly methylated promoter region in the ER gene [93]; thus, a correlation has been suggested with the downregulation of ER expression levels in TNBC patients and the absence of a response [94]. Histone H3 methylation and deacetylation lead to a less compact chromatin structure, which facilitates DNA access to transcription protein machineries. For example, one of the activated genes, due to histone modification in TNBC that provides proliferative features, is NF-κB and its NF-κB-inducing kinase (NIK) [95].

Table 1. Current clinical trials developed with epigenetic-based therapies in highly aggressive solid tumors in adulthood.

Identifier	Disease	Stage	Design	Drugs	Administration of ET	Epigenetic Target	Brief	Status
NCT02847000	Pancreatic cancer	Advanced	Early phase 1, single-arm, open-label, proof-of-concept clinical trial	**Decitabine**/tetra-hydrouridine	Orally	DNMT	Drug combination of decitabine and tetrahydrouridine in patients that have progressed through one or more lines of therapy. The most frequent adverse event was anemia and decitabine exhibited a limited systemic effect.	C
NCT01845805	Pancreatic cancer	Resected	Phase II trial, randomized, single group assignment, open label.	Oral **azacitidine** (CC-486)/nanoparticle albumin-bound paclitaxel or gemcitabine	Orally	DNMT	Azacitidine (CC-486) until recurrence, then first-line treatment: Abraxane or gemcitabine.	R
NCT04257448	Pancreatic cancer	Advanced	Open-label phase I/II study, non-randomized, sequential assignment, open label	**Romidepsin, azacitidine**, nab-paclitaxel, gemcitabine, durvalumab, lenalidomide	Subcutaneous	HDAC and DNMT	Azacitidine and/or romidepsin in combination with nab-paclitaxel/gemcitabine followed by sequential immune targeting with programmed death ligand (PD-L)1 blockade in combination with low-dose lenalidomide.	R
NCT02489903	SCLC, NSCLC, neuroendocrine tumors and ovarian epithelial cancer	Platinum refractory/resistant	Phase II study, randomized, parallel assignment, open label	**RRx-001**, cisplatin, etoposide, carboplatin, irinotecan, vinorelbine, Doxil, gemcitabine, taxane, Paclitaxel, nab-Paclitaxel, pemetrexed	Intravenously	DNMT	Participants with SCLC will receive one of the following: RRx-001 followed by platinum-doublet chemotherapy or platinum-based chemotherapy alone. Neuroendocrine, RRx-001 followed by platinum-doublet chemotherapy. NSCLC, RRx-001 followed by platinum-doublet chemotherapy. Participants with platinum refractory/resistant ovarian will receive one of the following: RRx-001 followed by platinum-doublet chemotherapy or chemotherapy alone.	A
NCT03901469	Triple-negative breast cancer	Without germline mutations of BRCA1 or BRCA2	Phase 2 study, non-randomized, single group assignment, open label	**ZEN-3694**, talazoparib	Orally	BET	Triple-negative breast cancer without germline mutations of BRCA1 or BRCA2	R

Table 1. *Cont.*

Identifier	Disease	Stage	Design	Drugs	Administration of ET	Epigenetic Target	Brief	Status
NCT01199908	Triple-negative breast cancer	Metastatic	Phase I/II trial, single group assignment, open label	**Decitabine, panobinostat**, tamoxifen	Intravenously	DNMT and HDAC	ER is silenced by methyl and histone groups. Reactivation of ER by demethylating inhibitors (such as decitabine) and histone deacetylase inhibitors (such as panobinostat) can remove these methyl and histone groups and reactivate ER with tamoxifen.	T
NCT01700569	Grade IV astrocytoma/glioblastoma	Complete or near-complete resection with unmethylated MGMT gene	A phase-1 dose-escalation study, single group assignment, open label,	Folinic acid concomitantly with temozolomide and radiation	Orally	DNMT	Temozolomide in combination with radiation therapy induces MGMT. Then, folinic Acid is able to lead MGMT methylation.	R
NCT00925132	Metastatic melanoma	Refractory/resistant to any prior treatment	Phase Ib/II trial with dose escalation, single group assignment, open label	Combination of temozolomide, **decitabine, panobinostat**	Orally	DNMT and HDAC	The treatment combination is proposed to unlock genes (Apaf-1) that may contribute to mechanisms that cause tumor growth. The triple agent was well tolerated.	T
NCT02816021	Metastatic melanoma	Unresectable stage III/IV metastatic melanoma	Phase II non-randomized, open label	**Oral azacitidine (CC-486)**, pembrolizumab	Orally	DNMT	The goal of this clinical research study is to learn if oral azacitidine (CC-486) and pembrolizumab (MK-3475) can help to control melanoma progression.	R
NCT01876641	Metastatic melanoma	BRAF-mutated tumors regardless of prior treatment	Phase 1/2 trial, single group assignment, open label	Vemurafenib, cobimetinib, **Decitabine**	Subcutaneous	DNMT	Improve the low therapy response rate with the combination of vemurafenib with decitabine plus cobimetinib.	T
NCT03765229	Metastatic melanoma	In non-Inflamed stage III/IV	An exploratory, open-label, single-arm, phase II study	**Entinostat**, pembrolizumab or any other PD-1/PD-L1 inhibitor	Orally	HDAC	Induction of epigenetic changes in tumor biology by entinostat to enhance treatment response, progression-free survival and incidence of adverse events.	R
NCT00715793	Metastatic melanoma	Unresectable stage IIIB/IV despite prior therapies	Single-arm phase I/II trial, single group assignment, open label	**Decitabine**, temozolomide	Intravenously	DNMT	The combination of decitabine and temozolomide may induce changes in DNA to improve clinical response. Determine the efficacy, safety and tolerability of the combination decitabine and temozolomide. This study obtained 18% ORR and 61% clinical benefit rate (CR + PR + SD)	C

Table 1. *Cont.*

Identifier	Disease	Stage	Design	Drugs	Administration of ET	Epigenetic Target	Brief	Status
NCT03903458	Metastatic melanoma	Refractory, locally advanced or metastatic	Open label, non-randomized, phase IB; single group assignment	**Tinostamustine**, nivolumab	N/A	HDAC	To assess the safety, tolerability and recommended dose of tinostamustine in combination with nivolumab and characterize potential predictive biomarkers of the combination treatment.	R
NCT00404508	Ovarian cancer and other solid tumors	Persistent or progression to first-line platinum-based chemotherapy	Randomized, double-blind phase II trial. Parallel assignment	Topotecan, **hydralazine, valproate**	Orally	DNMT and HDAC	Inhibitors of DNA methylation and HDAC inhibition may synergize the cytotoxicity of chemotherapy to improve response, progression-free survival and overall survival. A clinical benefit was observed in 80% patients and the main toxicity was hematologic.	C
NCT02159820	Ovarian cancer	Previously untreated	Open label, randomized, phase II to III, intergroup trial. Parallel assignment	**Decitabine**, paclitaxel, carboplatin	Intravenously	DNMT	Decitabine may trigger epigenetic reprogramming of tumor cells and possible immune cells could induce pronounced long-term clinical effect by chemosensitization and immunopotentiation.	R
NCT02900560	Ovarian cancer	Platinum-resistant/refractory	Open-label, non-randomized, four-cohort phase II. Parallel assignment	Pembrolizumab and **oral azacitidine (CC-486)**	Orally	DNMT	Four cohorts of combined oral azacitidine (CC-486) and intravenous pembrolizumab to evaluate the safety and efficacy. Mandatory tumor biopsies for DNA methylation analysis.	A

Drugs in **bold** are the epigenetic-based therapies. ET: epigenetic therapy. DNMT: DNA methyltransferases. HDAC: histone deacetylases. BET: bromodomain and extra-terminal motif proteins. ORR: overall response rate. CR: complete response. PR: partial response. SD: stable disease. A: active, not recruiting. C: completed. R: recruiting. T: terminated.

A high percentage of TNBC patients carry germline/somatic mutations or epigenetic silencing in *BRCA1*, which implies a deficient DNA repair machinery. Genome-wide DNA methylation analysis in TNBC supports that hypermethylation causes the downregulation of PRSS8, VAMP8 and CLDN4 factors, which confer mesenchymal features [96]. One study revealed a high incidence of *BRCA1* methylation in a TNBC basal-like subtype. This finding could imply resistance to PARP inhibitors for the treatment of *BRCA*-mutant basal-like TNBC [97]. As most of the cases carry mutations in *TP53*, one study has demonstrated that the use of zinc metallochaperones (ZMCs) is efficient to reactivate zinc-deficient mutant *TP53*, by restoring its zinc binding. The use of ZMC1 with a mutation in $TP53^{R175H}$ restores *TP53* reactivation [98]. Another mechanism altered by epigenetic modifications in TNBC is the epithelial-to-mesenchymal transition (EMT). The combination of the methyltransferase inhibitor, SGI-110, with the histone deacetylase inhibitor, MS275, has shown a high anti-tumor ability against TNBC, by epigenetically targeting EMT. Here, TNBC cells showed a marked upregulation of the epithelial protein E-cadherin, and WNT inhibition, and reduced nuclear translocation of EpCAM, which reversed the mesenchymal phenotype after treatment [99]. CD24 overexpression is associated with histone acetylation and is an independent poor prognostic factor in TNBC; importantly, CD24 may be a potential therapeutic target for this type of breast cancer [100]. Mutation analysis revealed that a novel carbazole, SH-I-14, disrupted the STAT3–DNMT1 interaction and led to the re-expression of tumor-suppressive genes such *PDLIM4* or *VHL*, through demethylation, and showed a high anti-proliferative effect in TNBC models [100].

Concerning histone acetylation, one study showed high levels of H3K9 acetylation in the *TGFβR2* promoter in the TNBC cell line, MDA-MB-231. Moreover, the inhibition of *TGFβR2* decreased migration of the cell line [101]. Another factor, the enhancer of zeste homolog 2 (EZH2), is a type of histone methyltransferase that is highly expressed in TNBCs, and its expression implies shorter disease-free survival in TNBC patients [102]. EZH2 works together with HDACs to mediate transcription repression, by increasing histone H3 Lys27 trimethylation (H3K27me3). One study reported that the inhibition of EZH2 increases H3 Lys27 acetylation, which promotes open chromatin transcription activation, and induces apoptosis in TNBC, through the upregulation of B-cell lymphoma-2-like 11 (BIM) [103].

In respect to ncRNA, the presence of hypermethylation at miR-31 loci in TNBC has been described. Moreover, miR-31 maps to the sequence of a novel long non-coding RNA, LAOT554202 [104]. Both are downregulated in TNBC; however, epigenetic treatment was shown to increase both miR-31 and LAOT554202 expression [104].

Also, the deregulation of some lncRNAs has been associated with the progression of different breast tumors [105]. It has been described that high levels of MALAT1 have correlated with tumor aggressiveness and poor survival of TNBC patients [106,107]. Another lncRNA, HOTAIR, is commonly upregulated in TNBC and associated with the invasive phenotype [108] and lymph node metastasis [109]. In contrast, GAS5 has a protective effect against TNBC, and its overexpression suppressed tumor progression [110], and increased sensitivity to paclitaxel and the subsequent apoptosis ratio [111]. A meta-analysis from 21 studies reported that patients with upregulation of HOTAIR and MALAT1, among others, and downregulation of GAS5 and another three lncRNAs, presented poor survival rates [112]. Another meta-analysis supported that the expression of some lncRNAs, such as MALAT1 and HOTAIR, are associated with positive lymph nodes, while the expression of GAS5 exhibited the opposite effect [113]. Although the FDA has approved epigenetic agents to overcome chemoresistance, to reverse DNA methylation (e.g., 5-azacytidine), and to reverse histone deacetylation (e.g., Trischostatin A and vorinostat (SAHA)), the efficacy of 5-azacytidine has not been consistent in breast cancers. Currently, a new BET inhibitor, ZEN-3694, is being tested in clinical trials because of its ability to prevent the interaction between the BET proteins and acetylated histones (Figure 2). ZEN-3694 is being evaluated in TNBC patients without germline mutations of *BRCA1* or *BRCA2* (NCT03901469; Table 1). Another phase I/II clinical trial is based on the reactivation of ER by decitabine and the histone deacetylase inhibitor, LBH589, in order to enhance the subsequent tamoxifen treatment (NCT01194908; Table 1).

Modification of the epigenetic machinery is a new tool for the treatment of TNBC, especially BET inhibitors. These drugs have already shown positive effects in preclinical models, and they have yet to be evaluated in clinical trials. These new drugs against epigenetic targets have the potential to decrease tumor aggressiveness and increase sensitivity to standard treatments. Maybe in the foreseeable future, these treatments will improve patient prognosis.

2.3. Epigenetic Modulation in Pancreatic Ductal Adenocarcinoma

Pancreatic ductal adenocarcinoma (PDAC) shows the lowest five-year survival rate, around 3%, and it is the fourth leading cause of cancer-related deaths in men and women [114]. It is often misdiagnosed and the symptoms are commonly treated by ambulatory care, leading to a late diagnosis; thus, patients present metastatic disease in ~80% of cases at diagnosis. Furthermore, it exhibits chemoresistance due to a complex link between the tumor cells and their microenvironment [115]. In PDAC, most of the studies are centered on mutations in *SMAD4*, *TP53*, *KRAS* or *CDKN2A*, which happen in more than 50% of patients [116]. Furthermore, the mutation in *MBD4* has been found in PDAC, with microsatellite instability [117]. A recent study discovered mutations and genetic variants in several epigenetic regulators, such as *ARID1B*, *PBRM1*, *SMARCA2*, *KDM6A*, *ARID1A*, *SMARCA4*, and *MLL2* [118]. In addition, PDAC has a broad epigenetic signature, which activates oncogenes and inactivates tumor-suppressive genes [119]. Both high- and low-grade PDAC exhibit specific epigenetic features associated with gene expression patterns. In low-grade PDAC, a highly enhanced H3K4me3 domain has been found, while in high-grade PDAC, a higher H3K4me1 signal was found [120]. Increased expression of DNMT1, DNMT3A and DNMT3B has been detected in PDAC, which suggests direct involvement in the epigenetic regulation of tumor progression [121]. In fact, hypermethylation has been found in *APC* (47.9% of cases), *BRCA1* (45.8%), P16/*INK4a* (35.4%), P15/*INK4b* (35.4%), *RARβ* (35.4%), and *P73* promoters (33.3%) in PDAC patients. Moreover, other genes are methylated to impair several signaling pathways, such as TGF-β, WNT, integrin or ROBO [122].

Concerning histone-modifying enzymes, aberrant HATs and HDACs have been found in PDAC. One study, performed in PDAC-derived cell lines, showed an inhibition of the expression of HAT, P300, and a secondary upregulation of several miRNAs [123]. The supplementary missense mutation in *P300* supports its role as a tumor-suppressive gene in PDAC [124]. The aberrant expression of HDACs is frequently observed in PDACs. For example, HDAC2 and HDAC7 expressions are increased in PDACs, especially in poorly differentiated cases [125,126]. Also, the overexpression of HDAC7 clearly differentiates PDAC from other benign pancreatic neoplasms. A study found that HDAC1 was overexpressed in 56% of PDAC and PanIN lesions [127]. Other studies suggest that RNF2 allows ubiquitination of H2A and downregulation of RNF2, which inhibits tumor proliferation in PDAC in vitro [128]. Histone acetyltransferase (HAT) inhibitors impact genome-wide H3K27ac patterns of PDAC cells [120]. The HAT inhibitors ICG-001 and C646 also impair gene expression and inhibit tumor growth in PDAC [129].

Concerning miRNA, one study with PDAC patients revealed a poor prognosis signature based on the deregulation of 64 miRNAs, and the upregulation of miR-21, miR-196a-2, miR-203, miR-155, miR-210, and miR-222 [130]. Further studies confirmed a decreased expression of miR-132 in PDAC by promoter methylation [131]. Also, lncRNAs have appeared as important regulators for PDAC tumorigenesis [132]. HOTAIR, HOTTIP, MALAT1, and PVT1 are the most studied oncogenic lncRNA in PDAC [133], while LINC00673 and H19 are potential tumor suppressors [134,135]. PIWI-interacting RNAs (piRNAs) and their association with the PIWI subfamily of Argonaute proteins are crucial in pancreatic cancer progression. Indeed, PIWIL1 and PIWIL2 proteins are downregulated in PDAC, probably due to CpG island methylation [136].

The impact of bromodomain inhibitors has also been evaluated in PDAC. BRD4770 is an inhibitor of G9a that induces PDAC autophagy [137]. Moreover, histone methylation regulatory genes, such as KDM6A, are expressed and considered a new candidate in PDAC tumorigenesis [118]. KDM6A is an H3K27me3 demethylase, which is necessary for endoderm differentiation [138]. Another study reported that regions with loss of KDM6A sensitize PDAC cells to bromodomain inhibitors [139]. Other factors have been involved in the progression of PDAC. For example, EZH2 is an H3K27 methyltransferase that has been shown to be overexpressed in PDAC cell lines and patients [140]. The high expression of EZH2 is associated with an aggressive, poorly differentiated subgroup, which shows a shorter survival of patients [141]. Treatments based on the EZH2 inhibitor, DZNep, enhanced the effect of gemcitabine in tumor-derived cell lines and primary cultures from PDAC [142]. Small-molecule inhibitors against EZH2, which are currently being investigated as target therapies against PDAC, are as follows: EPZ-6438, GSK126, CPI-169 and UNC-1999 [143]. High expression of KDM2B is found in PDAC, and it associates with $KRAS^{G12D}$ to promote tumor initiation in in vivo models [144]. It has been reported that histone H3 modification of the *MUC2* promoter region regulates *MUC2* gene expression, and this expression could be positively modulated by treatment with trichostatin A (TSA) and 5-aza [145]. Another significant treatment is based on the inhibition of telomerase, through the following epigenetic mechanism: methyl-2-cyano-3,12-dioxooleana-1,9(11)-dien-28-oate (CDDO-Me). This drug is able to decrease cell proliferation and induce apoptosis in PDAC, through the inhibition of the DNA methyl transferases DNMT1 and DNMT3a [146]. Another strategy with 5-aza-dC in combination with a MEK inhibitor is able to induce cell cycle arrest [147]. Interleukin-13 receptor α2 (IL-13Rα2) is a tumor-associated antigen and a potential target for cancer therapy. Indeed, histones at the IL-13Rα2 promoter region are highly- acetylated; thus, treatment with HDAC inhibitors enhanced the expression of IL-13Rα2 and allowed sensitization for a second treatment [148].

In clinical trials, a pilot study with relapsed patients (NCT02847000; Table 1) tested decitabine in combination with tetrahydrouridine, a cytidine deaminase inhibitor, to avoid catabolism of decitabine. In this study, investigators found scarce effect, due to the local and systemic overexpression of cytidine deaminase in metastatic patients; the resectable patients did not overexpress this protein. This suggested a need for even higher tetrahydrouridine doses in advanced stages [149]. Another phase II trial with resectable PDAC is ongoing, to improve survival with oral azacitidine (CC-486); it includes high-risk patients that have positive lymph nodes, positive margins and/or elevated CA19-9 levels (NCT01845805; Table 1; Figure 1). In another study, with advanced or metastatic PDAC patients, only the patients treated with the combination of azacitidine plus nab-paclitaxel completed the treatment [150]. Previously, other studies have set the bases for the use of romidepsin with small-molecule inhibitors, to target both the MAPK and PI3K signaling pathways to increase apoptosis in RAS-mutated tumors, such as PDAC [151]. Currently, a new clinical trial against PDAC is active, to determine the safety and tolerability of azacitidine and/or romidepsin, combined with nab-paclitaxel/gemcitabine, followed by anti-PD-L1 and lenalidomide (NCT04257448; Table 1). Despite the vast epigenetic landscape of PDAC, clinical and translational research is opening broad treatment perspectives with hopeful results, which involve modulation of the immune response, or administration of epigenetic therapies alone or in combination with standard chemotherapy, to improve patients survival.

2.4. Epigenetic Modulation in Glioblastoma

Glioblastoma (GBM) is the most commonly diagnosed tumor in elderly Caucasian men [152]. Unfortunately, there is no effective treatment for GBM and the standard treatment for such brain tumors comprises surgical resection with concomitant chemoradiotherapy with temozolomide, followed by adjuvant chemotherapy [153]. However, the main handicaps achieving a successful recovery are tumor heterogeneity, chemoresistance of cancer stem cells, and diffusion of drugs through the blood–brain barrier. Based on molecular profiling, GBMs are classified into the following three major groups: (1) the 1p/19q co-deletion status group, consisting of the IDH-mutant-1p/19q co-deletion status low-grade group; (2) the G-CIMP-low group, including IDH-mutant non-co-deletion status with low DNA methylation status; and (3) the G-CIMP-high group, including the IDH-mutant non-co-deletion group with higher global levels of DNA methylation. IDH mutants lead to major epigenetic changes, because they produce the onco-metabolite 2-hydroxyglutarate that hampers iron-dependent hydroxylases, which includes the 5′-methylcytosine hydroxylases belonging to the TET family [154]. Among these, the second group, G-CIMP-low, has the worst prognosis [155].

MGMT (O-6-methylguanine DNA methyltransferase) hypermethylation predicts BCNU (carmustine) and temozolomide response in gliomas [156,157]. Moreover, patients with hypermethylation of MGMT showed longer overall survival than patients without methylation (43 vs. 16 months, respectively), and a longer time to progress (36 vs. 11 months, respectively) [158]. Treatment with temozolomide combined with the HDAC inhibitor suberoylanilide hydroxamic acid (SAHA) delayed temozolomide resistance when compared with treatment with temozolomide alone, by MGMT overexpression [159]. Some HDAC inhibitory prodrugs of butyric acid and valproic acid increased the antitumor efficacy of doxorubicin, without cardiotoxicity, in mouse models of GBM (Figure 2) [160].

Recently, it has been described that a specific GBM subtype, with high levels of MGMT, expresses methyl-CpG binding domain 3 (MBD3) protein, which targets CK1A. Therefore, this subtype of patients may obtain benefit from CK1A activator pyrvinium pamoate (Pyr-Pam), leading to MBD3 degradation [161]. The new histone deacetylase inhibitor CKD5 is a derivative of 7-ureido-N-hydroxyheptanamide, and it revealed strong antitumor effects in GBM, both in in vitro and in vivo models. The use of the demethylases KDM1 and KDM5A was also evaluated as a potential therapeutic target [161]. A study demonstrated that the inhibition of KDM1 and KDM5A showed a significant antitumor effect in wild-type and temozolomide-resistant GBM cells [162]. Another study tested the multi-KDM inhibitor JIB-04, which has strong anti-clonogenic activity in wild-type and temozolomide-resistant GBM cell lines [163]. Another potent HDAC6 inhibitor, CAY-10603, is able to induce apoptosis in several GBM primary and stem cell-like cell lines [164]. Another study, with small molecules such as EZH2 and HDACi, achieved proliferation arrest of GBM [165]. Treatment with vorinostat (HDAC inhibitor) and tranylcypromine (histone lysine demethylase KDM1A inhibitor) (Figure 2) decreased GBM stem cell proliferation and led to significant tumor regression in mouse models [166]. Also, the use of bromodomain inhibitors have risen in popularity, due to enhanced tumor lethality [167]. In fact, the BET inhibitor caused downregulation of the lncRNA HOTAIR, which induced cell cycle arrest in GBM cells [168]. Several signaling pathways, such as WNT/β-catenin, mTOR, or P53-HIF, are found to be activated in gliomas, due to the downregulation of several lncRNAs [63]. The inhibition of HOTAIR leads to the increased expression of miR-326, which induces the expression of FGF-1 [169]. Another lncRNA, MALAT1, which is upregulated in temozolomide-resistant GBM, has been seen to promote miR-101, miR-203 and thymidylate synthase expression when downregulated [170,171].

Concerning clinical trials, the use of temsirolimus has obtained interesting improvement in 36% of treated patients; furthermore, the treatment achieved a significantly longer time to progress [172]. In contrast, panobinostat administration with bevacizumab did not show any significant improvement in progression-free survival compared to bevacizumab alone [173]. A phase I/II trial with a histone deacetylase inhibitor, romidepsin, found this drug to be inefficient for patients with recurrent GBM [174]. Currently, a phase I clinical trial is ongoing, to test whether folic acid is able to lead to MGMT methylation and improve temozolomide plus radiation treatment in grade IV tumors (NCT01700569; Table 1). This trial was based on the fact that folate could induce DNA methylation and increase the sensitivity to temozolomide in in vivo models [175].

In conclusion, although molecular diagnosis has brought new options to identify and treat patients, therapeutic options remain without any significant changes. Currently, the best standard treatment is the maximum safe resection, followed by chemoradiation and adjuvant chemotherapy. We hope that new clinical trials with epigenetic target therapies could improve the responses to conventional treatments.

2.5. Epigenetic Modulation in Metastatic Melanoma

The main issue with metastatic melanoma lies in its chemoresistance. Currently, the new immunecheckpoint inhibitors against CTLA-4, PD-1 or PD-L1 have improved patient outcome. However, secondary genomic aberrations make tumor cells acquire rapid resistance to these therapies [176]. One of the risk factors associated with melanoma is UV radiation; this is due to changes in DNA methyltransferase and in histone acetylation, which leads to silencing of tumor-suppressive genes. In contrast, some dietary consumption of green tea and proanthocyanidins from grape seeds has the ability to block UV-induced epigenetic modification in the skin of *CIP1*/P21 or *P16*/*INK4a* [177]. The epigenetic modifications of melanoma are well defined; in fact, malignant transformation of peritumoral skin is due to epigenetic changes [178]. CC chemokine receptor 7 (*CCR7*) and CXC chemokine receptor 4 (*CXCR4*) are epigenetically upregulated in melanoma cells, and have the ability to induce metastasis of melanoma [179]. The following four tumor-suppressive genes are frequently hypermethylated in advanced melanoma: death-associated protein kinase (*DAPK*), O6-methylguanine DNA methyl-transferase (*MGMT*), *RAS* association domain family protein 1A (*RASSF1A*), and retinoic acid receptor-β2 (*RAR-β2*). The hypermethylation of *DAPK*, *MGMT* and *RASSF1A* is significantly lower in the early stages than in the advanced stages, whereas the incidence of hypermethylation of *RAR-β2* is highly similar in the early and advanced stages [180]. The HDAC inhibitor dacinostat (LAQ824) is able to restore retinoid sensitivity by reverting *RAR-β2* methylation in melanoma cells, and it achieved the highest benefits in combination with retinoids [181]. Also, TET proteins have been reported to play a crucial role in melanoma, since their ectopic expression of TET2 eradicates tumor proliferation and increases survival in vivo [37]. It has been described that the loss of histone acetylation and H3K4 (histone H3 Lysine 4) methylation in *BRAFV600E* and *PTEN* promote malignant transformation of melanocytes [182]. EZH2 is another factor expressed in metastatic melanoma; its depletion has been shown to restore P21/*CDKN1A* expression and arrest cell proliferation [183].

Concerning ncRNA, several studies have reported the importance of miRNA regulation in melanoma. For example, miRNA-125b is involved in the regulation of vitamin D receptor (VDR), and in the resistance of 1,25-dihydroxyvitamin D_3, a potential therapy for metastatic melanoma [184]. Moreover, the expression of other miRNAs, from a large cluster of parentally imprinted regions located on chromosome 14q32, is significantly downregulated in melanoma, by epigenetic modulation. Interestingly, this miRNA cluster can be re-expressed with a combination of demethylating agents and histone deacetylase inhibitors. In this region, re-expression of mir-376a and mir-376c delayed cell growth and migration; moreover, one of the targets of both miRNAs is IGF1R, which is a tumor-prone factor in melanoma [185].

Since the largest clinical issue in the treatment of advanced melanoma patients is chemoresistance, the effort of researchers is centered around the discovery of a new treatment method to improve drug sensitivity. Interleukin-2 has exhibited potent antitumor activity in the fight against melanoma; nevertheless, its high toxicity has limited its use [186]. Treatment with SAHA is able to induce H3 and H4 hyperacetylation of P14/*ARF* promoter, and upregulate its expression [187]. Treatment with 5-aza-dC prevents the induction of DNMT1 and DNMT3b at the P16/*INK4A* promoter, leading to its subsequent activation [187]. Another treatment evaluated is allyl isothiocyanate (AITC), which has been reported to reduce cell proliferation and decrease the activation of HDACs, HATs, and other histone methyl transferases (HMTs). This approach is a very promising epigenetic therapy for advanced melanoma [188]. Some isothiocyanates, such as sulforaphane and iberin, could act over the epigenetic modulation of melanomas, and are currently under investigation [189]. Immune checkpoint-based therapy has improved patient lifespan from nine months to 2 years [190]. Perhaps, in the near future, the combination of anti-CTLA4 or anti-PD1 immune checkpoint inhibitors and epigenetic therapy could suppress the chemoresistance of metastatic melanoma [191].

Clinical trials with epigenetic therapy in metastatic melanoma have been mostly based on decitabine and other epigenetic modulating drugs, such as histone deacetylase inhibitors. A phase I clinical trial has explored the safety and tolerability of two epigenetic drugs, decitabine and panobinostat (a histone deacetylase inhibitor), in combination with temozolomide, to overcome chemoresistance in advanced melanoma (NCT00925132; Table 1). However, in this study, most of the patients exhibited disease progression [192]. Another clinical trial is testing the efficacy of oral azacitidine (CC-486) combined with pembrolizumab (NCT02816021; Table 1; Figure 1). Here, PD-1-naïve patients achieved a partial response (55% ORR), and accrual to this arm A continues; however, none of the patients with progression on prior PD-1 therapy, in arm B, have responded [193]. Other investigators have tested whether the action of vemurafenib (BRAF inhibitor) is more effective in combination with decitabine in low doses (NCT01876641; Table 1). Although the trial was terminated, due to a loss of funding, 3/14 patients achieved a complete response, 3/14 had a partial response, and 5/14 had stable disease. Moreover, its preclinical assessment demonstrated effectiveness of the combination, and a high potential in delaying chemoresistance [194]. Another clinical trial, performed in non-inflamed stage III/IV melanoma, is recruiting patients (NCT03765229; Table 1), and its clinical rationale is based on the induction of PD-L1 expression by the action of entinostat (HDAC inhibitor; Figure 2) [195]. The addition of anti-PD-1/anti-PD-L1 checkpoint inhibitors to HDAC inhibitors has been demonstrated to enhance the antitumor effect when compared to monotherapy, both in in vitro and in vivo models [196,197]. Another phase I clinical trial has evaluated the safety and efficacy of decitabine in combination with temozolomide (NCT00715793; Table 1). Here, there were 2/35 complete responses (CR), 4/35 partial responses (PR), 14/35 stable diseases (SD), 13/35 progressive diseases (PD), and the median overall survival was 12.4 months [198]. Another drug combination under investigation is tinostamustine with the anti-PD-L1 antibody nivolumab (NCT03903458; Table 1). Tinostamustine is an alkylating histone deacetylase inhibitor (HDACi), which resulted from the fusion of the alkylating agent bendamustine to the pan-HDACi vorinostat (Figure 2). This combination is expected to enhance the antineoplastic effect in refractory, locally advanced, or metastatic melanoma patients [199]. Also, the alkylating agent dacarbazine is the only drug approved by the Food and Drug Administration (FDA) as a therapy for advanced melanoma, with response rates between 7 and 13% [200].

Epigenetic therapies allow the reversibility of epigenetic modifications and are drawing attention to metastatic melanoma research, to prevent or delay the emergence of resistance to current standard treatments. Therefore, new discoveries in epigenetic therapies are expected to be evaluated in further clinical trials.

2.6. Epigenetic Modulation in Ovarian Cancer

Aggressive ovarian tumors (AOT) are the gynecological cancers with the highest mortality rate, probably because most AOT patients present advanced stages at diagnosis (stage III or IV), due to the lack of symptoms or unavailable specific screening biomarkers [201]. While response in the early stages is frequently acceptable, advanced tumors present a short progression driven by chemoresistance. Some translational research has shown that epigenetic aberrations are quite important in tumor initiation and development [202]. For example, the expression of HDAC2 hampers the DNA damage responses induced by platinum compounds, and contributes to the pathogenesis and chemoresistance of AOT [203]. In addition, the inhibition of H4K16 acetylation has been observed in AOT [204]. Further, hMOF, a member of the HATs family that acetylates H4K16, could also serve as an epigenetic biomarker for the diagnosis of malignant AOT, since patients with high expression levels of hMOF present improved survival when compared to those with low hMOF levels [205]. The presence of class I HDACs are able to induce the progression of AOT, and high expression of class I HDACs has also been detected in AOT patient samples. Furthermore, the expression of class I HDAC proteins has been considered a poor prognostic biomarker in AOT [206]. Cacan et al. have demonstrated that the downregulation of RGS2, an inhibitor of G-protein-coupled receptor proteins (GPCRs), confers chemoresistance of AOT cells, which is in part due to the repression of the promoter region of *RGS2* by class I HDACs [207]. Also, chemoresistance to platinum-based drugs has been associated with SIRT1 upregulation through the BRCA1–SIRT1–EGFR axis [208]. SIRT1 upregulation correlates to *TP53* inactivation by deacetylation [209]. SIRT3, in contrast, inhibits AOT cell migration via TWIST downregulation [210]. Other factors, such as EZH2, are overexpressed and have a direct positive correlation with AOT histological grade and tumor stage [211]. Further, 3-deazaneplanocin A (DZNEP) is a target for EZH2, with a promising anticancer efficacy against AOT [211]. Another EZH2 inhibitor, GSK126 (Figure 2), has demonstrated a better response in *ARID1A*-mutated patients [212]. Another study has associated LSD1 overexpression with AOT [213], and the combination of LSD1 with sodium butyrate increases most of the hallmarks of AOT [214,215]. Other factors, such as KDM3A, are crucial for AOT progression, undifferentiation, and platinum resistance, and have been identified as a potential target for AOT [216].

It is known that cancer modifies the microenvironment to inhibit the immune system. In this context, the overexpression of HLA-class I and II has been associated to AOT [217]. Epigenetically silenced hMLH1, together with cisplatin, could be an effective treatment, alongside decitabine and other HDAC inhibitors, such as belinostat (Figure 2), against AOT [218]. Chemoresistant tumor cells have inhibited the expression of OX-40L and 4-1BBL, two stimulator receptors of the immune system, with the concomitant overexpression of the immunosuppressive factor PD-L1 [219]. Indeed, HDAC1 and HDAC3 showed a strong association with OX-40L and 4-1BBL promoters, which contributes to OX-40L and 4-1BBL repression [219].

The inhibition of histone acetyltransferase is a new approach for the treatment of malignant AOT and its chemoresistance. The following three HDAC inhibitors have been approved by the FDA: romidepsin, panobinostat, and vorinostat (Figure 2). Trichostatin A (TSA), which exhibits a significant inhibition of class I and II HDACs, is able to activate P73 and trigger apoptosis in AOT cells [220]. Another study evaluated belinostat with carboplatin in platinum refractory AOT patients. However, the lack of drug activity concluded in the termination of the study [221]. Other authors initiated a phase Ib/II trial with recurrent AOT patients, to evaluate the clinical benefit of paclitaxel, carboplatin and belinostat [222]. Here, 3/35 patients presented a complete response, while 12/35 exhibited a partial response, with an ORR of 43%. It is remarkable that the median overall survival was not reached; thus, the results showed that paclitaxel + carboplatin + belinostat regimen demonstrated a clinical benefit. In a phase II study, vorinostat was evaluated for the treatment of recurrent AOT; however, vorinostat exhibited minimal activity as a single agent [223]. Another phase II trial evaluated the effect of hydralazine and magnesium valproate (NCT00404508; Table 1; Figures 1 and 2). The clinical benefit with these epigenetic agents was observed in 80% of patients, which supported their use as epigenetic therapy to overcome chemoresistance in recurrent patients [224]. Another study tested decitabine as an epigenetic chemosensitizer to carboplatin plus a paclitaxel regimen (NCT02159820; Table 1). The study is supported by the fact that 5-aza-dC treatment is able to restore P27 expression and increases the sensitivity of tumor cells to cisplatin [225]. Another study aims to determine the optimal dose of oral azacitidine (CC-486) in combination with pembrolizumab, for the treatment of platinum-resistant or refractory AOT (NCT02900560; Table 1; Figure 1).

AOC is strongly influenced by epigenetic changes that affected DNA methylation and histone modifications. The first attempts to modify the epigenetic of AOC with drugs have achieved low response rates as single agents; thus, their combination with targeted therapies, based on the mutational burden of tumors, must be evaluated.

3. Conclusions

In the clinic, patients with highly aggressive tumors are presented with different prognoses, despite having a similar stage and grade of cancer. These observations could be explained by the tumor heterogeneity that is characterized by several epigenetic modification profiles [226]. Firstly, we must highlight several oncogenic point mutations associated with epigenetic regulators, such as *IDH1/2, EZH2* or *DNMT3A*. Moreover, not all mutations are tumor-prone, and we must consider tumor-suppressive factors such as KDM6A and CREBBP/P300 [227]. Finally, another important element is when DNA epigenetic modifications emerge with histone modifications, to inactivate the action of tumor-suppressive factors [228]. All these actions are crucial in the regulation of tumor initiation and development. Overall, these alterations could serve as molecular biomarkers to stratify high-risk patients into different groups and provide the best treatment strategy in each case. We are confident that all the positive results, obtained in hematopoietic malignancies in preclinical studies, provide a strong rationale for further trials in highly aggressive solid tumors, to improve patient survival and prevent chemoresistance. Most of the clinical trials with epigenetic drugs are in combination with standard chemotherapies; however, further research is needed with the combination of epigenetic drugs and targeted therapies.

Author Contributions: Conceptualization, J.M.-U. and J.G.-F.; writing—original draft preparation, J.M.-U.; figures and tables, M.M.-G.; writing—review and editing, M.F.-C. and J.M.-U.; visualization, M.M.-G. and M.F.-C.; supervision, J.G.-F.; funding acquisition, J.M.-U. and J.G.-F. All authors have read and agreed to the published version of the manuscript.

Funding: This work has been carried out thanks to "V Becas de Investigación Carmen Delgado/Miguel Pérez-Mateo" (25791/001) by Asociación Cáncer de Páncreas (ACanPan) y la Asociación Española de Pancreatología (AESPANC).

Institutional Review Board Statement: Not applicable.

Informed Consent Statement: Not applicable.

Data Availability Statement: Not applicable.

Acknowledgments: We especially thank the oncologist Aberto Orta-Ruiz from the Medical Oncology Department (Fundacion Jimenez Diaz University Hospital) for his appreciated revision, suggestions and criticism for the present review article. All figures have been designed with BioRender.com.

Conflicts of Interest: The authors declare no conflict of interest.

References

1. Li, B.; Carey, M.; Workman, J.L. The Role of Chromatin during Transcription. *Cell* **2007**, *128*, 707–719. [CrossRef]
2. Lehninger, A.L.; Nelson, D.L.; Cox, M.M. *Lehninger Principles of Biochemistry*; W.H. Freeman: New York, NY, USA, 2005; ISBN 978-0-7167-4339-2.
3. Mariño-Ramírez, L.; Kann, M.G.; Shoemaker, B.A.; Landsman, D. Histone Structure and Nucleosome Stability. *Expert Rev. Proteom.* **2005**, *2*, 719–729. [CrossRef] [PubMed]
4. Becker, P.B.; Workman, J.L. Nucleosome Remodeling and Epigenetics. *Cold Spring Harb Perspect. Biol.* **2013**, *5*. [CrossRef] [PubMed]
5. Cheng, Y.; He, C.; Wang, M.; Ma, X.; Mo, F.; Yang, S.; Han, J.; Wei, X. Targeting Epigenetic Regulators for Cancer Therapy: Mechanisms and Advances in Clinical Trials. *Signal Transduct. Target. Ther.* **2019**, *4*, 62. [CrossRef] [PubMed]
6. Lee, E.; Wang, J.; Yumoto, K.; Jung, Y.; Cackowski, F.C.; Decker, A.M.; Li, Y.; Franceschi, R.T.; Pienta, K.J.; Taichman, R.S. DNMT1 Regulates Epithelial-Mesenchymal Transition and Cancer Stem Cells, Which Promotes Prostate Cancer Metastasis. *Neoplasia* **2016**, *18*, 553–566. [CrossRef]
7. Peng, K.; Su, G.; Ji, J.; Yang, X.; Miao, M.; Mo, P.; Li, M.; Xu, J.; Li, W.; Yu, C. Histone Demethylase JMJD1A Promotes Colorectal Cancer Growth and Metastasis by Enhancing Wnt/β-Catenin Signaling. *J. Biol. Chem.* **2018**, *293*, 10606–10619. [CrossRef] [PubMed]
8. Liu, W.-H.; Chang, L.-S. Arachidonic Acid Induces Fas and FasL Upregulation in Human Leukemia U937 Cells via Ca^{2+}/ROS-Mediated Suppression of ERK/c-Fos Pathway and Activation of P38 MAPK/ATF-2 Pathway. *Toxicol. Lett.* **2009**, *191*, 140–148. [CrossRef] [PubMed]

9. Esteller, M.; Gaidano, G.; Goodman, S.N.; Zagonel, V.; Capello, D.; Botto, B.; Rossi, D.; Gloghini, A.; Vitolo, U.; Carbone, A.; et al. Hypermethylation of the DNA Repair Gene O(6)-Methylguanine DNA Methyltransferase and Survival of Patients with Diffuse Large B-Cell Lymphoma. *J. Natl. Cancer Inst.* **2002**, *94*, 26–32. [CrossRef] [PubMed]
10. Qin, J.; Liu, Y.; Lu, Y.; Liu, M.; Li, M.; Li, J.; Wu, L. Hypoxia-Inducible Factor 1 Alpha Promotes Cancer Stem Cells-like Properties in Human Ovarian Cancer Cells by Upregulating SIRT1 Expression. *Sci. Rep.* **2017**, *7*, 10592. [CrossRef] [PubMed]
11. Tian, Y.-F.; Wang, H.-C.; Luo, C.-W.; Hung, W.-C.; Lin, Y.-H.; Chen, T.-Y.; Li, C.-F.; Lin, C.-Y.; Pan, M.-R. Preprogramming Therapeutic Response of PI3K/MTOR Dual Inhibitor via the Regulation of EHMT2 and P27 in Pancreatic Cancer. *Am. J. Cancer Res.* **2018**, *8*, 1812–1822.
12. Ghazi, T.; Arumugam, T.; Foolchand, A.; Chuturgoon, A.A. The Impact of Natural Dietary Compounds and Food-Borne Mycotoxins on DNA Methylation and Cancer. *Cells* **2020**, *9*, 2004. [CrossRef] [PubMed]
13. Holliday, R. A New Theory of Carcinogenesis. *Br. J. Cancer* **1979**, *40*, 513–522. [CrossRef] [PubMed]
14. Ramsahoye, B.H.; Biniszkiewicz, D.; Lyko, F.; Clark, V.; Bird, A.P.; Jaenisch, R. Non-CpG Methylation Is Prevalent in Embryonic Stem Cells and May Be Mediated by DNA Methyltransferase 3a. *Proc. Natl. Acad. Sci. USA* **2000**, *97*, 5237–5242. [CrossRef] [PubMed]
15. Saxonov, S.; Berg, P.; Brutlag, D.L. A Genome-Wide Analysis of CpG Dinucleotides in the Human Genome Distinguishes Two Distinct Classes of Promoters. *Proc. Natl. Acad. Sci. USA* **2006**, *103*, 1412–1417. [CrossRef]
16. Smith, Z.D.; Meissner, A. DNA Methylation: Roles in Mammalian Development. *Nat. Rev. Genet.* **2013**, *14*, 204–220. [CrossRef]
17. Schübeler, D. Function and Information Content of DNA Methylation. *Nature* **2015**, *517*, 321–326. [CrossRef]
18. El-Maarri, O.; Kareta, M.S.; Mikeska, T.; Becker, T.; Diaz-Lacava, A.; Junen, J.; Nüsgen, N.; Behne, F.; Wienker, T.; Waha, A.; et al. A Systematic Search for DNA Methyltransferase Polymorphisms Reveals a Rare DNMT3L Variant Associated with Subtelomeric Hypomethylation. *Hum. Mol. Genet.* **2009**, *18*, 1755–1768. [CrossRef] [PubMed]
19. Robertson, K.D.; Uzvolgyi, E.; Liang, G.; Talmadge, C.; Sumegi, J.; Gonzales, F.A.; Jones, P.A. The Human DNA Methyltransferases (DNMTs) 1, 3a and 3b: Coordinate MRNA Expression in Normal Tissues and Overexpression in Tumors. *Nucleic Acids Res.* **1999**, *27*, 2291–2298. [CrossRef]
20. Zhang, J.; Yang, C.; Wu, C.; Cui, W.; Wang, L. DNA Methyltransferases in Cancer: Biology, Paradox, Aberrations, and Targeted Therapy. *Cancers* **2020**, *12*, 2123. [CrossRef]
21. Klose, R.J.; Bird, A.P. Genomic DNA Methylation: The Mark and Its Mediators. *Trends Biochem. Sci.* **2006**, *31*, 89–97. [CrossRef]
22. Yildirim, O.; Li, R.; Hung, J.-H.; Chen, P.B.; Dong, X.; Ee, L.-S.; Weng, Z.; Rando, O.J.; Fazzio, T.G. Mbd3/NURD Complex Regulates Expression of 5-Hydroxymethylcytosine Marked Genes in Embryonic Stem Cells. *Cell* **2011**, *147*, 1498–1510. [CrossRef] [PubMed]
23. Kim, K.; Chadalapaka, G.; Lee, S.-O.; Yamada, D.; Sastre-Garau, X.; Defossez, P.-A.; Park, Y.-Y.; Lee, J.-S.; Safe, S. Identification of Oncogenic MicroRNA-17-92/ZBTB4/Specificity Protein Axis in Breast Cancer. *Oncogene* **2012**, *31*, 1034–1044. [CrossRef] [PubMed]
24. Mudbhary, R.; Hoshida, Y.; Chernyavskaya, Y.; Jacob, V.; Villanueva, A.; Fiel, M.I.; Chen, X.; Kojima, K.; Thung, S.; Bronson, R.T.; et al. UHRF1 Overexpression Drives DNA Hypomethylation and Hepatocellular Carcinoma. *Cancer Cell* **2014**, *25*, 196–209. [CrossRef] [PubMed]
25. Raynal, N.J.-M.; Lee, J.T.; Wang, Y.; Beaudry, A.; Madireddi, P.; Garriga, J.; Malouf, G.G.; Dumont, S.; Dettman, E.J.; Gharibyan, V.; et al. Targeting Calcium Signaling Induces Epigenetic Reactivation of Tumor Suppressor Genes in Cancer. *Cancer Res.* **2016**, *76*, 1494–1505. [CrossRef]
26. Krushkal, J.; Zhao, Y.; Hose, C.; Monks, A.; Doroshow, J.H.; Simon, R. Concerted Changes in Transcriptional Regulation of Genes Involved in DNA Methylation, Demethylation, and Folate-Mediated One-Carbon Metabolism Pathways in the NCI-60 Cancer Cell Line Panel in Response to Cancer Drug Treatment. *Clin. Epigenet.* **2016**, *8*, 73. [CrossRef] [PubMed]
27. Yamada, D.; Pérez-Torrado, R.; Filion, G.; Caly, M.; Jammart, B.; Devignot, V.; Sasai, N.; Ravassard, P.; Mallet, J.; Sastre-Garau, X.; et al. The Human Protein Kinase HIPK2 Phosphorylates and Downregulates the Methyl-Binding Transcription Factor ZBTB4. *Oncogene* **2009**, *28*, 2535–2544. [CrossRef]
28. Alhosin, M.; Omran, Z.; Zamzami, M.A.; Al-Malki, A.L.; Choudhry, H.; Mousli, M.; Bronner, C. Signalling Pathways in UHRF1-Dependent Regulation of Tumor Suppressor Genes in Cancer. *J. Exp. Clin. Cancer Res.* **2016**, *35*, 174. [CrossRef]
29. Giovinazzo, H.; Walker, D.; Wyhs, N.; Liu, J.; Esopi, D.M.; Vaghasia, A.M.; Jain, Y.; Bhamidipati, A.; Zhou, J.; Nelson, W.G.; et al. A High-Throughput Screen of Pharmacologically Active Compounds for Inhibitors of UHRF1 Reveals Epigenetic Activity of Anthracycline Derivative Chemotherapeutic Drugs. *Oncotarget* **2019**, *10*, 3040–3050. [CrossRef] [PubMed]
30. Wilting, R.H.; Dannenberg, J.-H. Epigenetic Mechanisms in Tumorigenesis, Tumor Cell Heterogeneity and Drug Resistance. *Drug Resist. Updates* **2012**, *15*, 21–38. [CrossRef]
31. Keshet, I.; Lieman-Hurwitz, J.; Cedar, H. DNA Methylation Affects the Formation of Active Chromatin. *Cell* **1986**, *44*, 535–543. [CrossRef]
32. Baylin, S.B.; Jones, P.A. A Decade of Exploring the Cancer Epigenome—Biological and Translational Implications. *Nat. Rev. Cancer* **2011**, *11*, 726–734. [CrossRef]
33. Pastor, W.A.; Aravind, L.; Rao, A. TETonic Shift: Biological Roles of TET Proteins in DNA Demethylation and Transcription. *Nat. Rev. Mol. Cell Biol.* **2013**, *14*, 341–356. [CrossRef] [PubMed]

34. Liu, C.; Liu, L.; Chen, X.; Shen, J.; Shan, J.; Xu, Y.; Yang, Z.; Wu, L.; Xia, F.; Bie, P.; et al. Decrease of 5-Hydroxymethylcytosine Is Associated with Progression of Hepatocellular Carcinoma through Downregulation of TET1. *PLoS ONE* **2013**, *8*, e62828. [CrossRef]
35. Rasmussen, K.D.; Helin, K. Role of TET Enzymes in DNA Methylation, Development, and Cancer. *Genes Dev.* **2016**, *30*, 733–750. [CrossRef]
36. Turcan, S.; Rohle, D.; Goenka, A.; Walsh, L.A.; Fang, F.; Yilmaz, E.; Campos, C.; Fabius, A.W.M.; Lu, C.; Ward, P.S.; et al. IDH1 Mutation Is Sufficient to Establish the Glioma Hypermethylator Phenotype. *Nature* **2012**, *483*, 479–483. [CrossRef] [PubMed]
37. Lian, C.G.; Xu, Y.; Ceol, C.; Wu, F.; Larson, A.; Dresser, K.; Xu, W.; Tan, L.; Hu, Y.; Zhan, Q.; et al. Loss of 5-Hydroxymethylcytosine Is an Epigenetic Hallmark of Melanoma. *Cell* **2012**, *150*, 1135–1146. [CrossRef]
38. Yang, H.; Liu, Y.; Bai, F.; Zhang, J.-Y.; Ma, S.-H.; Liu, J.; Xu, Z.-D.; Zhu, H.-G.; Ling, Z.-Q.; Ye, D.; et al. Tumor Development Is Associated with Decrease of TET Gene Expression and 5-Methylcytosine Hydroxylation. *Oncogene* **2013**, *32*, 663–669. [CrossRef]
39. Nacheva, G.A.; Guschin, D.Y.; Preobrazhenskaya, O.V.; Karpov, V.L.; Ebralidse, K.K.; Mirzabekov, A.D. Change in the Pattern of Histone Binding to DNA upon Transcriptional Activation. *Cell* **1989**, *58*, 27–36. [CrossRef]
40. Schneider, J.; Shilatifard, A. Histone Demethylation by Hydroxylation: Chemistry in Action. *ACS Chem. Biol.* **2006**, *1*, 75–81. [CrossRef]
41. Audia, J.E.; Campbell, R.M. Histone Modifications and Cancer. *Cold Spring Harb Perspect. Biol.* **2016**, *8*, a019521. [CrossRef]
42. Jenuwein, T.; Allis, C.D. Translating the Histone Code. *Science* **2001**, *293*, 1074–1080. [CrossRef] [PubMed]
43. Di Cerbo, V.; Schneider, R. Cancers with Wrong HATs: The Impact of Acetylation. *Brief. Funct. Genom.* **2013**, *12*, 231–243. [CrossRef]
44. Seligson, D.B.; Horvath, S.; McBrian, M.A.; Mah, V.; Yu, H.; Tze, S.; Wang, Q.; Chia, D.; Goodglick, L.; Kurdistani, S.K. Global Levels of Histone Modifications Predict Prognosis in Different Cancers. *Am. J. Pathol.* **2009**, *174*, 1619–1628. [CrossRef] [PubMed]
45. Fraga, M.F.; Ballestar, E.; Villar-Garea, A.; Boix-Chornet, M.; Espada, J.; Schotta, G.; Bonaldi, T.; Haydon, C.; Ropero, S.; Petrie, K.; et al. Loss of Acetylation at Lys16 and Trimethylation at Lys20 of Histone H4 Is a Common Hallmark of Human Cancer. *Nat. Genet.* **2005**, *37*, 391–400. [CrossRef] [PubMed]
46. Milazzo, G.; Mercatelli, D.; Di Muzio, G.; Triboli, L.; De Rosa, P.; Perini, G.; Giorgi, F.M. Histone Deacetylases (HDACs): Evolution, Specificity, Role in Transcriptional Complexes, and Pharmacological Actionability. *Genes* **2020**, *11*, 556. [CrossRef]
47. Kim, E.-J.; Kho, J.-H.; Kang, M.-R.; Um, S.-J. Active Regulator of SIRT1 Cooperates with SIRT1 and Facilitates Suppression of P53 Activity. *Mol. Cell* **2007**, *28*, 277–290. [CrossRef]
48. Singh, M.M.; Manton, C.A.; Bhat, K.P.; Tsai, W.-W.; Aldape, K.; Barton, M.C.; Chandra, J. Inhibition of LSD1 Sensitizes Glioblastoma Cells to Histone Deacetylase Inhibitors. *Neuro-Oncology* **2011**, *13*, 894–903. [CrossRef]
49. Pedersen, M.T.; Helin, K. Histone Demethylases in Development and Disease. *Trends Cell Biol.* **2010**, *20*, 662–671. [CrossRef]
50. Dhalluin, C.; Carlson, J.E.; Zeng, L.; He, C.; Aggarwal, A.K.; Zhou, M.M. Structure and Ligand of a Histone Acetyltransferase Bromodomain. *Nature* **1999**, *399*, 491–496. [CrossRef]
51. Xu, Y.; Vakoc, C.R. Targeting Cancer Cells with BET Bromodomain Inhibitors. *Cold Spring Harb Perspect. Med.* **2017**, *7*. [CrossRef]
52. Bernstein, E.; Caudy, A.A.; Hammond, S.M.; Hannon, G.J. Role for a Bidentate Ribonuclease in the Initiation Step of RNA Interference. *Nature* **2001**, *409*, 363–366. [CrossRef]
53. Martinez, J.; Patkaniowska, A.; Urlaub, H.; Lührmann, R.; Tuschl, T. Single-Stranded Antisense SiRNAs Guide Target RNA Cleavage in RNAi. *Cell* **2002**, *110*, 563–574. [CrossRef]
54. Zamore, P.D.; Tuschl, T.; Sharp, P.A.; Bartel, D.P. RNAi: Double-Stranded RNA Directs the ATP-Dependent Cleavage of MRNA at 21 to 23 Nucleotide Intervals. *Cell* **2000**, *101*, 25–33. [CrossRef]
55. Calin, G.A.; Sevignani, C.; Dumitru, C.D.; Hyslop, T.; Noch, E.; Yendamuri, S.; Shimizu, M.; Rattan, S.; Bullrich, F.; Negrini, M.; et al. Human MicroRNA Genes Are Frequently Located at Fragile Sites and Genomic Regions Involved in Cancers. *Proc. Natl. Acad Sci. USA* **2004**, *101*, 2999–3004. [CrossRef]
56. Han, J.; Lee, Y.; Yeom, K.-H.; Nam, J.-W.; Heo, I.; Rhee, J.-K.; Sohn, S.Y.; Cho, Y.; Zhang, B.-T.; Kim, V.N. Molecular Basis for the Recognition of Primary MicroRNAs by the Drosha-DGCR8 Complex. *Cell* **2006**, *125*, 887–901. [CrossRef] [PubMed]
57. Vagin, V.V.; Sigova, A.; Li, C.; Seitz, H.; Gvozdev, V.; Zamore, P.D. A Distinct Small RNA Pathway Silences Selfish Genetic Elements in the Germline. *Science* **2006**, *313*, 320–324. [CrossRef] [PubMed]
58. Liu, Y.; Dou, M.; Song, X.; Dong, Y.; Liu, S.; Liu, H.; Tao, J.; Li, W.; Yin, X.; Xu, W. The Emerging Role of the PiRNA/Piwi Complex in Cancer. *Mol. Cancer* **2019**, *18*, 123. [CrossRef]
59. Koch, L. Functional Genomics: Screening for LncRNA Function. *Nat. Rev. Genet.* **2017**, *18*, 70. [CrossRef]
60. Wang, Z.; Yang, B.; Zhang, M.; Guo, W.; Wu, Z.; Wang, Y.; Jia, L.; Li, S.; Cancer Genome Atlas Research Network; Xie, W.; et al. LncRNA Epigenetic Landscape Analysis Identifies EPIC1 as an Oncogenic LncRNA That Interacts with MYC and Promotes Cell-Cycle Progression in Cancer. *Cancer Cell* **2018**, *33*, 706–720.e9. [CrossRef] [PubMed]
61. Bhan, A.; Mandal, S.S. Long Noncoding RNAs: Emerging Stars in Gene Regulation, Epigenetics and Human Disease. *Chem. Med. Chem.* **2014**, *9*, 1932–1956. [CrossRef]
62. Tsai, M.-C.; Manor, O.; Wan, Y.; Mosammaparast, N.; Wang, J.K.; Lan, F.; Shi, Y.; Segal, E.; Chang, H.Y. Long Noncoding RNA as Modular Scaffold of Histone Modification Complexes. *Science* **2010**, *329*, 689–693. [CrossRef]
63. Shi, J.; Dong, B.; Cao, J.; Mao, Y.; Guan, W.; Peng, Y.; Wang, S. Long Non-Coding RNA in Glioma: Signaling Pathways. *Oncotarget* **2017**, *8*, 27582–27592. [CrossRef]

64. Wu, Y.; Xiong, Q.; Li, S.; Yang, X.; Ge, F. Integrated Proteomic and Transcriptomic Analysis Reveals Long Noncoding RNA HOX Transcript Antisense Intergenic RNA (HOTAIR) Promotes Hepatocellular Carcinoma Cell Proliferation by Regulating Opioid Growth Factor Receptor (OGFr). *Mol. Cell Proteom.* **2018**, *17*, 146–159. [CrossRef] [PubMed]
65. Chen, J.; Lin, C.; Yong, W.; Ye, Y.; Huang, Z. Calycosin and Genistein Induce Apoptosis by Inactivation of HOTAIR/p-Akt Signaling Pathway in Human Breast Cancer MCF-7 Cells. *Cell Physiol. Biochem.* **2015**, *35*, 722–728. [CrossRef] [PubMed]
66. Gutschner, T.; Hämmerle, M.; Eissmann, M.; Hsu, J.; Kim, Y.; Hung, G.; Revenko, A.; Arun, G.; Stentrup, M.; Gross, M.; et al. The Noncoding RNA MALAT1 Is a Critical Regulator of the Metastasis Phenotype of Lung Cancer Cells. *Cancer Res.* **2013**, *73*, 1180–1189. [CrossRef] [PubMed]
67. Tian, Y.; Zhang, X.; Hao, Y.; Fang, Z.; He, Y. Potential Roles of Abnormally Expressed Long Noncoding RNA UCA1 and Malat-1 in Metastasis of Melanoma. *Melanoma Res.* **2014**, *24*, 335–341. [CrossRef]
68. Schmidt, L.H.; Spieker, T.; Koschmieder, S.; Schäffers, S.; Humberg, J.; Jungen, D.; Bulk, E.; Hascher, A.; Wittmer, D.; Marra, A.; et al. The Long Noncoding MALAT-1 RNA Indicates a Poor Prognosis in Non-Small Cell Lung Cancer and Induces Migration and Tumor Growth. *J. Thorac. Oncol.* **2011**, *6*, 1984–1992. [CrossRef]
69. Ma, K.; Wang, H.; Li, X.; Li, T.; Su, G.; Yang, P.; Wu, J. Long Noncoding RNA MALAT1 Associates with the Malignant Status and Poor Prognosis in Glioma. *Tumour Biol.* **2015**, *36*, 3355–3359. [CrossRef]
70. Liu, W.; Zhou, Z.; Chen, L.; Wang, X. Comparison of Azacitidine and Decitabine in Myelodysplastic Syndromes and Acute Myeloid Leukemia: A Network Meta-Analysis. *Clin. Lymphoma Myeloma Leuk.* **2021**. [CrossRef]
71. Momparler, R.L. Epigenetic Therapy of Cancer with 5-Aza-2′-Deoxycytidine (Decitabine). *Semin Oncol.* **2005**, *32*, 443–451. [CrossRef]
72. Jung, Y.; Park, J.; Kim, T.Y.; Park, J.-H.; Jong, H.-S.; Im, S.-A.; Robertson, K.D.; Bang, Y.-J.; Kim, T.-Y. Potential Advantages of DNA Methyltransferase 1 (DNMT1)-Targeted Inhibition for Cancer Therapy. *J. Mol. Med.* **2007**, *85*, 1137–1148. [CrossRef]
73. Marks, P.A.; Richon, V.M.; Rifkind, R.A. Histone Deacetylase Inhibitors: Inducers of Differentiation or Apoptosis of Transformed Cells. *J. Natl. Cancer Inst.* **2000**, *92*, 1210–1216. [CrossRef] [PubMed]
74. Iannitti, T.; Palmieri, B. Clinical and Experimental Applications of Sodium Phenylbutyrate. *Drugs R D* **2011**, *11*, 227–249. [CrossRef]
75. Maleszewska, M.; Kaminska, B. Deregulation of Histone-Modifying Enzymes and Chromatin Structure Modifiers Contributes to Glioma Development. *Future Oncol.* **2015**, *11*, 2587–2601. [CrossRef]
76. Bruserud, Ø.; Stapnes, C.; Ersvaer, E.; Gjertsen, B.T.; Ryningen, A. Histone Deacetylase Inhibitors in Cancer Treatment: A Review of the Clinical Toxicity and the Modulation of Gene Expression in Cancer Cell. *Curr. Pharm. Biotechnol.* **2007**, *8*, 388–400. [CrossRef] [PubMed]
77. Jarred, E.G.; Bildsoe, H.; Western, P.S. Out of Sight, out of Mind? Germ Cells and the Potential Impacts of Epigenomic Drugs. *F1000 Res.* **2018**, *7*. [CrossRef]
78. Shah, M.H.; Binkley, P.; Chan, K.; Xiao, J.; Arbogast, D.; Collamore, M.; Farra, Y.; Young, D.; Grever, M. Cardiotoxicity of Histone Deacetylase Inhibitor Depsipeptide in Patients with Metastatic Neuroendocrine Tumors. *Clin. Cancer Res.* **2006**, *12*, 3997–4003. [CrossRef] [PubMed]
79. Riaz, S.P.; Lüchtenborg, M.; Coupland, V.H.; Spicer, J.; Peake, M.D.; Møller, H. Trends in Incidence of Small Cell Lung Cancer and All Lung Cancer. *Lung Cancer* **2012**, *75*, 280–284. [CrossRef]
80. He, Z.; Li, D.; Ma, J.; Chen, L.; Duan, H.; Zhang, B.; Gao, C.; Li, J.; Xing, X.; Zhao, J.; et al. TRIM36 Hypermethylation Is Involved in Polycyclic Aromatic Hydrocarbons-Induced Cell Transformation. *Environ. Pollut.* **2017**, *225*, 93–103. [CrossRef]
81. Morabito, A.; Rolfo, C. Small Cell Lung Cancer: A New Era Is Beginning? *Cancers* **2021**, *13*, 2646. [CrossRef]
82. Nikolaidis, G.; Raji, O.Y.; Markopoulou, S.; Gosney, J.R.; Bryan, J.; Warburton, C.; Walshaw, M.; Sheard, J.; Field, J.K.; Liloglou, T. DNA Methylation Biomarkers Offer Improved Diagnostic Efficiency in Lung Cancer. *Cancer Res.* **2012**, *72*, 5692–5701. [CrossRef] [PubMed]
83. Sakaeda, M.; Sato, H.; Ishii, J.; Miyata, C.; Kamma, H.; Shishido-Hara, Y.; Shimoyamada, H.; Fujiwara, M.; Endo, T.; Tanaka, R.; et al. Neural Lineage-Specific Homeoprotein BRN2 Is Directly Involved in TTF1 Expression in Small-Cell Lung Cancer. *Lab. Investig.* **2013**, *93*, 408–421. [CrossRef] [PubMed]
84. Kwei, K.A.; Kim, Y.H.; Girard, L.; Kao, J.; Pacyna-Gengelbach, M.; Salari, K.; Lee, J.; Choi, Y.-L.; Sato, M.; Wang, P.; et al. Genomic Profiling Identifies TITF1 as a Lineage-Specific Oncogene Amplified in Lung Cancer. *Oncogene* **2008**, *27*, 3635–3640. [CrossRef] [PubMed]
85. Powrózek, T.; Krawczyk, P.; Nicoś, M.; Kuźnar-Kamińska, B.; Batura-Gabryel, H.; Milanowski, J. Methylation of the DCLK1 Promoter Region in Circulating Free DNA and Its Prognostic Value in Lung Cancer Patients. *Clin. Transl. Oncol.* **2016**, *18*, 398–404. [CrossRef] [PubMed]
86. Wang, L.; Aakre, J.A.; Jiang, R.; Marks, R.S.; Wu, Y.; Chen, J.; Thibodeau, S.N.; Pankratz, V.S.; Yang, P. Methylation Markers for Small Cell Lung Cancer in Peripheral Blood Leukocyte DNA. *J. Thorac. Oncol.* **2010**, *5*, 778–785. [CrossRef]
87. Luszczek, W.; Cheriyath, V.; Mekhail, T.M.; Borden, E.C. Combinations of DNA Methyltransferase and Histone Deacetylase Inhibitors Induce DNA Damage in Small Cell Lung Cancer Cells: Correlation of Resistance with IFN-Stimulated Gene Expression. *Mol. Cancer Ther.* **2010**, *9*, 2309–2321. [CrossRef]

88. El-Khoury, V.; Breuzard, G.; Fourré, N.; Dufer, J. The Histone Deacetylase Inhibitor Trichostatin A Downregulates Human MDR1 (ABCB1) Gene Expression by a Transcription-Dependent Mechanism in a Drug-Resistant Small Cell Lung Carcinoma Cell Line Model. *Br. J. Cancer* **2007**, *97*, 562–573. [CrossRef]
89. Das, D.S.; Ray, A.; Das, A.; Song, Y.; Tian, Z.; Oronsky, B.; Richardson, P.; Scicinski, J.; Chauhan, D.; Anderson, K.C. A Novel Hypoxia-Selective Epigenetic Agent RRx-001 Triggers Apoptosis and Overcomes Drug Resistance in Multiple Myeloma Cells. *Leukemia* **2016**, *30*, 2187–2197. [CrossRef]
90. Morgensztern, D.; Rose, M.; Waqar, S.N.; Morris, J.; Ma, P.C.; Reid, T.; Brzezniak, C.E.; Zeman, K.G.; Padmanabhan, A.; Hirth, J.; et al. RRx-001 Followed by Platinum plus Etoposide in Patients with Previously Treated Small-Cell Lung Cancer. *Br. J. Cancer* **2019**, *121*, 211–217. [CrossRef]
91. Mathieu, L.; Shah, S.; Pai-Scherf, L.; Larkins, E.; Vallejo, J.; Li, X.; Rodriguez, L.; Mishra-Kalyani, P.; Goldberg, K.B.; Kluetz, P.G.; et al. FDA Approval Summary: Atezolizumab and Durvalumab in Combination with Platinum-Based Chemotherapy in Extensive Stage Small Cell Lung Cancer. *Oncologist* **2021**, *26*, 433–438. [CrossRef]
92. Herschkowitz, J.I.; Zhao, W.; Zhang, M.; Usary, J.; Murrow, G.; Edwards, D.; Knezevic, J.; Greene, S.B.; Darr, D.; Troester, M.A.; et al. Comparative Oncogenomics Identifies Breast Tumors Enriched in Functional Tumor-Initiating Cells. *Proc. Natl. Acad. Sci. USA* **2012**, *109*, 2778–2783. [CrossRef] [PubMed]
93. Benevolenskaya, E.V.; Islam, A.B.M.M.K.; Ahsan, H.; Kibriya, M.G.; Jasmine, F.; Wolff, B.; Al-Alem, U.; Wiley, E.; Kajdacsy-Balla, A.; Macias, V.; et al. DNA Methylation and Hormone Receptor Status in Breast Cancer. *Clin. Epigenet.* **2016**, *8*, 17. [CrossRef] [PubMed]
94. Martínez-Galán, J.; Torres-Torres, B.; Núñez, M.I.; López-Peñalver, J.; Del Moral, R.; Ruiz De Almodóvar, J.M.; Menjón, S.; Concha, A.; Chamorro, C.; Ríos, S.; et al. ESR1 Gene Promoter Region Methylation in Free Circulating DNA and Its Correlation with Estrogen Receptor Protein Expression in Tumor Tissue in Breast Cancer Patients. *BMC Cancer* **2014**, *14*, 59. [CrossRef] [PubMed]
95. Yamamoto, M.; Ito, T.; Shimizu, T.; Ishida, T.; Semba, K.; Watanabe, S.; Yamaguchi, N.; Inoue, J.-I. Epigenetic Alteration of the NF-KB-Inducing Kinase (NIK) Gene Is Involved in Enhanced NIK Expression in Basal-like Breast Cancer. *Cancer Sci.* **2010**, *101*, 2391–2397. [CrossRef]
96. Grigoriadis, A.; Mackay, A.; Noel, E.; Wu, P.J.; Natrajan, R.; Frankum, J.; Reis-Filho, J.S.; Tutt, A. Molecular Characterisation of Cell Line Models for Triple-Negative Breast Cancers. *BMC Genom.* **2012**, *13*, 619. [CrossRef] [PubMed]
97. Lee, J.S.; Fackler, M.J.; Lee, J.H.; Choi, C.; Park, M.H.; Yoon, J.H.; Zhang, Z.; Sukumar, S. Basal-like Breast Cancer Displays Distinct Patterns of Promoter Methylation. *Cancer Biol. Ther.* **2010**, *9*, 1017–1024. [CrossRef]
98. Na, B.; Yu, X.; Withers, T.; Gilleran, J.; Yao, M.; Foo, T.K.; Chen, C.; Moore, D.; Lin, Y.; Kimball, S.D.; et al. Therapeutic Targeting of BRCA1 and TP53 Mutant Breast Cancer through Mutant P53 Reactivation. *NPJ Breast Cancer* **2019**, *5*, 14. [CrossRef]
99. Su, Y.; Hopfinger, N.R.; Nguyen, T.D.; Pogash, T.J.; Santucci-Pereira, J.; Russo, J. Epigenetic Reprogramming of Epithelial Mesenchymal Transition in Triple Negative Breast Cancer Cells with DNA Methyltransferase and Histone Deacetylase Inhibitors. *J. Exp. Clin. Cancer Res.* **2018**, *37*, 314. [CrossRef]
100. Kwon, M.J.; Han, J.; Seo, J.H.; Song, K.; Jeong, H.M.; Choi, J.-S.; Kim, Y.J.; Lee, S.-H.; Choi, Y.-L.; Shin, Y.K. CD24 Overexpression Is Associated with Poor Prognosis in Luminal A and Triple-Negative Breast Cancer. *PLoS ONE* **2015**, *10*, e0139112. [CrossRef]
101. Dhasarathy, A.; Phadke, D.; Mav, D.; Shah, R.R.; Wade, P.A. The Transcription Factors Snail and Slug Activate the Transforming Growth Factor-Beta Signaling Pathway in Breast Cancer. *PLoS ONE* **2011**, *6*, e26514. [CrossRef]
102. Győrffy, B.; Surowiak, P.; Budczies, J.; Lánczky, A. Online Survival Analysis Software to Assess the Prognostic Value of Biomarkers Using Transcriptomic Data in Non-Small-Cell Lung Cancer. *PLoS ONE* **2013**, *8*, e82241. [CrossRef]
103. Huang, J.P.; Ling, K. EZH2 and Histone Deacetylase Inhibitors Induce Apoptosis in Triple Negative Breast Cancer Cells by Differentially Increasing H3 Lys27 Acetylation in the BIM Gene Promoter and Enhancers. *Oncol. Lett.* **2017**, *14*, 5735–5742. [CrossRef] [PubMed]
104. Augoff, K.; McCue, B.; Plow, E.F.; Sossey-Alaoui, K. MiR-31 and Its Host Gene LncRNA LOC554202 Are Regulated by Promoter Hypermethylation in Triple-Negative Breast Cancer. *Mol. Cancer* **2012**, *11*, 5. [CrossRef] [PubMed]
105. Diermeier, S.D.; Chang, K.-C.; Freier, S.M.; Song, J.; El Demerdash, O.; Krasnitz, A.; Rigo, F.; Bennett, C.F.; Spector, D.L. Mammary Tumor-Associated RNAs Impact Tumor Cell Proliferation, Invasion, and Migration. *Cell Rep.* **2016**, *17*, 261–274. [CrossRef] [PubMed]
106. Jin, C.; Yan, B.; Lu, Q.; Lin, Y.; Ma, L. Reciprocal Regulation of Hsa-MiR-1 and Long Noncoding RNA MALAT1 Promotes Triple-Negative Breast Cancer Development. *Tumour Biol.* **2016**, *37*, 7383–7394. [CrossRef]
107. Zuo, Y.; Li, Y.; Zhou, Z.; Ma, M.; Fu, K. Long Non-Coding RNA MALAT1 Promotes Proliferation and Invasion via Targeting MiR-129–5p in Triple-Negative Breast Cancer. *Biomed. Pharmacother.* **2017**, *95*, 922–928. [CrossRef]
108. Liang, H.; Huang, W.; Wang, Y.; Ding, L.; Zeng, L. Overexpression of MiR-146a-5p Upregulates LncRNA HOTAIR in Triple-Negative Breast Cancer Cells and Predicts Poor Prognosis. *Technol. Cancer Res. Treat.* **2019**, *18*, 1533033819882949. [CrossRef]
109. Collina, F.; Aquino, G.; Brogna, M.; Cipolletta, S.; Buonfanti, G.; De Laurentiis, M.; Di Bonito, M.; Cantile, M.; Botti, G. LncRNA HOTAIR Up-Regulation Is Strongly Related with Lymph Nodes Metastasis and LAR Subtype of Triple Negative Breast Cancer. *J. Cancer* **2019**, *10*, 2018–2024. [CrossRef]
110. Li, S.; Zhou, J.; Wang, Z.; Wang, P.; Gao, X.; Wang, Y. Long Noncoding RNA GAS5 Suppresses Triple Negative Breast Cancer Progression through Inhibition of Proliferation and Invasion by Competitively Binding MiR-196a-5p. *Biomed. Pharmacother.* **2018**, *104*, 451–457. [CrossRef]

111. Zheng, S.; Li, M.; Miao, K.; Xu, H. LncRNA GAS5-Promoted Apoptosis in Triple-Negative Breast Cancer by Targeting MiR-378a-5p/SUFU Signaling. *J. Cell Biochem.* **2020**, *121*, 2225–2235. [CrossRef] [PubMed]
112. Tuluhong, D.; Dunzhu, W.; Wang, J.; Chen, T.; Li, H.; Li, Q.; Wang, S. Prognostic Value of Differentially Expressed LncRNAs in Triple-Negative Breast Cancer: A Systematic Review and Meta-Analysis. *Crit. Rev. Eukaryot. Gene Expr.* **2020**, *30*, 447–456. [CrossRef] [PubMed]
113. Zhang, S.; Ma, F.; Xie, X.; Shen, Y. Prognostic Value of Long Non-Coding RNAs in Triple Negative Breast Cancer: A PRISMA-Compliant Meta-Analysis. *Medicine* **2020**, *99*, e21861. [CrossRef] [PubMed]
114. Siegel, R.L.; Miller, K.D.; Fuchs, H.E.; Jemal, A. Cancer Statistics, 2021. *CA Cancer J. Clin.* **2021**, *71*, 7–33. [CrossRef] [PubMed]
115. Zeng, S.; Pöttler, M.; Lan, B.; Grützmann, R.; Pilarsky, C.; Yang, H. Chemoresistance in Pancreatic Cancer. *Int. J. Mol. Sci.* **2019**, *20*, 4504. [CrossRef]
116. Singhi, A.D.; Wood, L.D. Early Detection of Pancreatic Cancer Using DNA-Based Molecular Approaches. *Nat. Rev. Gastroenterol. Hepatol.* **2021**. [CrossRef]
117. Riccio, A.; Aaltonen, L.A.; Godwin, A.K.; Loukola, A.; Percesepe, A.; Salovaara, R.; Masciullo, V.; Genuardi, M.; Paravatou-Petsotas, M.; Bassi, D.E.; et al. The DNA Repair Gene MBD4 (MED1) Is Mutated in Human Carcinomas with Microsatellite Instability. *Nat. Genet.* **1999**, *23*, 266–268. [CrossRef]
118. Waddell, N.; Pajic, M.; Patch, A.-M.; Chang, D.K.; Kassahn, K.S.; Bailey, P.; Johns, A.L.; Miller, D.; Nones, K.; Quek, K.; et al. Whole Genomes Redefine the Mutational Landscape of Pancreatic Cancer. *Nature* **2015**, *518*, 495–501. [CrossRef] [PubMed]
119. Jones, S.; Zhang, X.; Parsons, D.W.; Lin, J.C.-H.; Leary, R.J.; Angenendt, P.; Mankoo, P.; Carter, H.; Kamiyama, H.; Jimeno, A.; et al. Core Signaling Pathways in Human Pancreatic Cancers Revealed by Global Genomic Analyses. *Science* **2008**, *321*, 1801–1806. [CrossRef]
120. Gerrard, D.L.; Boyd, J.R.; Stein, G.S.; Jin, V.X.; Frietze, S. Disruption of Broad Epigenetic Domains in PDAC Cells by HAT Inhibitors. *Epigenomes* **2019**, *3*, 11. [CrossRef]
121. Gao, J.; Wang, L.; Xu, J.; Zheng, J.; Man, X.; Wu, H.; Jin, J.; Wang, K.; Xiao, H.; Li, S.; et al. Aberrant DNA Methyltransferase Expression in Pancreatic Ductal Adenocarcinoma Development and Progression. *J. Exp. Clin. Cancer Res.* **2013**, *32*, 86. [CrossRef]
122. Guo, M.; Jia, Y.; Yu, Z.; House, M.G.; Esteller, M.; Brock, M.V.; Herman, J.G. Epigenetic Changes Associated with Neoplasms of the Exocrine and Endocrine Pancreas. *Discov. Med.* **2014**, *17*, 67–73.
123. Mees, S.T.; Mardin, W.A.; Wendel, C.; Baeumer, N.; Willscher, E.; Senninger, N.; Schleicher, C.; Colombo-Benkmann, M.; Haier, J. EP300–a MiRNA-Regulated Metastasis Suppressor Gene in Ductal Adenocarcinomas of the Pancreas. *Int. J. Cancer* **2010**, *126*, 114–124. [CrossRef] [PubMed]
124. Gayther, S.A.; Batley, S.J.; Linger, L.; Bannister, A.; Thorpe, K.; Chin, S.F.; Daigo, Y.; Russell, P.; Wilson, A.; Sowter, H.M.; et al. Mutations Truncating the EP300 Acetylase in Human Cancers. *Nat. Genet.* **2000**, *24*, 300–303. [CrossRef] [PubMed]
125. Fritsche, P.; Seidler, B.; Schüler, S.; Schnieke, A.; Göttlicher, M.; Schmid, R.M.; Saur, D.; Schneider, G. HDAC2 Mediates Therapeutic Resistance of Pancreatic Cancer Cells via the BH3-Only Protein NOXA. *Gut* **2009**, *58*, 1399–1409. [CrossRef]
126. Ouaïssi, M.; Sielezneff, I.; Silvestre, R.; Sastre, B.; Bernard, J.-P.; Lafontaine, J.S.; Payan, M.J.; Dahan, L.; Pirrò, N.; Seitz, J.F.; et al. High Histone Deacetylase 7 (HDAC7) Expression Is Significantly Associated with Adenocarcinomas of the Pancreas. *Ann. Surg. Oncol.* **2008**, *15*, 2318–2328. [CrossRef] [PubMed]
127. Zhou, W.; Liang, I.-C.; Yee, N.S. Histone Deacetylase 1 Is Required for Exocrine Pancreatic Epithelial Proliferation in Development and Cancer. *Cancer Biol. Ther.* **2011**, *11*, 659–670. [CrossRef]
128. Chen, S.; Chen, J.; Zhan, Q.; Zhu, Y.; Chen, H.; Deng, X.; Hou, Z.; Shen, B.; Chen, Y.; Peng, C. H2AK119Ub1 and H3K27Me3 in Molecular Staging for Survival Prediction of Patients with Pancreatic Ductal Adenocarcinoma. *Oncotarget* **2014**, *5*, 10421–10433. [CrossRef] [PubMed]
129. Arensman, M.D.; Telesca, D.; Lay, A.R.; Kershaw, K.M.; Wu, N.; Donahue, T.R.; Dawson, D.W. The CREB-Binding Protein Inhibitor ICG-001 Suppresses Pancreatic Cancer Growth. *Mol. Cancer Ther.* **2014**, *13*, 2303–2314. [CrossRef]
130. Park, J.Y.; Helm, J.; Coppola, D.; Kim, D.; Malafa, M.; Kim, S.J. MicroRNAs in Pancreatic Ductal Adenocarcinoma. *World J. Gastroenterol.* **2011**, *17*, 817–827. [CrossRef]
131. Zhang, S.; Hao, J.; Xie, F.; Hu, X.; Liu, C.; Tong, J.; Zhou, J.; Wu, J.; Shao, C. Downregulation of MiR-132 by Promoter Methylation Contributes to Pancreatic Cancer Development. *Carcinogenesis* **2011**, *32*, 1183–1189. [CrossRef]
132. Han, T.; Hu, H.; Zhuo, M.; Wang, L.; Cui, J.-J.; Jiao, F.; Wang, L.-W. Long Non-Coding RNA: An Emerging Paradigm of Pancreatic Cancer. *Curr. Mol. Med.* **2016**, *16*, 702–709. [CrossRef] [PubMed]
133. Xie, Z.; Chen, X.; Li, J.; Guo, Y.; Li, H.; Pan, X.; Jiang, J.; Liu, H.; Wu, B. Salivary HOTAIR and PVT1 as Novel Biomarkers for Early Pancreatic Cancer. *Oncotarget* **2016**, *7*, 25408–25419. [CrossRef]
134. Zheng, J.; Huang, X.; Tan, W.; Yu, D.; Du, Z.; Chang, J.; Wei, L.; Han, Y.; Wang, C.; Che, X.; et al. Pancreatic Cancer Risk Variant in LINC00673 Creates a MiR-1231 Binding Site and Interferes with PTPN11 Degradation. *Nat. Genet.* **2016**, *48*, 747–757. [CrossRef] [PubMed]
135. Ma, C.; Nong, K.; Zhu, H.; Wang, W.; Huang, X.; Yuan, Z.; Ai, K. H19 Promotes Pancreatic Cancer Metastasis by Derepressing Let-7's Suppression on Its Target HMGA2-Mediated EMT. *Tumour Biol.* **2014**, *35*, 9163–9169. [CrossRef] [PubMed]
136. Li, W.; Martinez-Useros, J.; Garcia-Carbonero, N.; Fernandez-Aceñero, M.J.; Orta, A.; Ortega-Medina, L.; Garcia-Botella, S.; Perez-Aguirre, E.; Diez-Valladares, L.; Celdran, A.; et al. The Clinical Significance of PIWIL3 and PIWIL4 Expression in Pancreatic Cancer. *J. Clin. Med.* **2020**, *9*, 1252. [CrossRef] [PubMed]

137. A Small-Molecule Probe of the Histone Methyltransferase G9a Induces Cellular Senescence in Pancreatic Adenocarcinoma—PubMed. Available online: https://pubmed.ncbi.nlm.nih.gov/22536950/ (accessed on 27 October 2020).
138. Jiang, W.; Wang, J.; Zhang, Y. Histone H3K27me3 Demethylases KDM6A and KDM6B Modulate Definitive Endoderm Differentiation from Human ESCs by Regulating WNT Signaling Pathway. *Cell Res.* **2013**, *23*, 122–130. [CrossRef] [PubMed]
139. Andricovich, J.; Perkail, S.; Kai, Y.; Casasanta, N.; Peng, W.; Tzatsos, A. Loss of KDM6A Activates Super-Enhancers to Induce Gender-Specific Squamous-like Pancreatic Cancer and Confers Sensitivity to BET Inhibitors. *Cancer Cell* **2018**, *33*, 512–526.e8. [CrossRef] [PubMed]
140. Ougolkov, A.V.; Bilim, V.N.; Billadeau, D.D. Regulation of Pancreatic Tumor Cell Proliferation and Chemoresistance by the Histone Methyltransferase Enhancer of Zeste Homologue 2. *Clin. Cancer Res.* **2008**, *14*, 6790–6796. [CrossRef]
141. Toll, A.D.; Dasgupta, A.; Potoczek, M.; Yeo, C.J.; Kleer, C.G.; Brody, J.R.; Witkiewicz, A.K. Implications of Enhancer of Zeste Homologue 2 Expression in Pancreatic Ductal Adenocarcinoma. *Hum. Pathol.* **2010**, *41*, 1205–1209. [CrossRef]
142. Avan, A.; Crea, F.; Paolicchi, E.; Funel, N.; Galvani, E.; Marquez, V.E.; Honeywell, R.J.; Danesi, R.; Peters, G.J.; Giovannetti, E. Molecular Mechanisms Involved in the Synergistic Interaction of the EZH2 Inhibitor 3-Deazaneplanocin A with Gemcitabine in Pancreatic Cancer Cells. *Mol. Cancer Ther.* **2012**, *11*, 1735–1746. [CrossRef]
143. McGrath, J.; Trojer, P. Targeting Histone Lysine Methylation in Cancer. *Pharmacol. Ther.* **2015**, *150*, 1–22. [CrossRef]
144. Tzatsos, A.; Paskaleva, P.; Ferrari, F.; Deshpande, V.; Stoykova, S.; Contino, G.; Wong, K.-K.; Lan, F.; Trojer, P.; Park, P.J.; et al. KDM2B Promotes Pancreatic Cancer via Polycomb-Dependent and -Independent Transcriptional Programs. *J. Clin. Investig.* **2013**, *123*, 727–739. [CrossRef]
145. Yamada, N.; Hamada, T.; Goto, M.; Tsutsumida, H.; Higashi, M.; Nomoto, M.; Yonezawa, S. MUC2 Expression Is Regulated by Histone H3 Modification and DNA Methylation in Pancreatic Cancer. *Int. J. Cancer* **2006**, *119*, 1850–1857. [CrossRef] [PubMed]
146. Deeb, D.; Brigolin, C.; Gao, X.; Liu, Y.; Pindolia, K.R.; Gautam, S.C. Induction of Apoptosis in Pancreatic Cancer Cells by CDDO-Me Involves Repression of Telomerase through Epigenetic Pathways. *J. Carcinog. Mutagen.* **2014**, *5*, 177. [CrossRef] [PubMed]
147. Wang, X.; Wang, H.; Jiang, N.; Lu, W.; Zhang, X.F.; Fang, J.Y. Effect of Inhibition of MEK Pathway on 5-Aza-Deoxycytidine-Suppressed Pancreatic Cancer Cell Proliferation. *Genet. Mol. Res.* **2013**, *12*, 5560–5573. [CrossRef]
148. Fujisawa, T.; Joshi, B.H.; Puri, R.K. Histone Modification Enhances the Effectiveness of IL-13 Receptor Targeted Immunotoxin in Murine Models of Human Pancreatic Cancer. *J. Transl. Med.* **2011**, *9*, 37. [CrossRef]
149. Sohal, D.; Krishnamurthi, V.; Tohme, R.; Gu, X.; Lindner, D.; Landowski, T.H.; Pink, J.; Radivoyevitch, T.; Fada, S.; Lee, Z.; et al. A Pilot Clinical Trial of the Cytidine Deaminase Inhibitor Tetrahydrouridine Combined with Decitabine to Target DNMT1 in Advanced, Chemorefractory Pancreatic Cancer. *Am. J. Cancer Res.* **2020**, *10*, 3047–3060.
150. Cohen, A.L.; Ray, A.; Van Brocklin, M.; Burnett, D.M.; Bowen, R.C.; Dyess, D.L.; Butler, T.W.; Dumlao, T.; Khong, H.T. A Phase I Trial of Azacitidine and Nanoparticle Albumin Bound Paclitaxel in Patients with Advanced or Metastatic Solid Tumors. *Oncotarget* **2017**, *8*, 52413–52419. [CrossRef] [PubMed]
151. Bahr, J.C.; Robey, R.W.; Luchenko, V.; Basseville, A.; Chakraborty, A.R.; Kozlowski, H.; Pauly, G.T.; Patel, P.; Schneider, J.P.; Gottesman, M.M.; et al. Blocking Downstream Signaling Pathways in the Context of HDAC Inhibition Promotes Apoptosis Preferentially in Cells Harboring Mutant Ras. *Oncotarget* **2016**, *7*, 69804–69815. [CrossRef]
152. Aldape, K.; Zadeh, G.; Mansouri, S.; Reifenberger, G.; von Deimling, A. Glioblastoma: Pathology, Molecular Mechanisms and Markers. *Acta Neuropathol.* **2015**, *129*, 829–848. [CrossRef]
153. Alexander, B.M.; Cloughesy, T.F. Adult Glioblastoma. *J. Clin. Oncol.* **2017**, *35*, 2402–2409. [CrossRef] [PubMed]
154. Flavahan, W.A.; Drier, Y.; Liau, B.B.; Gillespie, S.M.; Venteicher, A.S.; Stemmer-Rachamimov, A.O.; Suvà, M.L.; Bernstein, B.E. Insulator Dysfunction and Oncogene Activation in IDH Mutant Gliomas. *Nature* **2016**, *529*, 110–114. [CrossRef]
155. Ceccarelli, M.; Barthel, F.P.; Malta, T.M.; Sabedot, T.S.; Salama, S.R.; Murray, B.A.; Morozova, O.; Newton, Y.; Radenbaugh, A.; Pagnotta, S.M.; et al. Molecular Profiling Reveals Biologically Discrete Subsets and Pathways of Progression in Diffuse Glioma. *Cell* **2016**, *164*, 550–563. [CrossRef] [PubMed]
156. Esteller, M.; Garcia-Foncillas, J.; Andion, E.; Goodman, S.N.; Hidalgo, O.F.; Vanaclocha, V.; Baylin, S.B.; Herman, J.G. Inactivation of the DNA-Repair Gene MGMT and the Clinical Response of Gliomas to Alkylating Agents. *N. Engl. J. Med.* **2000**, *343*, 1350–1354. [CrossRef]
157. Hegi, M.E.; Diserens, A.-C.; Gorlia, T.; Hamou, M.-F.; de Tribolet, N.; Weller, M.; Kros, J.M.; Hainfellner, J.A.; Mason, W.; Mariani, L.; et al. MGMT Gene Silencing and Benefit from Temozolomide in Glioblastoma. *N. Engl. J. Med.* **2005**, *352*, 997–1003. [CrossRef]
158. Smrdel, U.; Popovic, M.; Zwitter, M.; Bostjancic, E.; Zupan, A.; Kovac, V.; Glavac, D.; Bokal, D.; Jerebic, J. Long-Term Survival in Glioblastoma: Methyl Guanine Methyl Transferase (MGMT) Promoter Methylation as Independent Favourable Prognostic Factor. *Radiol. Oncol.* **2016**, *50*, 394–401. [CrossRef] [PubMed]
159. Kitange, G.J.; Mladek, A.C.; Carlson, B.L.; Schroeder, M.A.; Pokorny, J.L.; Cen, L.; Decker, P.A.; Wu, W.; Lomberk, G.A.; Gupta, S.K.; et al. Inhibition of Histone Deacetylation Potentiates the Evolution of Acquired Temozolomide Resistance Linked to MGMT Upregulation in Glioblastoma Xenografts. *Clin. Cancer Res.* **2012**, *18*, 4070–4079. [CrossRef] [PubMed]
160. Tarasenko, N.; Nudelman, A.; Rozic, G.; Cutts, S.M.; Rephaeli, A. Effects of Histone Deacetylase Inhibitory Prodrugs on Epigenetic Changes and DNA Damage Response in Tumor and Heart of Glioblastoma Xenograft. *Investig. New Drugs* **2017**, *35*, 412–426. [CrossRef]

161. Moon, B.-S.; Cai, M.; Lee, G.; Zhao, T.; Song, X.; Giannotta, S.L.; Attenello, F.J.; Yu, M.; Lu, W. Epigenetic Modulator Inhibition Overcomes Temozolomide Chemoresistance and Antagonizes Tumor Recurrence of Glioblastoma. *J. Clin. Investig.* **2020**. [CrossRef]
162. Choi, S.A.; Kwak, P.A.; Park, C.-K.; Wang, K.-C.; Phi, J.H.; Lee, J.Y.; Lee, C.S.; Lee, J.-H.; Kim, S.-K. A Novel Histone Deacetylase Inhibitor, CKD5, Has Potent Anti-Cancer Effects in Glioblastoma. *Oncotarget* **2017**, *8*, 9123–9133. [CrossRef]
163. Romani, M.; Daga, A.; Forlani, A.; Pistillo, M.P.; Banelli, B. Targeting of Histone Demethylases KDM5A and KDM6B Inhibits the Proliferation of Temozolomide-Resistant Glioblastoma Cells. *Cancers* **2019**, *11*, 878. [CrossRef] [PubMed]
164. Wang, Z.; Hu, P.; Tang, F.; Lian, H.; Chen, X.; Zhang, Y.; He, X.; Liu, W.; Xie, C. HDAC6 Promotes Cell Proliferation and Confers Resistance to Temozolomide in Glioblastoma. *Cancer Lett.* **2016**, *379*, 134–142. [CrossRef]
165. Grinshtein, N.; Rioseco, C.C.; Marcellus, R.; Uehling, D.; Aman, A.; Lun, X.; Muto, O.; Podmore, L.; Lever, J.; Shen, Y.; et al. Small Molecule Epigenetic Screen Identifies Novel EZH2 and HDAC Inhibitors That Target Glioblastoma Brain Tumor-Initiating Cells. *Oncotarget* **2016**, *7*, 59360–59376. [CrossRef] [PubMed]
166. Singh, M.M.; Johnson, B.; Venkatarayan, A.; Flores, E.R.; Zhang, J.; Su, X.; Barton, M.; Lang, F.; Chandra, J. Preclinical Activity of Combined HDAC and KDM1A Inhibition in Glioblastoma. *Neuro-Oncology* **2015**, *17*, 1463–1473. [CrossRef] [PubMed]
167. Ishida, C.T.; Bianchetti, E.; Shu, C.; Halatsch, M.-E.; Westhoff, M.A.; Karpel-Massler, G.; Siegelin, M.D. BH3-Mimetics and BET-Inhibitors Elicit Enhanced Lethality in Malignant Glioma. *Oncotarget* **2017**, *8*, 29558–29573. [CrossRef]
168. Pastori, C.; Kapranov, P.; Penas, C.; Peschansky, V.; Volmar, C.-H.; Sarkaria, J.N.; Bregy, A.; Komotar, R.; St Laurent, G.; Ayad, N.G.; et al. The Bromodomain Protein BRD4 Controls HOTAIR, a Long Noncoding RNA Essential for Glioblastoma Proliferation. *Proc. Natl. Acad. Sci. USA* **2015**, *112*, 8326–8331. [CrossRef]
169. Ke, J.; Yao, Y.; Zheng, J.; Wang, P.; Liu, Y.; Ma, J.; Li, Z.; Liu, X.; Li, Z.; Wang, Z.; et al. Knockdown of Long Non-Coding RNA HOTAIR Inhibits Malignant Biological Behaviors of Human Glioma Cells via Modulation of MiR-326. *Oncotarget* **2015**, *6*, 21934–21949. [CrossRef]
170. Cai, T.; Liu, Y.; Xiao, J. Long Noncoding RNA MALAT1 Knockdown Reverses Chemoresistance to Temozolomide via Promoting MicroRNA-101 in Glioblastoma. *Cancer Med.* **2018**, *7*, 1404–1415. [CrossRef]
171. Chen, W.; Xu, X.-K.; Li, J.-L.; Kong, K.-K.; Li, H.; Chen, C.; He, J.; Wang, F.; Li, P.; Ge, X.-S.; et al. MALAT1 Is a Prognostic Factor in Glioblastoma Multiforme and Induces Chemoresistance to Temozolomide through Suppressing MiR-203 and Promoting Thymidylate Synthase Expression. *Oncotarget* **2017**, *8*, 22783–22799. [CrossRef]
172. Galanis, E.; Buckner, J.C.; Maurer, M.J.; Kreisberg, J.I.; Ballman, K.; Boni, J.; Peralba, J.M.; Jenkins, R.B.; Dakhil, S.R.; Morton, R.F.; et al. Phase II Trial of Temsirolimus (CCI-779) in Recurrent Glioblastoma Multiforme: A North Central Cancer Treatment Group Study. *J. Clin. Oncol.* **2005**, *23*, 5294–5304. [CrossRef]
173. Lee, E.Q.; Reardon, D.A.; Schiff, D.; Drappatz, J.; Muzikansky, A.; Grimm, S.A.; Norden, A.D.; Nayak, L.; Beroukhim, R.; Rinne, M.L.; et al. Phase II Study of Panobinostat in Combination with Bevacizumab for Recurrent Glioblastoma and Anaplastic Glioma. *Neuro-Oncology* **2015**, *17*, 862–867. [CrossRef] [PubMed]
174. Iwamoto, F.M.; Lamborn, K.R.; Kuhn, J.G.; Wen, P.Y.; Yung, W.K.A.; Gilbert, M.R.; Chang, S.M.; Lieberman, F.S.; Prados, M.D.; Fine, H.A. A Phase I/II Trial of the Histone Deacetylase Inhibitor Romidepsin for Adults with Recurrent Malignant Glioma: North American Brain Tumor Consortium Study 03–03. *Neuro-Oncology* **2011**, *13*, 509–516. [CrossRef]
175. Hervouet, E.; Debien, E.; Campion, L.; Charbord, J.; Menanteau, J.; Vallette, F.M.; Cartron, P.-F. Folate Supplementation Limits the Aggressiveness of Glioma via the Remethylation of DNA Repeats Element and Genes Governing Apoptosis and Proliferation. *Clin. Cancer Res.* **2009**, *15*, 3519–3529. [CrossRef] [PubMed]
176. Winder, M.; Virós, A. Mechanisms of Drug Resistance in Melanoma. *Handb. Exp. Pharmacol.* **2018**, *249*, 91–108. [CrossRef]
177. Katiyar, S.K.; Singh, T.; Prasad, R.; Sun, Q.; Vaid, M. Epigenetic Alterations in Ultraviolet Radiation-Induced Skin Carcinogenesis: Interaction of Bioactive Dietary Components on Epigenetic Targets. *Photochem. Photobiol.* **2012**, *88*, 1066–1074. [CrossRef] [PubMed]
178. Uzdensky, A.; Demyanenko, S.; Bibov, M.; Sharifulina, S.; Kit, O.; Przhedetski, Y.; Pozdnyakova, V. Expression of Proteins Involved in Epigenetic Regulation in Human Cutaneous Melanoma and Peritumoral Skin. *Tumour Biol.* **2014**, *35*, 8225–8233. [CrossRef]
179. Mori, T.; Kim, J.; Yamano, T.; Takeuchi, H.; Huang, S.; Umetani, N.; Koyanagi, K.; Hoon, D.S.B. Epigenetic Up-Regulation of C-C Chemokine Receptor 7 and C-X-C Chemokine Receptor 4 Expression in Melanoma Cells. *Cancer Res.* **2005**, *65*, 1800–1807. [CrossRef]
180. Hoon, D.S.B.; Spugnardi, M.; Kuo, C.; Huang, S.K.; Morton, D.L.; Taback, B. Profiling Epigenetic Inactivation of Tumor Suppressor Genes in Tumors and Plasma from Cutaneous Melanoma Patients. *Oncogene* **2004**, *23*, 4014–4022. [CrossRef]
181. Kato, Y.; Salumbides, B.C.; Wang, X.-F.; Qian, D.Z.; Williams, S.; Wei, Y.; Sanni, T.B.; Atadja, P.; Pili, R. Antitumor Effect of the Histone Deacetylase Inhibitor LAQ824 in Combination with 13-Cis-Retinoic Acid in Human Malignant Melanoma. *Mol. Cancer Ther.* **2007**, *6*, 70–81. [CrossRef]
182. Fiziev, P.; Akdemir, K.C.; Miller, J.P.; Keung, E.Z.; Samant, N.S.; Sharma, S.; Natale, C.A.; Terranova, C.J.; Maitituoheti, M.; Amin, S.B.; et al. Systematic Epigenomic Analysis Reveals Chromatin States Associated with Melanoma Progression. *Cell Rep.* **2017**, *19*, 875–889. [CrossRef]
183. Fan, T.; Jiang, S.; Chung, N.; Alikhan, A.; Ni, C.; Lee, C.-C.R.; Hornyak, T.J. EZH2-Dependent Suppression of a Cellular Senescence Phenotype in Melanoma Cells by Inhibition of P21/CDKN1A Expression. *Mol. Cancer Res.* **2011**, *9*, 418–429. [CrossRef]

184. Essa, S.; Denzer, N.; Mahlknecht, U.; Klein, R.; Collnot, E.M.; Tilgen, W.; Reichrath, J. VDR MicroRNA Expression and Epigenetic Silencing of Vitamin D Signaling in Melanoma Cells. *J. Steroid Biochem. Mol. Biol.* **2010**, *121*, 110–113. [CrossRef]
185. Zehavi, L.; Avraham, R.; Barzilai, A.; Bar-Ilan, D.; Navon, R.; Sidi, Y.; Avni, D.; Leibowitz-Amit, R. Silencing of a Large MicroRNA Cluster on Human Chromosome 14q32 in Melanoma: Biological Effects of Mir-376a and Mir-376c on Insulin Growth Factor 1 Receptor. *Mol. Cancer* **2012**, *11*, 44. [CrossRef] [PubMed]
186. DeVore, R.F.; Hellerqvist, C.G.; Wakefield, G.B.; Wamil, B.D.; Thurman, G.B.; Minton, P.A.; Sundell, H.W.; Yan, H.P.; Carter, C.E.; Wang, Y.F.; et al. Phase I Study of the Antineovascularization Drug CM101. *Clin. Cancer Res.* **1997**, *3*, 365–372. [PubMed]
187. Venza, M.; Visalli, M.; Biondo, C.; Lentini, M.; Catalano, T.; Teti, D.; Venza, I. Epigenetic Regulation of P14ARF and P16INK4A Expression in Cutaneous and Uveal Melanoma. *Biochim. Biophys. Acta* **2015**, *1849*, 247–256. [CrossRef] [PubMed]
188. Mitsiogianni, M.; Mantso, T.; Trafalis, D.T.; Vasantha Rupasinghe, H.P.; Zoumpourlis, V.; Franco, R.; Botaitis, S.; Pappa, A.; Panayiotidis, M.I. Allyl Isothiocyanate Regulates Lysine Acetylation and Methylation Marks in an Experimental Model of Malignant Melanoma. *Eur. J. Nutr.* **2020**, *59*, 557–569. [CrossRef]
189. Mitsiogianni, M.; Trafalis, D.T.; Franco, R.; Zoumpourlis, V.; Pappa, A.; Panayiotidis, M.I. Sulforaphane and Iberin Are Potent Epigenetic Modulators of Histone Acetylation and Methylation in Malignant Melanoma. *Eur. J. Nutr.* **2020**. [CrossRef]
190. Luke, J.J.; Flaherty, K.T.; Ribas, A.; Long, G.V. Targeted Agents and Immunotherapies: Optimizing Outcomes in Melanoma. *Nat. Rev. Clin. Oncol.* **2017**, *14*, 463–482. [CrossRef]
191. Gallagher, S.J.; Shklovskaya, E.; Hersey, P. Epigenetic Modulation in Cancer Immunotherapy. *Curr. Opin. Pharmacol.* **2017**, *35*, 48–56. [CrossRef]
192. Xia, C.; Leon-Ferre, R.; Laux, D.; Deutsch, J.; Smith, B.J.; Frees, M.; Milhem, M. Treatment of Resistant Metastatic Melanoma Using Sequential Epigenetic Therapy (Decitabine and Panobinostat) Combined with Chemotherapy (Temozolomide). *Cancer Chemother. Pharm.* **2014**, *74*, 691–697. [CrossRef]
193. Burton, E.M.; Woody, T.; Glitza, I.C.; Amaria, R.N.; Keung, E.Z.-Y.; Diab, A.; Patel, S.P.; Wong, M.K.K.; Yee, C.; Hwu, P.; et al. A Phase II Study of Oral Azacitidine (CC-486) in Combination with Pembrolizumab (PEMBRO) in Patients (Pts) with Metastatic Melanoma (MM). *J. Clin. Oncol.* **2019**, *37*, 9560. [CrossRef]
194. Zakharia, Y.; Monga, V.; Swami, U.; Bossler, A.D.; Freesmeier, M.; Frees, M.; Khan, M.; Frydenlund, N.; Srikantha, R.; Vanneste, M.; et al. Targeting Epigenetics for Treatment of BRAF Mutated Metastatic Melanoma with Decitabine in Combination with Vemurafenib: A Phase Lb Study. *Oncotarget* **2017**, *8*, 89182–89193. [CrossRef]
195. Woods, D.M.; Sodré, A.L.; Villagra, A.; Sarnaik, A.; Sotomayor, E.M.; Weber, J. HDAC Inhibition Upregulates PD-1 Ligands in Melanoma and Augments Immunotherapy with PD-1 Blockade. *Cancer Immunol. Res.* **2015**, *3*, 1375–1385. [CrossRef] [PubMed]
196. Booth, L.; Roberts, J.L.; Poklepovic, A.; Kirkwood, J.; Dent, P. HDAC Inhibitors Enhance the Immunotherapy Response of Melanoma Cells. *Oncotarget* **2017**, *8*, 83155–83170. [CrossRef] [PubMed]
197. Jespersen, H.; Olofsson Bagge, R.; Ullenhag, G.; Carneiro, A.; Helgadottir, H.; Ljuslinder, I.; Levin, M.; All-Eriksson, C.; Andersson, B.; Stierner, U.; et al. Concomitant Use of Pembrolizumab and Entinostat in Adult Patients with Metastatic Uveal Melanoma (PEMDAC Study): Protocol for a Multicenter Phase II Open Label Study. *BMC Cancer* **2019**, *19*, 415. [CrossRef] [PubMed]
198. Tawbi, H.A.; Beumer, J.H.; Tarhini, A.A.; Moschos, S.; Buch, S.C.; Egorin, M.J.; Lin, Y.; Christner, S.; Kirkwood, J.M. Safety and Efficacy of Decitabine in Combination with Temozolomide in Metastatic Melanoma: A Phase I/II Study and Pharmacokinetic Analysis. *Ann. Oncol.* **2013**, *24*, 1112–1119. [CrossRef]
199. Gupta, S.; Janostiak, R.; Wajapeyee, N. Transcriptional Regulators and Alterations That Drive Melanoma Initiation and Progression. *Oncogene* **2020**. [CrossRef] [PubMed]
200. Middleton, M.R.; Grob, J.J.; Aaronson, N.; Fierlbeck, G.; Tilgen, W.; Seiter, S.; Gore, M.; Aamdal, S.; Cebon, J.; Coates, A.; et al. Randomized Phase III Study of Temozolomide versus Dacarbazine in the Treatment of Patients with Advanced Metastatic Malignant Melanoma. *J. Clin. Oncol.* **2000**, *18*, 158–166. [CrossRef]
201. Yang, Q.; Yang, Y.; Zhou, N.; Tang, K.; Lau, W.B.; Lau, B.; Wang, W.; Xu, L.; Yang, Z.; Huang, S.; et al. Epigenetics in Ovarian Cancer: Premise, Properties, and Perspectives. *Mol. Cancer* **2018**, *17*, 109. [CrossRef]
202. Jordan, S.; Steer, C.; DeFazio, A.; Quinn, M.; Obermair, A.; Friedlander, M.; Francis, J.; O'Brien, S.; Goss, G.; Wyld, D.; et al. Patterns of Chemotherapy Treatment for Women with Invasive Epithelial Ovarian Cancer—A Population-Based Study. *Gynecol. Oncol.* **2013**, *129*, 310–317. [CrossRef]
203. Huang, R.; Langdon, S.P.; Tse, M.; Mullen, P.; Um, I.H.; Faratian, D.; Harrison, D.J. The Role of HDAC2 in Chromatin Remodelling and Response to Chemotherapy in Ovarian Cancer. *Oncotarget* **2016**, *7*, 4695–4711. [CrossRef] [PubMed]
204. Liu, N.; Zhang, R.; Zhao, X.; Su, J.; Bian, X.; Ni, J.; Yue, Y.; Cai, Y.; Jin, J. A Potential Diagnostic Marker for Ovarian Cancer: Involvement of the Histone Acetyltransferase, Human Males Absent on the First. *Oncol. Lett.* **2013**, *6*, 393–400. [CrossRef]
205. Cai, M.; Hu, Z.; Liu, J.; Gao, J.; Tan, M.; Zhang, D.; Zhu, L.; Liu, S.; Hou, R.; Lin, B. Expression of HMOF in Different Ovarian Tissues and Its Effects on Ovarian Cancer Prognosis. *Oncol. Rep.* **2015**, *33*, 685–692. [CrossRef] [PubMed]
206. Weichert, W.; Denkert, C.; Noske, A.; Darb-Esfahani, S.; Dietel, M.; Kalloger, S.E.; Huntsman, D.G.; Köbel, M. Expression of Class I Histone Deacetylases Indicates Poor Prognosis in Endometrioid Subtypes of Ovarian and Endometrial Carcinomas. *Neoplasia* **2008**, *10*, 1021–1027. [CrossRef] [PubMed]
207. Cacan, E. Epigenetic Regulation of RGS2 (Regulator of G-Protein Signaling 2) in Chemoresistant Ovarian Cancer Cells. *J. Chemother.* **2017**, *29*, 173–178. [CrossRef] [PubMed]

208. Li, D.; Wu, Q.-J.; Bi, F.-F.; Chen, S.-L.; Zhou, Y.-M.; Zhao, Y.; Yang, Q. Effect of the BRCA1-SIRT1-EGFR Axis on Cisplatin Sensitivity in Ovarian Cancer. *Am. J. Transl. Res.* **2016**, *8*, 1601–1608. [PubMed]
209. Jang, K.Y.; Kim, K.S.; Hwang, S.H.; Kwon, K.S.; Kim, K.R.; Park, H.S.; Park, B.-H.; Chung, M.J.; Kang, M.J.; Lee, D.G.; et al. Expression and Prognostic Significance of SIRT1 in Ovarian Epithelial Tumours. *Pathology* **2009**, *41*, 366–371. [CrossRef] [PubMed]
210. Dong, X.-C.; Jing, L.-M.; Wang, W.-X.; Gao, Y.-X. Down-Regulation of SIRT3 Promotes Ovarian Carcinoma Metastasis. *Biochem. Biophys. Res. Commun.* **2016**, *475*, 245–250. [CrossRef] [PubMed]
211. Jones, B.A.; Varambally, S.; Arend, R.C. Histone Methyltransferase EZH2: A Therapeutic Target for Ovarian Cancer. *Mol. Cancer Ther.* **2018**, *17*, 591–602. [CrossRef]
212. Bitler, B.G.; Aird, K.M.; Garipov, A.; Li, H.; Amatangelo, M.; Kossenkov, A.V.; Schultz, D.C.; Liu, Q.; Shih, I.-M.; Conejo-Garcia, J.R.; et al. Synthetic Lethality by Targeting EZH2 Methyltransferase Activity in ARID1A-Mutated Cancers. *Nat. Med.* **2015**, *21*, 231–238. [CrossRef]
213. Chen, C.; Ge, J.; Lu, Q.; Ping, G.; Yang, C.; Fang, X. Expression of Lysine-Specific Demethylase 1 in Human Epithelial Ovarian Cancer. *J. Ovarian Res.* **2015**, *8*, 28. [CrossRef] [PubMed]
214. Shao, G.; Wang, J.; Li, Y.; Liu, X.; Xie, X.; Wan, X.; Yan, M.; Jin, J.; Lin, Q.; Zhu, H.; et al. Lysine-Specific Demethylase 1 Mediates Epidermal Growth Factor Signaling to Promote Cell Migration in Ovarian Cancer Cells. *Sci. Rep.* **2015**, *5*, 15344. [CrossRef] [PubMed]
215. Mrkvicova, A.; Chmelarova, M.; Peterova, E.; Havelek, R.; Baranova, I.; Kazimirova, P.; Rudolf, E.; Rezacova, M. The Effect of Sodium Butyrate and Cisplatin on Expression of EMT Markers. *PLoS ONE* **2019**, *14*, e0210889. [CrossRef] [PubMed]
216. Ramadoss, S.; Sen, S.; Ramachandran, I.; Roy, S.; Chaudhuri, G.; Farias-Eisner, R. Lysine-Specific Demethylase KDM3A Regulates Ovarian Cancer Stemness and Chemoresistance. *Oncogene* **2017**, *36*, 1537–1545. [CrossRef]
217. Kübler, K.; Arndt, P.F.; Wardelmann, E.; Landwehr, C.; Krebs, D.; Kuhn, W.; van der Ven, K. Genetic Alterations of HLA-Class II in Ovarian Cancer. *Int. J. Cancer* **2008**, *123*, 1350–1356. [CrossRef] [PubMed]
218. Steele, N.; Finn, P.; Brown, R.; Plumb, J.A. Combined Inhibition of DNA Methylation and Histone Acetylation Enhances Gene Re-Expression and Drug Sensitivity in Vivo. *Br. J. Cancer* **2009**, *100*, 758–763. [CrossRef]
219. Cacan, E. Epigenetic-Mediated Immune Suppression of Positive Co-Stimulatory Molecules in Chemoresistant Ovarian Cancer Cells. *Cell Biol. Int.* **2017**, *41*, 328–339. [CrossRef]
220. Muscolini, M.; Cianfrocca, R.; Sajeva, A.; Mozzetti, S.; Ferrandina, G.; Costanzo, A.; Tuosto, L. Trichostatin A Up-Regulates P73 and Induces Bax-Dependent Apoptosis in Cisplatin-Resistant Ovarian Cancer Cells. *Mol. Cancer Ther.* **2008**, *7*, 1410–1419. [CrossRef]
221. Dizon, D.S.; Blessing, J.A.; Penson, R.T.; Drake, R.D.; Walker, J.L.; Johnston, C.M.; DiSilvestro, P.A.; Fader, A.N. A Phase II Evaluation of Belinostat and Carboplatin in the Treatment of Recurrent or Persistent Platinum-Resistant Ovarian, Fallopian Tube, or Primary Peritoneal Carcinoma: A Gynecologic Oncology Group Study. *Gynecol. Oncol.* **2012**, *125*, 367–371. [CrossRef]
222. Dizon, D.S.; Damstrup, L.; Finkler, N.J.; Lassen, U.; Celano, P.; Glasspool, R.; Crowley, E.; Lichenstein, H.S.; Knoblach, P.; Penson, R.T. Phase II Activity of Belinostat (PXD-101), Carboplatin, and Paclitaxel in Women with Previously Treated Ovarian Cancer. *Int. J. Gynecol. Cancer* **2012**, *22*, 979–986. [CrossRef]
223. Modesitt, S.C.; Sill, M.; Hoffman, J.S.; Bender, D.P. Gynecologic Oncology Group A Phase II Study of Vorinostat in the Treatment of Persistent or Recurrent Epithelial Ovarian or Primary Peritoneal Carcinoma: A Gynecologic Oncology Group Study. *Gynecol. Oncol.* **2008**, *109*, 182–186. [CrossRef]
224. Candelaria, M.; Gallardo-Rincón, D.; Arce, C.; Cetina, L.; Aguilar-Ponce, J.L.; Arrieta, O.; González-Fierro, A.; Chávez-Blanco, A.; de la Cruz-Hernández, E.; Camargo, M.F.; et al. A Phase II Study of Epigenetic Therapy with Hydralazine and Magnesium Valproate to Overcome Chemotherapy Resistance in Refractory Solid Tumors. *Ann. Oncol.* **2007**, *18*, 1529–1538. [CrossRef]
225. Zhao, Y.; Li, Q.; Wu, X.; Chen, P. Upregulation of P27Kip1 by Demethylation Sensitizes Cisplatin-Resistant Human Ovarian Cancer SKOV3 Cells. *Mol. Med. Rep.* **2016**, *14*, 1659–1666. [CrossRef] [PubMed]
226. Seligson, D.B.; Horvath, S.; Shi, T.; Yu, H.; Tze, S.; Grunstein, M.; Kurdistani, S.K. Global Histone Modification Patterns Predict Risk of Prostate Cancer Recurrence. *Nature* **2005**, *435*, 1262–1266. [CrossRef] [PubMed]
227. Bird, A. DNA Methylation Patterns and Epigenetic Memory. *Genes Dev.* **2002**, *16*, 6–21. [CrossRef] [PubMed]
228. Fahrner, J.A.; Eguchi, S.; Herman, J.G.; Baylin, S.B. Dependence of Histone Modifications and Gene Expression on DNA Hypermethylation in Cancer. *Cancer Res.* **2002**, *62*, 7213–7218.

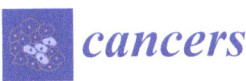

Review

Revisiting Mitochondria Scored Cancer Progression and Metastasis

Rohit Gundamaraju [1,*], Wenying Lu [2] and Rishya Manikam [3,*]

[1] ER Stress and Mucosal Immunology Lab, School of Health Sciences, College of Health and Medicine, University of Tasmania, Launceston, Tasmania, TAS 7248, Australia
[2] Respiratory Translational Research Group, Department of Laboratory Medicine, School of Health Sciences, University of Tasmania, Launceston, Tasmania, TAS 7248, Australia; wenying.lu@utas.edu.au
[3] Emergency and Acute Care Centre, Faculty of Medicine, University Malaya, Kuala Lumpur 59100, Malaysia
* Correspondence: rohit.gundamaraju@utas.edu.au (R.G.); rishya@ummc.edu.my (R.M.)

Simple Summary: The indispensible role of mitochondria has been described over a century ago by Otto Warburg which has been serving the fields of cell biology and cancer biology immensely. Mitochondria are the principal site for vital mechanisms which vastly dictate the physiology. The intricacy of mitochondria's role cancer have been noticed and well addressed in recent times. The underlying mechanisms are surfacing to unveil the nature of mitochondria and its participation in tumor cell motility and metastasis. This addressing may unravel novel therapeutic options. This review summarizes and reweighs the key aspects like underlying and emerging mechanisms which might be useful in designing novel chemotherapy.

Abstract: The Warburg effect has immensely succored the study of cancer biology, especially in highlighting the role of mitochondria in cancer stemness and their benefaction to the malignancy of oxidative and glycolytic cancer cells. Mitochondrial genetics have represented a focal point in cancer therapeutics due to the involvement of mitochondria in programmed cell death. The mitochondrion has been well established as a switch in cell death decisions. The mitochondrion's instrumental role in central bioenergetics, calcium homeostasis, and translational regulation has earned it its fame in metastatic dissemination in cancer cells. Here, we revisit and review mechanisms through which mitochondria influence oncogenesis and metastasis by underscoring the oncogenic mitochondrion that is capable of transferring malignant capacities to recipient cells.

Keywords: mitochondria; metastasis; OXPHOS; cancer; Warburg effect; cancer therapeutics

1. Good and Bad Mitochondria

Tumor cell metabolic reprogramming dictates the difference between normal and tumor cells. Mitochondria play a major role in metabolic reprogramming:It has been shown that tumor mitochondria not only change their structure but also decrease the potential of oxidative phosphorylation (OXPHOS) and apoptosis [1]. Considering the countless functions of mitochondria, including in the tricarboxylic acid (TCA) cycle, OXPHOS, etc., it is no surprise that mitochondria are directly involved in cancer progression (Figure 1) [2]. Metastasis is a hallmark of cancer and includes several steps: detachment of local tumors, intra-invasion, circulation in the blood, extra-invasion, and colonization in the secondary sites for survival. In all the above stages, mitochondrial metabolism is tuned for tumor cell adaptation to facilitate metastasis [3]. In addition, several postulations have been proposed on the vital role of mitochondria in metastasis, where mitochondria help overcome perturbations in metastasis environments. mtDNA single nucleotide polymorphisms (SNPs) and a few mutations might lead to distinctions in metastatic susceptibilities in cancer histotypes or patient groups. Many studies have revealed that mitochondria are involved in a chain of events including modulation of the the microenvironment, motility and invasion, plasticity, and consolidation [4]. Therefore, in the current review, we consolidated the essential contributing factors of mitochondria in cancer progression and, specifically, metastasis. We also discuss several questions that address the underlying mechanisms of context-dependent contributions of mitochondria in metastasis.

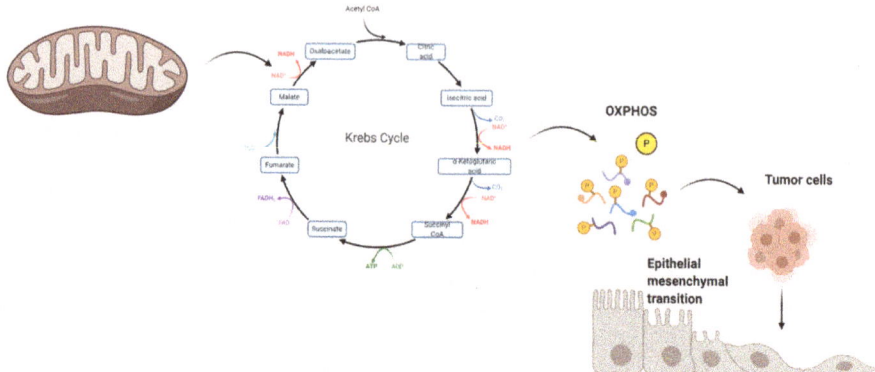

Figure 1. Epithelial–mesenchymal transition (EMT) by mitochondria. TCA: tricarboxylic acid; OXPHOS: oxidative phosphorylation. Mitochondrial metabolites are accumulated upon mutation of the indicated TCA cycle enzymes which activates the EMT. In cancer cells, the TCA cycle not only serve to produce reducing equivalents to fuel the electron transport chain, but also to generate biosynthetic intermediates that are necessary for cell proliferation and migration.

2. Can Mitochondrial Dynamics Dictate Cancer Spread?

The balance of mitochondrial fusion and fission is necessary for the regulation of various processes, including the quality of mitochondria, cell metabolism, cell death, proliferation, and cell migration, and is maintained by numerous mitochondrial-shaping proteins. Negative modulations or malfunctions in these processes resulting in changes in mitochondrial dynamics lead to diseases like cancer [5]. Mitochondrial dynamics are correlated with various diverse disease pathologies. For instance, a high nutrient-deprived state triggers mitochondrial fission and hence results in programmed cell death. A significant number of proteins such as the GTPases (Mfn1, Mfn2, Opa1, and Drp1) have strong regulatory effects in balancing mitochondrial fusion and fission. Any perturbations or failure in managing the correct dynamic state leads to cancer [6]. It is noteworthy that mitochondrial dynamics have a deep role in cancer cell migration (Figure 2). The discovery of susceptibility to cancer associated with altered or modulated mitochondrial dynamics could result in new targeted therapies. Some of these altered dynamics, such as mitochondrial fission, are discussed in this review.

Mitochondrial dynamics also massively impact apoptosis. Studies have correlated them to dynamic homeostasis and tumor growth. Strikingly, signaling downstream of mutant KRAS in pancreatic cancers leads to mitochondrial fragmentation and increased activation of Drp1, processes that are required for KRAS-driven tumor growth in vivo. In addition, recent studies also suggest that mitochondrial dynamics are important for regulating metastatic phenotypes such as invasion and migration in breast and thyroid cancers [7].

Examples of high-to-low expressions of Drp1 and Mfn1 have been implicated in metastatic breast cancer [8]. Moreover, Drp1 is regarded as crucial for apoptosis due to its informed role in releasing cytochrome-c. The Drp1/Mfn1 expression ratio correlates to aggressive cancers and cell proliferation. The Drp1/Mfn1 expression ratio was found to be increased in hepatocellular carcinoma (HCC) tissues and associated with poor prognosis. Escalated mitochondrial fission mediated by imbalanced reactive oxygen species (ROS) production was found to be the primary reason for the pro-survival ability of the HCC cells under both in vitro and in vivo conditions [9]. High Drp1 expression was also observed in ovarian cancers where Drp1 was found coexisting with cell cycle-related genes, thereby facilitating cancer cell proliferation [10]. Mitochondrial fission also aided in cisplatin resistance in ovarian cancers [11]. Drp1 inhibitors like Driptor1 were employed against breast cancer cells, which show not only that the mitochondrial dynamics-mediated pathway is useful in designing anti-cancer therapy [12] but also that mitochondrial fission facilitates the survival, apoptosis, and drug resistance of breast cancer cells [13].

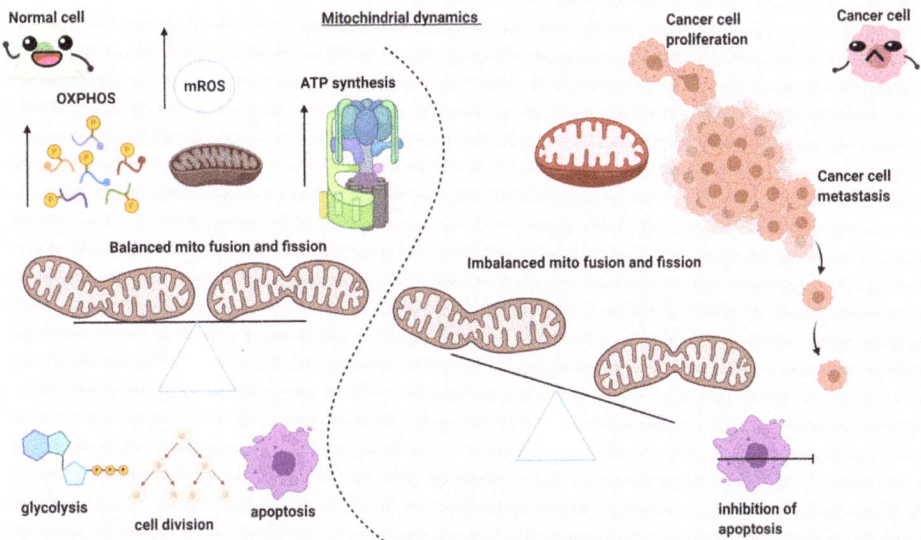

Figure 2. The differential role of mitochondrial dynamics in normal and cancer cells. OXPHOS: oxidative phosphorylation; ATP: adenosine tri phosphate; mROS: mitochondrial reactive oxygen species. The morphology and physiology of the mitochondria and its healthy functioning is governed by fission proteins. Mitochondria fission promotes glycolysis, mitophagy, and apoptosis and is also necessary for cell division. In contrast, mitochondria fusion promotes ATP and ROS production via OXPHOS. In normal cells (left area of the figure), mitochondria fusion and fission are well-balanced, which results in healthy homeostasis. Whereas in cancer cells, an imbalance of the fusion and fission is favored to drive proliferation, metastasis, and the maintenance of cancer stem cell phenotypes.

Mammalian target of rapamycin complex 1 (mTORC1), which is a trigger factor in cancers, stimulates translation of mitochondrial fission process 1 (MTFP1), which is coupled to pro-fission phosphorylation and mitochondrial recruitment of DRP1 in melanoma cells [14]. This shows that DRP1 couples with pro-cancer pathways. Other very recent evidence of mitochondrial dynamics and their role in cancer promotion was recorded in a study where Drp1 increased prostate cancer cell survival under metabolic stress conditions [15]. Further, knock down of Nestin, which is one of the classic markers in gastrointestinal cancers, downregulated recruitment of Drp1 to mitochondria in gastrointestinal stromal tumor cells [16]. To support this, another novel study consisting of Paris Saponin II (PSII), a major steroidal saponin extracted from Rhizoma Paris polyphylla, was employed against Drp1, which aided the modulation of Drp1-mediated mitochondrial fission [17]. The PSII in [17] surprisingly downsized the xenograft tumor size and impeded the phosphorylation of ERK1/2 and Drp1 at Ser616. Mitochondrial dynamics also enormously influence survival and stemness maintenance of cancer stem cells (CSCs), which are responsible for tumor recurrence and other malignant traits. Blockade of fission debilitated the self-renewal capacity of CSCs and led to CSC exhaustion. In addition, the reliability and functionality of T cells in the cancer microenvironment depend vastly on the mitochondrial dynamics balance, which hints at the essentiality and usefulness of targeting mitochondrial dynamics in anti-cancer treatment [18].

3. Mitochondria's Vital Role in Numerous Cancers

Mitochondria have been well-known as crucial factors in various characteristics of cancer biology, including cancer development, metastasis, and drug resistance [19,20]. The alteration of mitochondria dynamics can affect the regulation of cancer cells. Mitochondria duties in dynamic networks include changes in size and distribution of sub-cellular components, and these dynamics are maintained by two main opposing processes: fission and fusion [21], regulated by dynamin-related protein 1 (Drp1) and mitofusins (Mfns) [22], respectively. Unbalanced mitochondrial fission or fusion dysregulates the cellular processes that contribute to tumorigenesis [23,24]. In breast cancer, increased mitochondrial fragmentation intensifies the capabilities of breast cancer cells to metastasize by activating Drp1 or silencing Mfns [8].The imbalance of Drp1/Mfn expression has also been found to cause additional mitochondrial fission and impaired mitochondrial fusion inhuman lung cancer cell lines, which is a key process for cell cycle progression [25].In addition, cancer cells are involved in the mitochondrial respiration chain to gain an obvious increase in ATP production [26]. Cancer cells generate invasion or metastasis by utilizing energy, powered through the transcription co-activator, PGC-1α, to promote OXPHOS, mitochondrial biogenesis, and oxygen consumption rate [27]. The association between PGC-1α expression in the invasion and metastasis of human invasive breast cancer was found in previous study [27]. Furthermore, the dysregulation of mitochondrial respiratory chains prompts ROS-induced integrin β5 expression and results in an increase in tumor cell invasion and metastasis in gastric cancer cells [28]. In addition, mitochondrial respiratory chain complexes are involved in cell apoptosis processes, in particular, complexes I and III are key regulators of cell apoptosis and major sources of ROS generation [29]. In most aggressive breast cancer, the most remarkable activity of complexes is observed. ROS-associated signaling pathways can be a potential suppressor for the tumor treatment target. On the other hand, mitochondrial dysfunction is identified as being associated with cancer progression. mtDNA mutations have been frequently encountered in cancer cells. Mitochondrial fusion activity is essential for mtDNA maintenance, a loss of mtDNA has been correlated with the drug resistance of anti-estrogen therapy in breast cancer [30]. Moreover, the mutation of mtDNA is one of the key factors that stimulate mitochondrial-mediated metastasis. For instance, mutated ROS-generating mtDNA promotes invasion and metastasis in lung cancer cells and breast cancer cells [31,32]. In addition, declined OXPHOS gene expression was found to result in metastasis in cancer cell lines and in metastatic melanoma in renal cancer specimens [33].

Other aspects to be considered are cross-links with mitochondrial dysfunction and promotion of tumor cells metastasis. Epithelial–mesenchymal transition (EMT) enables cancer cells to obtain the migration abilities to move out of the primary tumor and translocate to new target organs [34,35]. EMT transfers the epithelial cell to mesenchymal phenotypes in many epithelial tumor cells that are affected by mitochondrial dysfunction [33]. Mitochondrial dysfunction initiates EMT via EMT signaling pathways. TGF-β is known as a key growth factor controlling EMT progression through TGF-β/SMAD/SNAIL, phosphatidylinositol-3-kinase (PI3K)/AKT signaling pathways [36]. TGF-β phosphorylates TGF-β receptor-regulated Smad2 and Smad3, then upregulates the expression of their downstream gene, Snail-1, which is a positive regulator of EMT and metastasis [36]. Activated PI3K/AKT signaling can also upregulate the intracellular expression of Snail, thereby inducing the EMT [37]. The depleted mtDNA induces mitochondrial dysfunction and further triggers EMT induction, the prostate and breast adenocarcinoma cells show mesenchymal phenotypes with TGF-β overexpression [38].Moreover, in hepatocellular carcinoma cells, mtDNA depletion induces EMT via TGF-β/SMAD/SNAIL signaling [39]. In the tumor microenvironment, the hypoxia-induced accumulation of HIF-1 alpha activates the expression of TWIST which ultimately induces EMT [40]. The co-expression of HIF-1 alpha, TWIST, and Snail in primary tumors of head and neck cancer patients correlates with the poorest prognosis [41]. mtDNA depletion also can induce mitochondrial dysfunction and promotes EMT induction via mitochondrial reversed signaling. Mitochondrial reversed signaling triggers transcriptional activation of EMT signaling pathways, such as SNAIL, TWIST, and mesenchymal markers, such as vimentin, N-cadherin, with a corresponding loss of epithelial marker E-cadherin [42]. mtDNA-depletioncan also cause a loss of mesenchymal phenotypes of ESPR, such as ESPR1 in breast cells and expressed stem-cell phenotypes, suggesting a generation of cancer stem cells [42]. On the other hand, mutated mitochondrial metabolic enzymes are closely correlated with EMT-induced metastasis, which contributes to the initiation of oncogenic signaling cascades in cancers [43,44]. Another link with mitochondria in cancer cell metastasis is epidermal growth factor receptor (EGFR). EGFR was found intensively expressed in the mitochondria of highly invasive non-small cell lung cancer (NSCLC) cells [45]. EGF is a growth factor that initiates the EMT by activating the RAS/RAF/MEK/ERK MAPK signaling cascade. The activated ERK1/2-MAPK induces EMT, promoting the regulation of cell motility and invasion [46]. EGF initiates cancer cell invasion by regulating mitochondrial functions. EGF activates the mitochondrial translocation of EGFR, mitochondrial fission, and redistribution, upregulates cellular ATP production, and enhances cancer cell motility in vitro and in vivo. Furthermore, EGFR can regulate mitochondrial dynamics by interchanging with Mfn1 and disturbing Mfn1 polymerization, therefore, overexpression of Mfn1 reverses the phenotypes resulting from EGFR mitochondrial translocation to induce mitochondrial fragmentation [45].

4. Multiple Mechanisms of Metastasis by Mitochondria

Deciphering the mechanisms of metastasis involving mitochondria is extremely important in establishing therapeutics. The tumor microenvironment plays a prominent role in the progression of cancer, and it has a similar role in cancer chemoresistance via a mechanism called mitochondrial transfer, which broadly favors further invasion and metastasis. Mitochondrial transfer occurs in cells that fail to perform aerobic respiration due to mtDNA malfunction [47]. On the other hand, a horizontal mitochondrial transfer is also associated with chemoresistance. In the tumor microenvironment, horizontal transfer is regarded as lethal, since the transfer of mtDNA from the host cell to the cancer cell leads to escalated tumor-initiation ability because the cancer cells possess reduced respiratory function, and horizontal transfer in such instances improves the aggressiveness of cancer cells. Studies have exhibited that mtDNA transfer protects the cells from chemotherapeutic drugs. In a study involving acute myelogenous leukemia (AML), cells took up functional mitochondria from the bone marrow-derived stromal cells, which lead to protection of the cells from the drug effect and evasion of cell death [48]. Mitochondrial transfer under an in vivo setting not only leads to chemoresistance but also disease relapse. This entire concept of mitochondrial transfer endorses the notion of tumor plasticity and highlights the ability of the tumor cells to overcome unfavorable conditions by altering energy metabolism [19]. Further, mitochondrial transfer has been implicated in murine tumor models with essential functional consequences for tumor growth and metastasis. This has also been supported by studies where the mitochondrial transfer rescued cancer cells that were suffering deficiencies in OXPHOS and were prone to therapeutic apoptosis [49]. It is a proven phenomenon that dysregulated mitochondrial trafficking leads to metastasis of cancer cells.

Ubiquitination of syntaphylin (SNPH) (Figure 3) is regarded as a vital regulator of mitochondrial trafficking. Studies show that SNPH aids in binding the mitochondria to the microtubule. Mechanistic studies hint that SNPH is modified by the ubiquitin ligase CHIP/STUB1 and deubiquitinated in a USP7-dependant manner, which suggeststhat ubiquitination of SNPH isa pivotal regulator of mitochondrial trafficking and tumor cell invasion [50]. Apart from the SNPH mechanics, hypoxia also governs mitochondria localization in cancer cells. Tumor cells under the influence of hypoxia downregulate

SNPH protein and mRNA levels, which inturn leads to increased invasiveness in glioblastoma cells. Surprisingly, tumors with stabilized HIFα or with deletions resulted in lower expression of SNPH, denoting SNPH's principal role in metastasis [50].

Mitochondria can enormously influence malignant transformation and dictate the tumor plasticity of cancer cells and govern several mechanisms to address tough environmental conditions. Mitochondria are the major source of ROS utilized in OXPHOS. Mitochondrial enzymes, such as pyruvate dehydrogenase (PDH), a-ketoglutarate-dehydrogenase (a-KGDH), acyl-CoA dehydrogenase, and glycerol-3-phosphate dehydrogenase, are involved in ROS generation [51]. The huge difference between normal cells and cancer cells is the controlled levels of mitochondrial ROS (mROS). The levels of mROS are properly regulated in cancer cells in order to play a role in essential cellular processes. On the other hand, cancer cells have functions like oncogene activation, tumor suppressor loss, and hypoxia, which lead to uncontrollable mROS levels that aid in sustaining cancer cell. mROS levels participate in multiple steps of oncogenesis and induce mtDNA mutations. They also influence apoptosis evasion, metabolic reprogramming, and cellular proliferation [52]. mROS is responsible for the activation of several important oncogenic signaling pathways such as the epidermal growth factor receptor (EGFR) signaling pathway [53]. Mitochondria help the epithelial cells in gaining migration speed by providing energy, as it was demonstrated that insufficient energy with deficiencies of mitochondria inhibited cell motility. Similarly, mitEGFR enhances mitochondria fission and cancer cell motility, independent of its phosphorylation status [45]. In order to drive towards a proliferative state and escape mitochondrial permeability transition-mediated cell death, cancer cells intelligently maintain high levels of anti-oxidant proteins to prevent ROS accumulation. On the other hand, the interrelationship between mROS and hypoxia inducible factor-1 (HIF-1) is complex. Hypoxia-mediated mROS leads to HIF-1 activation, which facilitates metastasis because of the metabolic shift from OXPHOS to glycolysis by increasing the expression of glycolyticenzymes. In contrast, HIF-1 decreases mROS production, promotes tumor growth, and facilitates the survival of metastatic cells, denoting the vibrant and functional role of mROS in various cancers [51].

Similar to the above, Sirtuin 3 (SIRT3) is involved in several key processes such as the response to oxidative stress and mitochondrial metabolism regulation. SIRT3, a NAD+-dependent mitochondrial deacetylase that promotes efficient oxidative metabolism, is a key regulator of mitochondrial ROS production and detoxification [54]. Literature suggests that SIRT3 has a role in regulating mitochondrial quality control and affects genes involved in homeostasis such as PGC-1α and TFAM. SIRT3 silencing results in making breast and colon cancer cell lines prone to cytotoxic treatment-mediated sensitivity via escalated oxidative stress and altered biogenesis [55]. SIRT3's role in malignancy was also assessed in a study where silencing of SIRT3 resulted in a reduction of visible clones by 64%, when assessed by a clonogenicity assay. This enumerates the fact that SIRT3 downregulation leads to compromised mitochondrial metabolism and increased sensitivity to oxidative stress [56]. Promotion of metastasis by ROS is tricky. High levels of ROS lead to inhibition of metastasis in melanoma, whereas in other cancers, ROS promotes metastasis [54]. Considering the role of SIRT3 in regulating ROS homeostasis, studies have shown that SIRT3 is essential in extinguishing Src oxidation and Src/Fak signaling to inhibit cell migration and metastasis in breast cancer cells via ROS adjustment [54].

Mitochondrial fission is a process commonly implicated in tumor progression, where dynamin-related protein-1 (Drp1) is bonded to one of its receptors, mitochondrial fission factor (MFF), on the mitochondrial outer membrane. Mitochondrial fission has been widely correlated with cell death and mitochondrial integrity [57]. MFF is overexpressed in numerous cancers. MFF is linked to VDAC1 in the mitochondrial outer membrane, which partially explains its association with cancer progression. However, mechanistically, MFF silencing leads to an upsurge of mitochondrial outer membrane permeability and oxidative stress, which inturn leads to the triggering of mitochondrial-mediated cell death, thereby impeding tumor proliferation and metastasis in mice [57]. A very recent study has determined the role of mitochondrial fission in cancer [58]. This study utilized phosphatidyl serine decarboxylase (PISD), an enzyme that orchestrates mitochondrial fission. It was evidenced that mitochondrial fission inhibits metastasis in triple-negative breast cancer cells. The study also enumerated that the alterations in mitochondrial fission not only inhibited cancer metastasis, cell migration, and cell invasion, but also repressed cancer cell signaling via ERK and Akt [58].

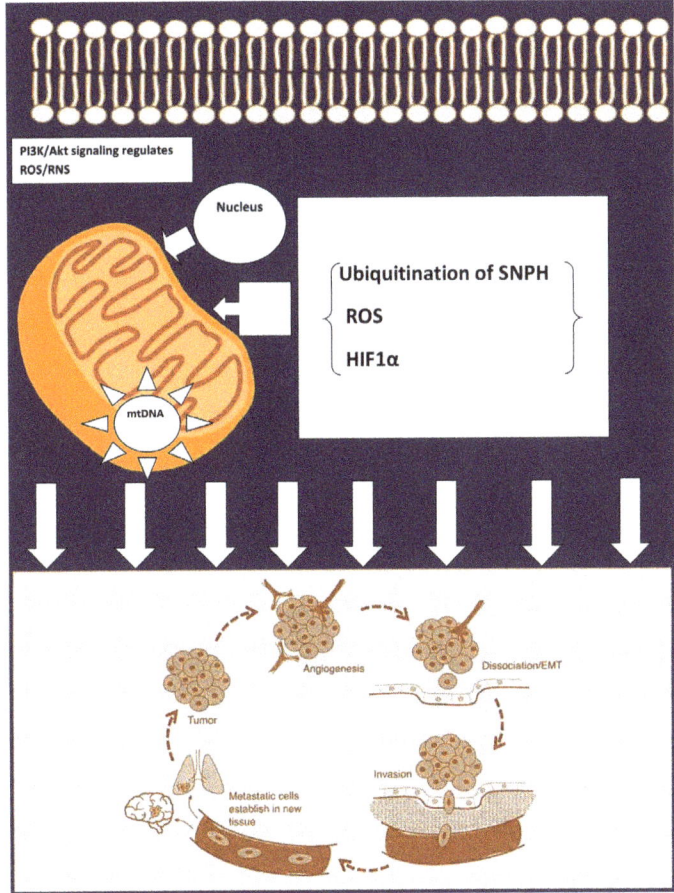

Figure 3. Regulation of EMT by mitochondria. ROS: reactive oxygen species; PI3K: Phosphoinositide 3-kinases; SNPH: syntaphilin; HIF: hypoxia inducible factor. Tumorigenesis calls for hypoxic-mediated reprogramming for metastasis. Bcl-2 family members regulate the PI3K pathway involved in metastasis progression. ROS generated during the metabolic process play a critical role in metastasis. Syntaphilin (SNPH), which generally arrests the mitochondrial trafficking in neurons, inhibits metastasis. In tumors with high expression of SNPH, mitochondria are anchored perinuclearly, resulting in lessened cell invasion and inhibited metastatic dissemination. In tumors with loss of SNPH expression, mitochondria are free to move to the cortical cytoskeleton via Kinesin/MIRO1 complexes. These cortical mitochondria fuel enhanced tumor cell invasion and correlate with poorer prognoses. Hypoxia can increase eNOS phosphorylation by activating the PI3K/AKT pathway. HIF-1α can also directly influence the expression of eNOS, which can be activated by phosphorylation of the serine 1177 residue, thereby, triggering migration and angiogenesis.

5. Mitochondrial Stress Response in Cancer Spread

Mitochondria are responsible for more than just energy production. Recently discovered mechanisms like mitochondrial unfolded protein response (mtUPR) and mitochondrial precursor over accumulation stress (mPOS) are paving new avenues for therapeutics and for understanding diseases better via mitochondria [59]. A genetic study in yeast denoted a novel protective mechanism named mPOS against mitochondrial protein import deficiency. mPOS is a newly-discovered pathway of proteostatic stress-mediated cell death due to mitochondrial dysfunction. mPOS is triggered by mitochondrial damage and the aberrant accumulation of mitochondrial precursors in the cytosol [60]. In parallel to this, mitoCPR was spotted in budding yeast. mitoCPR is a novel cellular response to defective mitochondrial protein import that protects mitochondrial functions [61]. The mitochondrion has an inherently stressful internal environment and it is speculated that dysregulation of stress signaling or an inability to switch on these adaptations during times of mitochondrial stress may underpin mitochondrial dysfunction and amount to pathological states overtime.

The role of mitochondrial chaperones in the cell stress response is quite intriguing. Gamitrinib, for instance, is a mitochondrial targeted HSP90 inhibitor with potential anti-cancer activity. Glioblastoma cells induced with low doses of gamitranib revealed accumulation of unfolded proteins in the mitochondria and a stress response gene characterized by upregulation of chaperones, especially Hsp70. Utilizing this target (mitoUPR) in mitochondria, TRAP-1 or CypD were ablated by genetic or chemical inhibitors. This resulted in the downregulation of NF-kB and related genes. Furthermore, there was an upregulation of pro-apoptotic genes, which aided in mitochondrial-mediated cell death. NF-kB has a wide role in tumor promotion and endorsement in the metastatic environment. Additionally, NF-kB plays a major role in treatment resistance and poor outcomes in cancer. Hence, targeting mitoUPR aids in concomitant loss of NF-kB, which inturn results in exposing the tumors to apoptosis-based therapies [62]. This clearly shows that mitoUPR can be a potential target for cancer therapy. Supplemental to this, new study evidence shows that mitoUPR under the absence of stress, as a part of an adaptive mechanism by cancer cells, results in reduced oxidative stress and is called mitohormesis. mitUPR has an axis with SIRT3, which supports invasion and metastasis. In addition, changes in the mtUPR gene resulted in poor clinical outcomes in patients with breast cancer [63].

6. Mitochondrial Ion Channels as a Target in Combating Cancer

The mitochondrial channels, characterized as either outer or inner membrane channels, are widely targeted in cancer therapies. The outer membrane channels include VDAC and the inner membrane channels include mtKATP, mtBKCa, mtIKCa, mtKv1.3, mtTASK-3, and the nonselective permeability transition pore (MPTP) [64]. Mitochondrial outer membrane channels participate in mitochondrial outer membrane permeabilization, while inner membrane channels modulate changes in membrane potential and thereby influence reactive oxygen (ROS) production and efficiency of the respiratory chain. ROS in turn may activate MPTP or the caspase-independent ROS-triggered parthanatos (poly (ADP-ribose) polymerase-1 dependent cell death). In addition, MPTP can also be triggered by Ca^{2+} overload in the mitochondrial matrix or by IMM depolarization and by several other factors (for example oxidative stress) [65].

The basis for mitochondrial ion channels being targeted is due to their role in cancer metastasis. A brief description of the role of potassium channels and their role in cancer progression is that channels like IKCa control OXPHOS. Inhibition of the channel has no or only minor effects on cell proliferation in the presence of glucose, but forcing the cells to generate ATP exclusively via oxidative phosphorylation by culturing them in galactose, allowed researchers to understand that inhibition of the channel decreased proliferation. Kv1.3 is another channel that modulates the cell cycle. Mitochondrial calcium fluxes have also been shown to regulate cancer proliferation. Additionally, calcium channels also drive proliferation. The constitutively active Ca^{2+} transfer from the endoplasmic reticulum (ER) to mitochondria plays a crucial role inensuring viability of tumorigenic cells, and defects in this uptake into mitochondria lead to cancer cell death. The crosstalk between potassium and calcium channels isnot completely clear, but a putative K+/H+transporter, LETM1, has been shown on calcium influx/efflux into/from mitochondria, and silencing ofLETM1 promoted AMPK activation, cell cycle arrest, and autophagy [66].

MPTP can be activated indirectly by different drugs eliciting changes in inner membrane potential, causing ROS production, or leading to calcium overload in the matrix. MPTP opening leads to rupture of the mitochondrial outer membrane (MOM), which contributes to cytochrome-c release, a process required for apoptosome formation and subsequent activation of effector caspases.

7. Mitochondria as a Therapeutic Target in Cancers

The energy required for cancer cell migration, invasion, and metastasis is supplied by mitochondria. Suppression of the mitochondrial energy function can reduce the frequency of tumor cell metastasis and invasion (Table 1). Targeting dysregulated Drp1-dependent mitochondrial fission could supply a novel scenario for defeating breast cancer metastasis [8]. On the other hand, another novel therapeutic strategy to limit or prevent cancer metastasis is by potentially blocking EMT through targeting specific EMT biomarker genes that are correlated with mitochondria health, signal proteins of the mitochondrial reverse signaling pathway, specific metabolic enzymes, or metabolism-dependent epigenetic reprogramming [33]. As proof, the PI3K/AKT signaling pathway plays a key role in EMT progress and is considered to be a principal signaling pathway in cancer that prompts extensive transcriptional and metabolic reprogramming, specifically in mitochondria. PI3K has been considered a potential target for the prevention and treatment of metastatic tumors. Inhibitors of PI3K have been utilized in tumor treatment to inhibit mitochondrial ATP production and diminish glycolysis [67–69]. A recent study highlighted a compound called NSC130362, which belongs to the class of 1,4-naphthoquinones (NQs) and has vibrant pharmacological properties [70]; it has been shown to possess anti-cancer effects, including anti-proliferative and anti-angiogenesis activity [71,72], suppress glycolysis and mitochondrial function [73], and inhibit NF-κB signaling [74]. Natural products on the other hand have also received attention in cancer chemotherapy. Honokiol (HNK) is a potent anti-tumor agent that affects EGFR and mitochondrial function to inhibit the cancer cells' genesis and metastasis. A study has shown that HNK inhibits mitochondrial respiration, which leads to the induction of apoptosis in lung cancer cells [75]. There are other natural products that have been identified with direct or indirect effects on mitochondrial function in cancers (Table 2 [76]).

Table 1. Treatment targets of mitochondria to suppress tumor cells metastasis.

Target Treatment	Mechanism	Cancers	References
Phosphatidylinositol-3 kinase (PI3K)	Inhibits mitochondrial transcription and metabolic reprogramming	Lung cancer cell lines	[68]
Adenomatous Polyposis Coli (APC) protein	Reverses mitochondrial trafficking by regulating Wnt signaling	Colorectal cancer	[77]
Drp1, Mnf1	Extends mitochondrial fission	Breast cancer	[8]
pSer9-GSK-3β;	Suppresses mitochondrial respiratory chain complexes	Breast cancer	[78]
Mito-TAM (derivative of Tamoxifen)	Disrupts mitochondrial respiratory chain complexes and OXPHOS	Breast cancer	[79]
PGC-1α	Impairs mitochondrial biogenesis and OXPHOS	shPGC-1α cells	[27]

Table 2. Natural compounds affecting mitochondrial function and acting as cancer therapeutics [76].

Compound	Source	Mode of Action	Cancers
Honokiol	*Magnolia grandifloris*	Induces mitochondrial apoptosis	Lung cancer, Breast cancer, Leukemia
Curcumin	Turmeric	Inducesapoptosis via multiple mechanisms	Skin cancer, Cervical cancer, NSCLC
Pancratistatin	Spider lily *Pancratiumlittorale*	Induces ROS stress, loss of mitochondrial potential, apoptosis	Breast cancer, Colon cancer, Lymphoma
OSW-1	*Ornithogalumsaudersiae*	Damages mitochondrial membranes, Ca2+ dependent apoptosis	Leukemia, Malignant brain tumor, Pancreatic cancer
Epigallocatechin-3-gallate (EGCG)	Green tea	Accumulates in mitochondria, inducing apoptosis	Breast cancer, Colon cancer, Pancreatic cancer, Melanoma
Vitamin K3	Synthetic vitamin K precursor	Inhibits mitochondrial pol γ, causing ROS stress	Leukemia and various solid tumors

8. Conclusions

Recent advances in the field of cancer biology have delineated mitochondrial dysfunctions in cancer. Tumors take advantage of the modulated mitochondrial function to escalate invasiveness. Key mechanisms like respiration are not only essential for tumor growth but also for navigating tumor cells into the circulatory system, facilitating metastasis. Mechanisms connecting mitochondrial dynamics to the development of metastasis remain a puzzle. Moreover, the capability of the mitochondria in allowing cancer cells to adapt to stress should be considered. Consequently, mitochondrial biogenesis might answer these questions and unravel the mechanisms useful for therapeutic strategies for cancer treatment.

Author Contributions: R.G. designed, conceptualized and drafted the review; W.L. drafted the review; R.M. reviewed, read and finalized the review. All authors have read and agreed to the published version of the manuscript.

Funding: This review received no funding.

Acknowledgments: Research Management Training Centre: RMTC-LKL- TAHMAZ Meditech; Dato Seri Harlem Shah-Lim Kon Lian (LKL Sinovac Genesis).

Conflicts of Interest: The authors declare no conflict of interest.

Abbreviations

OXPHOS	Oxidative phosphorylation
SNP	Single nucleotide polymorphisms
EMT	Epithelial mesenchymal transition
Drp1	Dynamin-related protein
Mfn	Mitofusion
ROS	Reactive oxygen species
EGFR	Epidermal growth factor receptor
NSCLC	Non-small cell lung cancer
AML	Acute myelogenous leukemia
STUB1	STIP1 homology and U-Box containing protein 1

USP7	Ubiquitin-specific-processing protease 7
PDH	Pyruvate dehydrogenase
a-KGDH	a-ketoglutarate-dehydrogenase
Drp1	Dynamin-related protein-1
VDAC	Voltage dependent anion channels
MFF	Mitochondrial fission factor
PISD	Phosphatidyl serine decarboxylase
SIRT	Sirtuin
PI3K	Phosphatidylinositol-3 kinase
HNK	Honokiol
MOM	Mitochondrial outer membrane

References

1. Fu, A.; Hou, Y.; Yu, Z.; Zhao, Z.; Liu, Z. Healthy mitochondria inhibit the metastatic melanoma in lungs. *Int. J. Biol. Sci.* **2019**, *15*, 2707–2718. [CrossRef] [PubMed]
2. Grasso, D.; Zampieri, L.X.; Capelôa, T.; Van De Velde, J.A.; Sonveaux, P. Mitochondria in cancer. *Cell Stress* **2020**, *4*, 114–146. [CrossRef] [PubMed]
3. Yu, D.; Liu, C.; Guo, L. Mitochondrial metabolism and cancer metastasis. *Ann. Transl. Med.* **2020**, *8*, 904. [CrossRef] [PubMed]
4. Scheid, A.D.; Beadnell, T.C.; Welch, D. Roles of mitochondria in the hallmarks of metastasis. *Br. J. Cancer* **2021**, *124*, 124–135. [CrossRef] [PubMed]
5. Simula, L.; Nazio, F.; Campello, S. The mitochondrial dynamics in cancer and immune-surveillance. *Semin. Cancer Biol.* **2017**, *47*, 29–42. [CrossRef]
6. Dai, W.; Jiang, L. Dysregulated Mitochondrial Dynamics and Metabolism in Obesity, Diabetes, and Cancer. *Front. Endocrinol.* **2019**, *10*, 570. [CrossRef]
7. Anderson, G.R.; Wardell, S.E.; Cakir, M.; Yip, C.; Ahn, Y.-R.; Ali, M.; Yllanes, A.P.; Chao, C.A.; McDonnell, D.P.; Wood, K.C. Dysregulation of mitochondrial dynamics proteins are a targetable feature of human tumors. *Nat. Commun.* **2018**, *9*, 1–13. [CrossRef]
8. Zhao, J.; Zhang, J.; Yu, M.; Xie, Y.; Huang, Y.; Wolff, D.W.; Abel, P.W.; Tu, Y. Mitochondrial dynamics regulates migration and invasion of breast cancer cells. *Oncogene* **2013**, *32*, 4814–4824. [CrossRef]
9. Huang, Q.; Yongzhan, N.; Cao, H.; Jinliang, X.; Lyu, Y.; Guo, X.; Zhang, J.; Jibin, L.; Ren, T.; Haiyan, C.; et al. Increased mitochondrial fission promotes autophagy and hepatocellular carcinoma cell survival through the ROS-modulated coordinated regulation of the NFKB and TP53 pathways. *Autophagy* **2016**, *12*, 999–1014. [CrossRef]
10. Tanwar, D.K.; Parker, D.J.; Gupta, P.; Spurlock, B.; Alvarez, R.D.; Basu, M.K.; Mitra, K. Crosstalk between the mitochondrial fission protein, Drp1, and the cell cycle is identified across various cancer types and can impact survival of epithelial ovarian cancer patients. *Oncotarget* **2016**, *7*, 60021–60037. [CrossRef]
11. Han, Y.; Kim, B.; Cho, U.; Park, I.S.; Kim, S.I.; Dhanasekaran, D.N.; Tsang, B.K.; Song, Y.J. Mitochondrial fission causes cisplatin resistance under hypoxic conditions via ROS in ovarian cancer cells. *Oncogene* **2019**, *38*, 7089–7105. [CrossRef] [PubMed]
12. Wu, D.; Dasgupta, A.; Chen, K.; Neuber-Hess, M.; Patel, J.; Hurst, T.E.; Mewburn, J.D.; Lima, P.D.A.; Alizadeh, E.; Martin, A.; et al. Identification of novel dynamin-related protein 1 (Drp1) GTPase inhibitors: Therapeutic potential of Drpitor1 and Drpitor1a in cancer and cardiac ischemia-reperfusion injury. *FASEB J.* **2019**, *34*, 1447–1464. [CrossRef] [PubMed]
13. Tomková, V.; Sandoval-Acuña, C.; Torrealba, N.; Truksa, J. Mitochondrial fragmentation, elevated mitochondrial superoxide and respiratory supercomplexes disassembly is connected with the tamoxifen-resistant phenotype of breast cancer cells. *Free Radic. Biol. Med.* **2019**, *143*, 510–521. [CrossRef] [PubMed]
14. Morita, M.; Prudent, J.; Basu, K.; Goyon, V.; Katsumura, S.; Hulea, L.; Pearl, D.; Siddiqui, N.; Strack, S.; McGuirk, S.; et al. mTOR Controls Mitochondrial Dynamics and Cell Survival via MTFP1. *Mol. Cell* **2017**, *67*, 922–935. [CrossRef] [PubMed]
15. Lee, Y.G.; Nam, Y.; Shin, K.J.; Yoon, S.; Park, W.S.; Joung, J.Y.; Seo, J.K.; Jang, J.; Lee, S.; Nam, D.; et al. Androgen-induced expression of DRP1 regulates mitochondrial metabolic reprogramming in prostate cancer. *Cancer Lett.* **2020**, *471*, 72–87. [CrossRef]
16. Wang, J.; Cai, J.; Huang, Y.; Ke, Q.; Wu, B.; Wang, S.; Han, X.; Wang, T.; Wang, Y.; Li, W.; et al. Nestin regulates proliferation and invasion of gastrointestinal stromal tumor cells by altering mitochondrial dynamics. *Oncogene* **2016**, *35*, 3139–3150. [CrossRef]
17. Chen, M.; Ye, K.; Zhang, B.; Xin, Q.; Li, P.; Kong, A.N.; Wen, X.; Yang, J. Paris Saponin II inhibits colorectal carcinogenesis by regulating mitochondrial fission and NF-κB pathway. *Pharmacol. Res.* **2019**, *139*, 273–285. [CrossRef]
18. Ma, Y.; Wang, L.; Jia, R. The role of mitochondrial dynamics in human cancers. *Am. J. Cancer Res.* **2020**, *10*, 1278–1293.
19. Guerra, F.; Arbini, A.A.; Moro, L. Mitochondria and cancer chemoresistance. *Biochim. Biophys. Acta Bioenerg.* **2017**, *1858*, 686–699. [CrossRef]
20. Vyas, S.; Zaganjor, E.; Haigis, M.C. Mitochondria and Cancer. *Cell* **2016**, *166*, 555–566. [CrossRef]
21. Westermann, B. Mitochondrial fusion and fission in cell life and death. *Nat. Rev. Mol. Cell Biol.* **2010**, *11*, 872–884. [CrossRef] [PubMed]
22. Chan, D.C. Dissecting Mitochondrial Fusion. *Dev. Cell* **2006**, *11*, 592–594. [CrossRef] [PubMed]

23. Gogvadze, V.; Orrenius, S.; Zhivotovsky, B. Mitochondria in cancer cells: What is so special about them? *Trends Cell Biol.* **2008**, *18*, 165–173. [CrossRef] [PubMed]
24. Grandemange, S.; Herzig, S.; Martinou, J.-C. Mitochondrial dynamics and cancer. *Semin. Cancer Biol.* **2009**, *19*, 50–56. [CrossRef] [PubMed]
25. Rehman, J.; Zhang, H.J.; Toth, P.T.; Zhang, Y.; Marsboom, G.; Hong, Z.; Salgia, R.; Husain, A.N.; Wietholt, C.; Archer, S.L. Inhibition of mitochondrial fission prevents cell cycle progression in lung cancer. *FASEB J.* **2012**, *26*, 2175–2186. [CrossRef] [PubMed]
26. Ward, P.S.; Thompson, C.B. Metabolic Reprogramming: A Cancer Hallmark Even Warburg Did Not Anticipate. *Cancer Cell* **2012**, *21*, 297–308. [CrossRef]
27. LeBleu, V.S.; O'Connell, J.T.; Herrera, K.N.G.; Wikman-Kocher, H.; Pantel, K.; Haigis, M.C.; De Carvalho, F.M.; Damascena, A.; Chinen, L.T.D.; Rocha, R.M.; et al. PGC-1α mediates mitochondrial biogenesis and oxidative phosphorylation in cancer cells to promote metastasis. *Nat. Cell Biol.* **2014**, *16*, 992–1003. [CrossRef]
28. Hung, W.-Y.; Huang, K.-H.; Wu, C.-W.; Chi, C.-W.; Kao, H.-L.; Li, A.F.-Y.; Yin, P.-H.; Lee, H.-C. Mitochondrial dysfunction promotes cell migration via reactive oxygen species-enhanced β5-integrin expression in human gastric cancer SC-M1 cells. *Biochim. Biophys. Acta Gen. Subj.* **2012**, *1820*, 1102–1110. [CrossRef]
29. Acín-Pérez, R.; Fernández-Silva, P.; Peleato, M.L.; Pérez-Martos, A.; Enríquez, J.A. Respiratory Active Mitochondrial Supercomplexes. *Mol. Cell* **2008**, *32*, 529–539. [CrossRef]
30. Naito, A.; Carcel-Trullols, J.; Xie, C.-H.; Evans, T.T.; Mizumachi, T.; Higuchi, M. Induction of acquired resistance to antiestrogen by reversible mitochondrial DNA depletion in breast cancer cell line. *Int. J. Cancer* **2007**, *122*, 1506–1511. [CrossRef]
31. Dasgupta, S.; Soudry, E.; Mukhopadhyay, N.; Shao, C.; Yee, J.; Lam, S.; Lam, W.; Zhang, W.; Gazdar, A.F.; Fisher, P.B.; et al. Mitochondrial DNA mutations in respiratory complex-I in never-smoker lung cancer patients contribute to lung cancer progression and associated with EGFR gene mutation. *J. Cell Physiol.* **2012**, *227*, 2451–2460. [CrossRef] [PubMed]
32. Kulawiec, M.; Owens, K.M.; Singh, K.K. mtDNA G10398A variant in African-American women with breast cancer provides resistance to apoptosis and promotes metastasis in mice. *J. Hum. Genet.* **2009**, *54*, 647–654. [CrossRef] [PubMed]
33. Guerra, F.; Guaragnella, N.; Arbini, A.A.; Bucci, C.; Giannattasio, S.; Moro, L. Mitochondrial Dysfunction: A Novel Potential Driver of Epithelial-to-Mesenchymal Transition in Cancer. *Front. Oncol.* **2017**, *7*, 295. [CrossRef] [PubMed]
34. Polyak, K.; Weinberg, R.A. Transitions between epithelial and mesenchymal states: Acquisition of malignant and stem cell traits. *Nat. Rev. Cancer* **2009**, *9*, 265–273. [CrossRef] [PubMed]
35. Thiery, J.P.; Acloque, H.; Huang, R.Y.J.; Nieto, M.A. Epithelial-Mesenchymal Transitions in Development and Disease. *Cell* **2009**, *139*, 871–890. [CrossRef] [PubMed]
36. Katsuno, Y.; Lamouille, S.; Derynck, R. TGF-β signaling and epithelial–mesenchymal transition in cancer progression. *Curr. Opin. Oncol.* **2013**, *25*, 76–84. [CrossRef] [PubMed]
37. Xu, W.; Yang, Z.; Lu, N.-H. A new role for the PI3K/Akt signaling pathway in the epithelial-mesenchymal transition. *Cell Adhes. Migr.* **2015**, *9*, 317–324. [CrossRef]
38. Naito, A.; Cook, C.C.; Mizumachi, T.; Wang, M.; Xie, C.-H.; Evans, T.T.; Kelly, T.; Higuchi, M. Progressive tumor features accompany epithelial-mesenchymal transition induced in mitochondrial DNA-depleted cells. *Cancer Sci.* **2008**, *99*, 1584–1588. [CrossRef]
39. Yi, E.Y.; Park, S.Y.; Jung, S.Y.; Jang, W.J.; Kim, Y.J. Mitochondrial dysfunction induces EMT through the TGF-β/Smad/Snail signaling pathway in Hep3B hepatocellular carcinoma cells. *Int. J. Oncol.* **2015**, *47*, 1845–1853. [CrossRef]
40. Tam, S.Y.; Wu, V.W.C.; Law, H.K.W. Hypoxia-Induced Epithelial-Mesenchymal Transition in Cancers: HIF-1α and Beyond. *Front. Oncol.* **2020**, *10*, 486. [CrossRef]
41. Yang, M.-H.; Wu, M.-Z.; Chiou, S.-H.; Chen, P.-M.; Chang, S.-Y.; Liu, C.-J.; Teng, S.-C.; Wu, K.-J. Direct regulation of TWIST by HIF-1α promotes metastasis. *Nat. Cell Biol.* **2008**, *10*, 295–305. [CrossRef] [PubMed]
42. Mani, S.A.; Guo, W.; Liao, M.J.; Eaton, E.N.; Ayyanan, A.; Zhou, A.Y.; Brooks, M.; Reinhard, F.; Zhang, C.C.; Shipitsin, M.; et al. The Epithelial-Mesenchymal Transition Generates Cells with Properties of Stem Cells. *Cell* **2008**, *133*, 704–715. [CrossRef] [PubMed]
43. Hsu, C.-C.; Tseng, L.-M.; Lee, H.-C. Role of mitochondrial dysfunction in cancer progression. *Exp. Biol. Med.* **2016**, *241*, 1281–1295. [CrossRef] [PubMed]
44. Sciacovelli, M.; Frezza, C. Metabolic reprogramming and epithelial-to-mesenchymal transition in cancer. *FEBS J.* **2017**, *284*, 3132–3144. [CrossRef] [PubMed]
45. Che, T.-F.; Lin, C.-W.; Wu, Y.-Y.; Chen, Y.-J.; Han, C.-L.; Chang, Y.-L.; Chang, Y.-L.; Hsiao, T.-H.; Hong, T.-M.; Yang, P.-C. Mitochondrial translocation of EGFR regulates mitochondria dynamics and promotes metastasis in NSCLC. *Oncotarget* **2015**, *6*, 37349–37366. [CrossRef] [PubMed]
46. Choudhary, K.S.; Rohatgi, N.; Halldorsson, S.; Briem, E.; Gudjonsson, T.; Gudmundsson, S.; Rolfsson, O. EGFR Signal-Network Reconstruction Demonstrates Metabolic Crosstalk in EMT. *PLoS Comput. Biol.* **2016**, *12*, e1004924. [CrossRef]
47. Cho, Y.M.; Kim, J.H.; Kim, M.; Park, S.J.; Koh, S.H.; Ahn, H.S.; Kang, G.H.; Lee, J.-B.; Park, K.S.; Lee, H.K. Mesenchymal Stem Cells Transfer Mitochondria to the Cells with Virtually No Mitochondrial Function but Not with Pathogenic mtDNA Mutations. *PLoS ONE* **2012**, *7*, e32778. [CrossRef]

48. Moschoi, R.; Imbert, V.; Nebout, M.; Chiche, J.; Mary, D.; Prebet, T.; Saland, E.; Castellano, R.; Pouyet, L.; Collette, Y.; et al. Protective mitochondrial transfer from bone marrow stromal cells to acute myeloid leukemic cells during chemotherapy. *Blood* **2016**, *128*, 253–264. [CrossRef]
49. Berridge, M.V.; Crasso, C.; Neuzil, J. Mitochondrial Genome Transfer to Tumor Cells Breaks The Rules and Establishes a New Precedent in Cancer Biology. *Mol. Cell. Oncol.* **2018**, *5*, e1023929. [CrossRef]
50. Furnish, M.; Caino, M.C. Altered mitochondrial trafficking as a novel mechanism of cancer metastasis. *Cancer Rep.* **2020**, *3*, e1157. [CrossRef]
51. Missiroli, S.; Perrone, M.; Genovese, I.; Pinton, P.; Giorgi, C. Cancer metabolism and mitochondria: Finding novel mechanisms to fight tumours. *EBioMedicine* **2020**, *59*, 102943. [CrossRef] [PubMed]
52. Sabharwal, S.S.; Schumacker, P.T. Mitochondrial ROS in cancer: Initiators, amplifiers or an Achilles' heel? *Nat. Rev. Cancer* **2014**, *14*, 709–721. [CrossRef] [PubMed]
53. Liou, G.-Y.; Döppler, H.; DelGiorno, K.E.; Zhang, L.; Leitges, M.; Crawford, H.C.; Murphy, M.P.; Storz, P. Mutant KRas-Induced Mitochondrial Oxidative Stress in Acinar Cells Upregulates EGFR Signaling to Drive Formation of Pancreatic Precancerous Lesions. *Cell Rep.* **2016**, *14*, 2325–2336. [CrossRef] [PubMed]
54. Lee, J.J.; van de Ven, R.A.H.; Zaganjor, E.; Ng, M.R.; Barakat, A.; Demmers, J.J.P.G.; Finley, L.W.S.; Gonzalez Herrera, K.N.; Hung, Y.P.; Harris, I.S.; et al. Inhibition of epithelial cell migration and Src/FAK signaling by SIRT3. *Proc. Natl. Acad. Sci. USA* **2018**, *115*, 7057–7062. [CrossRef] [PubMed]
55. Torrens-Mas, M.; Hernández-López, R.; Oliver, J.; Roca, P.; Sastre-Serra, J. Sirtuin 3 silencing improves oxaliplatin efficacy through acetylation of MnSOD in colon cancer. *J. Cell. Physiol.* **2018**, *233*, 6067–6076. [CrossRef] [PubMed]
56. Torrens-Mas, M.; Hernández-López, R.; Pons, D.-G.; Roca, P.; Oliver, J.; Sastre-Serra, J. Sirtuin 3 silencing impairs mitochondrial biogenesis and metabolism in colon cancer cells. *Am. J. Physiol. Physiol.* **2019**, *317*, C398–C404. [CrossRef]
57. Seo, J.H.; Agarwal, E.; Chae, Y.C.; Lee, Y.G.; Garlick, D.S.; Storaci, A.M.; Ferrero, S.; Gaudioso, G.; Gianelli, U.; Vaira, V.; et al. Mitochondrial fission factor is a novel Myc-dependent regulator of mitochondrial permeability in cancer. *EBioMedicine* **2019**, *48*, 353–363. [CrossRef]
58. Humphries, B.A.; Cutter, A.C.; Buschhaus, J.M.; Chen, Y.-C.; Qyli, T.; Palagama, D.S.W.; Eckley, S.; Robison, T.H.; Bevoor, A.; Chiang, B.; et al. Enhanced mitochondrial fission suppresses signaling and metastasis in triple-negative breast cancer. *Breast Cancer Res.* **2020**, *22*, 1–18. [CrossRef]
59. Tang, M.; Luo, X.; Huang, Z.; Chen, L. MitoCPR: A novel protective mechanism in response to mitochondrial protein import stress. *Acta Biochim. Biophys. Sin.* **2018**, *50*, 1072–1074. [CrossRef]
60. Wang, X.; Chen, X.J. A cytosolic network suppressing mitochondria-mediated proteostatic stress and cell death. *Nature* **2015**, *524*, 481–484. [CrossRef]
61. Weidberg, H.; Amon, A. MitoCPR-A surveillance pathway that protects mitochondria in response to protein import stress. *Science* **2018**, *360*. [CrossRef] [PubMed]
62. Altieri, D.C. Mitochondrial compartmentalized protein folding and tumor cell survival. *Oncotarget* **2011**, *2*, 347–351. [CrossRef] [PubMed]
63. Kenny, T.C.; Craig, A.J.; Villanueva, A.; Germain, D. Mitohormesis Primes Tumor Invasion and Metastasis. *Cell Rep.* **2019**, *27*, 2292–2303. [CrossRef] [PubMed]
64. Leanza, L.; Zoratti, M.; Gulbins, E.; Szabo, I. Mitochondrial ion channels as oncological targets. *Oncogene* **2014**, *33*, 5569–5581. [CrossRef] [PubMed]
65. Peruzzo, R.; Szabo, I. Contribution of Mitochondrial Ion Channels to Chemo-Resistance in Cancer Cells. *Cancers* **2019**, *11*, 761. [CrossRef]
66. Bachmann, M.; Pontarin, G.; Szabo, I. The Contribution of Mitochondrial Ion Channels to Cancer Development and Progression. *Cell. Physiol. Biochem.* **2019**, *53*, 63–78.
67. Engelman, J.A.; Chen, L.; Tan, X.; Crosby, K.; Guimaraes, A.R.; Upadhyay, R.; Maira, M.; McNamara, K.; Perera, S.A.; Song, Y.; et al. Effective use of PI3K and MEK inhibitors to treat mutant Kras G12D and PIK3CA H1047R murine lung cancers. *Nat. Med.* **2008**, *14*, 1351–1356. [CrossRef]
68. Caino, M.C.; Ghosh, J.C.; Chae, Y.C.; Vaira, V.; Rivadeneira, D.B.; Faversani, A.; Rampini, P.; Kossenkov, A.V.; Aird, K.M.; Zhang, R.; et al. PI3K therapy reprograms mitochondrial trafficking to fuel tumor cell invasion. *Proc. Natl. Acad. Sci. USA* **2015**, *112*, 8638–8643. [CrossRef]
69. Ghosh, J.C.; Siegelin, M.D.; Vaira, V.; Faversani, A.; Tavecchio, M.; Chae, Y.C.; Lisanti, S.; Rampini, P.; Giroda, M.; Caino, M.C.; et al. Adaptive mitochondrial reprogramming and resistance to PI3K therapy. *J. Natl. Cancer Inst.* **2015**, *107*. [CrossRef]
70. Rozanov, D.; Cheltsov, A.; Nilsen, A.; Boniface, C.; Forquer, I.; Korkola, J.; Gray, J.; Tyner, J.; Tognon, C.E.; Mills, G.B.; et al. Targeting mitochondria in cancer therapy could provide a basis for the selective anti-cancer activity. *PLoS ONE* **2019**, *14*, e0205623. [CrossRef]
71. Hafeez, B.B.; Zhong, W.; Fischer, J.W.; Mustafa, A.; Shi, X.; Meske, L.; Hong, H.; Cai, W.; Havighurst, T.; Kim, K.; et al. Plumbagin, a medicinal plant (lumbago zeylanica)-derived 1,4-naphthoquinone, inhibits growth and metastasis of human prostate cancer PC-3M-luciferase cells in an orthotopic xenograft mouse model. *Mol. Oncol.* **2013**, *7*, 428–439. [CrossRef] [PubMed]
72. Kayashima, T.; Mori, M.; Yoshida, H.; Mizushina, Y.; Matsubara, K. 1,4-Naphthoquinone is a potent inhibitor of human cancer cell growth and angiogenesis. *Cancer Lett.* **2009**, *278*, 34–40. [CrossRef] [PubMed]

73. O'Brien, P.J. Molecular mechanisms of quinone cytotoxicity. *Chem. Biol. Interact.* **1991**, *80*, 1–41. [CrossRef]
74. Sandur, S.K.; Ichikawa, H.; Sethi, G.; Ahn, K.S.; Aggarwal, B.B. Plumbagin (5-hydroxy-2-methyl-1,4-naphthoquinone) suppresses NF-kappaB activation and NF-kappaB-regulated gene products through modulation of p65 and IkappaBalpha kinase activation, leading to potentiation of apoptosis induced by cytokine and chemotherapeutic agents. *J. Biol. Chem.* **2006**, *281*, 17023–17033. [PubMed]
75. Pan, J.; Zhang, Q.; Liu, Q.; Komas, S.M.; Kalyanaraman, B.; Lubet, R.A.; Wang, Y.; You, M. Honokiol Inhibits Lung Tumorigenesis through Inhibition of Mitochondrial Function. *Cancer Prev. Res.* **2014**, *7*, 1149–1159. [CrossRef] [PubMed]
76. Chen, G.; Wang, F.; Trachootham, D.; Huang, P. Preferential killing of cancer cells with mitochondrial dysfunction by natural compounds. *Mitochondrion* **2010**, *10*, 614–625. [CrossRef]
77. Mills, K.M.; Brocardo, M.G.; Henderson, B.R. APC binds the Miro/Milton motor complex to stimulate transport of mitochondria to the plasma membrane. *Mol. Biol. Cell* **2016**, *27*, 466–482. [CrossRef]
78. Jin, F.; Wu, Z.; Hu, X.; Zhang, J.; Gao, Z.; Han, X.; Qin, J.; Li, C.; Wang, Y. The PI3K/Akt/GSK-3β/ROS/eIF2B pathway promotes breast cancer growth and metastasis via suppression of NK cell cytotoxicity and tumor cell susceptibility. *Cancer Biol. Med.* **2019**, *16*, 38–54.
79. Rohlenova, K.; Sachaphibulkij, K.; Stursa, J.; Bezawork-Geleta, A.; Blecha, J.; Endaya, B.; Werner, L.; Cerny, J.; Zobalova, R.; Goodwin, J.; et al. Selective Disruption of Respiratory Supercomplexes as a New Strategy to Suppress Her2high Breast Cancer. *Antioxid. Redox Signal.* **2017**, *26*, 84–103. [CrossRef]

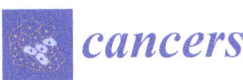

Review

Oncogenic Effects of HIV-1 Proteins, Mechanisms Behind

Maria Isagulants [1,2,3,4,*], Ekaterina Bayurova [1,2], Darya Avdoshina [1,2], Alla Kondrashova [2], Francesca Chiodi [3] and Joel M. Palefsky [5]

1. Gamaleya Research Center for Epidemiology and Microbiology, 123098 Moscow, Russia; bayurova_eo@chumakovs.su (E.B.); avdoshina_dv@chumakovs.su (D.A.)
2. M.P. Chumakov Federal Scientific Center for Research and Development of Immune-and-Biological Products of Russian Academy of Sciences, 108819 Moscow, Russia; kondrashova_as@chumakovs.su
3. Department of Microbiology, Tumor and Cell Biology, Karolinska Institutet, 17177 Stockholm, Sweden; francesca.chiodi@ki.se
4. Department of Research, Riga Stradins University, LV-1007 Riga, Latvia
5. Department of Medicine, University of California, San Francisco, CA 94117, USA; joel.palefsky@ucsf.edu
* Correspondence: maria.issagouliantis@ki.se or maria.issagouliantis@rsu.lv

Citation: Isagulants, M.; Bayurova, E.; Avdoshina, D.; Kondrashova, A.; Chiodi, F.; Palefsky, J.M. Oncogenic Effects of HIV-1 Proteins, Mechanisms Behind. *Cancers* 2021, 13, 305. https://doi.org/10.3390/cancers13020305

Received: 1 December 2020
Accepted: 4 January 2021
Published: 15 January 2021

Publisher's Note: MDPI stays neutral with regard to jurisdictional claims in published maps and institutional affiliations.

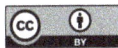

Copyright: © 2021 by the authors. Licensee MDPI, Basel, Switzerland. This article is an open access article distributed under the terms and conditions of the Creative Commons Attribution (CC BY) license (https://creativecommons.org/licenses/by/4.0/).

Simple Summary: People living with human immunodeficiency virus type 1 (HIV-1) (PLWH) are at increased risk of developing cancer despite successful antiretroviral therapy (ART). Here, authors suggest novel mechanism behind this phenomenon. HIV proteins, namely envelope protein gp120, accessory protein negative factor Nef, matrix protein p17, transactivator of transcription Tat and reverse transcriptase RT, are known to be oncogenic per se, to induce oxidative stress and to be released from the infected or expressing cells. These properties are proposed to underlie their capacity to affect bystander epithelial cells causing their malignant transformation, and to enhance tumorigenic potential of already transformed/cancer cells. HIV proteins can act alone or in collaboration with other known oncoproteins, specifically originating from the oncogenic human viruses such as human hepatitis B and C viruses, and human papilloma viruses of high carcinogenic risk, which cause the bulk of malignancies in people living with HIV-1 on ART.

Abstract: People living with human immunodeficiency virus (HIV-1) are at increased risk of developing cancer, such as Kaposi sarcoma (KS), non-Hodgkin lymphoma (NHL), cervical cancer, and other cancers associated with chronic viral infections. Traditionally, this is linked to HIV-1-induced immune suppression with depletion of CD4+ T-helper cells, exhaustion of lymphopoiesis and lymphocyte dysfunction. However, the long-term successful implementation of antiretroviral therapy (ART) with an early start did not preclude the oncological complications, implying that HIV-1 and its antigens are directly involved in carcinogenesis and may exert their effects on the background of restored immune system even when present at extremely low levels. Experimental data indicate that HIV-1 virions and single viral antigens can enter a wide variety of cells, including epithelial. This review is focused on the effects of five viral proteins: envelope protein gp120, accessory protein negative factor Nef, matrix protein p17, transactivator of transcription Tat and reverse transcriptase RT. Gp120, Nef, p17, Tat, and RT cause oxidative stress, can be released from HIV-1-infected cells and are oncogenic. All five are in a position to affect "innocent" bystander cells, specifically, to cause the propagation of (pre)existing malignant and malignant transformation of normal epithelial cells, giving grounds to the direct carcinogenic effects of HIV-1.

Keywords: human immunodeficiency virus type 1; epithelial cells; carcinogenicity; oxidative stress; reactive oxygen species; gp120; Tat; Nef; matrix protein p17; reverse transcriptase

1. Introduction

Immune suppression and related dysfunctions result in a high prevalence in people living with human immunodeficiency virus (PLWH) of HIV-1/AIDS-associated disorders, including so called AIDS-defining cancers (ADC)—Kaposi sarcoma (KS), non-Hodgkin lymphoma (NHL) and cervical cancer. In the era of antiretroviral therapy (ART), their rates have sharply declined: KS by 60–70% and NHL, by 30–50% compared to the pre-ART era. Still, the incidence of KS in PLWH remains elevated 800-fold, of NHL 10-fold and of ADC 4-fold, compared to their rates in the general population. There is also a significant increase in the number of yearly diagnosed cases of non-AIDS-defining cancers [1].

The incidence of these malignancies among PLWH remains elevated compared to that in uninfected population despite successful ART. Traditionally, this is linked to HIV-induced immune suppression with depletion of CD4+ T-helper cells, and exhaustion of lymphopoiesis, however, the immune suppression is much more complex than HIV-1 induced loss of CD4+ T cells. HIV-1 causes dysregulation of the innate immune system, persistent immune activation, dysfunction of the inflammatory response and immune system aging (senescence) early in HIV-1 infection. Successful ART ameliorates, but does not completely correct the major immune dysfunctions [2–6], substantial immunological impairment pertains even on the background of the successful ART [7,8] (for the latest review, see [9]). Hyper-immunoactivation and inflammation persisting in PLWH is recognized as a major cause of HIV-1 associated malignances. This abnormal immunoactivation emerges as the cumulative effect of thymic dysfunction, ART toxicity, persistent antigen stimulation caused by co-infections, microbial translocation, residual viremia and dysbiosis [10], aggravated by incomplete recovery of CD4+ T cell functions and intrinsic B and T cell defects on the background of persistent aberrant activation of monocytes, natural killer cells (NK) and innate lymphoid cells [7,11,12].The immune deficiency and dysfunction of the immune system may not be the only cause [13]. Under successful ART, HIV-1 should become latent, however, a study of HIV-1 integration sites in latently infected cell lines evidenced an ongoing viral replication [14], demonstrating that ART cannot fully suppress the process. Massive data have accumulated on the crucial role in high incidence of malignancies among PLWH of the residual virus production and circulating viral proteins. This review concentrates on their role in the high prevalence of cancers among individuals living with HIV-1.

2. Prevalence of Non-AIDS Defining Cancers Increases Despite Successful Antiretroviral Therapy

The category of non-AIDS-defining cancers (NADC) includes liver cancer related to infections with hepatitis B and C viruses (HBV and HCV), brain cancer, and cancers associated with infection with human papillomaviruses of high oncogenic risk (HR HPVs), specifically, the anal cancer.

2.1. Liver Cancer

Hepatocellular carcinoma (HCC) is the third-largest cause of cancer-related mortality on a global scale. It constitutes nearly the majority of liver cancer cases, followed by intrahepatic cholangiocellular carcinomas [15]. HCC is a recognized complication of liver cirrhosis, developing stepwise from regenerative to low-grade, then high-grade dysplastic nodules, although in some cases it may also develop de novo [15]. The burden of HCC is expected to increase worldwide in the next few decades, due to the population growth and aging expected in coming years [16]. Treated HIV-1 infection is associated with decreased survival in HCC, independent of stage, anticancer treatment, and geographical origins of the patients [16]. HIV-1 is not sufficient to cause liver cancer on its own, but may promote development of liver cancer by multiple mechanisms not yet fully understood [17]. Although the role of immune suppression in HCV-related HCC is not clear [17], mechanistic evidence suggests an accelerated progression of chronic liver disease to fibrosis and ultimately malignancy mediated by HIV-1-mediated impairment of antiviral CD4+ and CD8+ T-cell responses [18–20].

HIV-1 infection is characterized by increased microbial translocation resulting in elevated levels of circulating lipopolysaccharides (LPS) in the portal and systemic circulations [21]. LPS are well-known inducers of the innate immune activation. Increased levels of LPS and/or soluble CD14 (sCD14; reflects LPS-induced monocyte activation) in PLWH on ART correlate with impaired recovery of CD4+ T cells. They also tightly correlated with multiple markers of immune activation, specifically, high levels of type I interferons and activated CD8+ T cells. In HIV-1 infection, these two parameters strongly predict disease progression [21]. In the liver, LPS activate hepatic stellate (HSC) and Kupffer cells (KFC), resulting in the generation of superoxide and release of proinflammatory and profibrogenic cytokines such as TNF-α, IL-1, IL-6, and IL-12 that induce liver damage and accelerated liver fibrosis [22]. Activation of Kupffer cells by LPS involves signaling through TLR-4, shown to govern the transition from chronic hepatic inflammation to hepatocellular carcinoma [23]. Another product released from bacterial cell walls, (1→3)-β-D-Glucan (βDG), emerges as an additional significant source of monocyte and NK cell activation, further contributing to immune dysfunction and inflammation [24].

Growing evidence accumulates of HIV-1 grossly affecting the liver. HIV-1-monoinfected patients demonstrate markers of liver fibrinogenesis/liver injury (by transient liver elastography) correlated with high plasma levels of HIV-1 RNA [25]. HIV-1 RNA has been detected in primary human hepatocytes both ex vivo and in vitro [26,27]. Also many hepatocyte cell lines are permissive to a low level HIV-1 infection although the nature of receptor(s) for HIV-1 on liver cells is unclear [28]. HIV-1 can also directly infect Kupffer cells; infectious replication-competent HIV-1 has been isolated from KFC obtained from liver at autopsy from three HIV-1-infected individuals who died while on ART [29]. Another target of HIV-1 are hepatic stellate cells (HSC), the primary cells involved in liver fibrogenesis, affected through both direct HIV-1 infection and HIV-1 exposure [30]. Interactions of HIV-1, specifically its envelope protein gp120, with chemokine receptors CCR5 and CXCR4 induce cell signaling in HSCs and immune cells within the liver promoting inflammatory responses [31,32]. Direct HIV-1 infection of KFC results in the amplification of proinflammatory responses to LPS [33], enhanced fibrosis and cirrhosis, and exhaustion of virus-specific T-cells. HIV-1-infected HSCs produce collagen I and release monocyte chemoattractant protein-1 (MCP-1) [34]. Exposure of HSCs to HIV-1 results in the production of reactive oxygen species (ROS), and expression of collagen and tissue inhibitor of matrix metalloproteinases-1 (TIMP1) [35]. These events, together with abnormalities in the gut microbial communities, significantly contribute to the high rates of liver cancer in PLWH [36] (Figure 1).

Even more important driving force of hepatocellular carcinogenesis in PLWH is co-infection with HBV and HCV [37]. In HIV-1/HBV and HIV-1/HCV co-infected patients, HIV-1 infection decreases the rate of spontaneous viral clearance from the liver, accelerates fibrogenesis and increases the rates of liver-related morbidity and mortality, including the development of HCC [30,38]. In HIV-1/HCV co-infected individuals HCC occurs at a younger age and after a shorter period of HCV infection than in HIV-1 negative individuals [39], with the risk to develop HCC increasing each year by 11% [19]. Important risk factors for the progression to liver cancer are high HBV and HCV viral loads [18,19,40]. They are associated with (over)expression of viral oncoproteins known to induce oxidative stress and chromosomal instability/genomic damage, promote chronic inflammation with liver damage resulting in the malignant transformation of liver cells [41,42] (Figure 1).

2.2. Brain Cancer

PLWH are highly predisposed to developing brain cancer, including primary central nervous system lymphomas (PCNSL) and glioblastomas (GBM) [43,44]. In pre-ART era, brain tumors were registered in 10% of PLWH [43]. Prevalence of PCNSL in AIDS patients was 3600-fold greater than in the general population, reaching 12% in AIDS patients [44]. ART has dramatically reduced these rates, possibly due to the effect of protease inhibitors [45]. Still, the prevalence of brain tumors in PLWH appears to be higher than in general population: in USA; recorded prevalence of PCNSL in HIV-1 infected is 8.4% compared to <3.3% in the general US population [45,46] Also GBM occurs in PLWH (in various stages of HIV-1 infection) at a younger age and at a frequency 5.4- to 45-fold higher than in the general population [47]. Furthermore, the median survival rate in patients with GBM for PLWH is shorter than for HIV-1-negative patients receiving same treatment (an average of 8 compared to 14 months, respectively) [48].

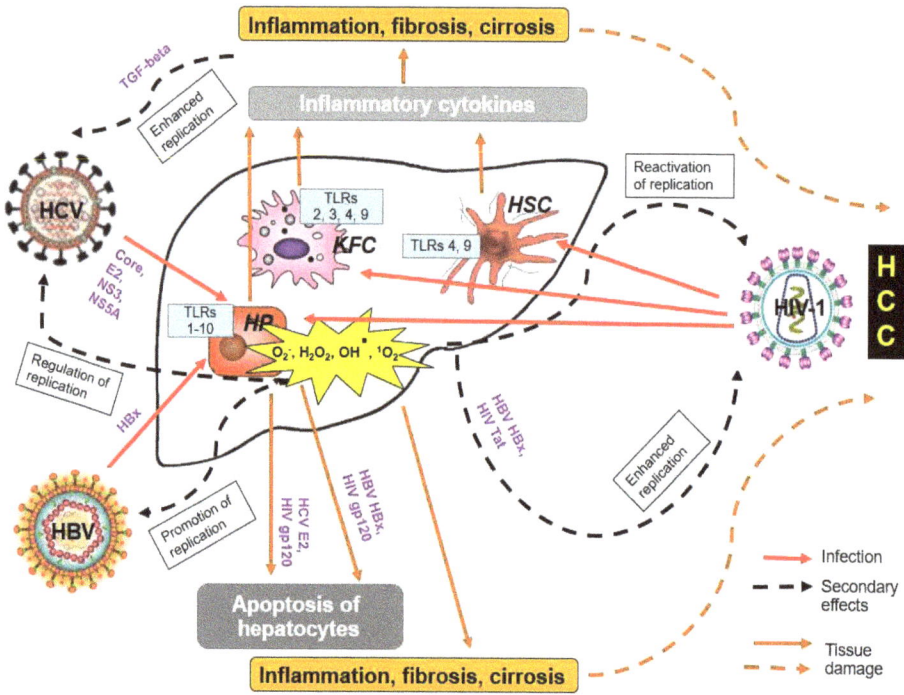

Figure 1. The effect of HIV-1 on cells of the liver. Infection with HIV-1 and even exposition of hepatocytes (HP), hepatic stellate cells (HSC), Kupffer cells (KFC) to HIV-1 leads to production of reactive oxygen species (ROS) and induction of proinflammatory microenvironment, which in turn, promote/enhance replication of HBV, HCV, as well as HIV-1 itself, resulting in enhanced fibrosis, cirrhosis and development of hepatocellular carcinoma (HCC). Infections are depicted in red, secondary effects in dashed black, and events leading to tissue damage in ochre-colored lines.

The nature of the brain tumor-HIV-1 relationship is not fully understood. The majority of these tumors are central nervous system lymphomas but gliomas may develop as well. GBM tumors appear approximately three years after HIV-1 infection [43]. The stimulatory effect of HIV-1 infection on the development of GBM has been associated with reduced immune surveillance. However, survival of PLWH after GBM diagnosis is not associated with CD4+ cell counts [47]. The absence of a correlation between GBM development & progression with immune incompetence [47,49–51] indicates that aggressive tumor behavior is not a direct consequence of the immune deficiency and suggests direct involvement of HIV-1 in the initiation and progression of brain cancers. Importantly, HIV-1 infection in the brain is not limited to microglia/macrophages, but also affects astrocytes, which can then serve as a potential reservoir for further productive infection, viral persistence, and latency [52,53].

2.3. Squamous Cell Carcinomas

PLWH suffer from squamous carcinomas at numerous sites including the lung, anogenital region, oral cavity, epiglottis and cervix. Many of these malignancies are associated with infection by human papillomaviruses of high carcinogenic risk (HR HPVs). Similar to the rates of liver and brain cancer, the rates of HR HPV-associated cancers in PLWH are steadily growing despite successful ART [54–56]. CD4+ levels and resulting immune suppression play a prominent role in controlling HPV replication and development of early disease, particularly, the development of pre-cancerous intraepithelial neoplasia: in PLWH, the probabilities of HPV acquisition and development of intraepithelial neoplasia increase in proportion to the loss of CD4 T cells [57]. However, progression to high-grade lesions and further to cancer is not predetermined by CD4+ depletion, i.e., is not a straightforward outcome of HIV-1-induced immune suppression [58,59], but rather an outcome of the accumulated changes in the host cell genome and transcriptome involving tumor suppressor genes, apoptosis-related genes, DNA damage-repair genes, and cell cycle regulatory genes [58,60,61].

Question arises how could this rely to the epithelial cells which are considered to be non-susceptible to HIV-1 infection and non-permissive to HIV-1 replication? HIV-1 infects a variety of immune cells, such as CD4+ T lymphocytes and monocytes/macrophages. However, several studies show that it may also infect or rather "trespass" other cell types, in which HIV-1 virions and individual HIV-1 proteins were repeatedly detected. In primate models, application of HIV-1 to the surfaces of oropharyngeal [62], anal/rectal [63], cervicovaginal and foreskin/penile [62,64–66] epithelia was shown to lead to subsequent systemic infection of HIV-1-susceptible immune cells, indicating that HIV-1 travels through these tissues to reach its targets. Indeed, application of HIV-1 to human foreskin, vaginal and cervical tissue explants ex vivo leads to the transmission of HIV-1 across these epithelia [64,66–71].

These findings are not restricted to the epithelial cells of the reproductive tract. HIV-1 antigens and RNA were detected in gastric epithelial cells in the biopsy and autopsy samples of HIV-1-infected patients; furthermore, TEM analysis visualized HIV-1 particles in the cytoplasm of gastric epithelial cells [72]. Interestingly, HIV-1 load in blood positively correlated with the number of HIV-1-infected gastric epithelial cells. The latter increased with progression of chronic infection, being significantly higher at the AIDS compared to the asymptomatic stage. HIV-1 infection of gastric epithelial cells associated with a severe inflammatory response in the gastric mucosa manifested by infiltration and aberrant activation of the immune cells [72].

Another example is presented by human mammary epithelial cells (MEC). MEC express HIV-1 receptors CD4, CCR5, CXCR4, and galactosyl ceramide (GalCer). Although the evidence for direct MEC infection by HIV-1 was missing, HIV-1 virions were found in the endosomal compartments of these cells. Furthermore, activated CD4+ T cells co-cultured with HIV-1-exposed MEC were productively infected with HIV-1 [73]. This confirmed that mammary epithelial cells can endocytose HIV-1 and facilitate its transfer to CD4+ T lymphocytes [73]. At the other end, a contact-dependent HIV-1 transfer was shown from HIV-1-infected macrophages to both primary and immortalized renal tubule epithelial cells (RTE). Live imaging of HIV-1 infected RTE cells revealed four different fates: latency, hypertrophy, cell death, and proliferation [74]. HIV-1 can also enter airway epithelial cells and alter their function by increasing the expression of inflammatory mediators [75]. This data unequivocally demonstrate that HIV-1 could be internalized and/or sequestered by human epithelial cells of different origins.

3. Mechanisms Underlying HIV-1 Pathogenicity in Epithelial Cells

In CD4+ cells HIV-1 was reported to preferably integrate into cancer-associated genes or cell cycle regulation genes dysregulation of which can lead to cancer formation as was described for other retroviruses [76–78]. Replication of HIV-1 in epithelial cells has not been shown except for the early findings of human uterine epithelial cells productively infected by HIV-1 with reverse transcription of viral RNA, transcription of viral DNA, and secretion of infectious virus [79]. Of note, co-cultivation of human CD4+ T cell lines with HIV-1-infected uterine epithelial cells (and also by virions released by these cells) led to HIV-1 infection of the CD4+ T cells [79]. Bulk of data accumulated so far evidence sequestration of HIV-1 by human epithelial cells of different origins without evidence of productive replication or integration. However, a "real" infection can take place as well.

HIV-1 was shown to hijack other viral Envs to directly enter CD4-negative cells through pseudotyping [80–82]. Lately, Tang Y. et al. have shown that HIV-1 infected T cells can fuse to and transfer the virus to placental trophoblasts, if the later express on their surfaces the envelope glycoprotein of human endogenous retrovirus family W1, syncytin [83]. This leads to the formation of an HIV-1 reservoir in the epithelial cells [83]. Syncytin-1 derives from a family of endogenous retroviruses and originates from HERVW1 infection of human germ cells [84]. Expression of syncytin could be a common feature of an epithelial cell which make them susceptible to HIV-1 via a "non-canonical" route of HIV-1 infection. These are not necessarily the epithelial cells of placenta. According to the recent preliminary report published in bioRxiv, HIV-1 can infect human bronchial epithelial cells; after exposition to HIV-1 they were shown to express p24 and contain latent HIV-1 provirus [85]. These findings along with the data by Asin SN et al. [79] indicate that in certain cases epithelial cells can be infected with HIV-1, possibly as a one-round abortive infection with reverse transcription of RNA and integration of the proviral DNA governed by respective enzymes constituting HIV-1 virion. Such integrated proviral HIV-1 DNA would not only serve as an HIV-1 reservoir, but would also give progeny to the genetically modified cells (with proviral DNA inserts) susceptible to malignant transformation. The observation by Hughes K et al. of a proliferation of HIV-1 infected epithelial cells consistent with clonal expansion of individual cells ideally fits this scenario [74].

HIV-1 antigens may also affect epithelial cells without infecting them. Epithelial cells may respond to the defective virions incapable of productive infection or freely circulating HIV-1 antigens shed by the infectious or defective virions. Addition of HIV-1/HIV-1 antigens to the epithelial cells generates an inflammatory microenvironment or rather microenvironmental immune abnormalities [86–88] (as those associated with HR HPV infection). Microenvironment of B-cell lymphomas in PLWH is characterized by expression of CD3, CD4, CD8, CD56, CD68, CD163, FOXP3, TIA1, granzyme B, perforin, CD57, CD34 and PD-1 [89], and enrichment with soluble factors, including cytokines IL-1, IL-2, IL6, IL10, and chemokines of the CCL and CXCL families [89,90]. Such microenvironment was also found in the intraepithelial cancerous lesions of PLWH [91]. Studies on the mucosa-associated lymphoid tissue system (MALT) in PLWH have shown abnormal immune responses in the mucosal milieu, including upregulation of expression of multiple regulatory cytokines such as IL-8, IL-23, TNF-α, IL-17A, and IFN-γ (TNF-α/IL-17A/IFN-γ triad), the depletion of Langerhans cells and CD3+ lymphocytes, increases in Foxp3+ T-regulatory cells, and in local lymphocyte infiltrates composed by CD8+ T cells, associated with the development of high-grade squamous intraepithelial lesions (HSILs) [91–94].

Furthermore, presence in the epithelial cells of HIV-1/HIV-1 proteins modulates their capacity to express E-cadherin, a marker of epithelial to mesenchymal transition (EMT) [69,75,95]. HIV-1 interaction with the surface of mucosal epithelial cells was also shown to activate the transforming growth factor-beta (TGF-β) and mitogen-activated protein kinase signaling pathways [96]. When activated, these pathways may lead to the disruption of epithelial junctions and EMT [97]. Indeed, EMT was induced by exposure of oral keratinocytes from HIV-1-negative individuals to HIV-1 virions as well as Tat and gp120 proteins [98]. Within premalignant cells or in the environment of the malignant cells, HIV-1 driven EMT would promote motile/migratory cells and accelerate the neoplastic process.

Altogether these observations imply direct carcinogenic effect(s) of HIV-1 virions and/or antigens. This concept, proposed in 2002 by B Clarke & R Chetty [58] and four years later by Palefsky JM [59], is now supported by considerable experimental proof. It brings up several issues of importance for epithelial cells: (i) could malignant transformation be promoted by cooperation of HIV-1 with other oncogenic viruses; (ii) which HIV-1 antigens are implicated; and finally (iii) what are the underlying molecular mechanisms?

4. Potentiation of Carcinogenesis by Interactions of HIV-1 with Other Oncogenic Viruses

Oncogenic transformation associated with virus infection was for a long time considered to result from a mono-infection (infection with a single virus). However, it is now established that in many cases induction of cancer depends on the simultaneous presence and interactions of multiple viral agents in diverse combinations. Viruses co-infecting human tissues may have synergistic or regulatory effects on carcinogenesis, targeting existing neoplastic cells as well as their microenvironment including reactive T-cells, B cells and macrophages, and non-immune cells such as endothelial cells. HIV-1, in particular, potentiates the effects of EBV, KSHV, HCV, and HPV oncogenes, promoting carcinogenesis in individuals co-infected with HIV-1 and EBV, KSHV, HCV, HBV, and HPV. Here, we will focus on molecular interactions of HIV-1 with HBV, HCV, and HPVs.

Progression to liver cancer/HCC in HIV-1/HBV and HIV-1/HCV co-infected patients is promoted by direct and indirect interactions between these viruses and their antigens within the cells harboring HIV-1 due to infection or sequestration of the virion (viral proteins). HIV-1 infection of hepatic cell lines increases the expression of HBV antigens [27]. HIV-1 gp120 causes intracellular accumulation of HBV DNA as well as HBsAg causing hepatotoxicity [99]. Direct interaction of HIV-1 and HBV in liver cells has been demonstrated, with the HBV X protein interacting with HIV-1 Tat to facilitate HIV-1 replication [99]. Upon co-cultivation of HIV-1 infected Jurkat cells with hepatocytes, up-to 16% of the latter acquire Nef. Sequestered Nef alters the size and numbers of lipid droplets (LD), inducing 1.5 to 2.5 fold up-regulation of replication of HCV subgenomic replicon, a remarkable finding in relation to the initially indolent viral replication. Nef also dramatically enhances the ethanol-mediated up-regulation of HCV replication accelerating progression to HCC [100]. HIV-1 gp 120 also causes TGF-β mediated up-regulation of HCV replication [86]. Taken together, these data indicate that HIV-1 and single HIV-1 proteins are critical elements in accelerating progression of liver pathogenesis by enhancing HBV and HCV replication and coordinating production of key intra- and extra-cellular molecules that orchestrate liver decay [100].

One of the mechanisms of HIV-1 potentiation of liver cancer is the induction of oxidative stress. HCV, HIV-1 (and antiretroviral therapy) act together to activate production of ROS in HSCs and hepatocytes. ROS promote phosphorylation of the major mitogen-activated protein kinases active in human cells, p38 kinase, c-JUN N-terminal kinase (JNK) and extracellular signal-regulated kinase (ERK) that control cell growth, differentiation and apoptosis. In their turn, the phosphorylated p38 MAPK, JNK, and p42/44 ERK phosphorylate nuclear factor kappa-light-chain-enhancer of activated B cells (NF-κB) protein complex, mastering transcriptional regulation of inflammation and cell death [31]. Following these events, phosphorylated NF-κB translocates to the nucleus, and where it normally modulates the production of both pro- and antifibrogenic/antiapoptotic genes, ensuring that liver cells are protected from apoptosis, but are capable to build the required inflammatory and immune responses [101]. In the presence of LPS, NF-κB can upregulate the expression of profibrogenic genes, such as procollagen α1, transforming growth factor β1 (TGF-β1) and tissue inhibitor of MMPs (TIMP-1) [31,101]. This process is accelerated by HIV-1/HIV-1 proteins: exposure of hepatocytes to HIV-1/HIV-1 proteins results in the elevated production of ROS and increased expression of collagen and TIMP1, further amplified by HCV infection, and even exposure to infectious HCV [35]. Taken together, these data indicate that HIV-1-mediated potentiation of hepatocellular carcinogenesis reflects a concerted action of HIV-1, HBV and HCV as viruses and/or individual viral proteins (Figure 1). Based on compelling data, McGivern & Lemon even suggested that the path to hepatocellular carcinoma in chronic hepatitis C shares important features with the carcinogenesis induced by HPV [102].

The increased risk of PLWH developing HPV-associated cancer can also, at least in part, be due to the interactions between HIV-1 and HPV. In general, epithelial cells of PLWH show loss of E-cadherin, and upregulation of vimentin and TGF-b1 expression with spindle-like morphology indicating induction of TGF-b1-dependent EMT, critical for malignant transformation. As noted above, EMT is induced not only due to HIV-1 infection, but also through exposition of epithelial cells to HIV-1 proteins [69,75,95,97]. EMT-induced keratinocytes can then be infected with pseudoviral HPV16 particles (HPV-16 PsVs) and whole HPV16 virus, with infected cells expressing viral oncogenes E6/E7, whereas unexposed keratinocytes could not be infected with either PsVs, or infectious HPV16. Furthermore, "HIV-1-induced" EMT keratinocytes could be transformed with HPV16 DNA, transformed cells showing active proliferation and migration [103]. This confirms that prolonged exposure to and interaction of HIV-1 with oral and anal epithelial cells induces EMT. EMT-induced loss of cell adhesion and increased proliferation and mobility of epithelial cells play a critical role in HPV infection and HPV-associated transformation. HIV-1-induced EMT in the orogenital mucosa may promote progression of pre-cancerous HPV-associated neoplasia to cancer in HIV-1-infected individuals [103].

"Molecular" cooperation between HIV-1 and HPV has not been sufficiently well characterized, but there are relevant examples in this field. Tat protein was shown to transactivate the HPV long control region and increase expression of oncoprotein E7 of HPV18 in HeLa cells [104,105]. Tat can upregulate the expression of E6 and E7 oncoproteins of HPV type 16 in HPV 16-infected human oral keratinocytes, notably enhancing the in vitro proliferative capacity of these cells [106,107], and increase the transcription of E2 modulating HPV replication [108]. The direct angiogenic effects of Tat [109] or its capacity to up-regulate the expression of E6 and E7 of HR-HPVs [110] allows Tat to favor the angiogenic switch in high-grade CIN. We have shown that gp120 and reverse transcriptases (RT) derived from various HIV-1 strains, can increase the expression of HPV 16 E6 in a cervical cancer cell line containing full-length HPV 16 genome Ca Ski (Figure 2), while HIV-1 p24 exerts no effect. In similar conditions, gp120 increases the expression of HPV16 E6 also in HPV16 immortalized anal epithelial AKC2 cells [104,106,111,112]. Furthermore, Tugizov et al. have shown that in the HPV-immortalized anal and cervical epithelial cells Tat and gp120 proteins induce the EMT phenotype, leading to increased migration of cells via collagen membranes [103]. The data on the interaction(s) between HPV and other HIV-1 proteins is missing.

Overall, these findings indicate that the increased incidence of AIDS-defining and non-AIDS defining forms of cancer in PLWH may reflect the direct or indirect, often concerted, carcinogenic effect(s) of HIV-1 and/or individual HIV-1 proteins on diverse infected as well as uninfected bystander cells. Furthermore, some HIV-1 proteins appear to be directly involved in cell transformation and propagation of malignant cells.

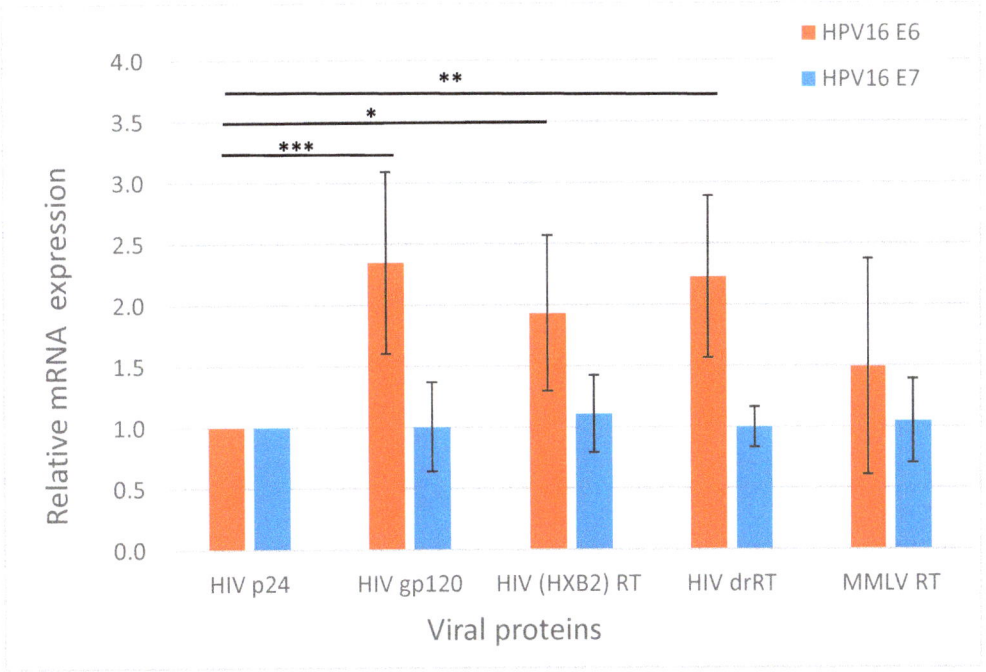

Figure 2. Transcription of oncoproteins E6 and E7 of HPV 16 in Ca Ski cells treated with HIV-1 proteins. Ca Ski cells harboring 600 full genomic copies of HPV 16 (ATCC CRL-1550) were cultured in RPMI-1640 medium (PanEco, Moscow, Russia) supplemented with 10% FBS and 100 mg/mL penicillin/streptomycin mix at 37 °C in an 5% CO_2 and split every 4 days. A panel of recombinant HIV-1 proteins: gp120 [113]; p24 (NIBSC ARP 694.1); RT of HIV-1-1 clade B HXB2 strain [114], drug resistant (dr) RT of HIV-1-1 clade B isolated from patient with multiple drug resistance mutation (RT1.14; [114]) and RT of Moloney murine leukemia virus (MMTV) (CRIE, Moscow, Russia) were added to the culture medium, typically in concentration of 1 ng/mL, and incubated for 48 h, according to the methodology described previously by Lein K. et al. [115] Total RNA was extracted and reverse transcribed as described by Jansons et al. 2020 [116]. Gene-specific PCRs were performed on Rotor-Gene 6000 (Qiagen, Darmstadt, Germany) with SYBR Green kit (Evrogen, Moscow, Russia) with primers specific to HPV 16 E6 and E7 [117]. Expression of mRNA, assessed by the standard ddCt method, was normalized to expression of 18S RNA (18Srna_rt_f: GTAACCCGTTGAACCCCATT; 18Srna_rt_r: CCATCCAATCGGTAGTAGCG), and presented as fold change compared to cells treated with p24, as was recommended earlier [118]. Values represent mean ± SD from two independent assays run in duplicates. *** $p < 0.001$, ** $p < 0.01$, * $p < 0.05$ by the ordinary two-way ANOVA with Sidak's multiple comparisons test.

5. HIV-1 Antigens Involved in Cell Transformation and Tumor Propagation

5.1. Transactivator of Transcription (Tat)

Tat has long since been known to influence cell cycle progression. In HeLa cells, Tat induces a significant increase in the levels of proliferation markers together with the reduction in the expression of cell cycle inhibitors of transcription [119]; it inhibits epithelial differentiation, blocks apoptosis in vitro and accelerates tumor formation in vivo [119]. In addition, Tat significantly increases in vitro migration in the absence of fetal calf serum [119]. These results suggest that HIV-1 may enhance carcinogenesis by promoting cell cycle progression [111]. Furthermore, it has been shown that binding of Tat to Tat-interacting promoter 30 (TIP30) enhanced EMT and metastasis of non-small cells lung cancer cells by regulating the nuclear translocation of Snail [120]. One of the possible mechanisms of Tat induced carcinogenesis is blocking at the mRNA level of the expression of a Rb family member pRb2/130 and cyclin-dependent kinase inhibitors p21 and p17 [111]. The transduction domain of Tat specifically attenuates growth of polyamine-deprived tumor cells [121]. Tat is also known to modulate VEGF and targets VEGFRs which increases angiogenesis and supports tumor growth [122]. Furthermore, Tat alters DNA repair in host cells, potentially leading to genomic instability [123,124]. Specifically, Tat induces expression of the DNA polymerase beta gene, which codes for a central mediator in the DNA base-excision repair pathway [125]. It also interferes with double-strand break DNA repair, as cellular extracts containing Tat possess a reduced capacity to re-join linearized DNA [126], indicating that Tat, as well as cellular co-factors of Tat, interfere with repair of double-stranded DNA breaks [123].

5.2. Envelope Glycoprotein gp120

Glioma cells were shown to interact with the HIV-1 envelope protein gp120. This interaction promotes proliferation, migration, survival and stimulates glycolysis in glioma cell lines and tumor growth in animal models [127]. Increased glycolysis, also known as the Warburg effect characteristic of malignancy [128], results in increased protein and lipid synthesis, and promotes uncontrolled propagation (both proliferation and invasion) of tumor cells, as it provides them with glycolytic intermediary precursors required for the synthesis of DNA, proteins and lipids [127,129]. As Tat, gp120 induces EMT and cell migration through the TGF-β1 and MAPK signaling pathways [115,130].

5.3. Accessory Protein Negative Factor (Nef)

Nef is one of the earliest and most abundantly expressed HIV-1 proteins. Nef has the ability to modulate multiple cellular signaling pathways in both CD4+ lymphocytes and macrophages. Nef inhibits the apoptotic function of p53 due to its ability to decrease p53 protein half-life and, consequently, p53 DNA binding activity and transcriptional activation [131]. Both internalized and ectopic expression of Nef in endothelial cells synergizes with Kaposi's sarcoma (KS) KSHV oncoprotein K1 to facilitate vascular tube formation and cell proliferation, and enhance angiogenesis in the chicken chorioallantoic membrane (CAM) model. In vivo experiments further indicate that Nef can accelerate K1-induced angiogenesis and tumorigenesis in athymic nu/nu mice [132]. On non-small lung cancer A549 cells, Nef promotes cell proliferation, migration, anchor independent growth and reduces the levels of expression of p53, increasing the aggressiveness of cancer cells [133].

5.4. Reverse Transcriptase (RT)

We have shown that constitutive expression of HIV-1 RT in murine mammary gland adenocarcinoma 4T1 cells leads to upregulation, in a concentration-dependent manner, of the expression of the transcription factors Twist and Snail tightly involved in EMT [134]. In vivo, expression of RT by 4T1 cells results in enhanced tumor growth and potentiates formation of metastasis in distal organs of immunocompetent syngenic mice [134]. Interestingly, this is not a common property of the reverse transcriptases, as constitutive expression of enzymatically active reverse transcriptase domain of telomerase reverse transcriptase, on contrary, suppressed both tumor growth and metastatic activity of 4T1 cells [116].

5.5. Matrix Protein p17

Matrix/p17 protein induces expression of chemokines [135], exerts pro-angiogenic [136] and lymphangiogenic [137] activities, and deregulates the biological activity of diverse cells of the immune system [138]. Overall, p17 generates a prolymphangiogenic microenvironment, predisposes the lymph node to lymphoma growth and metastasis [137] and promotes the aggressiveness (propagation) of human triple-negative breast cancer cells [139]. In a HIV-1 transgenic mouse model of lymphoma, only expression of HIV-1 p17, but not of other HIV-1 proteins, induced spontaneous B-cell lymphomas in HIV-1 transgenic mice, with p17 expressed at high levels in the early stages of the disease [140]. Murine lymphoma tissues exhibited enrichment in expression of the recombination-activating genes (Rag1/2) [140].

The latter suggests that intracellular signaling induced by p17 leads to genomic instability and promotes the transformation [140].

Thus, several HIV-1 proteins are directly or indirectly oncogenic, stimulating transformation of healthy cells and propagation and aggressiveness of already existing cancer cells. These oncogenic properties are linked to two essential characteristics of these proteins: their capacity to induce oxidative stress with production of reactive oxygen species and their ability to exit HIV-1-infected cells (active or passive transport).

6. Oncogenic HIV-1 Proteins Induce Oxidative Stress

Virally-induced cancer evolves over long periods of time in the context of a strongly oxidative microenvironment, on the background of chronic inflammation. Oxidative stress induced by chronic viral infection is one of the factors driving neoplastic transformation, ultimately leading to oncogenic mutations in many cellular signaling cascades that drive cell growth and proliferation [42,141]. Oxidative damage of chromosomal DNA and chronic immune-mediated inflammation are key features of HBV, HCV, HPV, and HIV-1 infections [42,141]. As we have earlier reviewed, numerous lines of evidence show that HIV-1 infection triggers pronounced oxidative stress in both laboratory models and the context of in vivo infection by deregulation of oxidative stress pathways with escalation of ROS production and by inducing mitochondrial dysfunction [141]. As a result, PLWH exhibit multiple markers of oxidative stress including DNA damage [134,142]. The enhancement of ROS production is mediated by the envelope protein Gp120, Tat, Nef, RT, and p17 [141–146].

6.1. Transactivator of Transcription

Tat induces oxidative stress both directly and indirectly via several independent mechanisms. The first involves the NADPH oxidases [147], and in the second, an enzyme involved in the catabolism of biogenic polyamines, spermine oxidase (SMO) [148], and the third, a mitochondrial dysfunction [149]. A detailed analysis of the levels of ROS in different subcellular compartments of the HIV-1 infected cells revealed a strong increase in the levels of H_2O_2 in the endoplasmic reticulum (ER), demonstrating with the help of genetically encoded ratiometric sensor HyPER [150,151]. This indicated the involvement in H_2O_2 production of NOX4 which primarily resides in ER [152]. The levels of H_2O_2 in the cytoplasm and mitochondria were not elevated [151]. The above activities of Tat are thought to underlie the onset of HIV-1-associated dementia [109,150].

6.2. Envelope Protein Gp120

Early findings indicated that gp120 increases free radical production from monocyte-derived macrophages (MDM) detected by spin-trapping methods, and that the spin trap adduct results from a reaction involving nitrogen oxide NO or its closely related oxidized derivatives [153]. We have earlier summarized a profound role of gp120 in the induction of oxidative stress [141], namely gp120 induces ROS production in cell lines of lymphoid origin, in the endothelial brain cells, astrocytes, neurons and microglia. In astrocytes, it enhances ROS production by several parallel mechanisms: via Fenton–Weiss–Haber reaction, NOX2 and NOX4, and cytochrome P450 2E1 (CYP2E1) [154,155]. The latter is mediated through the upregulation of CYP2E1 expression. In cancer (neuroblastoma) cells, gp120 induces proline oxidase that synthesized pyroline-5-carboxylate with concomitant generation of ROS (reviewed in [141]).

The effect of HIV-1/HIV-1 proteins on the cellular antioxidant defense system is controversial. They can both suppress and enhance antioxidant defense pathways [141]. Gp120 was shown to induce oxidative stress response. It up-regulates functional expression in cultured astrocytes of multidrug resistance protein 1 (Mrp1) which effluxes endogenous substrates glutathione and glutathione disulphide involved in cellular defense against oxidative stress [156]. It also upregulates the expression of nuclear factor erythroid derived 2-related factor 2 (Nrf2), a basic leucine zipper transcription factor which is known to regulate antioxidant defensive mechanisms) in human astrocytes, stimulating expression of key antioxidant defensive enzymes hemoxygenase (HO-1) and NAD(P)H dehydrogenase quinone1 (Nqo1) [157]. Pre-treatment of astrocytes with antioxidants or a specific calcium chelator BAPTA-AM, significantly blocks the upregulation of Nrf2, HO-1 and Nqo1 [157].

6.3. Accessory Protein Negative Factor

Nef protein has pro-oxidant activity in microglial cells and in neutrophils. It first induces phosphorylation and then translocation of the cytosolic subunit of NADPH oxidase complex p47(phox) into the plasma membrane which in turn induces superoxide anion release from macrophages [158,159]. As a multifunctional HIV-1 protein, Nef also activates the Vav/Rac/p21-activated kinase (PAK) signaling pathway involved in activation of phagocyte NADPH oxidase (thus, Nef indirectly activates NADPH oxidase) [160]. This leads to the dramatic augmentation of the production of ROS [100], and enhancement of cell responses to a variety of stimuli (Ca(2+) ionophore, formyl peptide, endotoxin) [160]. It also leads to decreased tolerance of the cells to hydrogen peroxide, specifically in astrocytes which normally support neuronal function and protects them against cytotoxic substances including ROS [161]. Rac1-dependent NOX2-mediated reactive oxygen species production was shown to contribute to ongoing HIV-1-related vascular dysfunction [162].

6.4. Reverse Transcriptase

We have previously demonstrated that expression of RT by human cells induces production of ROS [163]. Later studies demonstrated that this is a property of different RT variants, including drug resistant variants, and variants retargeted for lysosomal processing and secretion [114,163]. Expression of all RT variants led to an increase in the levels of expression of Phase II detoxifying enzymes HO-1 and Nqo-1. Artificial secretion of RT resulted in a decrease of RT capacity to induce oxidative stress with a decrease in the production of ROS compared to the parental enzyme [114].

6.5. Matrix Protein p17

There is no direct evidence of p17-induced oxidative stress. However, p17 possesses specific structural motifs defined as *"coiled coil"* sequences, and has a high propensity to form multimers, mis-fold and aggregate, forming amyloidogenic assemblies [164,165]. This is typical to amyloidogenic proteins actively involved in the pathogenesis of many human diseases, such as Alzheimer's disease and Parkinson' disease. Amyloidogenic assemblies are toxic, specifically to neural cells. Experiments in the invertebrate nematode *Caenorhabditis elegans* as a "biosensor" demonstrated that p17 significantly inhibits its pharyngeal contractions as do the amyloidogenic proteins [166]. Intrahippocampally injected into mice, p17 induced neurocognitive disorders, comparable in strenght to the effects of other known amyloidogenic proteins [166]. Interestingly, amyloidogenic proteins (typically amyloid-beta peptide Aβ) bound to redox active metal ions, such as copper, catalyse the production of ROS, in particular the most reactive one, hydroxyl radical. This effect may underlie the observed oxidative damage exerted by Aβ peptide on itself and on the surrounding molecules (proteins, lipids, DNA) [167]. One can hypothesize that matrix protein p17 with its amyloidogenic assemblies may trigger the production of ROS through a similar mechanism.

Thus, HIV-1 proteins with known oncogenic/mitogenic potential, Tat, gp120, Nef, RT, and potentially p17, have a potential to directly or indirectly induce oxidative stress, which could be one of the mechanisms by which they induce and potentiate carcinogenesis (Figure 3). Interestingly, HIV-1 proteins with an oncogenic potential involved in the induction of oxidative stress, such as Tat, gp120, Nef, RT, and possibly p17, can be found outside of the cells in which they are expressed.

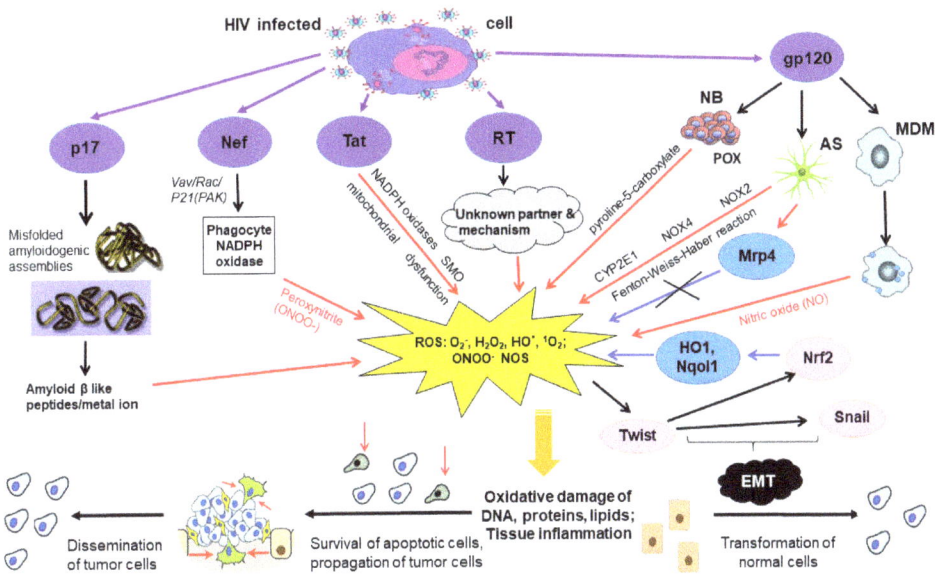

Figure 3. Suggestive mechanism of direct carcinogenic effects of HIV-1 proteins. HIV-1 infected cells express and release gp120, Tat, Nef, p17, RT, each capable of the induction of oxidative stress. (1) p17 may trigger the production of ROS through binding of redox active metal ions by its amyloidogenic assemblies [167]. (2) Nef may indirectly activate NADPH oxidase by activating the Vav/Rac/p21-activated kinase (PAK) signaling pathway involved in phagocytic NADPH oxidase activation and produce peroxynitrite [160]. (3) Tat induces oxidative action through several independent mechanisms via NADPH oxidase, spermine oxidase (SMO) induction and mitochondrial dysfunction [148]. (4) RT induces ROS through unknown mechanisms. There is ROS –dependent activation of the Twist [134], which regulates the expression of Nrf2, which stimulating the expression of antioxidant enzymes (HO1, Nqol1). In addition, the Twist regulates the expression of the Snail. Both transcription factors, Twist and Snail, are involved in epithelial to mesenchymal transduction (EMT). (5) Gp120 increases free radical production from monocyte-derived macrophages (MDM) inducing nitrogen oxide (NO). In astrocytes (AS), it enhances ROS production by several parallel mechanisms: via cytochrome P450 2E1 (CYP2E1), NOX2 and NOX4, and the Fenton-Weiss-Haber reaction. Multidrug resistance proteins (Mrps) involved in cellular defense against oxidative stress. Mrp4 (isoform of Mrp) involved in the regulation of ROS and it acts against ROS [156]. In neuroblastoma cells (NB) gp120 was shown to induce proline oxidase that produces pyroline-5-carboxylate with a concomitant generation of ROS [141]. Production of ROS, which damage of bystander cells inducing oxidative damage of DNA, proteins and lipids, apoptosis and inflammation. DNA damage drives genomic instability and promotes transformation of healthy cells, and propagation and dissemination of malignant cells [168]. Arrows indicate: purple arrows—secretion/entering the intercellular space; black arrows—relationships and interactions; red arrows—production of ROS; blue arrows—oxidative stress response. Text above arrows designates the processes leading to the production of ROS, and text below the arrows, forms of ROS.

7. Oncogenic HIV-1 Proteins Inducing Oxidative Stress Are Found in the Extracellular Space

7.1. Transactivator of Transcription

Tat protein can be produced and released into the extracellular space by cells harboring actively replicating HIV-1 as well as by latently infected cells, with further uptake by the neighboring uninfected cells. Uptake of Tat would result in upregulation of inflammatory genes and cytotoxicity; this scenario was observed in a number of HIV-1 associated comorbidities, specifically, in neurocognitive disorders, cardiovascular impairment and accelerated aging [169]. Dangerously, the process may occur on the background of successful ART, in the absence of active HIV-1 replication and viral production. Considering that approximately 2/3 of all Tat expressed by infected T cells is secreted [170], the activities of Tat described above make a considerable contribution into HIV-1 associated pathologies [171,172].

Soluble Tat, in the absence of the virus, has been shown to cause induction of apoptosis, release of neurotransmitters, oxidative stress and inflammation [169]. Uptake of Tat has been shown to lead to activation of several transcription factors [173,174] including Sp1, NF-κB, and others, resulting in the modulation of expression of both HIV-1 and host genes, including pro-inflammatory cytokines (like TNF-α, CCL2, IL-2, IL-6, and IL-8), adhesion molecules and sometimes, and pro- and anti-apoptotic factors [175–179], p53 and HPV oncoprotein E6 [107].

7.2. Envelope Protein gp120

Envelope protein gp120 is known to be secreted by chronically infected cells [180,181], particularly from the intraepithelial immune cells even in presence of ART [98]. A subset of PLWH demonstrate persistent circulation in plasma of gp120 [182] and in saliva [98]. Moreover, gp120 was found in tissues of PLWH [183]. Brain cells can be directly exposed to gp120 secreted by infiltrated and infected microglia and astrocytes [127]. Gp120 is internalized by bystander cells through receptor-independent mechanisms [184]. Internalization of gp120 leads to the release of several proinflammatory, angiogenic, and lymphangiogenic factors from affected cells [185].

7.3. Accessory Protein Negative Factor

Accessory protein negative factor Nef is found in the serum of PLWH [186,187]. Nef can stimulate its own export via the release of extracellular vesicles (exosomes) from HIV-1 infected cells [188]. Of note, exosomes serve as a marker and confirmation of the systemic oxidative stress [189]. Secreted in exosomes, Nef triggers apoptosis in bystander cells. Extracellular Nef has deleterious effects on CD4+ T cells [188,190]; on bystander B cells by suppressing immunoglobulin class switching [191]; and on astrocytes [192] and endothelial cells [162].

7.4. Reverse Transcriptase (RT)

In our lab, we have shown secretion of RT into cell culture fluids of cells transiently expressing RT [114]. Recently, RT was also detected in the exosomes detected in the uterine of PLWH [193].

7.5. Matrix Protein p17

Matrix protein p17 is continuously released into the extracellular space from HIV-1-infected cells, and can be detected in the plasma of PLWH and in different organs and tissue specimens [138]. Cellular aspartyl proteases promote the unconventional secretion of biologically active p17 [194]. HIV-1 secretion of biologically active p17 takes place at the plasma membrane and occurs following its interaction with phosphatidylinositol-(4,5)-bisphosphate and its subsequent cleavage from precursor Gag (Pr55Gag) by cellular aspartyl proteases [194]. Extracellularly, p17 deregulates the function of different cells involved in AIDS pathogenesis. Importantly, p17 accumulates and persists in different organs and tissues of PLWH on ART, even in the absence of any replicative activity [136,195,196]. These findings strongly suggest that p17 may be chronically present in HIV-1-I infected cells and tissues, even under ART-associated suppression of HIV-1 replication.

Thus, gp120 and Tat are actively secreted into the endothelial cell micro-environment, Nef can be neighboring uninfected cells including cells which cannot be infected with HIV-1, modulating their metabolism, cell cycle progression, ability to differentiate, motility, and, importantly, the genomic stability, through induction of ROS. Some HIV-1 proteins such as matrix p17 and gp120 can accumulate and persist in lymphoid tissues for at least 1 year after the on-start of ART on the background of successful suppression of viral replication [196]. These proteins are involved in different processes associated with malignant transformation and tumor growth with significant direct and indirect adverse effects on the epithelial cells.

These include a range of responses that contribute to endothelial dysfunction, including enhanced adhesiveness, permeability, cell proliferation, apoptosis, as well as activation of cytokine secretion [86], eventually leading to malignant transformation (Figure 3). In this respect, their effect would resemble oncogenesis mediated by known viral oncoproteins originating from EBV, HTLV-1, KSHV, HCV, HBV, HPV, and identified as causative agents of both AIDS-defining and non-AIDS defining forms of cancer.

8. Conclusions

People living with human immunodeficiency virus receiving antiretroviral therapy are characterized by high prevalence of different forms of cancer affecting epithelial cells. HIV-1 does not infect epithelial cells, however both HIV virions and proteins were shown to be sequestered into epithelial cells and affect their functions. These proteins have three specific properties:

- First, HIV proteins Tat, Nef, gp120, matrix protein p17, reverse transcriptase/RT induce oxidative stress with serious consequences in the form of DNA, protein and lipid damage, as well as changes in the intracellular signaling.
- Second, Tat, Nef, gp120, matrix protein p17, RT have a direct carcinogenic potential as demonstrated in the series of in vitro experiments and experiments in the laboratory animals.
- Third, Tat, Nef, gp120, matrix protein p17, reverse transcriptase/RT were shown to exit HIV expressing cells by different mechanisms, and, once present in the extracellular space, can be up-taken by innocent neighbor cells.

Sequestered/internalized by innocent bystander cells, these proteins modulate their metabolism, cell cycle progression, ability to differentiate, motility, redox balance (induce ROS) and genomic stability. Through this, they can trigger malignant transformation of normal cells. Another outcome is propagation (proliferation and dissemination) of already existing precancerous and cancer cells, and enhanced growth and metastatic activity of tumors expressing or exposed to HIV-1 proteins.

Altogether, we present a new mechanism of HIV-associated malignant transformation of epithelial cells driven by individual HIV proteins through the induction of reactive oxygen species. In this scenario, HIV-1 proteins act in a manner similar to the known viral oncogenes, and can cooperate with them promoting KSHV, EBV, HBV, HCV, and HPV-associated carcinogenesis. Such pathway of HIV associated carcinogenesis can co-occur together with carcinogenesis driven by persistent immune inflammation, and dysfunction of B cells, T cells and cellular components of the innate immune system.

Funding: This study was supported the Russian Fund for Basic Research grants 17_54_30002 and 20-04-01034 to M.I., Latvian Science Council grants LZP-2018/2-0308 and LZP-2020/2-0376 to M.I., and NCI R01CA 217715 to J.P. The work of Francesca Chiodi is supported by a grant from the Swedish Medical Research Council (Francesca Chiodi; Vetenskapsrådet 2019-01169).

Conflicts of Interest: The authors declare no conflict of interest.

References

1. Shiels, M.S.; Engels, E.A. Evolving epidemiology of HIV-associated malignancies. *Curr. Opin. HIV AIDS* **2017**, *12*, 6–11. [CrossRef] [PubMed]
2. Borrow, P. Innate immunity in acute HIV-1 infection. *Curr. Opin. HIV AIDS* **2011**, *6*, 353–363. [CrossRef] [PubMed]
3. Jenabian, M.A.; El-Far, M.; Vyboh, K.; Kema, I.; Costiniuk, C.T.; Thomas, R.; Baril, J.G.; LeBlanc, R.; Kanagaratham, C.; Radzioch, D.; et al. Immunosuppressive Tryptophan Catabolism and Gut Mucosal Dysfunction Following Early HIV Infection. *J. Infect. Dis.* **2015**, *212*, 355–366. [CrossRef] [PubMed]
4. Boasso, A.; Shearer, G.M.; Chougnet, C. Immune dysregulation in human immunodeficiency virus infection: Know it, fix it, prevent it? *J. Intern. Med.* **2009**, *265*, 78–96. [CrossRef]
5. Titanji, K.; Chiodi, F.; Bellocco, R.; Schepis, D.; Osorio, L.; Tassandin, C.; Tambussi, G.; Grutzmeier, S.; Lopalco, L.; De Milito, A. Primary HIV-1 infection sets the stage for important B lymphocyte dysfunctions. *AIDS* **2005**, *19*, 1947–1955. [CrossRef]

6. De Milito, A.; Nilsson, A.; Titanji, K.; Thorstensson, R.; Reizenstein, E.; Narita, M.; Grutzmeier, S.; Sonnerborg, A.; Chiodi, F. Mechanisms of hypergammaglobulinemia and impaired antigen-specific humoral immunity in HIV-1 infection. *Blood* **2004**, *103*, 2180–2186. [CrossRef]
7. Amu, S.; Lantto Graham, R.; Bekele, Y.; Nasi, A.; Bengtsson, C.; Rethi, B.; Sorial, S.; Meini, G.; Zazzi, M.; Hejdeman, B.; et al. Dysfunctional phenotypes of CD4 + and CD8 + T cells are comparable in patients initiating ART during early or chronic HIV-1 infection. *Medicine* **2016**, *95*, e3738. [CrossRef]
8. Lemma, M.; Petkov, S.; Bekele, Y.; Petros, B.; Howe, R.; Chiodi, F. Profiling of Inflammatory Proteins in Plasma of HIV-1-Infected Children Receiving Antiretroviral Therapy. *Proteomes* **2020**, *8*, 24. [CrossRef]
9. Yang, X.; Su, B.; Zhang, X.; Liu, Y.; Wu, H.; Zhang, T. Incomplete immune reconstitution in HIV/AIDS patients on antiretroviral therapy: Challenges of immunological non-responders. *J. Leukoc. Biol.* **2020**, *107*, 597–612. [CrossRef]
10. Zicari, S.; Sessa, L.; Cotugno, N.; Ruggiero, A.; Morrocchi, E.; Concato, C.; Rocca, S.; Zangari, P.; Manno, E.C.; Palma, P. Immune Activation, Inflammation, and Non-AIDS Co-Morbidities in HIV-Infected Patients under Long-Term ART. *Viruses* **2019**, *11*, 200. [CrossRef]
11. Nabatanzi, R.; Cose, S.; Joloba, M.; Jones, S.R.; Nakanjako, D. Effects of HIV infection and ART on phenotype and function of circulating monocytes, natural killer, and innate lymphoid cells. *AIDS Res. Ther.* **2018**, *15*, 7. [CrossRef] [PubMed]
12. Amu, S.; Ruffin, N.; Rethi, B.; Chiodi, F. Impairment of B-cell functions during HIV-1 infection. *AIDS* **2013**, *27*, 2323–2334. [CrossRef] [PubMed]
13. Silverberg, M.J.; Lau, B.; Achenbach, C.J.; Jing, Y.; Althoff, K.N.; D'Souza, G.; Engels, E.A.; Hessol, N.A.; Brooks, J.T.; Burchell, A.N. Cumulative incidence of cancer among persons with HIV in North America: A cohort study. *Ann. Intern. Med.* **2015**, *163*, 507–518. [CrossRef] [PubMed]
14. Symons, J.; Chopra, A.; Malatinkova, E.; De Spiegelaere, W.; Leary, S.; Cooper, D.; Abana, C.O.; Rhodes, A.; Rezaei, S.D.; Vandekerckhove, L.; et al. HIV integration sites in latently infected cell lines: Evidence of ongoing replication. *Retrovirology* **2017**, *14*, 1–11. [CrossRef] [PubMed]
15. Schawkat, K.; Reiner, C.S. Diffuse liver disease: Cirrhosis, focal lesions in cirrhosis, and vascular liver disease. *IDKD Springer Ser.* **2018**, 229–236.
16. Pinato, D.J.; Allara, E.; Chen, T.Y.; Trevisani, F.; Minguez, B.; Zoli, M.; Harris, M.; Dalla Pria, A.; Merchante, N.; Platt, H.; et al. Influence of HIV Infection on the Natural History of Hepatocellular Carcinoma: Results From a Global Multicohort Study. *J. Clin. Oncol.* **2019**, *37*, 296–304. [CrossRef]
17. Clifford, G.M.; Rickenbach, M.; Polesel, J.; Dal Maso, L.; Steffen, I.; Ledergerber, B.; Rauch, A.; Probst-Hensch, N.M.; Bouchardy, C.; Levi, F. Influence of HIV-related immunodeficiency on the risk of hepatocellular carcinoma. *AIDS* **2008**, *22*, 2135–2141. [CrossRef]
18. Pinato, D.J.; Dalla Pria, A.; Sharma, R.; Bower, M. Hepatocellular carcinoma: An evolving challenge in viral hepatitis and HIV coinfection. *AIDS* **2017**, *31*, 603–611. [CrossRef]
19. Gjærde, L.I.; Shepherd, L.; Jablonowska, E.; Lazzarin, A.; Rougemont, M.; Darling, K.; Battegay, M.; Braun, D.; Martel-Laferriere, V.; Lundgren, J.D. Trends in Incidences and Risk Factors for Hepatocellular Carcinoma and Other Liver Events in HIV and Hepatitis C Virus–coinfected Individuals From 2001 to 2014: A Multicohort Study. *Clin. Infect. Dis.* **2016**, *63*, 821–829. [CrossRef]
20. Joshi, D.; O'Grady, J.; Dieterich, D.; Gazzard, B.; Agarwal, K. Increasing burden of liver disease in patients with HIV infection. *Lancet* **2011**, *377*, 1198–1209. [CrossRef]
21. Brenchley, J.M.; Price, D.A.; Schacker, T.W.; Asher, T.E.; Silvestri, G.; Rao, S.; Kazzaz, Z.; Bornstein, E.; Lambotte, O.; Altmann, D.; et al. Microbial translocation is a cause of systemic immune activation in chronic HIV infection. *Nat. Med.* **2006**, *12*, 1365–1371. [CrossRef] [PubMed]
22. Marchetti, G.; Tincati, C.; Silvestri, G. Microbial translocation in the pathogenesis of HIV infection and AIDS. *Clin. Microbiol. Rev.* **2013**, *26*, 2–18. [CrossRef] [PubMed]
23. Soares, J.B.; Pimentel-Nunes, P.; Roncon-Albuquerque, R.; Leite-Moreira, A. The role of lipopolysaccharide/toll-like receptor 4 signaling in chronic liver diseases. *Hepatol. Int.* **2010**, *4*, 659–672. [CrossRef] [PubMed]
24. Ramendra, R.; Isnard, S.; Mehraj, V.; Chen, J.; Zhang, Y.; Finkelman, M.; Routy, J.P. Circulating LPS and (1–>3)-beta-D-Glucan: A Folie a Deux Contributing to HIV-Associated Immune Activation. *Front. Immunol.* **2019**, *10*, 465. [CrossRef] [PubMed]
25. Kovari, H.; Ledergerber, B.; Battegay, M.; Rauch, B.; Hirschel, B.; Foguena, A.K.; Vernazza, P.; Bernasconi, E.; Mueller, N.J.; Weber, R. Incidence and risk factors for chronic elevation of alanine aminotransferase levels in HIV-infected persons without hepatitis b or c virus co-infection. *Clin. Infect. Dis.* **2010**, *50*, 502–511. [CrossRef] [PubMed]
26. Crane, M.; Visvanathan, K.; Lewin, S.R. HIV Infection and TLR Signalling in the Liver. *Gastroenterol. Res. Pr.* **2012**, *2012*, 473925. [CrossRef] [PubMed]
27. Iser, D.M.; Warner, N.; Revill, P.A.; Solomon, A.; Wightman, F.; Saleh, S.; Crane, M.; Cameron, P.U.; Bowden, S.; Nguyen, T.; et al. Coinfection of hepatic cell lines with human immunodeficiency virus and hepatitis B virus leads to an increase in intracellular hepatitis B surface antigen. *J. Virol.* **2010**, *84*, 5860–5867. [CrossRef]
28. Ganesan, M.; Poluektova, L.Y.; Kharbanda, K.K.; Osna, N.A. Liver as a target of human immunodeficiency virus infection. *World J. Gastroenterol.* **2018**, *24*, 4728–4737. [CrossRef]
29. Kandathil, A.; Durand, C.; Quinn, J.; Cameron, A.; Thomas, D.; Balagopal, A. Liver macrophages and HIV-1 persistence. In Proceedings of the CROI, Seattle, WA, USA, 23–26 February 2015.

30. Chew, K.W.; Bhattacharya, D. Virologic and immunologic aspects of HIV-hepatitis C virus coinfection. *AIDS* **2016**, *30*, 2395–2404. [CrossRef]
31. Lin, W.; Weinberg, E.M.; Chung, R.T. Pathogenesis of accelerated fibrosis in HIV/HCV co-infection. *J. Infect. Dis.* **2013**, *207*, S13–S18. [CrossRef]
32. Hong, F.; Saiman, Y.; Si, C.; Mosoian, A.; Bansal, M.B. X4 Human immunodeficiency virus type 1 gp120 promotes human hepatic stellate cell activation and collagen I expression through interactions with CXCR4. *PLoS ONE* **2012**, *7*, e33659. [CrossRef] [PubMed]
33. Mosoian, A.; Zhang, L.; Hong, F.; Cunyat, F.; Rahman, A.; Bhalla, R.; Panchal, A.; Saiman, Y.; Fiel, M.I.; Florman, S.; et al. Frontline Science: HIV infection of Kupffer cells results in an amplified proinflammatory response to LPS. *J. Leukoc. Biol.* **2017**, *101*, 1083–1090. [CrossRef] [PubMed]
34. Tuyama, A.C.; Hong, F.; Saiman, Y.; Wang, C.; Ozkok, D.; Mosoian, A.; Chen, P.; Chen, B.K.; Klotman, M.E.; Bansal, M.B. Human immunodeficiency virus (HIV)-1 infects human hepatic stellate cells and promotes collagen I and monocyte chemoattractant protein-1 expression: Implications for the pathogenesis of HIV/hepatitis C virus–induced liver fibrosis. *Hepatology* **2010**, *52*, 612–622. [CrossRef] [PubMed]
35. Lin, W.; Wu, G.; Li, S.; Weinberg, E.M.; Kumthip, K.; Peng, L.F.; Mendez-Navarro, J.; Chen, W.C.; Jilg, N.; Zhao, H.; et al. HIV and HCV cooperatively promote hepatic fibrogenesis via induction of reactive oxygen species and NFkappaB. *J. Biol. Chem.* **2011**, *286*, 2665–2674. [CrossRef] [PubMed]
36. Herrera, S.; Martinez-Sanz, J.; Serrano-Villar, S. HIV, Cancer, and the Microbiota: Common Pathways Influencing Different Diseases. *Front. Immunol.* **2019**, *10*, 1466. [CrossRef]
37. Koziel, M.J.; Peters, M.G. Viral hepatitis in HIV infection. *N. Engl. J. Med.* **2007**, *356*, 1445–1454. [CrossRef]
38. Sun, H.Y.; Sheng, W.H.; Tsai, M.S.; Lee, K.Y.; Chang, S.Y.; Hung, C.C. Hepatitis B virus coinfection in human immunodeficiency virus-infected patients: A review. *World J. Gastroenterol.* **2014**, *20*, 14598–14614. [CrossRef]
39. Garcia-Samaniego, J.; Rodriguez, M.; Berenguer, J.; Rodriguez-Rosado, R.; Carbo, J.; Asensi, V.; Soriano, V. Hepatocellular carcinoma in HIV-infected patients with chronic hepatitis C. *Am. J. Gastroenterol.* **2001**, *96*, 179–183. [CrossRef]
40. Nabih, H.K. The Significance of HCV Viral Load in the Incidence of HCC: A Correlation Between Mir-122 and CCL2. *J. Gastrointest. Cancer* **2020**, *51*, 412–417. [CrossRef]
41. Lemon, S.M.; McGivern, D.R. Is hepatitis C virus carcinogenic? *Gastroenterology* **2012**, *142*, 1274–1278. [CrossRef]
42. Ivanov, A.V.; Valuev-Elliston, V.T.; Tyurina, D.A.; Ivanova, O.N.; Kochetkov, S.N.; Bartosch, B.; Isaguliants, M.G. Oxidative stress, a trigger of hepatitis C and B virus-induced liver carcinogenesis. *Oncotarget* **2017**, *8*, 3895. [CrossRef] [PubMed]
43. Hall, J.; Short, S. Management of glioblastoma multiforme in HIV patients: A case series and review of published studies. *Clin. Oncol.* **2009**, *21*, 591–597. [CrossRef] [PubMed]
44. Del Valle, L.; Piña-Oviedo, S. HIV disorders of the brain: Pathology and pathogenesis. *Front. Biosci.* **2006**, *11*, 718–732. [CrossRef] [PubMed]
45. Cedeno-Laurent, F.; Trujillo, J.R. Gliomas and brain lymphomas in HIV-1/AIDS patients: Reflections from a 20-year follow up in Mexico and Brazil. *Microbiol. Res.* **2011**, *2*, 11. [CrossRef]
46. Patel, A.P.; Fisher, J.L.; Nichols, E.; Abd-Allah, F.; Abdela, J.; Abdelalim, A.; Abraha, H.N.; Agius, D.; Alahdab, F.; Alam, T. Global, regional, and national burden of brain and other CNS cancer, 1990–2016: A systematic analysis for the Global Burden of Disease Study 2016. *Lancet Neurol.* **2019**, *18*, 376–393. [CrossRef]
47. Choy, W.; Lagman, C.; Lee, S.J.; Bui, T.T.; Safaee, M.; Yang, I. Impact of human immunodeficiency virus in the pathogenesis and outcome of patients with glioblastoma multiforme. *Brain Tumor Res. Treat.* **2016**, *4*, 77–86. [CrossRef]
48. Acevedo, N.; Pillai, C.; Welch, M. HCP-01diagnosis and management of high-grade glioma in patients with HIV. *Neuro Oncol.* **2015**, *17*, v101. [CrossRef]
49. Tacconi, L.; Stapleton, S.; Signorelli, F.; Thomas, D. Acquired immune deficiency syndrome (AIDS) and cerebral astrocytoma. *Clin. Neurol. Neurosurg.* **1996**, *98*, 149–151. [CrossRef]
50. Chamberlain, M.C. Gliomas in patients with acquired immune deficiency syndrome. *Cancer* **1994**, *74*, 1912–1914. [CrossRef]
51. Wolff, R.; Zimmermann, M.; Marquardt, G.; Lanfermann, H.; Nafe, R.; Seifert, V. Glioblastoma multiforme of the brain stem in a patient with aquired immunodeficiency syndrome. *Acta Neurochir.* **2002**, *144*, 941–945. [CrossRef]
52. Chiodi, F.; Fuerstenberg, S.; Gidlund, M.; Asjo, B.; Fenyo, E.M. Infection of brain-derived cells with the human immunodeficiency virus. *J. Virol.* **1987**, *61*, 1244–1247. [CrossRef] [PubMed]
53. Messam, C.A.; Major, E.O. Stages of restricted HIV-1 infection in astrocyte cultures derived from human fetal brain tissue. *J. Neurovirol.* **2000**, *6*, S90–S94. [PubMed]
54. Robbins, H.A.; Shiels, M.S.; Pfeiffer, R.M.; Engels, E.A. Epidemiologic contributions to recent cancer trends among HIV-infected people in the United States. *AIDS* **2014**, *28*, 881–890. [CrossRef]
55. Palefsky, J.M. HPV-associated anal and cervical cancers in HIV-infected individuals: Incidence and prevention in the antiretroviral therapy era. *Curr. Opin. HIV AIDS* **2017**, *12*, 26. [CrossRef] [PubMed]
56. Osazuwa-Peters, N.; Massa, S.T.; Simpson, M.C.; Adjei Boakye, E.; Varvares, M.A. Survival of human papillomavirus-associated cancers: Filling in the gaps. *Cancer* **2018**, *124*, 18–20. [CrossRef]

57. Strickler, H.D.; Burk, R.D.; Fazzari, M.; Anastos, K.; Minkoff, H.; Massad, L.S.; Hall, C.; Bacon, M.; Levine, A.M.; Watts, D.H. Natural history and possible reactivation of human papillomavirus in human immunodeficiency virus–positive women. *J. Natl. Cancer Inst.* **2005**, *97*, 577–586. [CrossRef]
58. Clarke, B.; Chetty, R. Postmodern cancer: The role of human immunodeficiency virus in uterine cervical cancer. *Mol. Pathol.* **2002**, *55*, 19–24. [CrossRef] [PubMed]
59. Palefsky, J. Biology of HPV in HIV infection. *Adv. Dent. Res.* **2006**, *19*, 99–105. [CrossRef]
60. Palefsky, J.M.; Holly, E.A. Chapter 6: Immunosuppression and co-infection with HIV. *J. Natl. Cancer Inst. Monogr.* **2003**, *2003*, 41–46. [CrossRef]
61. Chambuso, R.; Gray, C.M.; Kaambo, E.; Rebello, G.; Ramesar, R. Impact of Host Molecular Genetic Variations and HIV/HPV Co-infection on Cervical Cancer Progression: A Systematic review. *Oncomedicine* **2018**, *3*, 82–93. [CrossRef]
62. Joag, S.V.; Adany, I.; Li, Z.; Foresman, L.; Pinson, D.M.; Wang, C.; Stephens, E.B.; Raghavan, R.; Narayan, O. Animal model of mucosally transmitted human immunodeficiency virus type 1 disease: Intravaginal and oral deposition of simian/human immunodeficiency virus in macaques results in systemic infection, elimination of CD4+ T cells, and AIDS. *J. Virol.* **1997**, *71*, 4016–4023. [CrossRef] [PubMed]
63. Bosch, M.L.; Schmidt, A.; Agy, M.B.; Kimball, L.E.; Morton, W.R. Infection of Macaca nemestrina neonates with HIV-1 via different routes of inoculation. *AIDS* **1997**, *11*, 1555–1563. [CrossRef] [PubMed]
64. Carias, A.M.; McCoombe, S.; McRaven, M.; Anderson, M.; Galloway, N.; Vandergrift, N.; Fought, A.J.; Lurain, J.; Duplantis, M.; Veazey, R.S. Defining the interaction of HIV-1 with the mucosal barriers of the female reproductive tract. *J. Virol.* **2013**, *87*, 11388–11400. [CrossRef] [PubMed]
65. Girard, M.; Mahoney, J.; Wei, Q.; Van Der Ryst, E.; Muchmore, E.; Barré-Sinoussi, F.; Fultz, P.N. Genital infection of female chimpanzees with human immunodeficiency virus type 1. *AIDS Res. Hum. Retrovir.* **1998**, *14*, 1357–1367. [CrossRef]
66. Dinh, M.H.; Anderson, M.R.; McRaven, M.D.; Cianci, G.C.; McCoombe, S.G.; Kelley, Z.L.; Gioia, C.J.; Fought, A.J.; Rademaker, A.W.; Veazey, R.S.; et al. Visualization of HIV-1 interactions with penile and foreskin epithelia: Clues for female-to-male HIV transmission. *PLoS Pathog.* **2015**, *11*, e1004729. [CrossRef] [PubMed]
67. Ganor, Y.; Zhou, Z.; Tudor, D.; Schmitt, A.; Vacher-Lavenu, M.C.; Gibault, L.; Thiounn, N.; Tomasini, J.; Wolf, J.P.; Bomsel, M. Within 1 h, HIV-1 uses viral synapses to enter efficiently the inner, but not outer, foreskin mucosa and engages Langerhans-T cell conjugates. *Mucosal Immunol.* **2010**, *3*, 506–522. [CrossRef]
68. Hladik, F.; Sakchalathorn, P.; Ballweber, L.; Lentz, G.; Fialkow, M.; Eschenbach, D.; McElrath, M.J. Initial events in establishing vaginal entry and infection by human immunodeficiency virus type-1. *Immunity* **2007**, *26*, 257–270. [CrossRef]
69. Maher, D.; Wu, X.; Schacker, T.; Horbul, J.; Southern, P. HIV binding, penetration, and primary infection in human cervicovaginal tissue. *Proc. Natl. Acad. Sci. USA* **2005**, *102*, 11504–11509. [CrossRef]
70. Stoddard, E.; Ni, H.; Cannon, G.; Zhou, C.; Kallenbach, N.; Malamud, D.; Weissman, D. gp340 promotes transcytosis of human immunodeficiency virus type 1 in genital tract-derived cell lines and primary endocervical tissue. *J. Virol.* **2009**, *83*, 8596–8603. [CrossRef]
71. Zhou, Z.; De Longchamps, N.B.; Schmitt, A.; Zerbib, M.; Vacher-Lavenu, M.-C.; Bomsel, M.; Ganor, Y. HIV-1 efficient entry in inner foreskin is mediated by elevated CCL5/RANTES that recruits T cells and fuels conjugate formation with Langerhans cells. *PLoS Pathog.* **2011**, *7*, e1002100. [CrossRef]
72. Liu, R.; Huang, L.; Li, J.; Zhou, X.; Zhang, H.; Zhang, T.; Lei, Y.; Wang, K.; Xie, N.; Zheng, Y.; et al. HIV Infection in gastric epithelial cells. *J. Infect. Dis.* **2013**, *208*, 1221–1230. [CrossRef] [PubMed]
73. Dorosko, S.M.; Connor, R.I. Primary human mammary epithelial cells endocytose HIV-1 and facilitate viral infection of CD4+ T lymphocytes. *J. Virol.* **2010**, *84*, 10533–10542. [CrossRef] [PubMed]
74. Hughes, K.; Akturk, G.; Gnjatic, S.; Chen, B.; Klotman, M.; Blasi, M. Proliferation of HIV-infected renal epithelial cells following virus acquisition from infected macrophages. *AIDS* **2020**, *34*, 1581–1591. [CrossRef] [PubMed]
75. Brune, K.A.; Ferreira, F.; Mandke, P.; Chau, E.; Aggarwal, N.R.; D'Alessio, F.R.; Lambert, A.A.; Kirk, G.; Blankson, J.; Drummond, M.B.; et al. HIV Impairs Lung Epithelial Integrity and Enters the Epithelium to Promote Chronic Lung Inflammation. *PLoS ONE* **2016**, *11*, e0149679. [CrossRef]
76. Wagner, T.A.; McLaughlin, S.; Garg, K.; Cheung, C.Y.; Larsen, B.B.; Styrchak, S.; Huang, H.C.; Edlefsen, P.T.; Mullins, J.I.; Frenkel, L.M. HIV latency. Proliferation of cells with HIV integrated into cancer genes contributes to persistent infection. *Science* **2014**, *345*, 570–573. [CrossRef]
77. Fan, H.; Johnson, C. Insertional oncogenesis by non-acute retroviruses: Implications for gene therapy. *Viruses* **2011**, *3*, 398–422. [CrossRef]
78. Maldarelli, F. The role of HIV integration in viral persistence: No more whistling past the proviral graveyard. *J. Clin. Investig.* **2016**, *126*, 438–447. [CrossRef]
79. Asin, S.N.; Wildt-Perinic, D.; Mason, S.I.; Howell, A.L.; Wira, C.R.; Fanger, M.W. Human immunodeficiency virus type 1 infection of human uterine epithelial cells: Viral shedding and cell contact-mediated infectivity. *J. Infect. Dis.* **2003**, *187*, 1522–1533. [CrossRef]
80. Aiken, C. Pseudotyping human immunodeficiency virus type 1 (HIV-1) by the glycoprotein of vesicular stomatitis virus targets HIV-1 entry to an endocytic pathway and suppresses both the requirement for Nef and the sensitivity to cyclosporin A. *J. Virol.* **1997**, *71*, 5871–5877. [CrossRef]

81. King, B.; Daly, J. Pseudotypes: Your flexible friends. *Futur. Microbiol.* **2014**, *9*, 135–137. [CrossRef]
82. Tang, Y.; George, A.; Nouvet, F.; Sweet, S.; Emeagwali, N.; Taylor, H.E.; Simmons, G.; Hildreth, J.E. Infection of female primary lower genital tract epithelial cells after natural pseudotyping of HIV-1: Possible implications for sexual transmission of HIV-1. *PLoS ONE* **2014**, *9*, e101367. [CrossRef]
83. Tang, Y.; Woodward, B.O.; Pastor, L.; George, A.M.; Petrechko, O.; Nouvet, F.J.; Haas, D.W.; Jiang, G.; Hildreth, J.E.K. Endogenous Retroviral Envelope Syncytin Induces HIV-1 Spreading and Establishes HIV Reservoirs in Placenta. *Cell Rep.* **2020**, *30*, 4528–4539. [CrossRef] [PubMed]
84. Grandi, N.; Tramontano, E. Type W Human Endogenous Retrovirus (HERV-W) Integrations and Their Mobilization by L1 Machinery: Contribution to the Human Transcriptome and Impact on the Host Physiopathology. *Viruses* **2017**, *9*, 162. [CrossRef] [PubMed]
85. Devadoss, D.; Singh, S.P.; Acharya, A.; Do, K.C.; Periyasamy, P.; Manevski, M.; Mishra, N.; Tellez, C.; Ramakrishnan, S.; Belinsky, S. Lung Bronchial Epithelial Cells are HIV Targets for Proviral Genomic Integration. *bioRxiv* **2020**. [CrossRef]
86. Anand, A.R.; Rachel, G.; Parthasarathy, D. HIV Proteins and Endothelial Dysfunction: Implications in Cardiovascular Disease. *Front. Cardiovasc. Med.* **2018**, *5*, 185. [CrossRef]
87. De Paoli, P.; Carbone, A. Microenvironmental abnormalities induced by viral cooperation: Impact on lymphomagenesis. *Semin. Cancer Biol.* **2015**, *34*, 70–80. [CrossRef]
88. Mazzuca, P.; Caruso, A.; Caccuri, F. Endothelial Cell Dysfunction in HIV-1 Infection. *Endothel. Dysfunct. Old Concepts New Chall.* **2018**, 347. [CrossRef]
89. Liapis, K.; Clear, A.; Owen, A.; Coutinho, R.; Greaves, P.; Lee, A.M.; Montoto, S.; Calaminici, M.; Gribben, J.G. The microenvironment of AIDS-related diffuse large B-cell lymphoma provides insight into the pathophysiology and indicates possible therapeutic strategies. *Blood* **2013**, *122*, 424–433. [CrossRef]
90. Taylor, J.G.; Liapis, K.; Gribben, J.G. The role of the tumor microenvironment in HIV-associated lymphomas. *Biomark. Med.* **2015**, *9*, 473–482. [CrossRef]
91. Liu, Y.; Gaisa, M.M.; Wang, X.; Swartz, T.H.; Arens, Y.; Dresser, K.A.; Sigel, C.; Sigel, K. Differences in the Immune Microenvironment of Anal Cancer Precursors by HIV Status and Association With Ablation Outcomes. *J. Infect. Dis.* **2018**, *217*, 703–709. [CrossRef]
92. Paiardini, M.; Frank, I.; Pandrea, I.; Apetrei, C.; Silvestri, G. Mucosal immune dysfunction in AIDS pathogenesis. *AIDS Rev.* **2008**, *10*, 36–46. [PubMed]
93. Yaghoobi, M.; Le Gouvello, S.; Aloulou, N.; Duprez-Dutreuil, C.; Walker, F.; Sobhani, I. FoxP3 overexpression and CD1a+ and CD3 + depletion in anal tissue as possible mechanisms for increased risk of human papillomavirus-related anal carcinoma in HIV infection. *Color. Dis.* **2011**, *13*, 768–773. [CrossRef] [PubMed]
94. Guimaraes, A.G.; da Costa, A.G.; Martins-Filho, O.A.; Pimentel, J.P.; Zauli, D.A.; Peruhype-Magalhaes, V.; Teixeira-Carvalho, A.; Bela, S.R.; Xavier, M.A.; Coelho-Dos-Reis, J.G.; et al. CD11c + CD123Low dendritic cell subset and the triad TNF-alpha/IL-17A/IFN-gamma integrate mucosal and peripheral cellular responses in HIV patients with high-grade anal intraepithelial neoplasia: A systems biology approach. *JAIDS J. Acquir. Immune Defic. Syndr.* **2015**, *68*, 112–122. [CrossRef] [PubMed]
95. Micsenyi, A.M.; Zony, C.; Alvarez, R.A.; Durham, N.D.; Chen, B.K.; Klotman, M.E. Postintegration HIV-1 infection of cervical epithelial cells mediates contact-dependent productive infection of T cells. *J. Infect. Dis.* **2013**, *208*, 1756–1767. [CrossRef] [PubMed]
96. Yasen, A.; Herrera, R.; Rosbe, K.; Lien, K.; Tugizov, S.M. HIV internalization into oral and genital epithelial cells by endocytosis and macropinocytosis leads to viral sequestration in the vesicles. *Virology* **2018**, *515*, 92–107. [CrossRef]
97. Tugizov, S.M. Human immunodeficiency virus interaction with oral and genital mucosal epithelia may lead to epithelial-mesenchymal transition and sequestration of virions in the endosomal compartments. *Oral Dis.* **2020**, *26*, 40–46. [CrossRef] [PubMed]
98. Tugizov, S.M.; Herrera, R.; Chin-Hong, P.; Veluppillai, P.; Greenspan, D.; Michael Berry, J.; Pilcher, C.D.; Shiboski, C.H.; Jay, N.; Rubin, M.; et al. HIV-associated disruption of mucosal epithelium facilitates paracellular penetration by human papillomavirus. *Virology* **2013**, *446*, 378–388. [CrossRef] [PubMed]
99. Parvez, M.K. HBV and HIV co-infection: Impact on liver pathobiology and therapeutic approaches. *World J. Hepatol.* **2015**, *7*, 121–126. [CrossRef] [PubMed]
100. Park, I.W.; Fan, Y.; Luo, X.; Ryou, M.G.; Liu, J.; Green, L.; He, J.J. HIV-1 Nef is transferred from expressing T cells to hepatocytic cells through conduits and enhances HCV replication. *PLoS ONE* **2014**, *9*, e99545. [CrossRef] [PubMed]
101. Luedde, T.; Schwabe, R.F. NF-kappaB in the liver—Linking injury, fibrosis and hepatocellular carcinoma. *Nat. Rev. Gastroenterol. Hepatol.* **2011**, *8*, 108–118. [CrossRef] [PubMed]
102. McGivern, D.R.; Lemon, S.M. Tumor suppressors, chromosomal instability, and hepatitis C virus–associated liver cancer. *Annu. Rev. Pathol. Mech. Dis.* **2009**, *4*, 399–415. [CrossRef] [PubMed]
103. Tugizov, S.M.; Herrera, R.; Veluppillai, P.; Greenspan, D.; Palefsky, J.M. 46. HIV-induced epithelial–mesenchymal transition in mucosal epithelium facilitates HPV paracellular penetration. *Sex. Health* **2013**, *10*, 592. [CrossRef]
104. Tornesello, M.L.; Buonaguro, F.M.; Beth-Giraldo, E.; Giraldo, G. Human immunodeficiency virus type 1 tat gene enhances human papillomavirus early gene expression. *Intervirology* **1993**, *36*, 57–64. [CrossRef]

105. Buonaguro, F.M.; Tornesello, M.L.; Buonaguro, L.; Del Gaudio, E.; Beth-Giraldo, E.; Giraldo, G. Role of HIV as Cofactor in HPV Oncogenesis: In Vitro Evidences of Virus Interactions. In *Advanced Technologies in Research, Diagnosis and Treatment of AIDS and in Oncology*; Karger Publishers: Basel, Switzerland, 1994; Volume 46, pp. 102–109.
106. Kim, R.H.; Yochim, J.M.; Kang, M.K.; Shin, K.-H.; Christensen, R.; Park, N.-H. HIV-1 Tat enhances replicative potential of human oral keratinocytes harboring HPV-16 genome. *Int. J. Oncol.* **1992**, *33*, 777–782. [CrossRef]
107. Barillari, G.; Palladino, C.; Bacigalupo, I.; Leone, P.; Falchi, M.; Ensoli, B. Entrance of the Tat protein of HIV-1 into human uterine cervical carcinoma cells causes upregulation of HPV-E6 expression and a decrease in p53 protein levels. *Oncol. Lett.* **2016**, *12*, 2389–2394. [CrossRef]
108. Vernon, S.D.; Hart, C.E.; Reeves, W.C.; Icenogle, J.P. The HIV-1 tat protein enhances E2-dependent human papillomavirus 16 transcription. *Virus Res.* **1993**, *27*, 133–145. [CrossRef]
109. Barillari, G.; Ensoli, B. Angiogenic effects of extracellular human immunodeficiency virus type 1 Tat protein and its role in the pathogenesis of AIDS-associated Kaposi's sarcoma. *Clin. Microbiol. Rev.* **2002**, *15*, 310–326. [CrossRef] [PubMed]
110. Krill, L.S.; Tewari, K.S. Exploring the therapeutic rationale for angiogenesis blockade in cervical cancer. *Clin. Ther.* **2015**, *37*, 9–19. [CrossRef]
111. Nyagol, J.; Leucci, E.; Omnis, A.; De Falco, G.; Tigli, C.; Sanseverino, F.; Torricelli, M.; Palummo, N.; Pacenti, L.; Santopietro, R. The effects of HIV-1 Tat protein on cell cycle during cervical carcinogenesis. *Cancer Biol. Ther.* **2006**, *5*, 684–690. [CrossRef] [PubMed]
112. Bayurova, E. (Gamaleya Research Center for Epidemiology and Microbiology, M.P. Chumakov Federal Scientific Center for Research and Development of Immune-and-Biological Products of Russian Academy of Sciences, Moscow, Russia); Isagulants, M. (Gamaleya Research Center for Epidemiology and Microbiology; M.P. Chumakov Federal Scientific Center for Research and Development of Immune-and-Biological Products of Russian Academy of Sciences; Department of Microbiology, Tumor and Cell Biology, Karolinska Institutet; Department of Research, Riga Stradins University, Riga, Latvia); Tugizov, S. (Department of Medicine, University of California, San Francisco, CA, USA); Palefsky, J. (Department of Medicine, University of California, San Francisco, CA, USA). Personal communication, 2020.
113. Collini, P.J.; Bewley, M.A.; Mohasin, M.; Marriott, H.M.; Miller, R.F.; Geretti, A.M.; Beloukas, A.; Papadimitropoulos, A.; Read, R.C.; Noursadeghi, M.; et al. HIV gp120 in the Lungs of Antiretroviral Therapy-treated Individuals Impairs Alveolar Macrophage Responses to Pneumococci. *Am. J. Respir. Crit. Care Med.* **2018**, *197*, 1604–1615. [CrossRef]
114. Latanova, A.; Petkov, S.; Kuzmenko, Y.; Kilpelainen, A.; Ivanov, A.; Smirnova, O.; Krotova, O.; Korolev, S.; Hinkula, J.; Karpov, V.; et al. Fusion to Flaviviral Leader Peptide Targets HIV-1 Reverse Transcriptase for Secretion and Reduces Its Enzymatic Activity and Ability to Induce Oxidative Stress but Has No Major Effects on Its Immunogenic Performance in DNA-Immunized Mice. *J. Immunol. Res.* **2017**, *2017*, 7407136. [CrossRef] [PubMed]
115. Lien, K.; Mayer, W.; Herrera, R.; Rosbe, K.; Tugizov, S.M. HIV-1 proteins gp120 and tat induce the epithelial-mesenchymal transition in oral and genital mucosal epithelial cells. *PLoS ONE* **2019**, *14*, e0226343. [CrossRef] [PubMed]
116. Jansons, J.; Bayurova, E.; Skrastina, D.; Kurlanda, A.; Fridrihsone, I.; Kostyushev, D.; Kostyusheva, A.; Artyuhov, A.; Dashinimaev, E.; Avdoshina, D. Expression of the Reverse Transcriptase Domain of Telomerase Reverse Transcriptase Induces Lytic Cellular Response in DNA-Immunized Mice and Limits Tumorigenic and Metastatic Potential of Murine Adenocarcinoma 4T1 Cells. *Vaccines* **2020**, *8*, 318. [CrossRef]
117. Wechsler, E.I.; Tugizov, S.; Herrera, R.; Da Costa, M.; Palefsky, J.M. E5 can be expressed in anal cancer and leads to epidermal growth factor receptor-induced invasion in a human papillomavirus 16-transformed anal epithelial cell line. *J. Gen. Virol.* **2018**, *99*, 631–644. [CrossRef] [PubMed]
118. Aerts, J.L.; Gonzales, M.I.; Topalian, S.L. Selection of appropriate control genes to assess expression of tumor antigens using real-time RT-PCR. *BioTechniques* **2004**, *36*, 84–86, 88, 90–91. [CrossRef]
119. Huynh, D.; Vincan, E.; Mantamadiotis, T.; Purcell, D.; Chan, C.-K.; Ramsay, R. Oncogenic properties of HIV-Tat in colorectal cancer cells. *Curr. HIV Res.* **2007**, *5*, 403–409. [CrossRef]
120. Liu, Y.P.; Chen, C.H.; Yen, C.H.; Tung, C.W.; Chen, C.J.; Chen, Y.A.; Huang, M.S. Human immunodeficiency virus Tat-TIP30 interaction promotes metastasis by enhancing the nuclear translocation of Snail in lung cancer cell lines. *Cancer Sci.* **2018**, *109*, 3105–3114. [CrossRef]
121. Mani, K.; Sandgren, S.; Lilja, J.; Cheng, F.; Svensson, K.; Persson, L.; Belting, M. HIV-Tat protein transduction domain specifically attenuates growth of polyamine deprived tumor cells. *Mol. Cancer Ther.* **2007**, *6*, 782–788. [CrossRef]
122. Dandachi, D.; Moron, F. Effects of HIV on the Tumor Microenvironment. *Adv. Exp. Med. Biol.* **2020**, *1263*, 45–54. [CrossRef]
123. Nunnari, G.; Smith, J.A.; Daniel, R. HIV-1 Tat and AIDS-associated cancer: Targeting the cellular anti-cancer barrier? *J. Exp. Clin. Cancer Res.* **2008**, *27*, 3. [CrossRef]
124. Loarca, L.; Fraietta, J.A.; Pirrone, V.; Szep, Z.; Wigdahl, B. Human immunodeficiency and Virus (HIV) Infection and Cancer. *HIV/AIDS Contemp. Chall.* **2017**, *1*, 9. [CrossRef]
125. Srivastava, D.K.; Tendler, C.L.; Milani, D.; English, M.A.; Licht, J.D.; Wilson, S.H. The HIV-1 transactivator protein Tat is a potent inducer of the human DNA repair enzyme beta-polymerase. *AIDS* **2001**, *15*, 433–440. [CrossRef] [PubMed]
126. Chipitsyna, G.; Slonina, D.; Siddiqui, K.; Peruzzi, F.; Skorski, T.; Reiss, K.; Sawaya, B.E.; Khalili, K.; Amini, S. HIV-1 Tat increases cell survival in response to cisplatin by stimulating Rad51 gene expression. *Oncogene* **2004**, *23*, 2664–2671. [CrossRef] [PubMed]

127. Valentin-Guillama, G.; Lopez, S.; Kucheryavykh, Y.V.; Chorna, N.E.; Perez, J.; Ortiz-Rivera, J.; Inyushin, M.; Makarov, V.; Valentin-Acevedo, A.; Quinones-Hinojosa, A.; et al. HIV-1 Envelope Protein gp120 Promotes Proliferation and the Activation of Glycolysis in Glioma Cell. *Cancers* **2018**, *10*, 301. [CrossRef] [PubMed]
128. Warburg, O. On the origin of cancer cells. *Science* **1956**, *123*, 309–314. [CrossRef] [PubMed]
129. Gatenby, R.A.; Gillies, R.J. Why do cancers have high aerobic glycolysis? *Nat. Rev. Cancer* **2004**, *4*, 891–899. [CrossRef]
130. Yuan, Z.; Petree, J.R.; Lee, F.E.; Fan, X.; Salaita, K.; Guidot, D.M.; Sadikot, R.T. Macrophages exposed to HIV viral protein disrupt lung epithelial cell integrity and mitochondrial bioenergetics via exosomal microRNA shuttling. *Cell Death Dis.* **2019**, *10*, 580. [CrossRef]
131. Greenway, A.L.; McPhee, D.A.; Allen, K.; Johnstone, R.; Holloway, G.; Mills, J.; Azad, A.; Sankovich, S.; Lambert, P. Human immunodeficiency virus type 1 Nef binds to tumor suppressor p53 and protects cells against p53-mediated apoptosis. *J. Virol.* **2002**, *76*, 2692–2702. [CrossRef]
132. Xue, M.; Yao, S.; Hu, M.; Li, W.; Hao, T.; Zhou, F.; Zhu, X.; Lu, H.; Qin, D.; Yan, Q.; et al. HIV-1 Nef and KSHV oncogene K1 synergistically promote angiogenesis by inducing cellular miR-718 to regulate the PTEN/AKT/mTOR signaling pathway. *Nucleic Acids Res.* **2014**, *42*, 9862–9879. [CrossRef]
133. Santerre, M.; Chatila, W.; Wang, Y.; Mukerjee, R.; Sawaya, B.E. HIV-1 Nef promotes cell proliferation and microRNA dysregulation in lung cells. *Cell Cycle* **2019**, *18*, 130–142. [CrossRef]
134. Bayurova, E.; Jansons, J.; Skrastina, D.; Smirnova, O.; Mezale, D.; Kostyusheva, A.; Kostyushev, D.; Petkov, S.; Podschwadt, P.; Valuev-Elliston, V. HIV-1 Reverse Transcriptase Promotes Tumor Growth and Metastasis Formation via ROS-Dependent Upregulation of Twist. *Oxidative Med. Cell. Longev.* **2019**, *2019*, 1–28. [CrossRef] [PubMed]
135. Giagulli, C.; Magiera, A.K.; Bugatti, A.; Caccuri, F.; Marsico, S.; Rusnati, M.; Vermi, W.; Fiorentini, S.; Caruso, A. HIV-1 matrix protein p17 binds to the IL-8 receptor CXCR1 and shows IL-8-like chemokine activity on monocytes through Rho/ROCK activation. *Blood* **2012**, *119*, 2274–2283. [CrossRef]
136. Caccuri, F.; Giagulli, C.; Bugatti, A.; Benetti, A.; Alessandri, G.; Ribatti, D.; Marsico, S.; Apostoli, P.; Slevin, M.A.; Rusnati, M.; et al. HIV-1 matrix protein p17 promotes angiogenesis via chemokine receptors CXCR1 and CXCR2. *Proc. Natl. Acad. Sci. USA* **2012**, *109*, 14580–14585. [CrossRef] [PubMed]
137. Caccuri, F.; Rueckert, C.; Giagulli, C.; Schulze, K.; Basta, D.; Zicari, S.; Marsico, S.; Cervi, E.; Fiorentini, S.; Slevin, M.; et al. HIV-1 matrix protein p17 promotes lymphangiogenesis and activates the endothelin-1/endothelin B receptor axis. *Arter. Thromb. Vasc. Biol.* **2014**, *34*, 846–856. [CrossRef] [PubMed]
138. Fiorentini, S.; Giagulli, C.; Caccuri, F.; Magiera, A.K.; Caruso, A. HIV-1 matrix protein p17: A candidate antigen for therapeutic vaccines against AIDS. *Pharmacol. Ther.* **2010**, *128*, 433–444. [CrossRef] [PubMed]
139. Caccuri, F.; Giordano, F.; Barone, I.; Mazzuca, P.; Giagulli, C.; Ando, S.; Caruso, A.; Marsico, S. HIV-1 matrix protein p17 and its variants promote human triple negative breast cancer cell aggressiveness. *Infect. Agents Cancer* **2017**, *12*, 49. [CrossRef] [PubMed]
140. Carroll, V.A.; Lafferty, M.K.; Marchionni, L.; Bryant, J.L.; Gallo, R.C.; Garzino-Demo, A. Expression of HIV-1 matrix protein p17 and association with B-cell lymphoma in HIV-1 transgenic mice. *Proc. Natl. Acad. Sci. USA* **2016**, *113*, 13168–13173. [CrossRef] [PubMed]
141. Ivanov, A.V.; Valuev-Elliston, V.T.; Ivanova, O.N.; Kochetkov, S.N.; Starodubova, E.S.; Bartosch, B.; Isaguliants, M.G. Oxidative stress during HIV infection: Mechanisms and consequences. *Oxidative Med. Cell. Longev.* **2016**, *2016*. [CrossRef]
142. El-Amine, R.; Germini, D.; Zakharova, V.V.; Tsfasman, T.; Sheval, E.V.; Louzada, R.A.N.; Dupuy, C.; Bilhou-Nabera, C.; Hamade, A.; Najjar, F.; et al. HIV-1 Tat protein induces DNA damage in human peripheral blood B-lymphocytes via mitochondrial ROS production. *Redox Biol.* **2018**, *15*, 97–108. [CrossRef]
143. Estrada, V.; Monge, S.; Gomez-Garre, M.D.; Sobrino, P.; Masia, M.; Berenguer, J.; Portilla, J.; Vilades, C.; Martinez, E.; Blanco, J.R.; et al. Relationship between plasma bilirubin level and oxidative stress markers in HIV-infected patients on atazanavir- vs. efavirenz-based antiretroviral therapy. *HIV Med.* **2016**, *17*, 653–661. [CrossRef]
144. Kolgiri, V.; Nagar, V.; Patil, V. Association of serum total bilirubin and plasma 8-OHdG in HIV/AIDS patients. *Interv. Med. Appl. Sci.* **2018**, *10*, 76–82. [CrossRef] [PubMed]
145. Porter, K.M.; Sutliff, R.L. HIV-1, reactive oxygen species, and vascular complications. *Free Radic. Biol. Med.* **2012**, *53*, 143–159. [CrossRef] [PubMed]
146. Price, T.O.; Ercal, N.; Nakaoke, R.; Banks, W.A. HIV-1 viral proteins gp120 and Tat induce oxidative stress in brain endothelial cells. *Brain Res.* **2005**, *1045*, 57–63. [CrossRef] [PubMed]
147. Gu, Y.; Wu, R.F.; Xu, Y.C.; Flores, S.C.; Terada, L.S. HIV Tat activates c-Jun amino-terminal kinase through an oxidant-dependent mechanism. *Virology* **2001**, *286*, 62–71. [CrossRef]
148. Capone, C.; Cervelli, M.; Angelucci, E.; Colasanti, M.; Macone, A.; Mariottini, P.; Persichini, T. A role for spermine oxidase as a mediator of reactive oxygen species production in HIV-Tat-induced neuronal toxicity. *Free Radic. Biol. Med.* **2013**, *63*, 99–107. [CrossRef]
149. Perry, S.W.; Norman, J.P.; Litzburg, A.; Zhang, D.; Dewhurst, S.; Gelbard, H.A. HIV-1 transactivator of transcription protein induces mitochondrial hyperpolarization and synaptic stress leading to apoptosis. *J. Immunol.* **2005**, *174*, 4333–4344. [CrossRef]
150. Pocernich, C.B.; Sultana, R.; Mohmmad-Abdul, H.; Nath, A.; Butterfield, D.A. HIV-dementia, Tat-induced oxidative stress, and antioxidant therapeutic considerations. *Brain Res. Rev.* **2005**, *50*, 14–26. [CrossRef]

151. Wu, R.F.; Ma, Z.; Liu, Z.; Terada, L.S. Nox4-derived H_2O_2 mediates endoplasmic reticulum signaling through local Ras activation. *Mol. Cell. Biol.* **2010**, *30*, 3553–3568. [CrossRef]
152. Helmcke, I.; Heumuller, S.; Tikkanen, R.; Schroder, K.; Brandes, R.P. Identification of structural elements in Nox1 and Nox4 controlling localization and activity. *Antioxidants Redox Signal.* **2009**, *11*, 1279–1287. [CrossRef]
153. Pietraforte, D.; Tritarelli, E.; Testa, U.; Minetti, M. gp120 HIV envelope glycoprotein increases the production of nitric oxide in human monocyte-derived macrophages. *J. Leukoc. Biol.* **1994**, *55*, 175–182. [CrossRef]
154. Shah, A.; Kumar, S.; Simon, S.D.; Singh, D.P.; Kumar, A. HIV gp120- and methamphetamine-mediated oxidative stress induces astrocyte apoptosis via cytochrome P450 2E1. *Cell Death Dis.* **2013**, *4*, e850. [CrossRef] [PubMed]
155. Foga, I.O.; Nath, A.; Hasinoff, B.B.; Geiger, J.D. Antioxidants and dipyridamole inhibit HIV-1 gp120-induced free radical-based oxidative damage to human monocytoid cells. *J. Acquir. Immune Defic. Syndr. Hum. Retrovirol.* **1997**, *16*, 223–229. [CrossRef] [PubMed]
156. Ronaldson, P.T.; Bendayan, R. HIV-1 viral envelope glycoprotein gp120 produces oxidative stress and regulates the functional expression of multidrug resistance protein-1 (Mrp1) in glial cells. *J. Neurochem.* **2008**, *106*, 1298–1313. [CrossRef]
157. Reddy, P.V.; Gandhi, N.; Samikkannu, T.; Saiyed, Z.; Agudelo, M.; Yndart, A.; Khatavkar, P.; Nair, M.P. HIV-1 gp120 induces antioxidant response element-mediated expression in primary astrocytes: Role in HIV associated neurocognitive disorder. *Neurochem. Int.* **2012**, *61*, 807–814. [CrossRef] [PubMed]
158. Olivetta, E.; Pietraforte, D.; Schiavoni, I.; Minetti, M.; Federico, M.; Sanchez, M. HIV-1 Nef regulates the release of superoxide anions from human macrophages. *Biochem. J.* **2005**, *390*, 591–602. [CrossRef] [PubMed]
159. Olivetta, E.; Mallozzi, C.; Ruggieri, V.; Pietraforte, D.; Federico, M.; Sanchez, M. HIV-1 Nef induces p47(phox) phosphorylation leading to a rapid superoxide anion release from the U937 human monoblastic cell line. *J. Cell. Biochem.* **2009**, *106*, 812–822. [CrossRef] [PubMed]
160. Vilhardt, F.; Plastre, O.; Sawada, M.; Suzuki, K.; Wiznerowicz, M.; Kiyokawa, E.; Trono, D.; Krause, K.-H. The HIV-1 Nef protein and phagocyte NADPH oxidase activation. *J. Biol. Chem.* **2002**, *277*, 42136–42143. [CrossRef]
161. Masanetz, S.; Lehmann, M.H. HIV-1 Nef increases astrocyte sensitivity towards exogenous hydrogen peroxide. *Virol. J.* **2011**, *8*, 35. [CrossRef]
162. Chelvanambi, S.; Gupta, S.K.; Chen, X.; Ellis, B.W.; Maier, B.F.; Colbert, T.M.; Kuriakose, J.; Zorlutuna, P.; Jolicoeur, P.; Obukhov, A.G.; et al. HIV-Nef Protein Transfer to Endothelial Cells Requires Rac1 Activation and Leads to Endothelial Dysfunction Implications for Statin Treatment in HIV Patients. *Circ. Res.* **2019**, *125*, 805–820. [CrossRef]
163. Isaguliants, M.; Smirnova, O.; Ivanov, A.V.; Kilpelainen, A.; Kuzmenko, Y.; Petkov, S.; Latanova, A.; Krotova, O.; Engström, G.; Karpov, V. Oxidative stress induced by HIV-1 reverse transcriptase modulates the enzyme's performance in gene immunization. *Hum. Vacc. Immunother.* **2013**, *9*, 2111–2119. [CrossRef]
164. Massiah, M.A.; Starich, M.R.; Paschall, C.; Summers, M.F.; Christensen, A.M.; Sundquist, W.I. Three-dimensional structure of the human immunodeficiency virus type 1 matrix protein. *J. Mol. Biol.* **1994**, *244*, 198–223. [CrossRef] [PubMed]
165. Doherty, R.S.; De Oliveira, T.; Seebregts, C.; Danaviah, S.; Gordon, M.; Cassol, S. BioAfrica's HIV-1 proteomics resource: Combining protein data with bioinformatics tools. *Retrovirology* **2005**, *2*, 18. [CrossRef] [PubMed]
166. Zeinolabediny, Y.; Caccuri, F.; Colombo, L.; Morelli, F.; Romeo, M.; Rossi, A.; Schiarea, S.; Ciaramelli, C.; Airoldi, C.; Weston, R.; et al. HIV-1 matrix protein p17 misfolding forms toxic amyloidogenic assemblies that induce neurocognitive disorders. *Sci. Rep.* **2017**, *7*, 10313. [CrossRef]
167. Cheignon, C.; Tomas, M.; Bonnefont-Rousselot, D.; Faller, P.; Hureau, C.; Collin, F. Oxidative stress and the amyloid beta peptide in Alzheimer's disease. *Redox Biol.* **2018**, *14*, 450–464. [CrossRef] [PubMed]
168. Miller, I.P.; Pavlovic, I.; Poljsak, B.; Suput, D.; Milisav, I. Beneficial Role of ROS in Cell Survival: Moderate Increases in H_2O_2 Production Induced by Hepatocyte Isolation Mediate Stress Adaptation and Enhanced Survival. *Antioxidants* **2019**, *8*, 434. [CrossRef]
169. Ajasin, D.; Eugenin, E.A. HIV-1 Tat: Role in Bystander Toxicity. *Front. Cell. Infect. Microbiol.* **2020**, *10*, 61. [CrossRef]
170. Debaisieux, S.; Rayne, F.; Yezid, H.; Beaumelle, B. The ins and outs of HIV-1 Tat. *Traffic* **2012**, *13*, 355–363. [CrossRef]
171. Clark, E.; Nava, B.; Caputi, M. Tat is a multifunctional viral protein that modulates cellular gene expression and functions. *Oncotarget* **2017**, *8*, 27569–27581. [CrossRef]
172. Marino, J.; Wigdahl, B.; Nonnemacher, M.R. Extracellular HIV-1 Tat Mediates Increased Glutamate in the CNS Leading to Onset of Senescence and Progression of HAND. *Front. Aging Neurosci.* **2020**, *12*, 168. [CrossRef]
173. Montano, M.A.; Novitsky, V.A.; Blackard, J.T.; Cho, N.L.; Katzenstein, D.A.; Essex, M. Divergent transcriptional regulation among expanding human immunodeficiency virus type 1 subtypes. *J. Virol.* **1997**, *71*, 8657–8665. [CrossRef]
174. Karn, J.; Stoltzfus, C.M. Transcriptional and posttranscriptional regulation of HIV-1 gene expression. *Cold Spring Harb. Perspect. Med.* **2012**, *2*, a006916. [CrossRef] [PubMed]
175. Albini, A.; Ferrini, S.; Benelli, R.; Sforzini, S.; Giunciuglio, D.; Aluigi, M.G.; Proudfoot, A.E.; Alouani, S.; Wells, T.N.; Mariani, G.; et al. HIV-1 Tat protein mimicry of chemokines. *Proc. Natl. Acad. Sci. USA* **1998**, *95*, 13153–13158. [CrossRef] [PubMed]
176. Eugenin, E.A.; Dyer, G.; Calderon, T.M.; Berman, J.W. HIV-1 tat protein induces a migratory phenotype in human fetal microglia by a CCL2 (MCP-1)-dependent mechanism: Possible role in NeuroAIDS. *Glia* **2005**, *49*, 501–510. [CrossRef] [PubMed]

177. El-Hage, N.; Wu, G.; Wang, J.; Ambati, J.; Knapp, P.E.; Reed, J.L.; Bruce-Keller, A.J.; Hauser, K.F. HIV-1 Tat and opiate-induced changes in astrocytes promote chemotaxis of microglia through the expression of MCP-1 and alternative chemokines. *Glia* **2006**, *53*, 132–146. [CrossRef]
178. Lawrence, D.M.; Seth, P.; Durham, L.; Diaz, F.; Boursiquot, R.; Ransohoff, R.M.; Major, E.O. Astrocyte differentiation selectively upregulates CCL2/monocyte chemoattractant protein-1 in cultured human brain-derived progenitor cells. *Glia* **2006**, *53*, 81–91. [CrossRef]
179. Youn, G.S.; Ju, S.M.; Choi, S.Y.; Park, J. HDAC6 mediates HIV-1 tat-induced proinflammatory responses by regulating MAPK-NF-kappaB/AP-1 pathways in astrocytes. *Glia* **2015**, *63*, 1953–1965. [CrossRef]
180. Clouse, K.A.; Cosentino, L.M.; Weih, K.A.; Pyle, S.W.; Robbins, P.B.; Hochstein, H.D.; Natarajan, V.; Farrar, W.L. The HIV-1 gp120 envelope protein has the intrinsic capacity to stimulate monokine secretion. *J. Immunol.* **1991**, *147*, 2892–2901.
181. Kalyanaraman, V.S.; Rodriguez, V.; Veronese, F.; Rahman, R.; Lusso, P.; DeVico, A.L.; Copeland, T.; Oroszlan, S.; Gallo, R.C.; Sarngadharan, M.G. Characterization of the secreted, native gp120 and gp160 of the human immunodeficiency virus type 1. *AIDS Res. Hum. Retroviruses* **1990**, *6*, 371–380. [CrossRef]
182. Oh, S.-K.; Cruikshank, W.W.; Raina, J.; Blanchard, G.C.; Adler, W.H.; Walker, J.; Kornfeld, H. Identification of HIV-1 envelope glycoprotein in the serum of AIDS and ARC patients. *J. Acquir. Immune Defic. Syndr.* **1992**, *5*, 251–256. [CrossRef]
183. Jones, M.V.; Bell, J.E.; Nath, A. Immunolocalization of HIV envelope gp120 in HIV encephalitis with dementia. *AIDS* **2000**, *14*, 2709–2713. [CrossRef]
184. Berth, S.; Caicedo, H.H.; Sarma, T.; Morfini, G.; Brady, S.T. Internalization and axonal transport of the HIV glycoprotein gp120. *ASN Neuro* **2015**, *7*. [CrossRef] [PubMed]
185. Marone, G.; Rossi, F.W.; Pecoraro, A.; Pucino, V.; Criscuolo, G.; Paulis, A.; Spadaro, G.; Marone, G.; Varricchi, G. HIV gp120 Induces the Release of Proinflammatory, Angiogenic, and Lymphangiogenic Factors from Human Lung Mast Cells. *Vaccines* **2020**, *8*, 208. [CrossRef] [PubMed]
186. Caby, M.-P.; Lankar, D.; Vincendeau-Scherrer, C.; Raposo, G.; Bonnerot, C. Exosomal-like vesicles are present in human blood plasma. *Int. Immunol.* **2005**, *17*, 879–887. [CrossRef] [PubMed]
187. Ferdin, J.; Goricar, K.; Dolzan, V.; Plemenitas, A.; Martin, J.N.; Peterlin, B.M.; Deeks, S.G.; Lenassi, M. Viral protein Nef is detected in plasma of half of HIV-infected adults with undetectable plasma HIV RNA. *PLoS ONE* **2018**, *13*, e0191613. [CrossRef] [PubMed]
188. Lenassi, M.; Cagney, G.; Liao, M.; Vaupotič, T.; Bartholomeeusen, K.; Cheng, Y.; Krogan, N.J.; Plemenitaš, A.; Peterlin, B.M. HIV Nef is secreted in exosomes and triggers apoptosis in bystander CD4 + T cells. *Traffic* **2010**, *11*, 110–122. [CrossRef] [PubMed]
189. Chettimada, S.; Lorenz, D.R.; Misra, V.; Dillon, S.T.; Reeves, R.K.; Manickam, C.; Morgello, S.; Kirk, G.D.; Mehta, S.H.; Gabuzda, D. Exosome markers associated with immune activation and oxidative stress in HIV patients on antiretroviral therapy. *Sci. Rep.* **2018**, *8*, 7227. [CrossRef] [PubMed]
190. James, C.O.; Huang, M.-B.; Khan, M.; Garcia-Barrio, M.; Powell, M.D.; Bond, V.C. Extracellular Nef protein targets CD4 + T cells for apoptosis by interacting with CXCR4 surface receptors. *J. Virol.* **2004**, *78*, 3099–3109. [CrossRef]
191. Qiao, X.; He, B.; Chiu, A.; Knowles, D.M.; Chadburn, A.; Cerutti, A. Human immunodeficiency virus 1 Nef suppresses CD40-dependent immunoglobulin class switching in bystander B cells. *Nat. Immunol.* **2006**, *7*, 302–310. [CrossRef]
192. Saribas, A.S.; Cicalese, S.; Ahooyi, T.M.; Khalili, K.; Amini, S.; Sariyer, I.K. HIV-1 Nef is released in extracellular vesicles derived from astrocytes: Evidence for Nef-mediated neurotoxicity. *Cell Death Dis.* **2018**, *8*, e2542. [CrossRef]
193. Anyanwu, S.I.; Doherty, A.; Powell, M.D.; Obialo, C.; Huang, M.B.; Quarshie, A.; Mitchell, C.; Bashir, K.; Newman, G.W. Detection of HIV-1 and Human Proteins in Urinary Extracellular Vesicles from HIV+ Patients. *Adv. Virol.* **2018**, *2018*, 1–16. [CrossRef]
194. Caccuri, F.; Iaria, M.L.; Campilongo, F.; Varney, K.; Rossi, A.; Mitola, S.; Schiarea, S.; Bugatti, A.; Mazzuca, P.; Giagulli, C.; et al. Cellular aspartyl proteases promote the unconventional secretion of biologically active HIV-1 matrix protein p17. *Sci. Rep.* **2016**, *6*, 38027. [CrossRef] [PubMed]
195. Dolcetti, R.; Gloghini, A.; Caruso, A.; Carbone, A. A lymphomagenic role for HIV beyond immune suppression? *Blood* **2016**, *127*, 1403–1409. [CrossRef] [PubMed]
196. Popovic, M.; Tenner-Racz, K.; Pelser, C.; Stellbrink, H.J.; van Lunzen, J.; Lewis, G.; Kalyanaraman, V.S.; Gallo, R.C.; Racz, P. Persistence of HIV-1 structural proteins and glycoproteins in lymph nodes of patients under highly active antiretroviral therapy. *Proc. Natl. Acad. Sci. USA* **2005**, *102*, 14807–14812. [CrossRef] [PubMed]

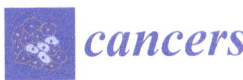

Review

The Complement System in Ovarian Cancer: An Underexplored Old Path

Yaiza Senent [1,2,3], Daniel Ajona [1,2,3,4,*], Antonio González-Martín [1,5], Ruben Pio [1,2,3,4,†] and Beatriz Tavira [1,3,6,†]

1. Translational Oncology Group, Program in Solid Tumors, Cima University of Navarra, 31008 Pamplona, Spain; ysenent@alumni.unav.es (Y.S.); agonzalezma@unav.es (A.G.-M.); rpio@unav.es (R.P.); btavirai@unav.es (B.T.)
2. Department of Biochemistry and Genetics, School of Sciences, University of Navarra, 31008 Pamplona, Spain
3. Navarra Institute for Health Research (IdISNA), 31008 Pamplona, Spain
4. Centro de Investigación Biomédica en Red de Cáncer (CIBERONC), 28029 Madrid, Spain
5. Department of Oncology, Clinica Universidad de Navarra, 28027 Madrid, Spain
6. Department of Pathology, Anatomy and Physiology, School of Medicine, University of Navarra, 31008 Pamplona, Spain
* Correspondence: dajonama@unav.es; Tel.: +34-948-19-47-00
† These authors contributed equally to this work.

Simple Summary: Ovarian cancer is one of the leading causes of death among women and the most lethal cause of death from gynecological malignancy in developed countries. The immune system plays an essential role in ovarian cancer progression, and its modulation may be used as an effective therapeutic tool. In this review, we examine the relevance of the cellular and humoral components of the adaptive and innate immune responses in ovarian cancer, focusing on the role of an essential component of innate immunity, the complement system. Elements of this system show tumor-promoting activities that impede the efficacy of developing treatment strategies. We discuss evidence that suggests a role of complement components in the progression of ovarian cancer and provide a rationale for evaluating the inhibition of complement components in combination with immunotherapies aimed to reactivate antitumor T-cell responses.

Abstract: Ovarian cancer is one of the most lethal gynecological cancers. Current therapeutic strategies allow temporary control of the disease, but most patients develop resistance to treatment. Moreover, although successful in a range of solid tumors, immunotherapy has yielded only modest results in ovarian cancer. Emerging evidence underscores the relevance of the components of innate and adaptive immunity in ovarian cancer progression and response to treatment. Particularly, over the last decade, the complement system, a pillar of innate immunity, has emerged as a major regulator of the tumor microenvironment in cancer immunity. Tumor-associated complement activation may support chronic inflammation, promote an immunosuppressive microenvironment, induce angiogenesis, and activate cancer-related signaling pathways. Recent insights suggest an important role of complement effectors, such as C1q or anaphylatoxins C3a and C5a, and their receptors C3aR and C5aR1 in ovarian cancer progression. Nevertheless, the implication of these factors in different clinical contexts is still poorly understood. Detailed knowledge of the interplay between ovarian cancer cells and complement is required to develop new immunotherapy combinations and biomarkers. In this context, we discuss the possibility of targeting complement to overcome some of the hurdles encountered in the treatment of ovarian cancer.

Keywords: ovarian cancer; adaptive immunity; innate immunity; complement system; immunotherapy; cancer immunology; tumor microenvironment

1. Current Status of Ovarian Cancer: Clinical Perspective and Needs

Ovarian cancer is the most lethal gynecological cancer in developed countries [1]. According to data from the US National Cancer Institute (NIH), the five-year survival rate for ovarian cancer is 49.1% [2]. This can be attributed to a delay in the diagnosis due to the lack of specific symptoms; 70% of cases are diagnosed in stage III or IV, making it difficult to treat with curative intent [3]. Ovarian cancer is a complex disease that comprises different tumor types, of which epithelial ovarian cancer represents 90–95% of all cases [4]. The current standard treatment includes surgery and platinum-based chemotherapy followed by a maintenance period with the anti-angiogenic therapy bevacizumab [5]. Initial responses to chemotherapy are frequently high, but unfortunately, up to 70% of patients experience recurrence within the first three years, especially patients who are late-diagnosed [5]. Survival rates have recently improved with the introduction of a new generation of poly (ADP-ribose) polymerase inhibitors (PARP inhibitors (PARPi)). These drugs, administered after chemotherapy, prolong the time during which the disease does not progress, mainly in patients carrying BRCA mutations [6]. Despite this great advance, the overall survival of patients with ovarian cancer is still low. There are a variety of factors associated with chemoresistance and relapse, including interactions between ovarian cancer cells and their surrounding immune microenvironment [7]. Ovarian cancers are considered "immunogenic tumors" in which spontaneous antitumor immune responses have been demonstrated [8,9]. The presence of tumors infiltrating $CD8^+$ lymphocytes in the tumor microenvironment (TME) is associated with longer recurrence-free and overall survival [10,11], whereas the recruitment of regulatory T (Treg) cells is correlated with a poor outcome [12]. These associations indicate that ovarian cancers could respond to immunotherapy. However, immune checkpoint inhibitors (anti-CTLA-4 or anti-PD-1/PD-L1) have yielded modest clinical results in ovarian cancer patients [13,14]. A better understanding of the interplay between ovarian tumor cells and the immunological players in innate and adaptive immunity is critical for developing strategies to overcome the resistance of ovarian cancers to immunotherapy [15,16].

A major effector of innate immunity is the complement system, which represents one of the first lines of defense that distinguish "self" from "non-self" [17]. This system is composed of more than 50 soluble or membrane-bound effectors, regulators, and receptors, and it plays a relevant role in numerous physiological and pathological processes, including cancer [18]. Some evidence suggests that the modulation of complement activation may be exploited for the development of successful treatments against cancer [19,20]. In this review, we discuss the role played by components of adaptive and innate immunity on the development and progression of ovarian cancer. We mainly focus on the complement system, its role in the TME, and the rationale behind the use of complement modulators for the treatment of ovarian cancer.

2. Cellular and Humoral Immune Components of the Ovarian Tumor Microenvironment

The continuous feedback between tumor cells and the immune system is now recognized as a distinguished cancer hallmark [21]. Neoplastic transformation is characterized by the acquisition of tumor-associated molecular patterns that can be detected by the immune system. It is believed that upon recognition, innate and adaptive immunity can eliminate the vast majority of incipient cancer cells, avoiding tumor formation. However, the immune system is unable to eliminate all emerging malignant cells. When transforming cells escape from immune-mediated elimination, a dynamic interplay is established between tumor cells and the immune system, resulting in tumor-associated immune responses that may facilitate the development and progression of cancer [22]. In the case of ovarian tumors, a plethora of immune and non-immune cell types and non-cellular elements are found in the TME, not only in primary tumors but also in ascites and metastases [23]. The co-existence of multiple distinct tumor immune microenvironments within a single individual highlights the high plasticity and adaptability of ovarian cancers [24]. Herein, we summarize the main roles of the cellular and humoral elements of the immune system in ovarian tumor progression.

2.1. Cellular Immune Components

Tumor cells co-exist with non-immune and immune cells, and this relationship determines the natural history of the tumor and its resistance or response to therapy. The cellular immune components of the ovarian TME include T and B lymphocytes, natural killer (NK) cells, dendritic cells (DCs), polymorphonuclear cells, and macrophages.

T cells are a prominent component of the ovarian TME. Infiltration by $CD8^+$ T cells is indicative of an ongoing immune response and is associated with a favorable prognosis [25]. Upon activation, tumor-specific $CD8^+$ T cells secrete IFN-γ, tumor necrosis factor (TNF)-α, and cytotoxic mediators. However, in the ovarian TME, $CD8^+$ T-cell responses are often dysfunctional. The autologous recognition of ovarian tumor antigens is limited to approximately 10% of the intratumoral $CD8^+$ T receptor (TCR) repertoire [26]. This state can be attributed to the upregulation of T-cell exhaustion molecules by persistent antigen exposure and the existence of a hostile TME characterized by nutrient deprivation, hypoxia, oxidative stress, high concentrations of pro-inflammatory molecules, and the presence of immunosuppressive cell subsets [27]. In fact, ovarian cancers are highly enriched in Treg cells [28], a subset of lymphocytes that hamper tumor immunosurveillance by fostering peripheral tolerance to tumor antigens. Treg cells release and metabolize ATP to adenosine by the action of CD39 and CD73, a process that mediates immunosuppression via the adenosine and A_{2A} pathways [29]. Consequently, depletion of Treg cells in ovarian cancer-bearing mice effectively restores antitumor antigen-specific T-cell responses [30]. Other lymphoid subsets are important elements of the ovarian cancer immune infiltrate. In an orthotopic syngeneic mouse model, antitumor immunity was driven by $CD4^+$ T cells [15]. A study identified a novel tumor-infiltrating NK subset characterized by a high expression of PD-1, reduced proliferative capability in response to cytokines, low degranulation, and impaired cytokine production upon interaction with tumor targets [31]. The presence of $CD20^+$ B cells was associated with increased survival in ovarian cancer patients [32]. In human metastases of high-grade serous ovarian cancer, B cells develop memory responses in the TME and promote antitumor immune responses [33].

DCs are a diverse group of innate immune cells that infiltrate tumors and present tumor-derived antigens to naïve T cells. High densities of tumor-infiltrating $DC-LAMP^+$ mature DCs suggest the establishment of an antitumor immune response, which is associated with a favorable prognosis in ovarian cancer patients [34]. However, this immune response is often rendered dysfunctional because of a variety of mechanisms, such as the upregulation of B7-H1 [35], the activation of the endoplasmic reticulum stress response factor X-box binding protein 1 (XBP1) [36], the attenuation of the toll-like receptor-mediated DC activation [37], and the activation of the cyclooxygenase 2 (COX2)/prostaglandin E_2 (PGE_2) axis to redirect the development of DCs toward the formation of myeloid-derived suppressor cells (MDSCs) [38].

MDSCs represent a heterogeneous population of immature myeloid cells that fail to differentiate into granulocytes, macrophages, or DCs. Two main subsets of MDSCs have been identified: polymorphonuclear MDSC (PMN-MDSC; $CD11b^+Ly6G^+Ly6C^{lo}$ in mice and $CD11b^+CD14^-CD15^+CD66b^+LOX-1^+$ in humans) and monocytic MDSC (M-MDSC; $CD11b^+Ly6G^-Ly6C^{hi}$ in mice and $CD14^+CD15^-HLA-DR^{-/lo}$ in humans). PMN-MDSCs and M-MDSCs are morphologically and phenotypically similar to neutrophils and monocytes, respectively [39]. These cells potently inhibit the anti-tumor immune response and reshape the TME to promote tumor growth and metastatic spread. The differentiation of myeloid precursors toward an MDSC phenotype is mediated by the inflammatory factor PGE_2 via DNA methyltransferase 3A (DNMT3A)-dependent hypermethylation and the downregulation of a subset of myeloid genes [40]. The infiltration of MDSCs into ovarian tumors is associated with the Snail-mediated upregulation of CXCL1 and CXCL2 chemokines that attract MDSCs to the tumor via CXCR2 [41]. In the tumor niche, granulocyte–monocyte colony-stimulating factor (GM-CSF), through the signal transducer and activator of transcription 5 (STAT-5) pathway, upregulates AMP-activated protein kinase alpha 1 (AMPKα-1) in MDSCs to suppress antitumor CD8$^+$ T-cell responses [42]. Both the presence of TNF-α and the production of NO by MDSCs sustain Th17 responses in the TME and myeloid cell recruitment in an IL-17-dependent manner [43,44].

Tumor-associated neutrophils, a cell population difficult to distinguish from PMN-MDSCs, are also involved in ovarian cancer-associated immune responses. In a KRAS-driven ovarian cancer mouse model, neutrophils reduced the amount of tumor-associated Treg cells and M-MDSCs while increasing the antitumor immune response via the upregulation of CD8$^+$ T-cell function [45]. By contrast, the activation of neutrophils by mitochondrial DNA from ascites obstructs anti-tumor immunity and is associated with worse outcomes in patients with advanced ovarian cancer [46]. This study also reported the formation of neutrophil extracellular traps (NETs), networks of neutrophil decondensed chromatin fibers that are capable of binding tumor cells to support metastatic progression [47]. These contrasting roles of neutrophils in ovarian cancer have been attributed to different polarization states induced by the presence of transforming growth factor (TGF)-β and type-1 interferons in the TME [48].

Tumor-associated macrophages (TAMs) play a major role in the pathogenesis of ovarian cancer [49]. Macrophages constitute over 50% of the cells in peritoneal ovarian tumor nodules and malignant ascites and are involved in ovarian cancer initiation, progression, and metastasis [50]. TAMs are highly plastic cells that can exhibit two main phenotypes: anti-tumorigenic M1-like (F4/80^{hi} and CD86$^+$ or CD80$^+$ or iNOS$^+$ in mice; CD68$^+$HLA-DR$^+$CD11c$^-$ and CD86$^+$ or CD80$^+$ or iNOS$^+$ in humans) and pro-tumorigenic M2-like (F4/80^{hi} and CD163$^+$ or CD206$^+$ or arginase$^+$ in mice; CD68$^+$HLA-DR$^+$CD11c$^-$ and CD163$^+$ or CD206$^+$ in humans). Analyses of TAM polarization in ovarian cancer show that M2 TAMs are associated with a poor prognosis [51,52]. Malignant cells direct TAM differentiation to facilitate tumor progression. The activation of the ovarian TAM pro-tumor phenotype requires the expression of zinc finger E-box binding homeobox 1 (ZEB1), a driver of the epithelial-mesenchymal transition (EMT), and involves direct crosstalk with tumor cells [53]. Tumor-expressed CD24 interacts with the inhibitory receptor sialic-acid-binding Ig-like lectin 10 (Siglec-10) expressed by ovarian cancer-inhibiting TAMs to avoid their antitumor effects [54]. Ovarian cancer cells skew co-cultured macrophages to a phenotype similar to that found in ovarian tumors [55]. Ovarian cancer cells promote membrane-cholesterol efflux and depletion of lipid rafts to polarize TAMs toward a tumor-promoting phenotype characterized by the upregulation of IL-4 signaling [56]. In return, TAMs enhance the malignant potential of ovarian cancer cells. Endothelial growth factor (EGF) secreted from TAMs promoted tumor growth at early stages of transcoelomic metastasis in a mouse model of ovarian cancer [57]. Moreover, TAMs enhance ovarian cancer invasiveness through activation of the nuclear factor kappa B (NF-kB) and Jun N-terminal kinase (JNK) pathways in tumor cells [58].

2.2. Humoral Immune Components

The crosstalk between the different cellular components of the TME is essential to reprogram tumor-associated immune responses. This process is orchestrated by complex networks interconnected by sets of soluble factors and extracellular structures, such as cytokines, chemokines, small metabolites, and microvesicles, among others [59]. In particular, cytokines mediate key interactions between immune and non-immune cells in the TME [60], and cytokine-based immunotherapy is a promising strategy to modulate the host's immune response toward the induction of apoptosis in tumor cells [61]. To date, there are two FDA-approved treatments for melanoma and metastatic renal cell cancer based on the administration of TNF-α and interleukin (IL)-2 [62]. In the case of ovarian cancer, the proinflammatory cytokine IL-6 has been established as a key immunoregulator [63]. IL-6, along with other cytokines, activates pathways such as STAT and NF-kB, whose modulation could be used as a potential therapeutic tool [63].

Many years ago, Bjørge et al. found elevated levels of complement C1q, C3, C3a, and soluble C5b-9 in ascites from ovarian cancer patients, suggesting that local complement activation may constitute an important soluble component of the ovarian TME [64]. More recently, ovarian cancer has been classified as a cancer type with "upregulated complement" [65]. Interestingly, over the last decade, the complement system has emerged as a major non-cellular regulator of the TME in cancer immunity. Tumor-associated complement activation may support chronic inflammation, promote an immunosuppressive microenvironment, induce angiogenesis, and activate cancer-related signaling pathways [66]. In the case of ovarian cancer, complement dysregulation may even participate in the onset of tumors since complement molecules are already overexpressed in precursor lesions [67]. In the following section, we summarize the evidence supporting the involvement of the complement system in ovarian cancer progression.

3. The Complement System and Its Dual Role in Ovarian Cancer

In 1896, the complement system was first described as a heat-labile component in the serum able to "complement" heat-stable factors (antibodies). Now, the complement system is broadly known as a central part of the innate immune response composed of soluble and membrane-bound proteins that can coordinate a nonspecific inflammatory response against microbes and unwanted host elements [18]. Complement-circulating effectors are predominantly synthesized in the liver and are distributed throughout the body in an inactivated state. Complement can be activated by three main distinctive pathways: the classical pathway (CP), the lectin pathway (LP), and the alternative pathway (AP) (Figure 1). The three pathways converge in the cleavage of the complement component C3 into C3a and C3b. The CP is initiated in foreign, damaged, or dying cells when the C1 complex, which includes C1q, C1r, and C1s, recognizes antibody clusters, pathogen-associated molecular patterns (PAMPs), or danger-associated molecular patterns (DAMPs), among other molecules [68]. The LP is initiated by the recognition of carbohydrate patterns by mannose-binding lectin (MBL) or ficolins, along with the mannan-binding lectin serine proteases MASP1 and MASP2 [68]. The initiation of both the CP and the LP leads to the cleavage of C4 into C4a and C4b and, subsequently, C2 into C2a and C2b. The complex formed by C4b and C2b (C4bC2b, formerly C4b2a) constitutes the classical C3 convertase, which is responsible for the cleavage of C3 into C3a and C3b [68]. The AP is initiated by the spontaneous hydrolysis of C3 into $C3(H_2O)$, followed by its binding to factor B. This complex is recognized by factor D, which catalyzes the cleavage of factor B to form the fluid-phase alternative C3 convertase $C3(H_2O)Bb$. This convertase can mediate the cleavage of C3 into C3a and C3b to form the membrane-bound alternative C3 convertase C3bBb [69]. Subsequently, C3b is able to bind to C4bC2b (in the CP and LP) or C3bBb (in the AP), leading to the formation of C5 convertase. This complex catalyzes the cleavage of C5 into C5a and C5b. The later fragment sequentially binds to C6, C7, C8, and C9 to form the cytolytic membrane attack complex (MAC) [18,68]. Many complement functions are mediated by the anaphylatoxins C3a and C5a, which act as potent inflammatory modulators [70]. These peptides signal through their respective G-protein-coupled receptors C3aR and C5aR1 [71]. A second, lesser-known C5a receptor, C5aR2, also participates in C5a responses, though its role remains unclear. Finally, an array of membrane and soluble complement regulatory proteins (CRPs) protects normal cells from the overactivation of complement [68] (Figure 1).

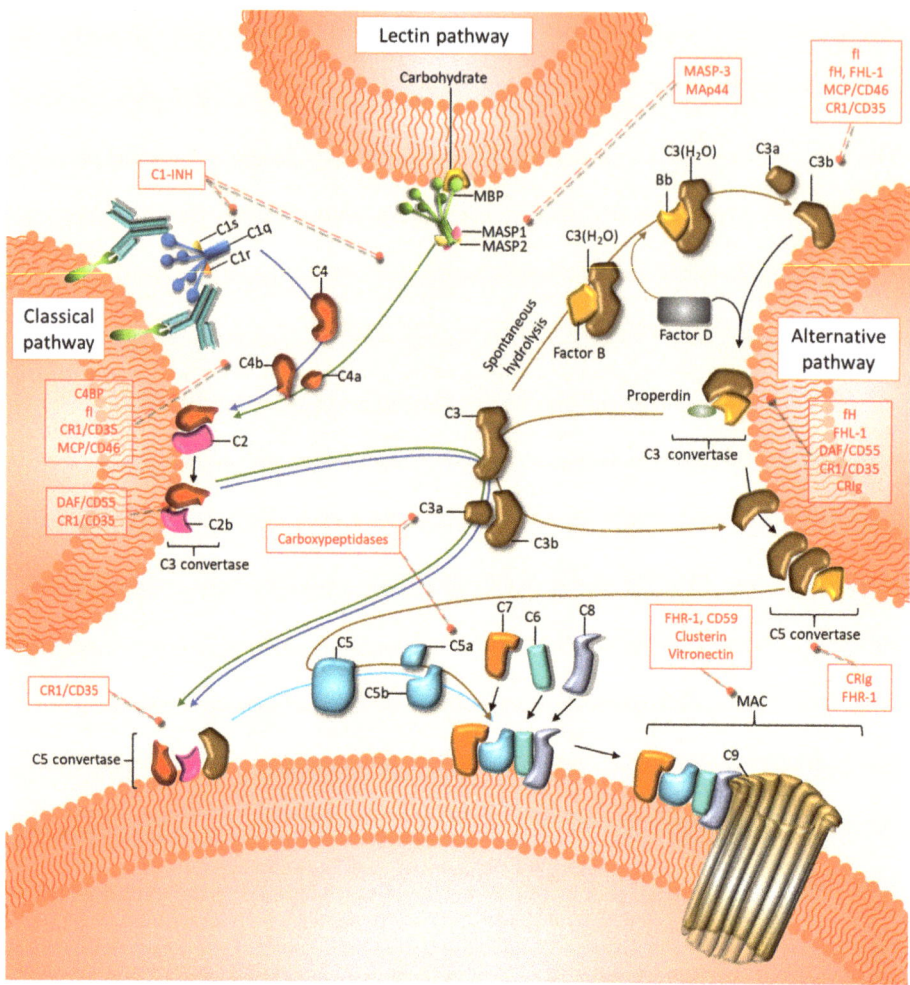

Figure 1. Schematic representation of the effectors and regulators of the complement cascade. Complement is initiated by three distinctive pathways: the classical (blue arrows), the lectin (green arrows), and the alternative (brown arrows) pathways. All three pathways converge in the formation of C3 and C5 convertases, which in turn generate the inflammation modulators C3a and C5a. The terminal steps, which culminate in the assembly of the membrane attack complex (MAC), are common to the three pathways. Inhibitory proteins of the three pathways are shown in red boxes.

Complement plays an essential role in the control of cellular immunity [18], participating in the regulation, differentiation, and trafficking of several immune cell types [17,72]. C3 and C4 depletion impair humoral immune responses in vivo [73–75]. It has been postulated that antigen–antibody clusters interact with complement and are recognized by DCs, B lymphocytes, and macrophages [76]. Further evidence of the interplay between adaptive and innate immunity is the CD21(CR2)-CD19-CD81 complex on B cells, which enhances B-cell receptor function [77,78], partially by recognizing C3d-tagged surfaces [79]. Anaphylatoxins also play an important role in immune regulation. Most immune cell types express C3aR and/or C5aR1 on their surfaces [65]. On B cells, C3a impairs polyclonal immune responses and TNF-α and IL-6 production [80,81]. C5a has been extensively reported to induce the migration of several cell types [82–86]. Interestingly, C5a fosters antigen cross-presentation and the maturation of DCs [87–89]. Moreover, C3a-C3aR and C5a-C5aR1 signaling promote the activation [90] and expansion [91] of T cells and divert their differentiation from Treg cells [92,93]. Complement inhibitory proteins, such as CD46, have been shown to modulate T-cell fate depending on the isoform expressed and the presence of IL-2 [94,95]. Moreover, negative modulation of the inhibitor CD59 was demonstrated to ameliorate antigen-specific T-cell responses [96]. Overall, the information gathered during the past few decades illustrates the interconnections between the complement system and adaptive and innate immunity and endorses the hypothesis that complement's role extends beyond its traditional non-specific, first-defense function.

Dysregulation of complement can lead to the development of several pathologies. Kidney diseases, such as atypical hemolytic uremic syndrome (aHUS) and C3 glomerulopathies, are closely related to complement anomalies. C3 glomerulopathies are characterized by the production of C3 fragments in the fluid phase via the alternative pathway and abnormal complement consumption that leads to the damage of the glomerular basement membrane [97]. Activation of the complement system is also involved in the pathogenesis of systemic autoimmune diseases [98]. Alterations in regulatory proteins can trigger serious conditions as well. Paroxysmal nocturnal hemoglobinuria (PNH) is a hematological disorder caused by a deficiency in glycosylphosphatidylinositol anchor synthesis that negatively affects the expression of the CRPs CD55 and CD59 [99]. More recently, cancer progression has been associated with complement activation [66].

In the next sections, we review studies that have reported the participation of components of the complement system in the biology of ovarian cancer or its potential clinical use. The findings of these studies are summarized in Tables 1 and 2.

Table 1. Summary of the studies in ovarian cancer cell lines and mouse models reporting tumor-promoting or tumor-suppressing activities mediated by complement components.

Component Type	Complement Component (s)	Role in Cancer	Experimental Setting	Cell Line(s)	In Vivo Model	Mechanism	Ref
Complement effectors and receptors	C1q	Anti-tumor	In vitro	SKOV3	-	Induction of apoptosis	[100]
	gC1qR	Anti-tumor	In vitro	C33a, SiHa	-	Induction of apoptosis	[101]
	gC1qR	Anti-tumor	In vitro	SKOV3, CAOV-3	-	Induction of apoptosis after paclitaxel treatment	[102]
	C3 and C5aR1	Pro-tumor	In vivo	-	Spontaneous model in C57BL/6 TgMISIIR-Tag mice	Inhibition of angiogenesis	[103]
	C3aR and C5aR1	Pro-tumor	In vivo	ID-8 VEGF	Syngenic model in C57BL/6 mice	Autocrine stimulation of tumor growth	[104]
	C3	Pro-tumor	In vivo	ID-8 VEGF	Syngenic model in C57BL/6 mice	Autocrine promotion of EMT	[105]
	C3 and C5aR1	Anti-tumor	In vivo	TC-1	Syngenic model in B6.SJL-PtprcaPep3b/BoyJ mice	Promotion of T-cell homing	[106]
	C5a	Anti-tumor Pro-tumor	In vivo	SKOV-3	Xenograft model in SCID mice	Dose-dependent effect on tumor growth	[107]

Table 1. Cont.

Component Type	Complement Component (s)	Role in Cancer	Experimental Setting	Cell Line(s)	In Vivo Model	Mechanism	Ref
Complement regulators	CD59, CD46, FH, and FHL-1	Pro-tumor	In vitro	Caov-3, SK-OV-3, SW626, PA-1, HUV-EC-C	-	Functional complement activation and regulation occurs locally in ascites	[64]
	CD55	Pro-tumor	In vivo	SK-OV-3	Xenograft model in SCID* mice	Blockade of CD55 leads to improved efficacy of mAb therapy	[108]
	CD55	Pro-tumor	In vivo	A2780, TOV112, CP70, HEC1a	Xenograft model in SCID mice	Silencing of CD55 restores sensitivity to chemotherapy	[109]
	CD59	Pro-tumor	In vivo	A2780	Xenograft model in SCID mice	Silencing of CD59 reduces tumor growth	[110]
	CD59	Pro-tumor	In vitro	SK-OV-3	-	Neutralization improves CDC mediated by mAb therapy	[111]
	CD46 and CD59	Pro-tumor	In vitro	IGROV1, OVCAR3, SKOV3, OAW42, INTOV1, INTOV2	-	Neutralization improves CDC mediated by mAb therapy	[112]
	CD46, CD55, and CD59	Pro-tumor	In vitro	SK-OV-3	-	Silencing of CRPs leads to improved efficacy of mAbs	[113]
	FH, FHL-1, and sCD46	Pro-tumor	In vitro	SK-OV-3, Caov-3, PA-1, SW626	-	Resistance to CDC	[114]

EMT: epithelial-mesenchymal transition, SCID: severe combined immunodeficient, mAb: monoclonal antibody, CDC: complement-dependent cytotoxicity.

Table 2. Summary of the studies performed with clinical samples reporting the potential clinical use of the determination of complement components.

Component Type	Complement Component(s)	Role in Cancer	Type of Sample	Methodology	Stage(s)	Mechanism	Ref
Complement effectors and receptors	C1q	Diagnosis	Serum	Mass spectrometry	III–IV	Overexpression	[115]
	gC1qR	Prognosis	Tissue	IHC	III–IV	Overexpression associated with shorter overall survival	[116]
	MBL and MASP-2	Diagnosis	Serum	ELISA	I–IV	Overexpression	[117]
	Ficolin-2 and ficolin-3	Diagnosis	Serum	ELISA	I–IV	Overexpression	[118]
	C3 and C4	Prediction of response	Plasma	Mass spectrometry	III–IV	Downregulation (C3) or upregulation (C4) in platinum-resistant patients	[119]
	C3	Diagnosis	Serum	Mass spectrometry	I–IV	Downregulation	[120]
	C3 and C5aR1	Prognosis	Tissue	Real-time PCR	I–II	mRNA levels associated with decreased overall survival	[104]

Table 2. Cont.

Component Type	Complement Component(s)	Role in Cancer	Type of Sample	Methodology	Stage(s)	Mechanism	Ref
Complement regulators	CD59, CD46, FH, and FHL-1	Pro-tumor	Ascitic fluid	Immunoblotting, ELISA, IHC	I, III, IV	Complement activation and regulation occurs locally in ascites	[64]
	CD46	Prognosis	Tissue	IHC	I–III	Expression associated with shorter survival	[121]
	CD46 and CD59	Therapy	Tissue	cDNA microarray, IHC	Advanced stage	Neutralization improves CDC mediated by mAb therapy	[112]
	CD46, CD55, and CD59	Pro-tumor	Tissue	IHC	Not specified	Overexpression in malignant tissue	[122]
	FH, FHL-1, and sCD46	Pro-tumor	Ascitic fluid, tissue	ELISA, IHC	III–IV	Overexpression in malignant tissue	[114]

IHC: immunohistochemistry, mAb: monoclonal antibody, CDC: complement-dependent cytotoxicity.

3.1. Complement Initiation Components in Ovarian Cancer

C1q, the first component of the classical complement activation pathway, links innate and adaptive immunity [123]. Both promoting and inhibitory roles have been reported for C1q in cancer progression, but most studies associate C1q expression with poor clinical outcomes in cancer, as is the case for gliomas and osteosarcomas [124,125]. C1q may act as a tumor-promoting factor through both complement-dependent and complement-independent mechanisms [126,127]. In ovarian cancer, the role of C1q appears to be context-dependent. In vitro, C1q displays an anti-tumor effect in SKOV3 cells by promoting apoptosis through the upregulation of the TNF-α pathway and the downregulation of the mammalian target of rapamycin (mTOR) survival pathway [100]. Conversely, expression levels of C1q in circulating extracellular vesicles isolated from ovarian cancer patients in stages III–IV are significantly elevated compared with those isolated from healthy individuals [115]. Discrepancies have also been observed in the case of the globular C1q receptor (gC1qR), a cell surface receptor for C1q. This molecule is upregulated in tumor cells [128], and its overexpression induces mitochondrial dysfunction and p53-dependent apoptosis in human cervical squamous carcinoma cells in vitro [101]. Consistently, the induction of gC1qR expression by paclitaxel in ovarian cancer cell lines SKOV3 and CAOV3 results in mitochondrial dysfunction and cell apoptosis [102]. However, this consistency observed in vitro disappears when clinical samples from ovarian cancer patients at different stages of the disease are analyzed. gC1qR downregulation was observed in ovarian cancer patients in the early stages of the disease (stages I–II) [102]. By contrast, gC1qR seems to be overexpressed in tumor tissue from ovarian cancer patients in stages III and IV, and this is associated with a poor prognosis and cisplatin resistance [116]. These data suggest an increase in complement activation during ovarian cancer progression. Consistent with this assumption, C4 was detected in ascitic fluid from late-stage patients, while it was undetectable in ascitic fluid from healthy donors [64]. Moreover, C4 levels were found to be upregulated in plasma samples from chemoresistant compared with chemosensitive ovarian cancer patients [119]. In the same study, complement factor I and C3 were found to be downregulated [119]. Finally, MBL and MASP2 serum levels are altered in ovarian cancer patients, and MBL levels are associated with advanced disease stages [117]. The ovarian tumor antigen cancer antigen 125 (CA-125), a highly glycosylated protein, may be a target for pattern recognition molecules, such as collectins and ficolins, which may mediate the interaction with MBL and the activation of the lectin pathway [129]. Serum ficolins have been reported to be elevated in ovarian cancer patients despite their lower tumor expression [118]. In conclusion, several studies have reported the presence of complement initiation factors in ovarian cancer. However, the contribution of these factors to ovarian cancer progression and response to treatment is still unclear and requires further investigation.

3.2. C3 and C5 in Ovarian Cancer

The C3- and C5-derived fragments C3a and C5a participate in the establishment of a chronic inflammatory state that may favor tumorigenesis and cancer progression [70]. In ovarian cancer, the implication of C3a and C5a seems to depend on multiple factors, although most of the evidence suggests a tumor-promoting effect. Nuñez-Cruz et al. assessed the role of complement in ovarian tumor progression using C3 and C5aR1-deficient mice. Complement inhibition impaired both tumor vascularization and growth [103]. Some molecular mechanisms have been associated with the tumor-promoting function of C3 and C5 in ovarian cancer tumor cells. These mechanisms include the activation of the phosphatidylinositol-3-kinase (PI3K) pathway and the induction of EMT [104,105]. C3 and C5 and their effector fragments also influence tumor progression by acting on immune cells. Circulating polymorphonuclear cells from ovarian cancer patients can acquire an immunosuppressive phenotype capable of restraining T-cell proliferation after exposure to ascites in a process dependent on C3 [130]. This T-cell non-responsiveness is associated with the production of C5a and is mediated by mTOR signaling and nuclear factor of activated T-cells (NFAT) translocation [131]. Interestingly, C5a may function in a dose-dependent manner. Thus, in a SKOV-3 tumor model, low local doses of C5a reduced tumor growth in association with the recruitment of M1 TAMs and NK cells, while high doses promoted tumor progression [107]. Ovarian cancer cells overexpress ribosomal protein S19 (RPS19), which leads to tumor growth through its interaction with C5aR1 in MDSCs [132]. By contrast, the local production of C3 and the release of C5a disrupt the tumor endothelial barrier, facilitating the homing of T cells and their tumor recruitment [106]. This study further stresses the contrasting effects associated with complement effectors in different models of ovarian cancer. Unfortunately, the results reported in patients do not clarify the matter. High levels of C3 or C5aR1 have been associated with decreased overall survival [104,133]. By contrast, reduced expression of C3 was observed in the blood of ovarian cancer patients [134], and this factor was downregulated in the serum of platinum-resistant patients [119].

3.3. Complement Regulatory Proteins in Ovarian Cancer

CRPs protect host cells from autologous complement attack, but they can render complement ineffective at eliminating cancer cells. Membrane-bound CRPs (mCRPs), such as CD46, CD55, and CD59, are expressed by ovarian cancer tumors [121,135] and cell lines [108,122,135]. These regulators are linked to worse clinical outcomes and may constitute an obstacle for cancer immunotherapy [121,136–138]. Their presence has also been associated with the development of multi-drug resistance in ovarian cancer cells [139]. Neutralization of mCRPs increases the sensitivity to complement-dependent cytotoxicity [111,113,139], reduces ovarian tumor growth [110], and enhances the anti-tumor efficacy of therapeutic antibodies [108,112]. In line with these findings, CD55 silencing restores cisplatin sensitivity to chemotherapy in resistant ovarian cancer cells [109]. Regarding soluble complement regulators, a range of studies has demonstrated their importance in several tumor types [140–143]. In ovarian cancer, some soluble complement inhibitors, such as factor H and factor H-like 1 (FHL-1), have been found in ascitic fluid and primary tumors [64,114]. However, the role of these regulators in ovarian cancer progression has not been defined yet.

In conclusion, the evidence suggests that complement dysregulation drives ovarian cancer progression. Complement effectors, receptors, and regulators have been implicated in different aspects of ovarian cancer biology (Figure 2). Although there are inconsistencies in the description of the role of complement components in some clinical or experimental contexts, the majority of studies point toward a tumor-promoting activity of complement in well-established tumors. These findings have paved the way for studies aimed to potentiate cancer therapies through the modulation of the complement system.

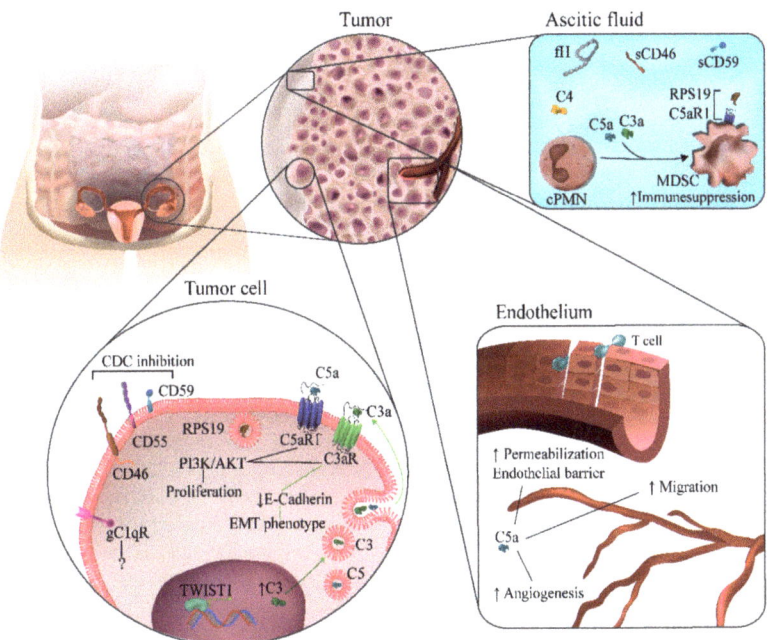

Figure 2. Complement-related mechanisms associated with ovarian cancer progression. Complement components have been implicated in different biological processes associated with ovarian cancer progression. They include modulation of immunosuppression in the tumor microenvironment; regulation of angiogenesis and endothelial permeabilization; autocrine and paracrine effects in tumor cells mediated by C1q, C3a, or C5a; and inhibition of complement-dependent cytotoxicity (CDC) by membrane-bound complement regulators.

4. Therapeutic Potential of Targeting Complement in Ovarian Cancer

Complement inhibition may be a useful therapeutic strategy against cancer [19]. Agonists of C5aR1 and C3aR increase ovarian tumor cell proliferation, migration, and invasion, suggesting that receptor antagonists could be used to block cancer growth [104]. Complement targeting may also impair angiogenesis, a highly relevant biological process in ovarian cancer. Elevated levels of serum VEGF after chemotherapy treatment have been associated with lower overall survival in ovarian cancer patients [144], and the anti-VEGF antibody bevacizumab has shown therapeutic activity in both patients and animal models [145–147]. Genetic or pharmacological inhibition of C3 or C5aR1 results in smaller and poorly vascularized ovarian tumors in vivo [103], and C5a is able to promote endothelial cell tube formation and migration [103,148]. Therefore, it can be speculated that inhibition of complement may potentiate the efficacy of anti-angiogenic agents.

Another scenario in which complement modulation may be of special relevance is immunotherapy. We previously described the implication of effectors and regulators of the complement system in the ability of T cells to infiltrate tumors and the response against tumor-associated antigens [149]. Using various models of lung cancer, we proposed that the modulation of complement activation can improve the antitumor efficacy of monoclonal antibodies targeting the PD-1/PD-L1 pathway [150]. This synergistic effect has also been reported in other tumor models targeting C5a/C5aR1 [151,152] or C3a/C3aR [151,153]. To our knowledge, these combinations have not been tested yet in models of ovarian cancer, and we can only hypothesize about the outcome of these studies. The inhibition of C3 or C5aR1 abrogates the suppressor phenotype of MDSCs in the ovarian TME [130,131], suggesting that complement inhibition may have a positive effect on the efficacy of anti-PD-1/PD-L1 therapies. Conversely, antitumor T cells require the production of C3 and the release of C5a in the endothelium in order to infiltrate ovarian tumors [106]. The targeting of mCRPs should also be considered in light of their relevance in the TME [136]. The inhibition of mCRPs may be used to sensitize tumors to other drugs. In ovarian cancer, the neutralization of CD46, CD55, and CD59 in combination with the anti-HER2 monoclonal antibodies trastuzumab and pertuzumab induces tumor cell killing in vitro [113]. Nevertheless, considering the dual role of complement molecules in ovarian tumors, in vivo studies are needed to determine whether complement inhibition has any impact on the response to checkpoint-based or antibody-based immunotherapies, and in which direction.

5. The Need for Preclinical Models to Better Delineate the Role of Complement in Ovarian Cancer

In this review, we discussed the functions that complement components exert in the biology of ovarian tumors. Many questions remain regarding the conflicting results observed in different experimental settings. To address these questions, in vivo models that faithfully recapitulate the complexity of the disease are needed. Currently, there are a few animal models established for the study of ovarian cancer. These include genetically engineered mouse models, xenograft cell transplants of human cell lines, and patient-derived xenografts [154]. These models have facilitated the study of many mechanisms associated with ovarian cancer progression and have allowed the evaluation of many therapeutic molecules [155]. For the study of complement-related mechanisms or treatments, mouse models that capture the complexity of the TME are required. Models based on syngeneic tumor cells injected intraperitoneally in immunocompetent mice represent a practical option. Some studies have used the syngeneic intraperitoneal injection of ID-8-MOSEC, a mouse epithelial ovarian cancer cell line originating in C57BL/6 mice, to evaluate the roles of C3, C5, and C5aR1 in ovarian cancer development and progression (Table 1) [104,106]. This cell line was developed by Dr. Katherine F. Roby in the Department of Anatomy and Cell Biology of the University of Kansas in the early 2000s, and it is one of the most frequently used ovarian cancer cell lines since it has the capacity to induce tumor peritoneal implants observed in stages III and IV [156]. Because of its slow growth rate, some strategies have been developed to increase the aggressiveness of this cell line, including the overexpression of dendritic cell chemoattractant beta-defensin 29 (Defb29) or VEGF [157], two factors associated with increased invasiveness. Nevertheless, this model does not completely recapitulate the human pathophysiology of the disease and does not exactly reproduce the TME [154]. The development of better ovarian cancer models is needed to unravel the mechanisms by which complement components modulate ovarian cancer progression and to evaluate complement-based therapeutic combinations.

6. Conclusions

A growing body of literature suggests that the complement system is involved in ovarian cancer progression. Nevertheless, the specific role of the different complement components in different clinical scenarios has just started to be unraveled, and many answers remain elusive. The molecular heterogeneity of ovarian cancers and the complexity of the biological interactions in the ovarian TME pose a challenge to our understanding of the mechanisms underlying the complement-associated immune responses and the identification of adequate therapeutic targets. The situation is aggravated by the lack of preclinical models that reliably recreate ovarian cancer traits. Therefore, further studies are needed to better delineate the complement-related mechanisms associated with ovarian cancer progression as well as to determine how complement activation should be modulated to treat ovarian cancer patients.

Author Contributions: Y.S., D.A., R.P., and B.T. conceived and designed the manuscript. All authors (Y.S., D.A., A.G.-M., R.P., and B.T.) wrote the manuscript. Y.S. prepared the figures. All authors have read and agreed to the published version of the manuscript.

Funding: The authors' work was supported by the Foundation for Applied Medical Research (FIMA), Centro de Investigación Biomédica en Red Cáncer (CIBERONC), Grupo Español de Investigación en Cáncer de Ovario (GEICO), Fundación Ramón Areces, and Instituto de Salud Carlos III-EU FEDER "Una manera de hacer Europa" (PI20/00419 and PI20/00959). YS was supported by a predoctoral fellowship from Ministerio de Ciencia, Innovación y Universidades (FPU18/02638).

Conflicts of Interest: D.A. and R.P. are authors of patents and patent applications claiming the determination of complement fragments for lung cancer diagnosis. No potential competing interests are disclosed by the other authors.

References

1. Wild, C.; Weiderpass, E.; Stewart, B.W. (Eds.) *World Cancer Report: Cancer Research for Cancer Prevention*; IARC Press: Lyon, France, 2020; ISBN 9789283204299.
2. National Cancer Institute. Cancer Stat Facts: Ovarian Cancer. Available online: https://seer.cancer.gov/statfacts/html/ovary.html (accessed on 15 July 2021).
3. Jayson, G.C.; Kohn, E.C.; Kitchener, H.C.; Ledermann, J.A. Ovarian cancer. *Lancet* **2014**, *384*, 1376–1388. [CrossRef]
4. Torre, L.A.; Trabert, B.; DeSantis, C.E.; Miller, K.D.; Samimi, G.; Runowicz, C.D.; Gaudet, M.M.; Jemal, A.; Siegel, R.L. Ovarian cancer statistics, 2018. *CA Cancer J. Clin.* **2018**, *68*, 284–296. [CrossRef]
5. Marth, C.; Reimer, D.; Zeimet, A.G. Front-line therapy of advanced epithelial ovarian cancer: Standard treatment. *Ann. Oncol.* **2017**, *28*, viii36–viii39. [CrossRef]
6. Lampert, E.J.; Zimmer, A.; Padget, M.; Cimino-Mathews, A.; Nair, J.R.; Liu, Y.; Swisher, E.M.; Hodge, J.W.; Nixon, A.B.; Nichols, E.; et al. Combination of PARP inhibitor Olaparib, and PD-L1 inhibitor Durvalumab, in recurrent ovarian cancer: A proof-of-concept phase II study. *Clin. Cancer Res.* **2020**, *26*, 4268–47279. [CrossRef]
7. Jain, S.; Annett, S.L.; Morgan, M.P.; Robson, T. The cancer stem cell niche in ovarian cancer and its impact on immune surveillance. *Int. J. Mol. Sci.* **2021**, *22*, 4091. [CrossRef]
8. Ghisoni, E.; Imbimbo, M.; Zimmermann, S.; Valabrega, G. Ovarian cancer immunotherapy: Turning up the heat. *Int. J. Mol. Sci.* **2019**, *20*, 2927. [CrossRef]
9. Kandalaft, L.E.; Motz, G.T.; Duraiswamy, J.; Coukos, G. Tumor immune surveillance and ovarian cancer: Lessons on immune mediated tumor rejection or tolerance. *Cancer Metastasis Rev.* **2011**, *30*, 141–151. [CrossRef]
10. Hamanishi, J.; Mandai, M.; Iwasaki, M.; Okazaki, T.; Tanaka, Y.; Yamaguchi, K.; Higuchi, T.; Yagi, H.; Takakura, K.; Minato, N.; et al. Programmed cell death 1 ligand 1 and tumor-infiltrating CD8+ T lymphocytes are prognostic factors of human ovarian cancer. *Proc. Natl. Acad. Sci. USA* **2007**, *104*, 3360–3365. [CrossRef]
11. Zhang, L.; Conejo-Garcia, J.R.; Katsaros, D.; Gimotty, P.A.; Massobrio, M.; Regnani, G.; Makrigiannakis, A.; Gray, H.; Schlienger, K.; Liebman, M.N.; et al. Intratumoral T cells, recurrence, and survival in epithelial ovarian cancer. *N. Engl. J. Med.* **2003**, *348*, 203–213. [CrossRef]
12. Curiel, T.J.; Coukos, G.; Zou, L.; Alvarez, X.; Cheng, P.; Mottram, P.; Evdemon-Hogan, M.; Conejo-Garcia, J.R.; Zhang, L.; Burow, M.; et al. Specific recruitment of regulatory T cells in ovarian carcinoma fosters immune privilege and predicts reduced survival. *Nat. Med.* **2004**, *10*, 942–949. [CrossRef]
13. Disis, M.L.; Taylor, M.H.; Kelly, K.; Beck, J.T.; Gordon, M.; Moore, K.M.; Patel, M.R.; Chaves, J.; Park, H.; Mita, A.C.; et al. Efficacy and safety of Avelumab for patients with recurrent or refractory ovarian cancer: Phase 1b results from the JAVELIN solid tumor trial. *JAMA Oncol.* **2019**, *5*, 393–401. [CrossRef] [PubMed]
14. Hamanishi, J.; Mandai, M.; Ikeda, T.; Minami, M.; Kawaguchi, A.; Murayama, T.; Kanai, M.; Mori, Y.; Matsumoto, S.; Chikuma, S.; et al. Safety and antitumor activity of Anti-PD-1 antibody, nivolumab, in patients with platinum-resistant ovarian cancer. *J. Clin. Oncol.* **2015**, *33*, 4015–4022. [CrossRef]
15. Hartl, C.A.; Bertschi, A.; Puerto, R.B.; Andresen, C.; Cheney, E.M.; Mittendorf, E.A.; Guerriero, J.L.; Goldberg, M.S. Combination therapy targeting both innate and adaptive immunity improves survival in a pre-clinical model of ovarian cancer. *J. Immunother. Cancer* **2019**, *7*, 199. [CrossRef] [PubMed]
16. Baci, D.; Bosi, A.; Gallazzi, M.; Rizzi, M.; Noonan, D.M.; Poggi, A.; Bruno, A.; Mortara, L. The Ovarian Cancer Tumor Immune Microenvironment (TIME) as target for therapy: A focus on innate immunity cells as therapeutic effectors. *Int. J. Mol. Sci.* **2020**, *21*, 3125. [CrossRef]
17. Dunkelberger, J.R.; Song, W.-C. Complement and its role in innate and adaptive immune responses. *Cell Res.* **2010**, *20*, 34–50. [CrossRef]
18. Ricklin, D.; Hajishengallis, G.; Yang, K.; Lambris, J.D. Complement: A key system for immune surveillance and homeostasis. *Nat. Immunol.* **2010**, *11*, 785–797. [CrossRef]
19. Pio, R.; Ajona, D.; Lambris, J.D. Complement inhibition in cancer therapy. *Semin. Immunol.* **2013**, *25*, 54–64. [CrossRef]

20. Ajona, D.; Ortiz-Espinosa, S.; Pio, R.; Lecanda, F. Complement in metastasis: A comp in the camp. *Front. Immunol.* **2019**, *10*, 669. [CrossRef]
21. Hanahan, D.; Weinberg, R.A. Hallmarks of cancer: The next generation. *Cell* **2011**, *144*, 646–674. [CrossRef]
22. Vesely, M.D.; Schreiber, R.D. Cancer immunoediting: Antigens, mechanisms, and implications to cancer immunotherapy. *Ann. N. Y. Acad. Sci.* **2013**, *1284*, 1–5. [CrossRef] [PubMed]
23. Rodriguez, G.; Galpin, K.; McCloskey, C.; Vanderhyden, B. The tumor microenvironment of epithelial ovarian cancer and its influence on response to immunotherapy. *Cancers* **2018**, *10*, 242. [CrossRef]
24. Jiménez-Sánchez, A.; Memon, D.; Pourpe, S.; Veeraraghavan, H.; Li, Y.; Vargas, H.A.; Gill, M.B.; Park, K.J.; Zivanovic, O.; Konner, J.; et al. Heterogeneous tumor-immune microenvironments among differentially growing metastases in an ovarian cancer patient. *Cell* **2017**, *170*, 927–938.e20. [CrossRef]
25. Hendry, S.; Salgado, R.; Gevaert, T.; Russell, P.A.; John, T.; Thapa, B.; Christie, M.; van de Vijver, K.; Estrada, M.V.; Gonzalez-Ericsson, P.I.; et al. Assessing tumor-infiltrating lymphocytes in solid tumors: A practical review for pathologists and proposal for a standardized method from the international immuno-oncology biomarkers working group: Part 2: TILs in melanoma, gastrointestinal tract carcinoma. *Adv. Anat. Pathol.* **2017**, *24*, 311–335. [CrossRef]
26. Scheper, W.; Kelderman, S.; Fanchi, L.F.; Linnemann, C.; Bendle, G.; de Rooij, M.A.J.; Hirt, C.; Mezzadra, R.; Slagter, M.; Dijkstra, K.; et al. Low and variable tumor reactivity of the intratumoral TCR repertoire in human cancers. *Nat. Med.* **2019**, *25*, 89–94. [CrossRef]
27. Wherry, E.J.; Kurachi, M. Molecular and cellular insights into T cell exhaustion. *Nat. Rev. Immunol.* **2015**, *15*, 486–499. [CrossRef]
28. Zhang, S.; Ke, X.; Zeng, S.; Wu, M.; Lou, J.; Wu, L.; Huang, P.; Huang, L.; Wang, F.; Pan, S. Analysis of CD8+ Treg cells in patients with ovarian cancer: A possible mechanism for immune impairment. *Cell. Mol. Immunol.* **2015**, *12*, 580–591. [CrossRef]
29. Maj, T.; Wang, W.; Crespo, J.; Zhang, H.; Wang, W.; Wei, S.; Zhao, L.; Vatan, L.; Shao, I.; Szeliga, W.; et al. Oxidative stress controls regulatory T cell apoptosis and suppressor activity and PD-L1-blockade resistance in tumor. *Nat. Immunol.* **2017**, *18*, 1332–1341. [CrossRef] [PubMed]
30. Chen, Y.L.; Chang, M.C.; Chen, C.A.; Lin, H.W.; Cheng, W.F.; Chien, C.L. Depletion of regulatory T lymphocytes reverses the imbalance between pro- and anti-tumor immunities via enhancing antigen-specific T cell immune responses. *PLoS ONE* **2012**, *7*, e47190. [CrossRef]
31. Pesce, S.; Greppi, M.; Tabellini, G.; Rampinelli, F.; Parolini, S.; Olive, D.; Moretta, L.; Moretta, A.; Marcenaro, E. Identification of a subset of human natural killer cells expressing high levels of programmed death 1: A phenotypic and functional characterization. *J. Allergy Clin. Immunol.* **2017**, *139*, 335–346.e3. [CrossRef]
32. Milne, K.; Köbel, M.; Kalloger, S.E.; Barnes, R.O.; Gao, D.; Gilks, C.B.; Watson, P.H.; Nelson, B.H. Systematic analysis of immune infiltrates in high-grade serous ovarian cancer reveals CD20, FoxP3 and TIA-1 as positive prognostic factors. *PLoS ONE* **2009**, *4*, e6412. [CrossRef]
33. Montfort, A.; Pearce, O.; Maniati, E.; Vincent, B.G.; Bixby, L.; Böhm, S.; Dowe, T.; Wilkes, E.H.; Chakravarty, P.; Thompson, R.; et al. A strong B-cell response is part of the immune landscape in human high-grade serous ovarian metastases. *Clin. Cancer Res.* **2017**, *23*, 250–262. [CrossRef] [PubMed]
34. Truxova, I.; Kasikova, L.; Hensler, M.; Skapa, P.; Laco, J.; Pecen, L.; Belicova, L.; Praznovec, I.; Halaska, M.J.; Brtnicky, T.; et al. Mature dendritic cells correlate with favorable immune infiltrate and improved prognosis in ovarian carcinoma patients. *J. Immunother. Cancer* **2018**, *6*, 139. [CrossRef]
35. Curiel, T.J.; Wei, S.; Dong, H.; Alvarez, X.; Cheng, P.; Mottram, P.; Krzysiek, R.; Knutson, K.L.; Daniel, B.; Zimmermann, M.C.; et al. Blockade of B7-H1 improves myeloid dendritic cell-mediated antitumor immunity. *Nat. Med.* **2003**, *9*, 562–567. [CrossRef]
36. Cubillos-Ruiz, J.R.; Silberman, P.C.; Rutkowski, M.R.; Chopra, S.; Perales-Puchalt, A.; Song, M.; Zhang, S.; Bettigole, S.E.; Gupta, D.; Holcomb, K.; et al. ER stress sensor XBP1 controls anti-tumor immunity by disrupting dendritic cell homeostasis. *Cell* **2015**, *161*, 1527–1538. [CrossRef]
37. Brencicova, E.; Jagger, A.L.; Evans, H.G.; Georgouli, M.; Laios, A.; Montalto, S.A.; Mehra, G.; Spencer, J.; Ahmed, A.A.; Raju-Kankipati, S.; et al. Interleukin-10 and prostaglandin E2 have complementary but distinct suppressive effects on Toll-like receptor-mediated dendritic cell activation in ovarian carcinoma. *PLoS ONE* **2017**, *12*, e0175712. [CrossRef]
38. Obermajer, N.; Muthuswamy, R.; Lesnock, J.; Edwards, R.P.; Kalinski, P. Positive feedback between PGE2 and COX2 redirects the differentiation of human dendritic cells toward stable myeloid-derived suppressor cells. *Blood* **2011**, *118*, 5498–5505. [CrossRef] [PubMed]
39. Veglia, F.; Perego, M.; Gabrilovich, D. Myeloid-derived suppressor cells coming of age review-article. *Nat. Immunol.* **2018**, *19*, 108–119. [CrossRef]
40. Rodríguez-Ubreva, J.; Català-Moll, F.; Obermajer, N.; Álvarez-Errico, D.; Ramirez, R.N.; Company, C.; Vento-Tormo, R.; Moreno-Bueno, G.; Edwards, R.P.; Mortazavi, A.; et al. Prostaglandin E2 leads to the acquisition of DNMT3A-dependent tolerogenic functions in human myeloid-derived suppressor cells. *Cell Rep.* **2017**, *21*, 154–167. [CrossRef] [PubMed]
41. Taki, M.; Abiko, K.; Baba, T.; Hamanishi, J.; Yamaguchi, K.; Murakami, R.; Yamanoi, K.; Horikawa, N.; Hosoe, Y.; Nakamura, E.; et al. Snail promotes ovarian cancer progression by recruiting myeloid-derived suppressor cells via CXCR2 ligand upregulation. *Nat. Commun.* **2018**, *9*, 1685. [CrossRef]

42. Trillo-Tinoco, J.; Sierra, R.A.; Mohamed, E.; Cao, Y.; de Mingo-Pulido, A.; Gilvary, D.L.; Anadon, C.M.; Costich, T.L.; Wei, S.; Flores, E.R.; et al. AMPK alpha-1 intrinsically regulates the function and differentiation of tumor myeloid-derived suppressor cells. *Cancer Res.* **2019**, *79*, 5034–5047. [CrossRef]
43. Charles, K.A.; Kulbe, H.; Soper, R.; Escorcio-Correia, M.; Lawrence, T.; Schultheis, A.; Chakravarty, P.; Thompson, R.G.; Kollias, G.; Smyth, J.F.; et al. The tumor-promoting actions of TNF-α involve TNFR1 and IL-17 in ovarian cancer in mice and humans. *J. Clin. Investig.* **2009**, *119*, 3011–3023. [CrossRef] [PubMed]
44. Obermajer, N.; Wong, J.L.; Edwards, R.P.; Chen, K.; Scott, M.; Khader, S.; Kolls, J.K.; Odunsi, K.; Billiar, T.R.; Kalinski, P. Induction and stability of human Th17 cells require endogenous NOS2 and cGMP-dependent NO signaling. *J. Exp. Med.* **2013**, *210*, 1433–1445. [CrossRef] [PubMed]
45. Yoshida, M.; Taguchi, A.; Kawana, K.; Ogishima, J.; Adachi, K.; Kawata, A.; Nakamura, H.; Sato, M.; Fujimoto, A.; Inoue, T.; et al. Intraperitoneal neutrophils activated by KRAS-induced ovarian cancer exert antitumor effects by modulating adaptive immunity. *Int. J. Oncol.* **2018**, *53*, 1580–1590. [CrossRef]
46. Singel, K.L.; Grzankowski, K.S.; Khan, A.N.M.N.H.; Grimm, M.J.; D'Auria, A.C.; Morrell, K.; Eng, K.H.; Hylander, B.; Mayor, P.C.; Emmons, T.R.; et al. Mitochondrial DNA in the tumour microenvironment activates neutrophils and is associated with worse outcomes in patients with advanced epithelial ovarian cancer. *Br. J. Cancer* **2019**, *120*, 207–217. [CrossRef] [PubMed]
47. Teijeira, A.; Garasa, S.; Ochoa, M.C.; Villalba, M.; Olivera, I.; Cirella, A.; Eguren-Santamaria, I.; Berraondo, P.; Schalper, K.A.; de Andrea, C.E.; et al. IL8, neutrophils, and NETs in a collusion against cancer immunity and immunotherapy. *Clin. Cancer Res.* **2021**, *27*, 2383–2393. [CrossRef]
48. Giese, M.A.; Hind, L.E.; Huttenlocher, A. Neutrophil plasticity in the tumor microenvironment. *Blood* **2019**, *133*, 2159–2167. [CrossRef]
49. Yousefzadeh, Y.; Hallaj, S.; Baghi Moornani, M.; Asghary, A.; Azizi, G.; Hojjat-Farsangi, M.; Ghalamfarsa, G.; Jadidi-Niaragh, F. Tumor associated macrophages in the molecular pathogenesis of ovarian cancer. *Int. Immunopharmacol.* **2020**, *84*, 106471. [CrossRef]
50. Gupta, V.; Yull, F.; Khabele, D. Bipolar tumor-associated macrophages in ovarian cancer as targets for therapy. *Cancers* **2018**, *10*, 366. [CrossRef] [PubMed]
51. Maccio, A.; Gramignano, G.; Cherchi, M.C.; Tanca, L.; Melis, L.; Madeddu, C. Role of M1-polarized tumor-associated macrophages in the prognosis of advanced ovarian cancer patients. *Sci. Rep.* **2020**, *10*, 6096. [CrossRef]
52. Reinartz, S.; Schumann, T.; Finkernagel, F.; Wortmann, A.; Jansen, J.M.; Meissner, W.; Krause, M.; Schwörer, A.M.; Wagner, U.; Müller-Brüsselbach, S.; et al. Mixed-polarization phenotype of ascites-associated macrophages in human ovarian carcinoma: Correlation of CD163 expression, cytokine levels and early relapse. *Int. J. Cancer* **2014**, *134*, 32–42. [CrossRef]
53. Cortés, M.; Sanchez-Moral, L.; de Barrios, O.; Fernández-Aceñero, M.J.; Martínez-Campanario, M.; Esteve-Codina, A.; Darling, D.S.; Győrffy, B.; Lawrence, T.; Dean, D.C.; et al. Tumor-associated macrophages (TAMs) depend on ZEB1 for their cancer-promoting roles. *EMBO J.* **2017**, *36*, 3336–3355. [CrossRef]
54. Barkal, A.A.; Brewer, R.E.; Markovic, M.; Kowarsky, M.; Barkal, S.A.; Zaro, B.W.; Krishnan, V.; Hatakeyama, J.; Dorigo, O.; Barkal, L.J.; et al. CD24 signalling through macrophage Siglec-10 is a target for cancer immunotherapy. *Nature* **2019**, *572*, 392–396. [CrossRef]
55. Hagemann, T.; Wilson, J.; Burke, F.; Kulbe, H.; Li, N.F.; Plüddemann, A.; Charles, K.; Gordon, S.; Balkwill, F.R. Ovarian cancer cells polarize macrophages toward a tumor-associated phenotype. *J. Immunol.* **2006**, *176*, 5023–5032. [CrossRef]
56. Goossens, P.; Rodriguez-Vita, J.; Etzerodt, A.; Masse, M.; Rastoin, O.; Gouirand, V.; Ulas, T.; Papantonopoulou, O.; Van Eck, M.; Auphan-Anezin, N.; et al. Membrane cholesterol efflux drives tumor-associated macrophage reprogramming and tumor progression. *Cell Metab.* **2019**, *29*, 1376–1389.e4. [CrossRef] [PubMed]
57. Yin, M.; Li, X.; Tan, S.; Zhou, H.J.; Ji, W.; Bellone, S.; Xu, X.; Zhang, H.; Santin, A.D.; Lou, G.; et al. Tumor-associated macrophages drive spheroid formation during early transcoelomic metastasis of ovarian cancer. *J. Clin. Investig.* **2016**, *126*, 4157–4173. [CrossRef] [PubMed]
58. Hagemann, T.; Wilson, J.; Kulbe, H.; Li, N.F.; Leinster, D.A.; Charles, K.; Klemm, F.; Pukrop, T.; Binder, C.; Balkwill, F.R. Macrophages induce invasiveness of epithelial cancer cells via NF-κB and JNK. *J. Immunol.* **2005**, *175*, 1197–1205. [CrossRef] [PubMed]
59. Gong, Y.; Yang, J.; Wang, Y.; Xue, L.; Wang, J. Metabolic factors contribute to T-cell inhibition in the ovarian cancer ascites. *Int. J. Cancer* **2020**, *147*, 1768–1777. [CrossRef] [PubMed]
60. Briukhovetska, D.; Dörr, J.; Endres, S.; Libby, P.; Dinarello, C.A.; Kobold, S. Interleukins in cancer: From biology to therapy. *Nat. Rev. Cancer* **2021**, *21*, 481–499. [CrossRef] [PubMed]
61. Chulpanova, D.S.; Kitaeva, K.V.; Green, A.R.; Rizvanov, A.A.; Solovyeva, V.V. Molecular aspects and future perspectives of cytokine-based anti-cancer immunotherapy. *Front. Cell Dev. Biol.* **2020**, *8*, 402. [CrossRef]
62. Conlon, K.C.; Miljkovic, M.D.; Waldmann, T.A. Cytokines in the treatment of cancer. *J. Interf. Cytokine Res.* **2019**, *39*, 6–21. [CrossRef]
63. Jiang, Y.; Wang, C.; Zhou, S. Targeting tumor microenvironment in ovarian cancer: Premise and promise. *Biochim. Biophys. Acta Rev. Cancer* **2020**, *1873*, 188361. [CrossRef]
64. Bjørge, L.; Hakulinen, J.; Vintermyr, O.K.; Jarva, H.; Jensen, T.S.; Iversen, O.E.; Meri, S. Ascitic complement system in ovarian cancer. *Br. J. Cancer* **2005**, *92*, 895–905. [CrossRef] [PubMed]

65. Roumenina, L.T.; Daugan, M.V.; Petitprez, F.; Sautès-Fridman, C.; Fridman, W.H. Context-dependent roles of complement in cancer. *Nat. Rev. Cancer* **2019**, *19*, 698–715. [CrossRef]
66. Pio, R.; Corrales, L.; Lambris, J.D. The role of complement in tumor growth. *Adv. Exp. Med. Biol.* **2014**, *772*, 229–262. [CrossRef]
67. Suryawanshi, S.; Huang, X.; Elishaev, E.; Budiu, R.A.; Zhang, L.; Kim, S.; Donnellan, N.; Mantia-Smaldone, G.; Ma, T.; Tseng, G.; et al. Complement pathway is frequently altered in endometriosis and endometriosis-associated ovarian cancer. *Clin. Cancer Res.* **2014**, *20*, 6163–6174. [CrossRef]
68. Merle, N.S.; Church, S.E.; Fremeaux-Bacchi, V.; Roumenina, L.T. Complement system part I-Molecular mechanisms of activation and regulation. *Front. Immunol.* **2015**, *6*, 262. [CrossRef] [PubMed]
69. Sarma, J.V.; Ward, P.A. The complement system. *Cell Tissue Res.* **2011**, *343*, 227–235. [CrossRef]
70. Ajona, D.; Ortiz-Espinosa, S.; Pio, R. Complement anaphylatoxins C3a and C5a: Emerging roles in cancer progression and treatment. *Semin. Cell Dev. Biol.* **2019**, *85*, 153–163. [CrossRef] [PubMed]
71. Hawksworth, O.A.; Li, X.X.; Coulthard, L.G.; Wolvetang, E.J.; Woodruff, T.M. New concepts on the therapeutic control of complement anaphylatoxin receptors. *Mol. Immunol.* **2017**, *89*, 36–43. [CrossRef]
72. Carroll, M.C. Complement and humoral immunity. *Vaccine* **2008**, *26*, I28–I33. [CrossRef]
73. Finco, O.; Li, S.; Cuccia, M.; Rosen, F.S.; Carroll, M.C. Structural differences between the two human complement C4 isotypes affect the humoral lmmune response. *J. Exp. Med.* **1992**, *175*, 537–543. [CrossRef]
74. O'Neil, K.M.; Ochs, H.D.; Heller, S.R.; Cork, L.C.; Morris, J.M.; Winkelstein, J.A. Role of C3 in humoral immunity. Defective antibody production in C3-deficient dogs. *J. Immunol.* **1988**, *140*, 1939–1945.
75. Pepys, M.B. Role of complement in induction of the allergic response. *Nat. New Biol.* **1972**, *237*, 157–159. [CrossRef]
76. Ochs, H.D.; Wedgwood, R.J.; Frank, M.M.; Heller, S.R.; Hosea, S.W. The role of complement in the induction of antibody responses. *Clin. Exp. Immunol.* **1983**, *53*, 208–216.
77. Fang, Y.; Xu, C.; Fu, Y.X.; Holers, V.M.; Molina, H. Expression of complement receptors 1 and 2 on follicular dendritic cells is necessary for the generation of a strong antigen-specific IgG response. *J. Immunol.* **1998**, *160*, 5273–5279.
78. Fearon, D.T.; Carroll, M.C.; Carroll, M.C. Regulation of B lymphocyte responses to foreign and self-antigens by the CD19/CD21 complex. *Annu. Rev. Immunol.* **2000**, *18*, 393–422. [CrossRef] [PubMed]
79. Barrington, R.A.; Zhang, M.; Zhong, X.; Jonsson, H.; Holodick, N.; Cherukuri, A.; Pierce, S.K.; Rothstein, T.L.; Carroll, M.C. CD21/CD19 coreceptor signaling promotes b cell survival during primary immune responses. *J. Immunol.* **2005**, *175*, 2859–2867. [CrossRef]
80. Fischer, W.H.; Hugli, T.E. Regulation of B cell functions by C3a and C3a(desArg): Suppression of TNF-alpha, IL-6, and the polyclonal immune response. *J. Immunol.* **1997**, *159*, 4279–4286. [PubMed]
81. Morgan, E.L.; Weigle, W.O.; Hugli, T.E. Anaphylatoxin-mediated regulation of the immune response. I. C3a-mediated suppression of human and murine humoral immune responses. *J. Exp. Med.* **1982**, *155*, 1412–1426. [CrossRef]
82. Kobayakawa, K.; Ohkawa, Y.; Yoshizaki, S.; Tamaru, T.; Saito, T.; Kijima, K.; Yokota, K.; Hara, M.; Kubota, K.; Matsumoto, Y.; et al. Macrophage centripetal migration drives spontaneous healing process after spinal cord injury. *Sci. Adv.* **2019**, *5*, eaav5086. [CrossRef] [PubMed]
83. Sozzoni, S.; Sallusto, F.; Luini, W.; Zhou, D.; Piemonti, L.; Allavena, P.; Van Damme, J.; Valitutti, S.; Lanzavecchia, A.; Mantovani, A. Migration of dendritic cells in response to formyl peptides, C5a, and a distinct set of chemokines. *J. Immunol.* **1995**, *155*, 3292–3295.
84. Riedemann, N.C.; Guo, R.-F.; Gao, H.; Sun, L.; Hoesel, M.; Hollmann, T.J.; Wetsel, R.A.; Zetoune, F.S.; Ward, P.A. Regulatory role of C5a on macrophage migration inhibitory factor release from neutrophils. *J. Immunol.* **2004**, *173*, 1355–1359. [CrossRef] [PubMed]
85. Markiewski, M.M.; DeAngelis, R.A.; Benencia, F.; Ricklin-Lichtsteiner, S.K.; Koutoulaki, A.; Gerard, C.; Coukos, G.; Lambris, J.D. Modulation of the antitumor immune response by complement. *Nat. Immunol.* **2008**, *9*, 1225–1235. [CrossRef] [PubMed]
86. Kupp, L.I.; Kosco, M.H.; Schenkein, H.A.; Tew, J.G. Chemotaxis of germinal centers B cells in response to C5a. *Eur. J. Immunol.* **1991**, *21*, 2697–2701. [CrossRef] [PubMed]
87. Yang, D.; Chen, Q.; Stoll, S.; Chen, X.; Howard, O.M.Z.; Oppenheim, J.J. Differential regulation of responsiveness to fMLP and C5a upon dendritic cell maturation: Correlation with receptor expression. *J. Immunol.* **2000**, *165*, 2694–2702. [CrossRef]
88. Kim, S.-H.; Cho, B.-H.; Kim, K.S.; Jang, Y.-S. Complement C5a promotes antigen cross-presentation by Peyer's patch monocyte-derived dendritic cells and drives a protective CD8+ T cell response. *Cell Rep.* **2021**, *35*, 108995. [CrossRef]
89. Soruri, A.; Riggert, J.; Schlott, T.; Kiafard, Z.; Dettmer, C.; Zwirner, J. Anaphylatoxin C5a induces monocyte recruitment and differentiation into dendritic cells by TNF-α and prostaglandin E2-dependent mechanisms. *J. Immunol.* **2003**, *171*, 2631–2636. [CrossRef]
90. Cravedi, P.; Leventhal, J.; Lakhani, P.; Ward, S.C.; Donovan, M.J.; Heeger, P.S. Immune cell-derived C3a and C5a costimulate human T cell alloimmunity. *Am. J. Transplant.* **2013**, *13*, 2530–2539. [CrossRef]
91. Lalli, P.N.; Strainic, M.G.; Yang, M.; Lin, F.; Medof, M.E.; Heeger, P.S. Locally produced C5a binds to T cell–expressed C5aR to enhance effector T-cell expansion by limiting antigen-induced apoptosis. *Blood* **2008**, *112*, 1759–1766. [CrossRef]
92. Kwan, W.; van der Touw, W.; Paz-Artal, E.; Li, M.O.; Heeger, P.S. Signaling through C5a receptor and C3a receptor diminishes function of murine natural regulatory T cells. *J. Exp. Med.* **2013**, *210*, 257–268. [CrossRef]

93. Strainic, M.G.; Shevach, E.M.; An, F.; Lin, F.; Medof, M.E. Absence of signaling into CD4+ cells via C3aR and C5aR enables autoinductive TGF-β1 signaling and induction of Foxp3+ regulatory T cells. *Nat. Immunol.* **2013**, *14*, 162–171. [CrossRef] [PubMed]
94. Le Friec, G.; Sheppard, D.; Whiteman, P.; Karsten, C.M.; Shamoun, S.A.-T.; Laing, A.; Bugeon, L.; Dallman, M.J.; Melchionna, T.; Chillakuri, C.; et al. The CD46-Jagged1 interaction is critical for human TH1 immunity. *Nat. Immunol.* **2012**, *13*, 1213–1221. [CrossRef]
95. Cardone, J.; Le Friec, G.; Vantourout, P.; Roberts, A.; Fuchs, A.; Jackson, I.; Suddason, T.; Lord, G.; Atkinson, J.P.; Cope, A.; et al. Complement regulator CD46 temporally regulates cytokine production by conventional and unconventional T cells. *Nat. Immunol.* **2010**, *11*, 862–871. [CrossRef] [PubMed]
96. Sivasankar, B.; Longhi, M.P.; Gallagher, K.M.E.; Betts, G.J.; Morgan, B.P.; Godkin, A.J.; Gallimore, A.M. CD59 blockade enhances antigen-specific CD4+ T cell responses in humans: A new target for cancer immunotherapy? *J. Immunol.* **2009**, *182*, 5203–5207. [CrossRef] [PubMed]
97. Ricklin, D.; Reis, E.S.; Lambris, J.D. Complement in disease: A defence system turning offensive. *Nat. Rev. Nephrol.* **2016**, *12*, 383–401. [CrossRef]
98. Chen, M.; Daha, M.R.; Kallenberg, C.G.M. The complement system in systemic autoimmune disease. *J. Autoimmun.* **2010**, *34*, J276–J286. [CrossRef] [PubMed]
99. Risitano, A.M. Paroxysmal nocturnal hemoglobinuria and other complement-mediated hematological disorders. *Immunobiology* **2012**, *217*, 1080–1087. [CrossRef]
100. Kaur, A.; Sultan, S.H.A.; Murugaiah, V.; Pathan, A.A.; Alhamlan, F.S.; Karteris, E.; Kishore, U. Human C1q induces apoptosis in an ovarian cancer cell line via tumor necrosis factor pathway. *Front. Immunol.* **2016**, *7*, 599. [CrossRef]
101. Chen, Z.; Gu, P.; Liu, K.; Su, Y.; Gao, L. The globular heads of the C1q receptor regulate apoptosis in human cervical squamous carcinoma cells via a p53-dependent pathway. *J. Transl. Med.* **2012**, *10*, 255. [CrossRef]
102. Lv, K.T.; Gao, L.J.; Hua, X.; Li, F.; Gu, Y.; Wang, W. The role of the globular heads of the C1q receptor in paclitaxel-induced human ovarian cancer cells apoptosis by a mitochondria-dependent pathway. *Anticancer Drugs* **2018**, *29*, 107–117. [CrossRef]
103. Nunez-Cruz, S.; Gimotty, P.A.; Guerra, M.W.; Connolly, D.C.; Wu, Y.-Q.; DeAngelis, R.A.; Lambris, J.D.; Coukos, G.; Scholler, N. Genetic and pharmacologic inhibition of complement impairs endothelial cell function and ablates ovarian cancer neovascularization. *Neoplasia* **2012**, *14*, 994-IN1. [CrossRef]
104. Cho, M.S.; Vasquez, H.G.; Rupaimoole, R.; Pradeep, S.; Wu, S.; Zand, B.; Han, H.D.; Rodriguez-Aguayo, C.; Bottsford-Miller, J.; Huang, J.; et al. Autocrine effects of tumor-derived complement. *Cell Rep.* **2014**, *6*, 1085–1095. [CrossRef]
105. Cho, M.S.; Rupaimoole, R.; Choi, H.-J.; Noh, K.; Chen, J.; Hu, Q.; Sood, A.K.; Afshar-Kharghan, V. Complement component 3 is regulated by TWIST1 and mediates epithelial–mesenchymal transition. *J. Immunol.* **2016**, *196*, 1412–1418. [CrossRef]
106. Facciabene, A.; De Sanctis, F.; Pierini, S.; Reis, E.S.; Balint, K.; Facciponte, J.; Rueter, J.; Kagabu, M.; Magotti, P.; Lanitis, E.; et al. Local endothelial complement activation reverses endothelial quiescence, enabling T-cell homing, and tumor control during T-cell immunotherapy. *Oncoimmunology* **2017**, *6*, e1326442. [CrossRef]
107. Gunn, L.; Ding, C.; Liu, M.; Ma, Y.; Qi, C.; Cai, Y.; Hu, X.; Aggarwal, D.; Zhang, H.; Yan, J. Opposing roles for complement component C5a in tumor progression and the tumor microenvironment. *J. Immunol.* **2012**, *189*, 2985–2994. [CrossRef]
108. Li, B.; Allendorf, D.J.; Hansen, R.; Marroquin, J.; Cramer, D.E.; Harris, C.L.; Yan, J. Combined yeast β-glucan and antitumor monoclonal antibody therapy requires C5a-mediated neutrophil chemotaxis via regulation of decay-accelerating factor CD55. *Cancer Res.* **2007**, *67*, 7421–7430. [CrossRef] [PubMed]
109. Saygin, C.; Wiechert, A.; Rao, V.S.; Alluri, R.; Connor, E.; Thiagarajan, P.S.; Hale, J.S.; Li, Y.; Chumakova, A.; Jarrar, A.; et al. CD55 regulates self-renewal and cisplatin resistance in endometrioid tumors. *J. Exp. Med.* **2017**, *214*, 2715–2732. [CrossRef] [PubMed]
110. Shi, X.; Zhang, B.; Zang, J.; Wang, G.; Gao, M. CD59 silencing via retrovirus-mediated RNA interference enhanced complement-mediated cell damage in ovary cancer. *Cell. Mol. Immunol.* **2009**, *6*, 61–66. [CrossRef] [PubMed]
111. Donin, N.; Jurianz, K.; Ziporen, L.; Schultz, S.; Kirschfink, M.; Fishelson, Z. Complement resistance of human carcinoma cells depends on membrane regulatory proteins, protein kinases and sialic acid. *Clin. Exp. Immunol.* **2003**, *131*, 254–263. [CrossRef] [PubMed]
112. Macor, P.; Mezzanzanica, D.; Cossetti, C.; Alberti, P.; Figini, M.; Canevari, S.; Tedesco, F. Complement activated by chimeric anti-folate receptor antibodies is an efficient effector system to control ovarian carcinoma. *Cancer Res.* **2006**, *66*, 3876–3883. [CrossRef] [PubMed]
113. Mamidi, S.; Cinci, M.; Hasmann, M.; Fehring, V.; Kirschfink, M. Lipoplex mediated silencing of membrane regulators (CD46, CD55 and CD59) enhances complement-dependent anti-tumor activity of trastuzumab and pertuzumab. *Mol. Oncol.* **2013**, *7*, 580–594. [CrossRef]
114. Junnikkala, S.; Hakulinen, J.; Jarva, H.; Manuelian, T.; Bjørge, L.; Bützow, R.; Zipfel, P.F.; Meri, S. Secretion of soluble complement inhibitors factor H and factor H-like protein (FHL-1) by ovarian tumour cells. *Br. J. Cancer* **2002**, *87*, 1119–1127. [CrossRef] [PubMed]
115. Zhang, W.; Peng, P.; Ou, X.; Shen, K.; Wu, X. Ovarian cancer circulating extracellular vesicles promote coagulation and have a potential in diagnosis: An iTRAQ based proteomic analysis. *BMC Cancer* **2019**, *19*, 1095. [CrossRef]
116. Yu, G.; Wang, J. Significance of hyaluronan binding protein (HABP1/P32/gC1qR) expression in advanced serous ovarian cancer patients. *Exp. Mol. Pathol.* **2013**, *94*, 210–215. [CrossRef]

117. Swierzko, A.S.; Szala, A.; Sawicki, S.; Szemraj, J.; Sniadecki, M.; Sokolowska, A.; Kaluzynski, A.; Wydra, D.; Cedzynski, M. Mannose-Binding Lectin (MBL) and MBL-associated serine protease-2 (MASP-2) in women with malignant and benign ovarian tumours. *Cancer Immunol. Immunother.* **2014**, *63*, 1129–1140. [CrossRef]
118. Szala, A.; Sawicki, S.; Swierzko, A.S.; Szemraj, J.; Sniadecki, M.; Michalski, M.; Kaluzynski, A.; Lukasiewicz, J.; Maciejewska, A.; Wydra, D.; et al. Ficolin-2 and ficolin-3 in women with malignant and benign ovarian tumours. *Cancer Immunol. Immunother.* **2013**, *62*, 1411–1419. [CrossRef] [PubMed]
119. Zhang, Z.; Qin, K.; Zhang, W.; Yang, B.; Zhao, C.; Zhang, X.; Zhang, F.; Zhao, L.; Shan, B. Postoperative recurrence of epithelial ovarian cancer patients and chemoresistance related protein analyses. *J. Ovarian Res.* **2019**, *12*, 29. [CrossRef]
120. Swiatly, A.; Horala, A.; Hajduk, J.; Matysiak, J.; Nowak-Markwitz, E.; Kokot, Z.J. MALDI-TOF-MS analysis in discovery and identification of serum proteomic patterns of ovarian cancer. *BMC Cancer* **2017**, *17*, 472. [CrossRef] [PubMed]
121. Surowiak, P.; Materna, V.; Maciejczyk, A.; Kaplenko, I.; Spaczynski, M.; Dietel, M.; Lage, H.; Zabel, M. CD46 expression is indicative of shorter revival-free survival for ovarian cancer patients. *Anticancer Res.* **2006**, *26*, 4943–4948. [PubMed]
122. Murray, K.P.; Mathure, S.; Kaul, R.; Khan, S.; Carson, L.F.; Twiggs, L.B.; Martens, M.G.; Kaul, A. Expression of complement regulatory proteins-CD35, CD46, CD55, and CD59-in benign and malignant endometrial tissue. *Gynecol. Oncol.* **2000**, *76*, 176–182. [CrossRef]
123. Reid, K.B.M. Complement component C1q: Historical perspective of a functionally versatile, and structurally unusual, serum protein. *Front. Immunol.* **2018**, *9*, 764. [CrossRef] [PubMed]
124. Mangogna, A.; Belmonte, B.; Agostinis, C.; Zacchi, P.; Iacopino, D.G.; Martorana, A.; Rodolico, V.; Bonazza, D.; Zanconati, F.; Kishore, U.; et al. Prognostic implications of the complement protein C1q in gliomas. *Front. Immunol.* **2019**, *10*, 2366. [CrossRef] [PubMed]
125. Chen, L.; Liu, J.-F.; Lu, Y.-; He, X.; Zhang, C.-; Zhou, H. Complement C1q (C1qA, C1qB, and C1qC) may be a potential prognostic factor and an index of tumor microenvironment remodeling in osteosarcoma. *Front. Oncol.* **2021**, *11*, 642144. [CrossRef]
126. Bonavita, E.; Gentile, S.; Rubino, M.; Maina, V.; Papait, R.; Kunderfranco, P.; Greco, C.; Feruglio, F.; Molgora, M.; Laface, I.; et al. PTX3 is an extrinsic oncosuppressor regulating complement-dependent inflammation in cancer. *Cell* **2015**, *160*, 700–714. [CrossRef]
127. Bulla, R.; Tripodo, C.; Rami, D.; Ling, G.S.; Agostinis, C.; Guarnotta, C.; Zorzet, S.; Durigutto, P.; Botto, M.; Tedesco, F. C1q acts in the tumour microenvironment as a cancer-promoting factor independently of complement activation. *Nat. Commun.* **2016**, *7*, 10346. [CrossRef]
128. Peerschke, E.I.B.; Ghebrehiwet, B. cC1qR/CR and gC1qR/p33: Observations in cancer. *Mol. Immunol.* **2014**, *61*, 100–109. [CrossRef]
129. Michalski, M.; Świerzko, A.S.; Sawicki, S.; Kałużyński, A.; Łukasiewicz, J.; Maciejewska, A.; Wydra, D.; Cedzyński, M. Interactions of ficolin-3 with ovarian cancer cells. *Immunobiology* **2019**, *224*, 316–324. [CrossRef]
130. Singel, K.L.; Emmons, T.R.; Khan, A.N.H.; Mayor, P.C.; Shen, S.; Wong, J.T.; Morrell, K.; Eng, K.H.; Mark, J.; Bankert, R.B.; et al. Mature neutrophils suppress T cell immunity in ovarian cancer microenvironment. *JCI Insight* **2019**, *4*, 122311. [CrossRef]
131. Emmons, T.R.; Giridharan, T.; Singel, K.L.; Khan, A.N.H.; Ricciuti, J.; Howard, K.; Silva-Del Toro, S.L.; Debreceni, I.L.; Aarts, C.E.M.; Brouwer, M.C.; et al. Mechanisms driving neutrophil-induced T-cell immunoparalysis in ovarian cancer. *Cancer Immunol. Res.* **2021**, *9*, 790–810. [CrossRef] [PubMed]
132. Markiewski, M.M.; Vadrevu, S.K.; Sharma, S.K.; Chintala, N.K.; Ghouse, S.; Cho, J.-H.; Fairlie, D.P.; Paterson, Y.; Astrinidis, A.; Karbowniczek, M. The ribosomal protein S19 suppresses antitumor immune responses via the complement C5a receptor 1. *J. Immunol.* **2017**, *198*, 2989–2999. [CrossRef]
133. Reese, B.; Silwal, A.; Daugherity, E.; Daugherity, M.; Arabi, M.; Daly, P.; Paterson, Y.; Woolford, L.; Christie, A.; Elias, R.; et al. Complement as prognostic biomarker and potential therapeutic target in renal cell carcinoma. *J. Immunol.* **2020**, *205*, 3218–3229. [CrossRef] [PubMed]
134. Lopez, M.F.; Mikulskis, A.; Kuzdzal, S.; Golenko, E.; Petricoin, E.F.; Liotta, L.A.; Patton, W.F.; Whiteley, G.R.; Rosenblatt, K.; Gurnani, P.; et al. A novel, high-throughput workflow for discovery and identification of serum carrier protein-bound peptide biomarker candidates in ovarian cancer samples. *Clin. Chem.* **2007**, *53*, 1067–1074. [CrossRef]
135. Bjørge, L.; Hakulinen, J.; Wahlström, T.; Matre, R.; Meri, S. Complement-regulatory proteins in ovarian malignancies. *Int. J. Cancer* **1997**, *70*, 14–25. [CrossRef]
136. Geller, A.; Yan, J. The role of membrane bound complement regulatory proteins in tumor development and cancer immunotherapy. *Front. Immunol.* **2019**, *10*, 1074. [CrossRef] [PubMed]
137. Durrant, L.G.; Chapman, M.A.; Buckley, D.J.; Spendlove, I.; Robins, R.A.; Armitage, N.C. Enhanced expression of the complement regulatory protein CD55 predicts a poor prognosis in colorectal cancer patients. *Cancer Immunol. Immunother.* **2003**, *52*, 638–642. [CrossRef]
138. Madjd, Z.; Pinder, S.E.; Paish, C.; Ellis, I.O.; Carmichael, J.; Durrant, L.G. Loss of CD59 expression in breast tumours correlates with poor survival. *J. Pathol.* **2003**, *200*, 633–639. [CrossRef]
139. Odening, K.E.; Li, W.; Rutz, R.; Laufs, S.; Fruehauf, S.; Fishelson, Z.; Kirschfink, M. Enhanced complement resistance in drug-selected P-glycoprotein expressing multi-drug-resistant ovarian carcinoma cells. *Clin. Exp. Immunol.* **2009**, *155*, 239–248. [CrossRef]

140. Okroj, M.; Hsu, Y.F.; Ajona, D.; Pio, R.; Blom, A.M. Non-small cell lung cancer cells produce a functional set of complement factor I and its soluble cofactors. *Mol. Immunol.* **2008**, *45*, 169–179. [CrossRef]
141. Pio, R.; Garcia, J.; Corrales, L.; Ajona, D.; Fleischhacker, M.; Pajares, M.J.; Cardenal, F.; Seijo, L.; Zulueta, J.J.; Nadal, E.; et al. Complement factor H is elevated in bronchoalveolar lavage fluid and sputum from patients with lung cancer. *Cancer Epidemiol. Biomarkers Prev.* **2010**, *19*, 2665–2672. [CrossRef]
142. Ajona, D.; Hsu, Y.-F.; Corrales, L.; Montuenga, L.M.; Pio, R. Down-regulation of human complement factor H sensitizes non-small cell lung cancer cells to complement attack and reduces in vivo tumor growth. *J. Immunol.* **2007**, *178*, 5991–5998. [CrossRef] [PubMed]
143. Ajona, D.; Castaño, Z.; Garayoa, M.; Zudaire, E.; Pajares, M.J.; Martinez, A.; Cuttitta, F.; Montuenga, L.M.; Pio, R. Expression of complement factor H by lung cancer cells: Effects on the activation of the alternative pathway of complement. *Cancer Res.* **2004**, *64*, 6310–6318. [CrossRef] [PubMed]
144. Mahner, S.; Woelber, L.; Eulenburg, C.; Schwarz, J.; Carney, W.; Jaenicke, F.; Milde-Langosch, K.; Mueller, V. TIMP-1 and VEGF-165 serum concentration during first-line therapy of ovarian cancer patients. *BMC Cancer* **2010**, *10*, 139. [CrossRef] [PubMed]
145. Perren, T.J.; Swart, A.M.; Pfisterer, J.; Ledermann, J.A.; Pujade-Lauraine, E.; Kristensen, G.; Carey, M.S.; Beale, P.; Cervantes, A.; Kurzeder, C.; et al. A phase 3 trial of Bevacizumab in ovarian cancer. *N. Engl. J. Med.* **2011**, *365*, 2484–2496. [CrossRef] [PubMed]
146. Gerber, H.P.; Ferrara, N. Pharmacology and pharmacodynamics of bevacizumab as monotherapy or in combination with cytotoxic therapy in preclinical studies. *Cancer Res.* **2005**, *65*, 671–680.
147. Mabuchi, S.; Terai, Y.; Morishige, K.; Tanabe-Kimura, A.; Sasaki, H.; Kanemura, M.; Tsunetoh, S.; Tanaka, Y.; Sakata, M.; Burger, R.A.; et al. Maintenance treatment with bevacizumab prolongs survival in an in vivo ovarian cancer model. *Clin. Cancer Res.* **2008**, *14*, 7781–7789. [CrossRef] [PubMed]
148. Corrales, L.; Ajona, D.; Rafail, S.; Lasarte, J.J.; Riezu-Boj, J.I.; Lambris, J.D.; Rouzaut, A.; Pajares, M.J.; Montuenga, L.M.; Pio, R. Anaphylatoxin C5a creates a favorable microenvironment for lung cancer progression. *J. Immunol.* **2012**, *189*, 4674–4683. [CrossRef]
149. Pio, R.; Ajona, D.; Ortiz-Espinosa, S.; Mantovani, A.; Lambris, J.D. Complementing the cancer-immunity cycle. *Front. Immunol.* **2019**, *10*, 774. [CrossRef]
150. Ajona, D.; Ortiz-Espinosa, S.; Moreno, H.; Lozano, T.; Pajares, M.J.; Agorreta, J.; Bértolo, C.; Lasarte, J.J.; Vicent, S.; Hoehlig, K.; et al. A combined PD-1/C5a blockade synergistically protects against lung cancer growth and metastasis. *Cancer Discov.* **2017**, *7*, 694–703. [CrossRef] [PubMed]
151. Wang, Y.; Sun, S.N.; Liu, Q.; Yu, Y.Y.; Guo, J.; Wang, K.; Xing, B.C.; Zheng, Q.F.; Campa, M.J.; Patz, E.F.; et al. Autocrine complement inhibits IL10-dependent T-cell-mediated antitumor immunity to promote tumor progression. *Cancer Discov.* **2016**, *6*, 1022–1035. [CrossRef]
152. Zha, H.; Han, X.; Zhu, Y.; Yang, F.; Li, Y.; Li, Q.; Guo, B.; Zhu, B. Blocking C5aR signaling promotes the anti-tumor efficacy of PD-1/PD-L1 blockade. *Oncoimmunology* **2017**, *6*, e1349587. [CrossRef] [PubMed]
153. Magrini, E.; Di Marco, S.; Mapelli, S.N.; Perucchini, C.; Pasqualini, F.; Donato, A.; Lopez, M.D.L.L.G.; Carriero, R.; Ponzetta, A.; Colombo, P.; et al. Complement activation promoted by the lectin pathway mediates C3aR-dependent sarcoma progression and immunosuppression. *Nat. Cancer* **2021**, *2*, 218–232. [CrossRef]
154. Bella, Á.; Di Trani, C.A.; Fernández-Sendin, M.; Arrizabalaga, L.; Cirella, A.; Teijeira, Á.; Medina-Echeverz, J.; Melero, I.; Berraondo, P.; Aranda, F. Mouse models of peritoneal carcinomatosis to develop clinical applications. *Cancers* **2021**, *13*, 963. [CrossRef] [PubMed]
155. Hasan, N.; Ohman, A.W.; Dinulescu, D.M. The promise and challenge of ovarian cancer models. *Transl. Cancer Res.* **2015**, *4*, 14–28. [CrossRef] [PubMed]
156. Roby, K.F.; Taylor, C.C.; Sweetwood, J.P.; Cheng, Y.; Pace, J.L.; Tawfik, O.; Persons, D.L.; Smith, P.G.; Terranova, P.F. Development of a syngeneic mouse model for events related to ovarian cancer. *Carcinogenesis* **2000**, *21*, 585–591. [CrossRef] [PubMed]
157. Conejo-Garcia, J.R.; Benencia, F.; Courreges, M.C.; Kang, E.; Mohamed-Hadley, A.; Buckanovich, R.J.; Holtz, D.O.; Jenkins, A.; Na, H.; Zhang, L.; et al. Tumor-infiltrating dendritic cell precursors recruited by a β-defensin contribute to vasculogenesis under the influence of Vegf-A. *Nat. Med.* **2004**, *10*, 950–958. [CrossRef]

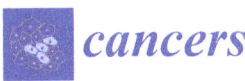

Review

Role of Oncogenic Pathways on the Cancer Immunosuppressive Microenvironment and Its Clinical Implications in Hepatocellular Carcinoma

Naoshi Nishida

Department of Gastroenterology and Hepatology, Kindai University Faculty of Medicine, 377-2 Ohno-Higashi, Osaka-Sayama 589-8511, Japan; naoshi@med.kindai.ac.jp; Tel.: +81-72-366-0221

Simple Summary: Hepatocellular carcinoma is known to become resistant to treatments easily by mutations in genes involved in the key cellular pathways targeted by current molecular targeted agents (MTAs). However, the immune checkpoint inhibitor (ICI) is a promising modality for cancer treatment, in which the cancer cells are made recognizable by the immune system. Blockade of the PD1/PDL1 proteins, which help cancers evade the immune system, is currently being tested in clinical trials in combination with MTAs. In this review, several cellular signaling pathways that can alter the immune processes within the tumor and can subsequently affect the patient's response to ICIs are detailed. This review may help scientists and clinicians to better understand the molecular factors that can influence ICI-based therapy and will help in identifying suitable cases for this type of treatment.

Abstract: The tumor immune microenvironment, including hepatocellular carcinoma (HCC), is complex, consisting of crosstalk among tumor components such as the cancer cells, stromal cells and immune cells. It is conceivable that phenotypic changes in cancer cells by genetic and epigenetic alterations affect the cancer–stroma interaction and anti-cancer immunity through the expression of immune checkpoint molecules, growth factors, cytokines, chemokines and metabolites that may act on the immune system in tumors. Therefore, predicting the outcome of ICI therapy requires a thorough understanding of the oncogenic signaling pathways in cancer and how they affect tumor immune evasion. In this review, we have detailed how oncogenic signaling pathways can play a role in altering the condition of the cellular components of the tumor immune microenvironment such as tumor-associated macrophages, regulatory T cells and myeloid-derived suppressor cells. The RAS/MAPK, PI3K/Akt, Wnt/β-catenin and JAK/STAT pathways have all been implicated in anti-tumor immunity. We also found that factors that reflect the immune microenvironment of the tumor, including the status of oncogenic pathways such as the volume of tumor-infiltrating T cells, expression of the immune checkpoint protein PD-1 and its ligand PD-L1, and activation of the Wnt/β-catenin signaling pathway, predict a response to ICI therapy in HCC cases.

Keywords: cancer; hepatocellular carcinoma; immune evasion; immunotherapy; immune checkpoint inhibitors; oncogenic signaling pathway; molecular targeted agents; genome; epigenome; tumor immune microenvironment

Citation: Nishida, N. Role of Oncogenic Pathways on the Cancer Immunosuppressive Microenvironment and Its Clinical Implications in Hepatocellular Carcinoma. *Cancers* **2021**, *13*, 3666. https://doi.org/10.3390/cancers13153666

Academic Editors: Ion Cristóbal and Marta Rodríguez

Received: 8 June 2021
Accepted: 19 July 2021
Published: 21 July 2021

Publisher's Note: MDPI stays neutral with regard to jurisdictional claims in published maps and institutional affiliations.

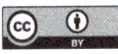

Copyright: © 2021 by the author. Licensee MDPI, Basel, Switzerland. This article is an open access article distributed under the terms and conditions of the Creative Commons Attribution (CC BY) license (https://creativecommons.org/licenses/by/4.0/).

1. Introduction

Hepatocellular carcinoma (HCC) is highly refractory and is the third leading cause of cancer-related deaths worldwide [1]. Recent advancements in molecular targeted agents (MTAs) for HCC have dramatically improved the prognosis for patients with this disease. Following the approval of sorafenib as the first MTA for advanced HCC, lenvatinib has also been applied as a first-line systemic chemotherapeutic for HCC, while regorafenib, cabozantinib and ramucirumab have been approved as second-line agents [2]. Because MTAs primarily target molecules involved in oncogenic signaling pathways that play an important role in the development of cancer cells, the development of clones resistant to MTAs can happen easily by genetic mutations and modifications in the specific molecular pathways [3,4]. Hence, additional chemotherapeutic agents would be required.

In contrast, immune checkpoint inhibitors (ICIs) play a role in tumor regression by a different mechanism from that of MTAs [5]. They are known to interfere with the immunosuppressive mechanism to enhance the anti-tumor immune response [6]. Because the target molecules of ICIs are primarily expressed in the stromal cells as well as the cancer cells, ICIs can be effective even for patients who fail to respond well to MTAs or acquire resistance to them, potentially enabling ICIs to complement treatment with MTAs [5,7–9]. Although the clinical trial of anti-programmed cell death-1 (PD-1) monotherapy failed to show a significant difference in the survival of patients with advanced HCC compared with conventional MTAs, synergic effects of the combination of different kinds of agents can be expected in several ongoing clinical trials of ICI-based therapy. Based on a successful Phase III clinical trial, the combination of the ICI atezolizumab (an anti-PD-1 antibody) with MTA bevacizumab (an anti-VEGF-A antibody) was approved as a first-line therapy for unresectable HCC [10,11].

Because of the complexity of cancer immunity, where immune cells, tumor cells and other types of stromal cells affect each other, understanding the immune microenvironment of the tumor is difficult [5]. While it has been considered that oncogenic mutations in tumor cells do not directly affect the outcome of ICI therapy, recent reports have suggested that mutation-induced changes in the tumor phenotype can affect the tumor–stroma interactions through alterations in the expression of immunosuppressive cytokines, chemokines, receptors and metabolites, thereby potentially affecting the tumor immune microenvironment [5]. Thus, the anti-tumor effect of MTAs in combination therapy with ICIs can be attributed to the direct action of MTAs on the HCC cells, as well as the reduction in the immunosuppressive nature of the tumor microenvironment through the inhibition of specific oncogenic signals [12].

To understand the significance of oncogenic signaling in the establishment of an immunosuppressive tumor microenvironment, and for the application of this knowledge to the treatment of HCC, this review focused on the role of specific genetic mutations involved in the oncogenic pathways responsible for anti-tumor immunity, and the current status of and perspectives on the combination of ICIs and MTAs for the treatment of HCC.

2. Cellular Components and Molecules Associated with an Inhibitory Tumor Immune Microenvironment

Oncogenic signals affect the expression of several immune-related molecules, including immune regulatory receptors, ligands, growth factors and other humoral factors, which affect diverse stromal cells as well as cancer cells. The cellular components of tumors and their states are major players in the regulation of the tumor immune microenvironment. Therefore, to better understand the impact of oncogenic signals on anti-cancer immunity, the functions of the stromal cells involved in the immune microenvironment of tumors are briefly discussed here.

2.1. Regulatory T-Cells

Regulatory T-cells (Tregs) are $CD4^+$ T-cells characterized by the expression of the transcription factor Foxp3. They can be induced in tumor tissues through growth factors and cytokines, such as transforming growth factor β (TGF-β), interleukin 10 (IL-10) and vascular endothelial growth factor (VEGF), and inhibit immune responses through various mechanisms [13]. In particular, Tregs express the inhibitory immune checkpoint molecule cytotoxic T-lymphocyte (associated) antigen 4 (CTLA-4), which plays a critical role in the regulation of T cell-mediated anti-tumor immunity. Generally, T cell activation occurs through binding of the co-stimulatory factor B7 (CD80/CD86) on antigen-presenting cells and CD28 on T-cells, in addition to T-cell receptor (TCR) recognition of major histocompatibility complex (MHC)-presented antigens. Binding of CD80/CD86 on dendritic cells (DCs) with CTLA-4 on Tregs results in the inhibition of DC maturation. In addition, the membrane molecule CD25 (IL-2 receptor subunit) on Tregs induces the depletion of IL-2 and suppression of cytotoxic T-cells (CTLs) by immunosuppressive cytokines such as TGF-β and IL-10, and cytotoxic secretions such as granzyme B and perforin released by Tregs [13]. A subtype of HCC that showed predominant expression of an mRNA related to Treg response has been reported [14]. Tregs also secrete the epidermal growth factor receptor (EGFR) ligand amphiregulin, which can promote the growth of HCC cells carrying EGFR in an autocrine manner [15]. Tregs also express VEGF receptor 2 on their surface, and the VEGF signal induces the expansion of this type of T cell [16].

2.2. Myeloid-Derived Suppresor Cells

Myeloid-derived suppressor cells (MDSCs) are a heterogeneous population of immature myeloid cells that suppress tumor immunity and can be induced by VEGF [16]. Via their increased arginase activity, degradation of arginine, and uptake of tryptophan, cysteine and other amino acids required for T-cell activation, MDSCs reduce the concentrations of these amino acids in the tissue microenvironment, thereby inhibiting the propagation and activation of T cells [17]. In addition, MDSCs produce TGF-β and IL-10, inducing Tregs and inhibiting natural killer (NK) cell function [18]. Furthermore, MDSCs induce the immunosuppressive M2 macrophages by secreting IL-10, which, in turn, downregulates IL-12 production by tumor-associated macrophages (TAMs) [19,20].

2.3. Tumor-Associated Macrophages

Generally, two types of macrophages exist in tumor tissues: M1 macrophages and M2 macrophages. Interferon-γ (IFN-γ) and Type 1 helper cell (Th1) cytokines induce the differentiation of inflammatory monocytes into M1 macrophages. Meanwhile, Type 2 helper cell (Th2) cytokines such as IL-4 and IL-13 promote the differentiation of tissue-resident monocytes into M2 macrophages [20]. In tumor immunity, M1 macrophages produce inflammatory cytokines such as tumor necrosis factor α (TNF-α), IL-6 and IL-12, and exert an anti-tumor effect, whereas M2 macrophages produce immunosuppressive cytokines such as IL-10 and TGF-β, and inhibit anti-tumor immune reactions [20]. The microenvironment in cancer is prone to inducing M2 polarization, which is a characteristic phenotype called tumor-associated macrophages (TAMs). The crosstalk between MDSCs and TAMs induces high IL-10 and low IL-12 levels. In addition, naïve $CD4^+$ T cells differentiate into Th2 cells that can produce IL-4 [21]. These processes result in the development of M2 macrophages, which is a disadvantageous state for tumor immunity. A high level of IL-10 induces the downregulation of human leukocyte antigen (HLA) Class II antigens and reduces the antigen presentation capacity of DCs [21]. It also expands the Treg population and inactivates natural killer (NK) cells. Additionally, the TGF-β secreted by MDSCs induces the expression of the inhibitory receptor T-cell immunoglobulin and mucin domain 3 (TIM-3) on TAMs [20].

2.4. Cancer-Associated Fibroblasts and Vascular Endothelial Cells

Cancer-associated fibroblasts (CAFs) have proangiogenic activity through the production of extracellular matrix and matrix metalloproteinases; they play a role in tissue remodeling [22]. They also inhibit NK cell function through the production of prostaglandin E2 (PGE2) and indoleamine-2,3-dioxygenase (IDO) [23]. Indoleamine-2,3-dioxygenase is an enzyme involved in tryptophan metabolism, and a reduced level of tryptophan in tumors inhibits local T-cell activation. Hence, crosstalk between CAFs and TAMs also plays a role in immunosuppression. CAFs produce IL-8 and cyclooxygenase-2 (COX2), which lead to the release of TNF and platelet-derived growth factor (PDGF) from TAMs, and further activation of CAFs.

2.5. Other Stromal Cells

The vascular endothelium is stimulated by angiogenic growth factors such as VEGF and PDGF. It stimulates Tregs and MDSCs in tumor tissues via the production of TGF-β,

VEGF and the chemokine C-X-C motif chemokine 12 (CXCL12) [20]. Hepatic satellite cells (HSCs), which generally play a critical role in liver fibrogenesis, also participate in the induction of Tregs and MDSCs by releasing hepatocyte growth factors [24,25]. HSCs also produce amphiregulin and CXCL12, which induce Tregs and MDSCs, respectively [26]. A subset of DCs with high expression of CTLA-4 was also observed in HCC tissues, which may carry immune tolerogenic effects through the production of IL-10 and IDO.

2.6. Immunosuppressive Metabolites

As shown above, the concentrations of metabolites from cancer cells and stromal cells strongly affect the immune state of the tumor. Cyclic adenosine monophosphate (cAMP), which accumulates in tumor tissues, inhibits $CD4^+$ and $CD8^+$ T-cell responses and macrophage activation, and enhances the Treg response by binding to adenosine A2A receptors [27]. In addition, due to the hypoxic environment in tumor tissues, cAMP upregulates the enzyme COX-2, which synthesizes PGE2 from arachidonic acid. Subsequently, PGE2 binds to prostaglandin E receptor 4 on T-cells and affects T-cell activation and cytokine production [20].

MDSC- and TAM-derived arginase hydrolyzes arginine in the urea cycle and inhibits the function of CTLs via this deficiency in L-arginine. In tumor tissues, a hypoxic environment results in the expression of hypoxia-inducible factor 1α (HIF-1α), which is known to activate arginase [17]. Additionally, IDO is reported to be produced by DCs, macrophages, CAFs, vascular endothelial cells and HCC cells via inflammatory cytokines [28]. As previously stated, IDO inhibits T-cell activation and amplification via depletion of tryptophan and stimulates the differentiation of naïve $CD4^+$ T-cells into Tregs [20,29].

2.7. Immune Checkpoint Molecules

Immune checkpoint molecules regulate excessive T-cell activation and help to maintain immune homeostasis. In cancer cells, however, these immune checkpoint molecules help tumors evade the immune response. Many immune checkpoint molecules and their ligands have been identified, as summarized in Figure 1. Of these, CTLA-4, programmed cell death-1 (PD-1) and its ligand, programmed cell death-ligand 1 (PD-L1), are believed to play central roles in tumors' immune evasion [5,20]. The induction of immune checkpoint molecules is regulated by environmental factors as well as cell signaling. For example, extracellular stimulation of IFN-γ and hypoxia-induced HIF-1 can enhance the expression of PD-L1 in cancer cells, MDSCs and TAMs [30]. The binding of PD-L1 to PD-1 on TAMs induces the release of the immunosuppressive cytokine IL-10. Additionally, activation of the phosphatidylinositol-3 kinase (PI3K)–Akt pathway also reportedly induces PD-L1, and the loss-of-function mutation of phosphatase and tensin homolog deleted from chromosome 10 (PTEN), a regulator of the PI3K–Akt pathway, is associated with the expression of PD-L1 in cancer [31,32]. We have also shown that activating mutations in PI3KCA are associated with PD-L1 expression in HCC cells [33]. TIM-3, lymphocyte-activation gene 3 (LAG-3) and the B- and T-lymphocyte attenuator (BTLA, CD272) are also known as co-inhibitory molecules on activated T-cells, based on their association with galectin-9, MHC Class II and herpesvirus entry mediator (HVME), respectively (Figure 1). These suppressive receptors are observed in tumor-infiltrating lymphocytes (TILs) in HCC tissues and are considered to be markers of exhausted T-cells [33–35].

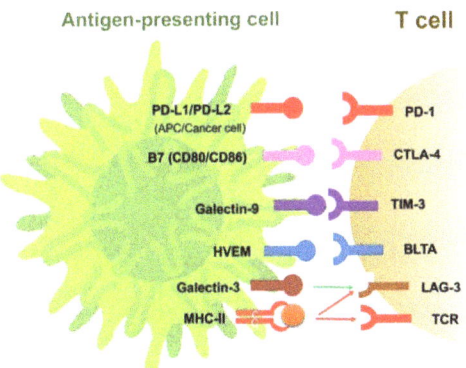

Figure 1. Immune checkpoint molecules and their ligands.

3. Unique Aspects of Immunological Characteristics in the Liver and Hepatocarcinogenesis

Although ICIs are becoming one of the key agents for the treatment of HCC, the response to this type of agent is still unsatisfactory in the majority of HCC cases compared with other types of malignancies [36]. The relatively low response rate to the ICIs can probably be attributed to the low antigenicity of HCC, as tumor mutation is not high in this type of tumor [36,37]. In addition, as the liver needs to be immunotolerant to nonpathological and persistent inflammation, it carries tolerance mechanisms to immune reactions, including cancer immunity.

The liver is continually exposed to the pathogen and microbe components from the gut via the blood supply of the portal vein. In this situation, the liver limits hypersensitivity to food-derived antigens and components of the intestinal flora to prevent excessive tissue damage and maintain systemic tolerance [38]. Chronic infection with hepatitis virus and persistent stimulation by metabolites further induce immune suppression in the liver, which is one of the unique characteristics of the underlying condition of hepatocarcinogenesis [39]. Resident macrophages (Kupffer cells) play a key role in hepatic tolerance through the production of anti-inflammatory cytokines, leading to downregulation of co-stimulatory molecules. This immunological environment of the liver results in the development of fully exhausted T-cells, where suppressive anti-tumor immunity is not susceptible to rescue by ICIs [36,39]. It has also been reported that $CD8^+$ $PD-1^+$ T-cells in NASH livers show a lack of immune surveillance and tissue-damaging function, which contribute to the increase in HCC emergence upon anti-PD-1 treatment in a NASH mouse model [40]. Augmentation of $CD8^+$ $PD-1^+$ T-cells was also observed in human NASH; a worse outcome in HCC patients treated with anti-PD-1 antibodies was observed [40]. Although the details of the difference in the response to ICIs between virally induced and NASH-induced HCCs are still unknown, it is possible that different amounts and quality of antigens and the difference in the liver microenvironment, such as the balance between partially exhausted and fully exhausted T-cells, may be involved in the outcome on ICIs [39,41,42].

In addition, ICI may not be effective or may even exacerbate the disease in some HCC patients. It is reported that blockade of the PD-1 and PD-L1 interaction may induce an expansion of $PD-1^+$ Tregs isolated from the liver of patients with chronic hepatitis C, because PD-1 on Tregs generally plays a role in the regulation of the $CD4^+CD25^+FoxP3^+$ T-cells [43]. Therefore, a blockade of the binding of the ligand with PD-1 on Tregs may result in further suppression of anti-tumor immunity [44]. More importantly, $PD-1^+$ Tregs may be involved in the hyperprogression of tumors in gastric cancer patients treated with anti-PD-1 antibodies [44]. As hyperprogression on anti-PD-1 antibodies has also been reported in HCC cases, ICI can be even detrimental in such cases [45].

4. Signaling Pathways and the Immune Microenvironment of Tumors

Alterations in oncogenic signaling in cancer not only trigger abnormal differentiation and cell proliferation, but also play a crucial role in the immune evasion of tumors [12]. Cancer-related signaling affects the state of the tumors' immune components via cytokine, chemokine and growth factor production. To date, genetic alterations in several signaling pathways observed in cancers have been reported to affect the tumor immune microenvironment.

4.1. RAS/MAPK Signaling Pathway

In malignant melanomas, activating mutations in BRAF (BRAF^{V600E}) induce constitutive activation of the mitogen-activated protein kinase (MAPK) pathway, which stimulates immune-tolerant DCs and inhibits CD8$^+$ T-cells via the expression of the immunosuppressive cytokines IL-6 and IL-10, as well as via VEGF [46]. This effect has been reported to be inhibited by BRAF inhibitors and VEGF inhibitors. Furthermore, RAS/MAPK signaling inhibits antigen presentation on tumor cells, and inhibition of this pathway is associated with the recovery of MHC expression by IFN-γ in malignant melanomas and breast cancer [47,48]. Meanwhile, in a murine model of pancreatic cancer, activating mutations in KRAS (KRAS^{G12D}) induced MDSCs via the production of granulocyte macrophage colony-stimulating factor (GM-CSF) and inhibition of CD8$^+$ T-cell infiltration into tumor tissues, which contributed to the establishment of an immunosuppressive tumor microenvironment [49]. In fact, GM-CSF is known to be upregulated in human pancreatic intraepithelial neoplasia and pancreatic cancer cells [49]. An association between activating mutations in KRAS and resistance to ICIs has also been reported in colorectal cancer. KRAS-mediated repression of interferon regulatory factor 2 (IRF) results in the high expression of the chemokine C-X-C motif ligand 3 (CXCL3), which induces MDSCs that express C-X-C motif chemokine receptor 2 (CXCR2) as the receptor of CXCL3 in tumor tissues [50]. In this manner, activation of KRAS induces MDSC-mediated resistance to antitumor immunity in patients with colorectal cancer (Figure 2).

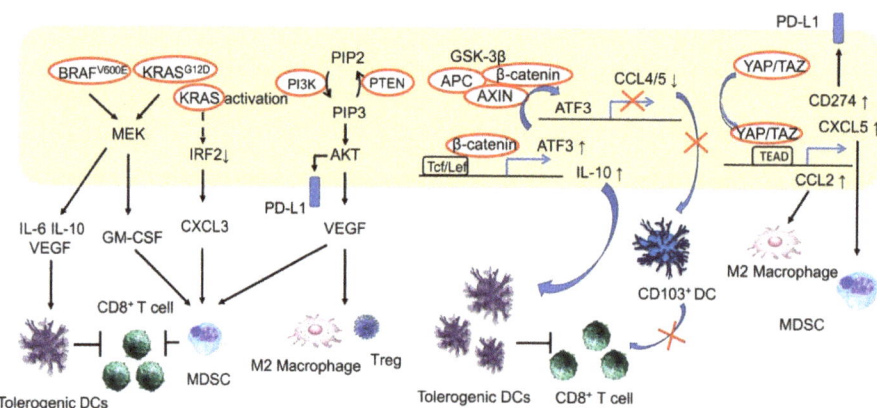

Figure 2. Effects of oncogenic signal activation on the tumor immune environment.

4.2. PI3K/Akt Signaling Pathway

Activation of the PI3K/AKT signaling pathway is involved in critical cellular functions, including survival, inhibition of apoptosis and proliferation. Activation of PI3K/AKT is one of the common features of cancer. PTEN, which regulates this pathway, demonstrates loss-of-function mutations in various cancers. In melanomas, mutations in PTEN are related to resistance to anti-PD-1 antibody treatment and are correlated with a reduced volume of CD8$^+$ TILs [51]. In a murine model, PI3K-β inhibitors improved sensitivity to treatment with anti-PD-1 antibodies and anti-CTLA4 antibodies when the resistance was induced by loss-of-function mutations in PTEN [51]. While loss of PTEN function is associated with the induction of various immunosuppressive cytokines, it also induces VEGF, which is presumed to be the mechanism by which immunosuppression is induced. In bladder cancer, activating mutations in PI3KCA are associated with a reduction in TIL volume, while PI3K inhibitors lead to an increase in TILs [52]. PI3K inhibitors have also been reported to inhibit Tregs and induce the differentiation of M2 macrophages into the M1 phenotype [53]. In addition, by inducing PD-L1 expression, both the RAS/MAPK and the PI3K/AKT signaling pathways can be involved in the suppression of anti-tumor immunity. We have previously reported that while activating mutations of the PI3K/AKT signaling pathway are associated with increased expression of PD-L1 in HCC, and the volume of TILs is generally high in PD-L1-positive HCC, TILs are deficient in HCCs with activating mutations of the PI3K/AKT signaling pathway [33]. Therefore, aside from external stimulation such as by IFN-γ, induction of PD-L1 is likely to be attributable to genetic mutations in the PI3K/AKT pathway in this setting (Figure 2).

BRAF^{V600E} induces immune-tolerant dendritic cells (DCs) via the induction of IL-6, IL-10 and VEGF, ultimately inhibiting the action of CD8$^+$ T-cells. In addition, KRAS^{G12D} induces MDSCs via GM-CSF production, thereby inhibiting CD8$^+$ T-cells from infiltrating tumor tissues. In colorectal cancer, KRAS activation is known to induce CXCL3 expression and the induction of MDSCs with CXCR2, the receptor of CXCL3. In contrast, PI3K/AKT signaling activation is associated with VEGF expression and a decrease in tumor-infiltrating lymphocyte (TIL) volume, and has been reported to induce Tregs and inhibit the shift of M2 macrophages into M1 macrophages. In addition, PI3K/AKT signaling induces PD-L1 expression. Under the activation of WNT/β-catenin signaling, activating transcription factor 3 (ATF3)-mediated CCL4 downregulation is considered to reduce the migration of CD103$^+$ dendritic cells into the tumor and reduce CD8$^+$ TILs in melanoma. CCL5 was suggested to be involved in HCC. The activation of the WNT/β-catenin signaling pathway has also been reported to be involved in the formation of an immune suppressive tumor microenvironment through the upregulation of IL-10. Activation of the transcription factors YAP/TAZ, which are regulated by Hippo signaling, upregulate PD-L1 and are involved in CXCL5-mediated induction of MDSCs. In addition, YAP is involved in the induction of M2 macrophages by enhancing the transcription of CCL2.

4.3. Wnt/β-Catenin Signaling Pathway

ICIs are presumed to be insufficiently effective in cases where infiltration of CD8$^+$ T-cells in tumors is lacking, and an analysis of human melanomas has revealed that activation of the Wnt/β-catenin signaling pathway is associated with reduced TILs in tumors. In melanomas with activating mutations in the Wnt/β-catenin signaling pathway, C-C chemokine ligand 4 (CCL4) is downregulated, which reduces the migration of CD103$^+$ DCs and leads to a deficiency in CD8$^+$ TILs. Furthermore, the transcriptional repression of CCL4 was attributed to the activation of activating transcription factor 3 (ATF3) as a result of the activation of the β-catenin signaling pathway [54]. Activating mutations of the Wnt/β-catenin pathway occur frequently in HCC, and immunosuppression in the tumor microenvironment based on activation of this signal in liver cancer is presumed to occur via downregulation of CCL5 [55]. In a murine HCC model, induction of CCL5 increased the number of DCs and CD8$^+$ T-cells in tumors (Figure 2). In melanomas, activation of Wnt/β-catenin signaling also reportedly led to the upregulation of IL-10 through the binding of β-catenin/T-cell factor (TCF) on the IL-10 promoter, thereby contributing to the formation of an immunosuppressive environment [56].

Aside from the altered Wnt/β-catenin signaling in tumor cells, activation of this signaling pathway reportedly disturbs the effector function of CD8$^+$ T-cells and induces the exhausted T-cell phenotype in HCC and colorectal cancers, which contributes to the establishment of immune suppressive tumor microenvironment [41]. Interestingly, neutralization of a canonical Wnt ligand, Wnt 3a, enhances the T-cell response through the rescue of DC activation, resulting in tumor regression in a mouse model [42].

4.4. MYC Gene

The transcription factor c-myc regulates the expression of genes necessary for cell proliferation and survival. In many cancers, amplification and overexpression of c-myc has been observed; these are involved in inducing the expression of immune checkpoint molecules such as PD-L1 and CD47 [57]. CD47 is a cell surface glycoprotein that regulates phagocytosis by binding to signal regulatory protein alpha (SIRP-α), which is specific to macrophages and DCs. Thus, overexpression of c-myc is involved in the immune evasion of cancer cells through CD47 and PD-L1.

4.5. Chromatin Remodeling Pathway

Genomic DNA is stored in the nucleus as chromatin. During transcription, replication or repair, alterations of the chromatin structure by chromatin remodeling regulate the access of transcription factors to the DNA. The SWItch/sucrose non-fermentable (SWI/SNF) complex is a chromatin remodeling factor that induces the alteration of nucleosomes via ATP hydrolysis. Genetic abnormalities in SWI/SNF complex subunits are frequently observed in HCC and other human tumors [33], and loss-of-function mutations in the polybromo 1 (PBRM1) gene involved in the SWI/SNF complex are common in renal cancer. Intriguingly, this PBRM1 mutation is associated with the therapeutic effect of ICIs in renal cancer. *PBRM1*-deficient renal cancers show altered transcriptional expression in the JAK/STAT (Janus kinase/signal transducers and activators of transcription) and immune signaling pathways [58].

4.6. JAK/STAT Signaling Pathway

The JAK/STAT pathway, which transmits signals that are crucial for growth, differentiation, survival and immunity, is altered in many types of malignancy. The downstream transcription factor, STAT3, acts on the PD-L1 promoter, thereby inducing upregulation of PD-L1 in cancer cells. In melanomas, JAK1 and JAK2 mutations inhibit signals from interferon receptors and reduce antigen presentation on tumor cells, which results in resistance to ICI therapy [59]. Meanwhile, β2-microglobulin gene mutations have been reported to induce resistance to ICI treatment via the loss of MHC Class I antigen expression on the cell surface [60].

4.7. Hippo Signaling Pathway

Hippo signaling, which is involved in the regulation of growth and differentiation as well as in controlling organ size, is dysfunctional in many malignancies. Reduced Hippo signaling is also associated with cancer's immune evasion. Hippo signaling regulates yes-associated protein (YAP) and "transcriptional coactivator with PDZ-binding motif" (TAZ), the activation of which leads to the expression of PD-L1 and stimulates MDSCs carrying CXCR2, by upregulation of its ligand, CXCL5 [61]. In a murine model of HCC, YAP was reported to be associated with tumor immunosuppression via the induction of M2 macrophages resulting from enhanced transcription of CCL2 (Figure 2) [62].

4.8. DNA Repair Pathway

It is well known that cancers carrying mutations in DNA mismatch genes induce a large number of neoantigens that are attributed to the emergence of a variety of passenger mutations that occur in the microsatellite sequences of the DNA, where anti-tumor immunity is enhanced. Therefore, microsatellite instability is a biomarker for efficacy in the treatment of ICIs [63]. Similarly, cancers with a high mutation burden (TMB) are also markers of tumors with an active immune microenvironment because of their high antigenicity [64]. Recently, it was reported that loss-of-function mutations in the breast cancer susceptibility (*BRCA*) 1 and *BRCA* 2 genes, which are involved in the homologous recombination pathway of DNA repair, are also markers of a high TMB and could be predictors of the outcome of ICI-based treatment [65]. From this perspective, alterations in DNA repair pathways are critical for the establishment of high antigenicity and "immune hot" status in cancer.

4.9. VEGF Signaling

In tumors, external stimulation can lead to the production of growth factors. In HCC, tissue hypoxia leads to the production of VEGF via the activation of hypoxia-inducible factor 1 (HIF-1), resulting in tumor angiogenesis. The cellular components of tumors that suppress tumor immune responses, such as MDSCs, Tregs and TAMs, express VEGF receptors; therefore, inhibition of VEGF/VEGFR can alter anti-tumor immunity [11]. Anti-PD-1 antibodies and anti-VEGFR-2 antibodies have been reported to have a synergistic effect in murine models of HCC. Anti-VEGFR-2 antibodies induce an increase in CTLs and a decrease in TAMs and Tregs [66]. Atezolizumab + bevacizumab is expected to combine the effects of ICIs with inhibition of VEGF signaling to alter immunity. Pembrolizumab + lenvatinib, a multikinase inhibitor (MKI) with a powerful antiangiogenic effect, and atezolizumab + cabozantinib, which is capable of blocking angiogenesis through the inhibition of VEGFR and AXL, and camrelizumab (an anti-PD-1 antibody) + apatinib (a selective VEGFR2-tyrosine kinase inhibitor) are in Phase III clinical trials, while avelumab (an anti-PD-L1 antibody) + axitinib (which strongly inhibits VEGFR) are undergoing Phase I/II trials (Table 1). ICIs and agents with an anti-VEGF/VEGFR effect are currently the most promising combination therapies for HCC because of their synergistic effect on cancer immunity [6,11].

Table 1. Clinical trials for combinations of molecular targeted agents and immune checkpoint inhibitors in hepatocellular carcinoma.

NCT Number [1] (Trial Name)	MTAs/ICIs [2]	Targets of MTAs	Setting
Phase I/II			
NCT03299946 (CaboNivo)	Cabozantinib/Nivolumab	TKI for VEGFR2, MET, AXL, etc.	neoadjuvant
NCT03170960 (COSMIC-021)	Cabozantinib/Atezolizumab	Same as above	First-line
NCT04442581	Cabozantinib/Pembrolizumab	Same as above	First-line
NCT01658878 (CheckMate 040)	Cabozantinib/Nivolumab±Ipilimumab	Same as above	First -and second-line
NCT03289533 (VEGF Liver 100)	Axitinib/Avelumab	TKI for VEGFR1-3, PDGFR, c-kit, etc.	First-line and AFP $\geq$ 400 ng/mL
NCT03841201, NCT03418922	Lenvatinib/Nivolumab	TKI for VEGFR1-3, FGFR1-4, etc.	First-line
NCT03347292 (Bayer 19497)	Regorafenib/Pembrolizumab	TKI for VEGFR1-3, TIE2, PDGFR, c-kit, RET, etc.	First-line
NCT04310709 (RENOBATE)	Regorafenib/Nivolumab	Same as above	First-line
NCT04183088	Regorafenib/Tislelizumab	Same as above	First-line
NCT03941873	Sitravatinib/Tislelizumab	TKI for VEGFR2, c-kit, AXL, etc.	First-line and later
NCT03475953 (REGOMUNE)	Regorafenib/Avelumab	TKI for VEGFR1-3, TIE2, PDGFR, c-kit, RET, etc.	Second-line
NCT04170556 (GOING)	Regorafenib/Followed by Nivolumab	Same as above	Second-line
NCT03539822 (CAMILLA)	Cabozantinib/Durvalumab	TKI for VEGFR2, MET, AXL, etc.	Second-line
NCT02572687	Ramucirumab/Durvalumab	Ab for VEGFR2	Second-line and AFP $\geq$ 1.5x ULN
NCT02423343	Galunisertib/Nivolumab	TKI for TGβR1	Second-line and AFP $\geq$ 200 ng/mL
Phase III			

Table 1. Cont.

NCT Number [1] (Trial Name)	MTAs/ICIs [2]	Targets of MTAs	Setting
NCT04102098 (IMbrave050)	Bevacizumab/Atezolizumab	Ab for VEGFA	Adjuvant
NCT03847428 (EMERALD-2)	Bevacizumab/±Durvalumab (vs. placebo)	Same as above	Adjuvant
NCT03713593 (LEAP-002)	Lenvatinib/Pembrolizumab (vs. Lenvatinib)	TKI for VEGFR1-3, FGFR1-4, etc.	First-line
NCT03755791 (COSMIC-312)	Cabozantinib/Atezolizumab (vs.orafenib or. Cabozantinib)	TKI for VEGFR2,MET, AXL, etc.	First-line
NCT03764293	Apatinib/Camrelizumab (vs. sorafenib)	TKI for VEGFR2	First-line

[1] National Clinical Trial number (ClinicalTrials.gov registry number). [2] MTA: molecular targeted agent; ICI: immune checkpoint inhibitor; TKI: tyrosine kinase inhibitor; Ab: antibody.

5. Signaling Pathway Abnormalities and the Immune Microenvironment in HCC

In a mouse model of HCC, it has been shown that activation of Wnt/β-catenin signaling induces reduced migration of CD103+ DCs and CD8+ TIL deficiency via downregulation of CCL5. Previous reports have also shown that Wnt/β-catenin activation is associated with the reduced expression of T cell-derived genes in HCC tissues. Therefore, HCC with activated Wnt/β-catenin signaling is unlikely to respond to ICIs because of the "immune cold" phenotype [67]. In fact, post-ICI therapy outcomes are reported to be poor in cases of HCC with Wnt/β-catenin activation [68]. Using a cohort of HCC cases from The Cancer Genome Atlas (TCGA), we determined that the expression of T cell-related genes was low in cases of HCC with activating mutations in Wnt/β-catenin (Figure 3). In addition, in an analysis of HCC tissues, we determined that HCCs with activating mutations in Wnt/β-catenin pathway genes are significantly deficient in CD8+ TILs [33]. However, we did not find CD8+ TILs to be associated with mutations in any other oncogenic signaling pathways (Table 2).

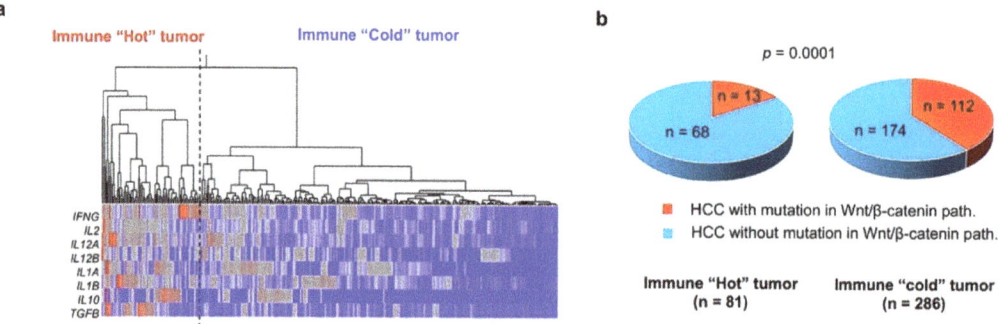

Figure 3. Tumor-infiltrating lymphocyte status and abnormal WNT/β-catenin activation. Hierarchical cluster analysis was used to classify HCCs based on the expression of eight T cell-related cytokine mRNAs obtained from the TCGA transcriptome dataset (RNA-seq V2 RSEM) (a) "Immune hot" and "immune cold" refer to HCCs with high and low levels of T cell-related gene expression, respectively. Thus, "immune hot" indicates a large volume of tumor-infiltrating lymphocytes (TILs), while "immune cold" suggests that TILs are deficient. (b) The presence or absence of activating mutations in WNT/β-catenin pathway genes are determined based on the presence or absence of *CTNNB1*, *AXIN1* and *APC* mutations in the TCGA provisional dataset obtained. Activating mutations in the WNT/β-catenin pathway are more frequently detected in "immune cold" HCCs than in "immune hot" tumors ($p = 0.0001$). The TCGA dataset used in the present study was downloaded in September 2019.

Table 2. Association between alterations in oncogenic signaling pathways and the degree of CD8+ tumor infiltrating lymphocytes.

Oncogenic Pathway	Mutation	CD8+ TILs		p Value [2]
		Median[1]	25–75th Percentile	
Wnt/β-catenin path.	with	6.18	1.30–26.9	0.0082
	without	17.6	5.77–38.0	
p53/cell cycle path.	with	18.7	5.70–32.7	0.7505
	without	12.9	3.60–38.3	
PI3K/Akt path.	with	1.14	0.17–2.03	0.5836
	without	1.16	0.36–2.88	
Chromatin remodeling	with	17.3	2.16–31.1	0.8056
	without	14.1	4.44–36.0	
Epigenetic regulator	with	0.75	0.15–1.81	0.1488
	without	1.29	0.42–2.88	
Oxidative/ER stress	with	1.63	0.53–5.74	0.1871
	without	1.11	0.28–2.72	
DNA repair	with	1.24	0.45–2.97	0.7392
	without	1.14	0.28–2.73	
TERT promoter	with	1.40	0.38–2.81	0.5093
	without	1.03	0.28–2.70	

Degree of tumor infiltrating lymphocytes (TILs) are compared between HCCs with mutations in each oncogenic pathway and those without mutations. In total, 154 HCCs were examined for mutations using the Ion AmpliSeq Comprehensive Cancer Panel, and the degree of CD8+ cells was examined using immunohistochemistry. [1] Median: median number of CD8+ TILs/high power field. [2] p value by Wilcoxon's rank-sum test.

In a transcriptome analysis, we reported that Wnt/β-catenin signaling activation was associated with the decreased expression of gene sets related to T-cell priming/activation, IFN-γ response, immunosuppression and Tregs; it was most significantly associated with the downregulation of genes related to the IFN-γ response in multivariate analysis [69]. These data are consistent with the deficiency in CD8+ T-cells in HCC tissues. In addition, we also reported that activating mutations in the Wnt/β-catenin pathway is negatively associated with PD-L1 expression in HCC [33]. As the expression of PD-L1 can be induced by the stimulation of IFN-γ, the lack of PD-L1 expression in HCC with Wnt/β-catenin activation can probably be attributed to the low degree of CD8+ TILs that should secrete IFN-γ [69]. On the other hand, a previous study found that mutations in genes involved in chromatin remodeling, such as AT-Rich Interaction Domain 2 (ARID2), were also associated with an immunosuppressive tumor microenvironment through the expression of genes involved in the induction of M2 macrophages [14], although there were no associations between mutations of the genes involved in chromatin remodeling and the degree of CD8+ TILs as well as PD-L1 expression [33]. As mutations of ARID2 are reportedly associated with the TAM subclass of HCC, the immune suppressive mechanism in HCCs with an ARID2 mutation should be different from that of CTNNB1 [14]. In contrast, PD-L1-positive HCCs often have high levels of CD8+ TILs [33]. This may be due to the fact that PD-L1 expression in HCC cells can be mainly attributed to stimulation by the IFN-γ from TILs. It is possible that, under continuous immune response to cancer cells, many CD8+ TILs are prone to expressing multiple inhibitory receptors (PD1, TIM-3, LAG-3) that result in the exhausted phenotype of T-cells [33]. In many cases, PD-L1 expression is considered to be a favorable prognostic factor of ICI therapy, suggesting that blockade of the PD-1/PD-L1 response could, at least partially, activate the T-cell immune response, even if the immune cells express additional inhibitory receptors. Indeed, we found that the absence of activating mutations in Wnt/β-catenin pathway genes, a high CD8+ TIL volume and

PD-L1 expression were associated with long progression-free survival of HCC patients on anti-PD-1 antibody therapy, regardless of the expression of other inhibitory receptors, such as TIM-3 and LAG-3 [69]. In this way, assessments of gene alterations in cellular signaling pathways are not only useful for finding suitable MTAs that act on the altered cellular signal, but may also, theoretically, serve to predict the response to ICI therapy, based on the tumor immune microenvironment.

6. Conclusions

Alterations of cell signaling pathways play a critical role not only in the development of a malignant phenotype in cancer cells but also in the determination of anti-cancer immunity. In a Phase III clinical trial with HCC patients, ICI monotherapy failed to yield a significant anti-cancer response, suggesting that ICIs will be used primarily in combination therapy [6]. It has been speculated that the "immune cold" phenotype of the tumor microenvironment is critical for poor prognosis with ICIs, where activation of the Wnt/β-catenin signaling pathway plays an important role. From this point of view, understanding the response of HCCs carrying Wnt/β-catenin mutations to combination therapy with ICI and MTA is clinically important but has not been clarified yet. Currently, a combination of atezolizumab + bevacizumab is applicable for unresectable HCC; the efficacy of this combination on HCCs showing the "immune cold" phenotype is now under investigation [36]. In addition, aside from atezolizumab + bevacizumab, many ongoing clinical trials have examined combinations of ICIs and MTAs for HCCs that are refractory upon ICI monotherapy, mainly with MTA showing an anti-angiogenic effect (Table 1). However, future trials are likely to examine combinations of ICIs with agents that inhibit other oncogenic pathways that are critical for hepatocarcinogenesis, such as the Wnt/β-catenin pathway, the RAS/MAPK pathway and the PI3K/AKT pathway.

Funding: This work was supported in part by a Grant-in-Aid for Scientific Research from the Japan Society for the Promotion of Science (KAKENHI: 21K07184, N. Nishida) and a grant from the Smoking Research Foundation (N. Nishida).

Conflicts of Interest: The author has not nothing to declare.

References

1. Villanueva, A. Hepatocellular Carcinoma. *N. Engl. J. Med.* **2019**, *380*, 1450–1462. [CrossRef]
2. Kudo, M. Recent Advances in Systemic Therapy for Hepatocellular Carcinoma in an Aging Society: 2020 Update. *Liver Cancer* **2020**, *9*, 640–662. [CrossRef]
3. Nishida, N.; Arizumi, T.; Hagiwara, S.; Ida, H.; Sakurai, T.; Kudo, M. MicroRNAs for the Prediction of Early Response to Sorafenib Treatment in Human Hepatocellular Carcinoma. *Liver Cancer* **2017**, *6*, 113–125. [CrossRef] [PubMed]
4. Nishida, N.; Nishimura, T.; Kaido, T.; Minaga, K.; Yamao, K.; Kamata, K.; Takenaka, M.; Ida, H.; Hagiwara, S.; Minami, Y.; et al. Molecular Scoring of Hepatocellular Carcinoma for Predicting Metastatic Recurrence and Requirements of Systemic Chemotherapy. *Cancers* **2018**, *10*, 367. [CrossRef]
5. Nishida, N.; Kudo, M. Immune checkpoint blockade for the treatment of human hepatocellular carcinoma. *Hepatol. Res.* **2018**, *48*, 622–634. [CrossRef]
6. Nishida, N.; Kudo, M. Immune Phenotype and Immune Checkpoint Inhibitors for the Treatment of Human Hepatocellular Carcinoma. *Cancers* **2020**, *12*, 1274. [CrossRef]
7. Nishida, N.; Kudo, M. Role of Immune Checkpoint Blockade in the Treatment for Human Hepatocellular Carcinoma. *Dig. Dis.* **2017**, *35*, 618–622. [CrossRef]
8. Nishida, N.; Kudo, M. Immunological Microenvironment of Hepatocellular Carcinoma and Its Clinical Implication. *Oncology* **2017**, *92* (Suppl. 1), 40–49. [CrossRef]
9. Aoki, T.; Kudo, M.; Ueshima, K.; Morita, M.; Chishina, H.; Takita, M.; Hagiwara, S.; Ida, H.; Minami, Y.; Tsurusaki, M.; et al. Exploratory Analysis of Lenvatinib Therapy in Patients with Unresectable Hepatocellular Carcinoma Who Have Failed Prior PD-1/PD-L1 Checkpoint Blockade. *Cancers* **2020**, *12*, 3048. [CrossRef]
10. Finn, R.S.; Qin, S.; Ikeda, M.; Galle, P.R.; Ducreux, M.; Kim, T.Y.; Kudo, M.; Breder, V.; Merle, P.; Kaseb, A.O.; et al. Atezolizumab plus Bevacizumab in Unresectable Hepatocellular Carcinoma. *N. Engl. J. Med.* **2020**, *382*, 1894–1905. [CrossRef] [PubMed]
11. Nishida, N. Clinical implications of the dual blockade of the PD-1/PD-L1 and vascular endothelial growth factor axes in the treatment of hepatocellular carcinoma. *Hepatobiliary Surg. Nutr.* **2020**, *9*, 640–643. [CrossRef]

12. Nishida, N.; Kudo, M. Oncogenic Signal and Tumor Microenvironment in Hepatocellular Carcinoma. *Oncology* **2017**, *93* (Suppl. 1), 160–164. [CrossRef]
13. Sprinzl, M.F.; Galle, P.R. Immune control in hepatocellular carcinoma development and progression: Role of stromal cells. *Semin. Liver Dis.* **2014**, *34*, 376–388. [CrossRef] [PubMed]
14. Fujita, M.; Yamaguchi, R.; Hasegawa, T.; Shimada, S.; Arihiro, K.; Hayashi, S.; Maejima, K.; Nakano, K.; Fujimoto, A.; Ono, A.; et al. Classification of primary liver cancer with immunosuppression mechanisms and correlation with genomic alterations. *EBioMedicine* **2020**, *53*, 102659. [CrossRef] [PubMed]
15. Zaiss, D.M.; van Loosdregt, J.; Gorlani, A.; Bekker, C.P.; Grone, A.; Sibilia, M.; van Bergen en Henegouwen, P.M.; Roovers, R.C.; Coffer, P.J.; Sijts, A.J. Amphiregulin enhances regulatory T cell-suppressive function via the epidermal growth factor receptor. *Immunity* **2013**, *38*, 275–284. [CrossRef] [PubMed]
16. Voron, T.; Colussi, O.; Marcheteau, E.; Pernot, S.; Nizard, M.; Pointet, A.L.; Latreche, S.; Bergaya, S.; Benhamouda, N.; Tanchot, C.; et al. VEGF-A modulates expression of inhibitory checkpoints on CD8+ T cells in tumors. *J. Exp. Med.* **2015**, *212*, 139–148. [CrossRef]
17. Hoechst, B.; Ormandy, L.A.; Ballmaier, M.; Lehner, F.; Kruger, C.; Manns, M.P.; Greten, T.F.; Korangy, F. A new population of myeloid-derived suppressor cells in hepatocellular carcinoma patients induces CD4(+)CD25(+)Foxp3(+) T cells. *Gastroenterology* **2008**, *135*, 234–243. [CrossRef]
18. Li, H.; Han, Y.; Guo, Q.; Zhang, M.; Cao, X. Cancer-expanded myeloid-derived suppressor cells induce anergy of NK cells through membrane-bound TGF-beta 1. *J. Immunol.* **2009**, *182*, 240–249. [CrossRef]
19. Arihara, F.; Mizukoshi, E.; Kitahara, M.; Takata, Y.; Arai, K.; Yamashita, T.; Nakamoto, Y.; Kaneko, S. Increase in CD14+HLA-DR-/low myeloid-derived suppressor cells in hepatocellular carcinoma patients and its impact on prognosis. *Cancer Immunol. Immunother* **2013**, *62*, 1421–1430. [CrossRef]
20. Prieto, J.; Melero, I.; Sangro, B. Immunological landscape and immunotherapy of hepatocellular carcinoma. *Nat. Rev. Gastroenterol. Hepatol.* **2015**, *12*, 681–700. [CrossRef] [PubMed]
21. Ostrand-Rosenberg, S.; Sinha, P.; Beury, D.W.; Clements, V.K. Cross-talk between myeloid-derived suppressor cells (MDSC), macrophages, and dendritic cells enhances tumor-induced immune suppression. *Semin. Cancer Biol.* **2012**, *22*, 275–281. [CrossRef]
22. Orimo, A.; Weinberg, R.A. Stromal fibroblasts in cancer: A novel tumor-promoting cell type. *Cell Cycle* **2006**, *5*, 1597–1601. [CrossRef]
23. Li, T.; Yang, Y.; Hua, X.; Wang, G.; Liu, W.; Jia, C.; Tai, Y.; Zhang, Q.; Chen, G. Hepatocellular carcinoma-associated fibroblasts trigger NK cell dysfunction via PGE2 and IDO. *Cancer Lett.* **2012**, *318*, 154–161. [CrossRef]
24. Neaud, V.; Faouzi, S.; Guirouilh, J.; Le Bail, B.; Balabaud, C.; Bioulac-Sage, P.; Rosenbaum, J. Human hepatic myofibroblasts increase invasiveness of hepatocellular carcinoma cells: Evidence for a role of hepatocyte growth factor. *Hepatology* **1997**, *26*, 1458–1466. [CrossRef]
25. Dunham, R.M.; Thapa, M.; Velazquez, V.M.; Elrod, E.J.; Denning, T.L.; Pulendran, B.; Grakoui, A. Hepatic stellate cells preferentially induce Foxp3+ regulatory T cells by production of retinoic acid. *J. Immunol.* **2013**, *190*, 2009–2016. [CrossRef] [PubMed]
26. Hochst, B.; Schildberg, F.A.; Sauerborn, P.; Gabel, Y.A.; Gevensleben, H.; Goltz, D.; Heukamp, L.C.; Turler, A.; Ballmaier, M.; Gieseke, F.; et al. Activated human hepatic stellate cells induce myeloid derived suppressor cells from peripheral blood monocytes in a CD44-dependent fashion. *J. Hepatol.* **2013**, *59*, 528–535. [CrossRef] [PubMed]
27. Gessi, S.; Merighi, S.; Sacchetto, V.; Simioni, C.; Borea, P.A. Adenosine receptors and cancer. *Biochim. Biophys. Acta* **2011**, *1808*, 1400–1412. [CrossRef] [PubMed]
28. Zhao, Q.; Kuang, D.M.; Wu, Y.; Xiao, X.; Li, X.F.; Li, T.J.; Zheng, L. Activated CD69+ T cells foster immune privilege by regulating IDO expression in tumor-associated macrophages. *J. Immunol.* **2012**, *188*, 1117–1124. [CrossRef]
29. Mezrich, J.D.; Fechner, J.H.; Zhang, X.; Johnson, B.P.; Burlingham, W.J.; Bradfield, C.A. An interaction between kynurenine and the aryl hydrocarbon receptor can generate regulatory T cells. *J. Immunol.* **2010**, *185*, 3190–3198. [CrossRef] [PubMed]
30. Chen, J.; Jiang, C.C.; Jin, L.; Zhang, X.D. Regulation of PD-L1: A novel role of pro-survival signalling in cancer. *Ann. Oncol.* **2016**, *27*, 409–416. [CrossRef]
31. Jiang, X.; Zhou, J.; Giobbie-Hurder, A.; Wargo, J.; Hodi, F.S. The activation of MAPK in melanoma cells resistant to BRAF inhibition promotes PD-L1 expression that is reversible by MEK and PI3K inhibition. *Clin. Cancer Res.* **2013**, *19*, 598–609. [CrossRef]
32. Song, M.; Chen, D.; Lu, B.; Wang, C.; Zhang, J.; Huang, L.; Wang, X.; Timmons, C.L.; Hu, J.; Liu, B.; et al. PTEN loss increases PD-L1 protein expression and affects the correlation between PD-L1 expression and clinical parameters in colorectal cancer. *PLoS ONE* **2013**, *8*, e65821. [CrossRef]
33. Nishida, N.; Sakai, K.; Morita, M.; Aoki, T.; Takita, M.; Hagiwara, S.; Komeda, Y.; Takenaka, M.; Minami, Y.; Ida, H.; et al. Association between Genetic and Immunological Background of Hepatocellular Carcinoma and Expression of Programmed Cell Death-1. *Liver Cancer* **2020**, *9*, 426–439. [CrossRef]
34. Yan, W.; Liu, X.; Ma, H.; Zhang, H.; Song, X.; Gao, L.; Liang, X.; Ma, C. Tim-3 fosters HCC development by enhancing TGF-beta-mediated alternative activation of macrophages. *Gut* **2015**, *64*, 1593–1604. [CrossRef]
35. Zheng, C.; Zheng, L.; Yoo, J.K.; Guo, H.; Zhang, Y.; Guo, X.; Kang, B.; Hu, R.; Huang, J.Y.; Zhang, Q.; et al. Landscape of Infiltrating T Cells in Liver Cancer Revealed by Single-Cell Sequencing. *Cell* **2017**, *169*, 1342–1356.e16. [CrossRef]

36. Sangro, B.; Sarobe, P.; Hervas-Stubbs, S.; Melero, I. Advances in immunotherapy for hepatocellular carcinoma. *Nat. Rev. Gastroenterol. Hepatol.* **2021**. [CrossRef] [PubMed]
37. Alexandrov, L.B.; Nik-Zainal, S.; Wedge, D.C.; Aparicio, S.A.; Behjati, S.; Biankin, A.V.; Bignell, G.R.; Bolli, N.; Borg, A.; Borresen-Dale, A.L.; et al. Signatures of mutational processes in human cancer. *Nature* **2013**, *500*, 415–421. [CrossRef] [PubMed]
38. Ringelhan, M.; Pfister, D.; O'Connor, T.; Pikarsky, E.; Heikenwalder, M. The immunology of hepatocellular carcinoma. *Nat. Immunol.* **2018**, *19*, 222–232. [CrossRef]
39. McLane, L.M.; Abdel-Hakeem, M.S.; Wherry, E.J. CD8 T Cell Exhaustion During Chronic Viral Infection and Cancer. *Annu. Rev. Immunol.* **2019**, *37*, 457–495. [CrossRef]
40. Pfister, D.; Nunez, N.G.; Pinyol, R.; Govaere, O.; Pinter, M.; Szydlowska, M.; Gupta, R.; Qiu, M.; Deczkowska, A.; Weiner, A.; et al. NASH limits anti-tumour surveillance in immunotherapy-treated HCC. *Nature* **2021**, *592*, 450–456. [CrossRef] [PubMed]
41. Schinzari, V.; Timperi, E.; Pecora, G.; Palmucci, F.; Gallerano, D.; Grimaldi, A.; Covino, D.A.; Guglielmo, N.; Melandro, F.; Manzi, E.; et al. Wnt3a/beta-Catenin Signaling Conditions Differentiation of Partially Exhausted T-effector Cells in Human Cancers. *Cancer Immunol. Res.* **2018**, *6*, 941–952. [CrossRef]
42. Pacella, I.; Cammarata, I.; Focaccetti, C.; Miacci, S.; Gulino, A.; Tripodo, C.; Rava, M.; Barnaba, V.; Piconese, S. Wnt3a Neutralization Enhances T-cell Responses through Indirect Mechanisms and Restrains Tumor Growth. *Cancer Immunol. Res.* **2018**, *6*, 953–964. [CrossRef]
43. Franceschini, D.; Paroli, M.; Francavilla, V.; Videtta, M.; Morrone, S.; Labbadia, G.; Cerino, A.; Mondelli, M.U.; Barnaba, V. PD-L1 negatively regulates CD4+CD25+Foxp3+ Tregs by limiting STAT-5 phosphorylation in patients chronically infected with HCV. *J. Clin. Investig.* **2009**, *119*, 551–564. [CrossRef] [PubMed]
44. Kamada, T.; Togashi, Y.; Tay, C.; Ha, D.; Sasaki, A.; Nakamura, Y.; Sato, E.; Fukuoka, S.; Tada, Y.; Tanaka, A.; et al. PD-1(+) regulatory T cells amplified by PD-1 blockade promote hyperprogression of cancer. *Proc. Natl. Acad. Sci. USA* **2019**, *116*, 9999–10008. [CrossRef] [PubMed]
45. Kim, C.G.; Kim, C.; Yoon, S.E.; Kim, K.H.; Choi, S.J.; Kang, B.; Kim, H.R.; Park, S.H.; Shin, E.C.; Kim, Y.Y.; et al. Hyperprogressive disease during PD-1 blockade in patients with advanced hepatocellular carcinoma. *J. Hepatol.* **2021**, *74*, 350–359. [CrossRef]
46. Sumimoto, H.; Imabayashi, F.; Iwata, T.; Kawakami, Y. The BRAF-MAPK signaling pathway is essential for cancer-immune evasion in human melanoma cells. *J. Exp. Med.* **2006**, *203*, 1651–1656. [CrossRef]
47. Boni, A.; Cogdill, A.P.; Dang, P.; Udayakumar, D.; Njauw, C.N.; Sloss, C.M.; Ferrone, C.R.; Flaherty, K.T.; Lawrence, D.P.; Fisher, D.E.; et al. Selective BRAFV600E inhibition enhances T-cell recognition of melanoma without affecting lymphocyte function. *Cancer Res.* **2010**, *70*, 5213–5219. [CrossRef]
48. Loi, S.; Dushyanthen, S.; Beavis, P.A.; Salgado, R.; Denkert, C.; Savas, P.; Combs, S.; Rimm, D.L.; Giltnane, J.M.; Estrada, M.V.; et al. RAS/MAPK Activation Is Associated with Reduced Tumor-Infiltrating Lymphocytes in Triple-Negative Breast Cancer: Therapeutic Cooperation Between MEK and PD-1/PD-L1 Immune Checkpoint Inhibitors. *Clin. Cancer Res.* **2016**, *22*, 1499–1509. [CrossRef]
49. Pylayeva-Gupta, Y.; Lee, K.E.; Hajdu, C.H.; Miller, G.; Bar-Sagi, D. Oncogenic Kras-induced GM-CSF production promotes the development of pancreatic neoplasia. *Cancer Cell* **2012**, *21*, 836–847. [CrossRef] [PubMed]
50. Liao, W.; Overman, M.J.; Boutin, A.T.; Shang, X.; Zhao, D.; Dey, P.; Li, J.; Wang, G.; Lan, Z.; Li, J.; et al. KRAS-IRF2 Axis Drives Immune Suppression and Immune Therapy Resistance in Colorectal Cancer. *Cancer Cell* **2019**, *35*, 559–572.e7. [CrossRef]
51. Peng, W.; Chen, J.Q.; Liu, C.; Malu, S.; Creasy, C.; Tetzlaff, M.T.; Xu, C.; McKenzie, J.A.; Zhang, C.; Liang, X.; et al. Loss of PTEN Promotes Resistance to T Cell-Mediated Immunotherapy. *Cancer Discov.* **2016**, *6*, 202–216. [CrossRef]
52. Borcoman, E.; De La Rochere, P.; Richer, W.; Vacher, S.; Chemlali, W.; Krucker, C.; Sirab, N.; Radvanyi, F.; Allory, Y.; Pignot, G.; et al. Inhibition of PI3K pathway increases immune infiltrate in muscle-invasive bladder cancer. *Oncoimmunology* **2019**, *8*, e1581556. [CrossRef]
53. Kaneda, M.M.; Messer, K.S.; Ralainirina, N.; Li, H.; Leem, C.J.; Gorjestani, S.; Woo, G.; Nguyen, A.V.; Figueiredo, C.C.; Foubert, P.; et al. PI3Kgamma is a molecular switch that controls immune suppression. *Nature* **2016**, *539*, 437–442. [CrossRef]
54. Spranger, S.; Bao, R.; Gajewski, T.F. Melanoma-intrinsic beta-catenin signalling prevents anti-tumour immunity. *Nature* **2015**, *523*, 231–235. [CrossRef]
55. Ruiz de Galarreta, M.; Bresnahan, E.; Molina-Sanchez, P.; Lindblad, K.E.; Maier, B.; Sia, D.; Puigvehi, M.; Miguela, V.; Casanova-Acebes, M.; Dhainaut, M.; et al. beta-Catenin Activation Promotes Immune Escape and Resistance to Anti-PD-1 Therapy in Hepatocellular Carcinoma. *Cancer Discov.* **2019**, *9*, 1124–1141. [CrossRef]
56. Yaguchi, T.; Goto, Y.; Kido, K.; Mochimaru, H.; Sakurai, T.; Tsukamoto, N.; Kudo-Saito, C.; Fujita, T.; Sumimoto, H.; Kawakami, Y. Immune suppression and resistance mediated by constitutive activation of Wnt/beta-catenin signaling in human melanoma cells. *J. Immunol.* **2012**, *189*, 2110–2117. [CrossRef]
57. Casey, S.C.; Tong, L.; Li, Y.; Do, R.; Walz, S.; Fitzgerald, K.N.; Gouw, A.M.; Baylot, V.; Gutgemann, I.; Eilers, M.; et al. MYC regulates the antitumor immune response through CD47 and PD-L1. *Science* **2016**, *352*, 227–231. [CrossRef]
58. Miao, D.; Margolis, C.A.; Gao, W.; Voss, M.H.; Li, W.; Martini, D.J.; Norton, C.; Bosse, D.; Wankowicz, S.M.; Cullen, D.; et al. Genomic correlates of response to immune checkpoint therapies in clear cell renal cell carcinoma. *Science* **2018**, *359*, 801–806. [CrossRef]

59. Zaretsky, J.M.; Garcia-Diaz, A.; Shin, D.S.; Escuin-Ordinas, H.; Hugo, W.; Hu-Lieskovan, S.; Torrejon, D.Y.; Abril-Rodriguez, G.; Sandoval, S.; Barthly, L.; et al. Mutations Associated with Acquired Resistance to PD-1 Blockade in Melanoma. *N. Engl. J. Med.* **2016**, *375*, 819–829. [CrossRef]
60. Romero, J.M.; Jimenez, P.; Cabrera, T.; Cozar, J.M.; Pedrinaci, S.; Tallada, M.; Garrido, F.; Ruiz-Cabello, F. Coordinated downregulation of the antigen presentation machinery and HLA class I/beta2-microglobulin complex is responsible for HLA-ABC loss in bladder cancer. *Int. J. Cancer* **2005**, *113*, 605–610. [CrossRef]
61. Wang, G.; Lu, X.; Dey, P.; Deng, P.; Wu, C.C.; Jiang, S.; Fang, Z.; Zhao, K.; Konaparthi, R.; Hua, S.; et al. Targeting YAP-Dependent MDSC Infiltration Impairs Tumor Progression. *Cancer Discov.* **2016**, *6*, 80–95. [CrossRef]
62. Guo, X.; Zhao, Y.; Yan, H.; Yang, Y.; Shen, S.; Dai, X.; Ji, X.; Ji, F.; Gong, X.G.; Li, L.; et al. Single tumor-initiating cells evade immune clearance by recruiting type II macrophages. *Genes Dev.* **2017**, *31*, 247–259. [CrossRef]
63. Le, D.T.; Durham, J.N.; Smith, K.N.; Wang, H.; Bartlett, B.R.; Aulakh, L.K.; Lu, S.; Kemberling, H.; Wilt, C.; Luber, B.S.; et al. Mismatch repair deficiency predicts response of solid tumors to PD-1 blockade. *Science* **2017**, *357*, 409–413. [CrossRef]
64. Gibney, G.T.; Weiner, L.M.; Atkins, M.B. Predictive biomarkers for checkpoint inhibitor-based immunotherapy. *Lancet Oncol.* **2016**, *17*, e542–e551. [CrossRef]
65. Zhou, Z.; Li, M. Evaluation of BRCA1 and BRCA2 as Indicators of Response to Immune Checkpoint Inhibitors. *JAMA Netw. Open* **2021**, *4*, e217728. [CrossRef]
66. Shigeta, K.; Datta, M.; Hato, T.; Kitahara, S.; Chen, I.X.; Matsui, A.; Kikuchi, H.; Mamessier, E.; Aoki, S.; Ramjiawan, R.R.; et al. Dual Programmed Death Receptor-1 and Vascular Endothelial Growth Factor Receptor-2 Blockade Promotes Vascular Normalization and Enhances Antitumor Immune Responses in Hepatocellular Carcinoma. *Hepatology* **2020**, *71*, 1247–1261. [CrossRef]
67. Sia, D.; Jiao, Y.; Martinez-Quetglas, I.; Kuchuk, O.; Villacorta-Martin, C.; Castro de Moura, M.; Putra, J.; Camprecios, G.; Bassaganyas, L.; Akers, N.; et al. Identification of an Immune-specific Class of Hepatocellular Carcinoma, Based on Molecular Features. *Gastroenterology* **2017**, *153*, 812–826. [CrossRef]
68. Harding, J.J.; Nandakumar, S.; Armenia, J.; Khalil, D.N.; Albano, M.; Ly, M.; Shia, J.; Hechtman, J.F.; Kundra, R.; El Dika, I.; et al. Prospective Genotyping of Hepatocellular Carcinoma: Clinical Implications of Next-Generation Sequencing for Matching Patients to Targeted and Immune Therapies. *Clin. Cancer Res.* **2019**, *25*, 2116–2126. [CrossRef]
69. Morita, M.; Nishida, N.; Sakai, K.; Aoki, T.; Chishina, H.; Takita, M.; Ida, H.; Hagiwara, S.; Minami, Y.; Ueshima, K.; et al. Immunological microenvironment predicts the survival of the patients with hepatocellular carcinoma treated with anti-PD-1 antibody. *Liver Cancer* **2021**, *10*, 380–393, in press. [CrossRef]

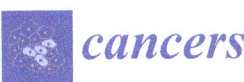

Systematic Review

A Broad Overview of Signaling in *Ph*-Negative Classic Myeloproliferative Neoplasms

Ana Guijarro-Hernández [1] and José Luis Vizmanos [1,2,*]

[1] Department of Biochemistry and Genetics, School of Sciences, University of Navarra, 31008 Pamplona, Spain; aguijarro@unav.es
[2] Navarra Institute for Health Research (IdiSNA), 31008 Pamplona, Spain
* Correspondence: jlvizmanos@unav.es

Simple Summary: There is growing evidence that *Ph*-negative myeloproliferative neoplasms are disorders in which multiple signaling pathways are significantly disturbed. The heterogeneous phenotypes observed among patients have highlighted the importance of having a comprehensive knowledge of the molecular mechanisms behind these diseases. This review aims to show a broad overview of the signaling involved in myeloproliferative neoplasms (MPNs) and other processes that can modify them, which could be helpful to better understand these diseases and develop more effective targeted treatments.

Abstract: *Ph*-negative myeloproliferative neoplasms (polycythemia vera (PV), essential thrombocythemia (ET) and primary myelofibrosis (PMF)) are infrequent blood cancers characterized by signaling aberrations. Shortly after the discovery of the somatic mutations in JAK2, MPL, and CALR that cause these diseases, researchers extensively studied the aberrant functions of their mutant products. In all three cases, the main pathogenic mechanism appears to be the constitutive activation of JAK2/STAT signaling and JAK2-related pathways (MAPK/ERK, PI3K/AKT). However, some other non-canonical aberrant mechanisms derived from mutant JAK2 and CALR have also been described. Moreover, additional somatic mutations have been identified in other genes that affect epigenetic regulation, tumor suppression, transcription regulation, splicing and other signaling pathways, leading to the modification of some disease features and adding a layer of complexity to their molecular pathogenesis. All of these factors have highlighted the wide variety of cellular processes and pathways involved in the pathogenesis of MPNs. This review presents an overview of the complex signaling behind these diseases which could explain, at least in part, their phenotypic heterogeneity.

Keywords: myeloproliferative neoplasms; signaling pathways; JAK2; CALR; MPL; TPOR

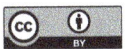

1. Introduction

Myeloproliferative neoplasms (MPNs) are rare hematological malignancies characterized by the clonal expansion of mature myeloid cells. MPNs arise from certain somatic mutations in hematopoietic stem cells (HSCs) which provide a selective advantage and lead to the expansion of aberrant clones.

Classic MPNs consist of chronic myeloid leukemia (CML), polycythemia vera (PV), essential thrombocythemia (ET) and primary myelofibrosis (PMF). In the last few years, the advances in molecular biology have provided key insights into the molecular mechanisms behind these diseases. CML is genetically defined by the *Philadelphia* (*Ph*) chromosome, the result of t(9;22)(q34;q11). This translocation leads to the production of a chimeric BCR-ABL1 protein with constitutive tyrosine kinase activity. The description of the *Ph* chromosome as a disease-initiating event in CML revolutionized the diagnosis and treatment of this disease [1]. The targeted therapy imatinib showed a specific inhibitory capacity against the tyrosine kinase activity of BCR-ABL1 [2–4] that, despite not being curative [5], increased the 10-year survival of CML patients in chronic phase to more than 83%–84% [6,7].

This review is focused on PV, ET and PMF, all of them *Ph*-negative MPNs that share similar and mostly mutually exclusive driver mutations affecting *JAK2*, *MPL* and *CALR*. The aberrant functions of the mutant products encoded by these genes have been extensively studied and the main mechanisms that lead to the myeloproliferation described. Currently, it is considered that the major hallmark of *Ph*-negative MPNs is the constitutive activation of JAK2-related signaling pathways. In fact, at this time, the only targeted therapy approved in MPNs is the JAK1/2 inhibitor ruxolitinib, which can reduce splenomegaly and other common symptoms in patients with PMF, post-PV/ET MF [8,9] and PV resistant or intolerant to hydroxyurea [9,10]. Although a reduction in the mutant allele burden is rare [9], it could be achieved in long-term treatment [11]. However, the improvement in the overall survival of ruxolitinib-treated patients has been questioned [12–14]. Actually, malignant cells can still survive in these patients and the clinical response could be mainly due to the downmodulation of proinflammatory cytokines derived from the JAK2 inhibition [15]. These arguments have led researchers to question whether JAK2 is really the best drug target in these diseases or not [16].

In the meantime, some non-canonical mechanisms of mutant JAK2 [17–24] and CALR [25–33] have been described. Chronic inflammation [34–62] and the bone marrow microenvironment [63–72] also seem to contribute to the heterogeneous phenotypes found among MPN patients.

Additionally, mutations in disease-modifying genes that seem to increase the risk of leukemic transformation or progression from ET to myelofibrosis have also been identified [73–75]. The products encoded by these genes are involved in epigenetic modification, tumor suppression, transcription regulation, splicing, and some other signaling pathways [76,77]. Other factors, such as genetic predisposition, age or environment have also been shown to influence the heterogeneity of MPN phenotypes [78].

This review presents an overview of the signaling behind *Ph*-negative MPNs attending not only to the activation of JAK2-related canonical signaling pathways, but also to other non-canonical pathways, disease-modifying signaling, and additional factors that have been found to be involved in the pathogenesis of these diseases.

2. JAK2-Related Canonical Signaling Pathways

JAK2 signaling is activated through a variety of receptors such as those for erythropoietin (EPOR), thrombopoietin (TPOR), and granulocyte/macrophage colony-stimulating factor (GM-CSFR). They regulate the production of the erythroid, megakaryocytic, and granulocytic lineages, respectively. When stimulated by ligands, receptors dimerize and bring JAK2 kinases into proximity. JAK2 is phosphorylated upon receptor binding and induces the phosphorylation of the cytoplasmic portion of the receptor and downstream factors.

In 2005, several research groups simultaneously published the presence of the somatic mutation p.V617F (JAK2^{V617F}) in the exon 14 of *JAK2* in patients with PV (96%), PMF (65%) and ET (55%) [79–84]. This mutation impairs the physiological inhibitory function of the JH2 pseudokinase domain upon the JH1 kinase domain, which acquires a constitutive activation that promotes JAK2 phosphorylation in the absence of ligand stimulation (Figure 1). In 2007, four additional gain-of-function somatic mutations in the exon 12 of *JAK2* were detected in 3% of patients with PV [84,85]: p.N542-E543del (30%), p.K539L (14%), p.E543-D544del (12%), and p.F537-K539delinsL (10%). All of them are located upstream of the JH2 pseudokinase domain and promote an increased phosphorylation of JAK2 compared to p.V617F [86].

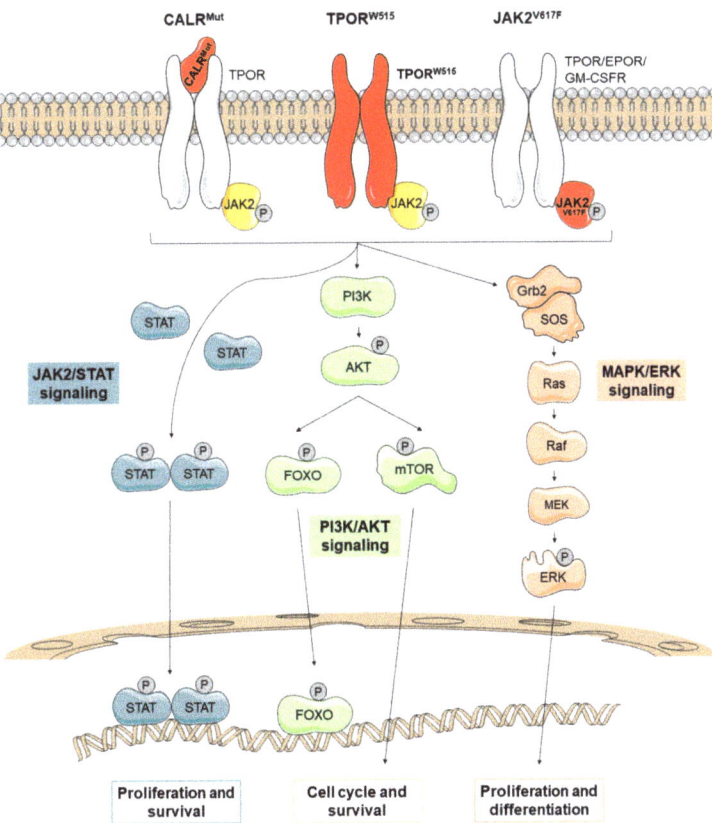

Figure 1. JAK2-related canonical signaling pathways active in *Ph*-negative myeloproliferative neoplasms (MPNs). Mutations in *CALR* (CALR^{MUT}), *JAK2* (JAK2^{V617F}), and *MPL* (TPOR^{W515}) lead to the constitutive activation of JAK2/STAT, PI3K/AKT, and MAPK/ERK signaling that promotes the transport to the nucleus of several transcription factors such as STATs and FOXO. There, they regulate transcription of their target genes, causing increased proliferation and survival of mutant cells. Mutant proteins are depicted in red.

In 2006, the gain-of-function mutation p.W515L in the exon 10 of *MPL* was identified in a minor proportion of MPN patients [87]. p.W515L and p.W515K are the most commonly reported mutations, identified in approximately 5% of PMF patients and 1% of ET patients [88]. *MPL* encodes the thrombopoietin receptor (TPOR), which depends on JAKs to mediate signal transduction. *MPL* mutations (TPOR^{W515}) promote the dimerization and activation of TPOR, leading to transphosphorylation and activation of the previously bound JAK2 proteins (Figure 1) [89].

The molecular alteration that causes the 60–90% of PMF and ET cases in patients not harboring *JAK2/MPL* mutations was described in 2013 [90]. During that year, two research groups identified mutations in *CALR* [91,92], a gene that encodes calreticulin, a ubiquitous protein found in the endoplasmic reticulum (ER) of all nucleated cells with multiple functions inside and outside this organelle. CALR is a Ca^{2+}-binding chaperone mainly involved in the regulation of intracellular Ca^{2+} homeostasis and a regulator of protein folding in the cellular response to ER stress (unfolding protein response (UPR)) [93]. However, this protein has been also found associated with other cytoplasmic, nuclear and extracellular proteins, so it could be involved in a wide variety of signaling pathways [94].

In fact, CALR has been associated with cellular stress responses, adipocyte differentiation, cardiogenesis, proliferation, wound healing, apoptosis and immunogenic cell death [90,94].

The structure of wild-type CALR consists of a signal peptide and three domains: an amino-terminal N-domain, a proline-rich P-domain and a carboxy-terminal C-domain, which contains an ER retention signal (KDEL). The *CALR* mutations described to date are insertions or deletions in exon 9 that shift the reading frame by one base pair (+1), mainly a 52-bp deletion (c.1902_1143del) or type 1 mutation (CALR^{del52}), and a 5-bp insertion (c.1154_1155insTTGTC) or type 2 mutation (CALR^{ins5}). As a result, mutant CALRs (CALR^{Mut}) show a novel C-terminal end that lacks the ER retention motif (KDEL) [91,92] and some Ca^{2+}-binding sites [95]. In 2016, it was published that CALR^{Mut} is transported to the cellular membrane where it activates TPOR in a ligand-independent manner (Figure 1) [96–99]. The characterization of the TPOR binding capacity has revealed that the C-terminal end of CALR^{Mut} blocks the P-domain of the protein, which constitutively exerts an inhibitory effect on the N-domain. Consequently, the N-domain can bind to immature N-glycans on TPOR [96]. This mechanism is consistent with the observation that the N-glycan binding motif located in N-domain of CALR^{Mut} is required for TPOR activation [97]. In fact, blocking N-glycosylation on asparagine 117 of TPOR diminishes CALR-dependent TPOR activation [97,100]. Both wild-type and mutant CALR recognize immature forms of N-glycans and fold the protein correctly, but CALR^{Mut} fails to dissociate from the targeted protein [101]. Thus, the CALR^{Mut}-TPOR complex moves from the ER to the plasma membrane through the Golgi apparatus and is secreted out of cells [102]. However, secreted CALR^{Mut} is only capable to activate TPOR on the cell surface of cells expressing CALR^{Mut} since only these cells have the immature N-glycans on TPOR [96,102,103]. Stimulation of TPOR leads to the activation of JAK2-dependent signaling in a similar way to the rest of the *Ph*-negative MPNs.

In conclusion, the mutations described to date in *JAK2*, *MPL* and *CALR* lead to a constitutive activation of JAK2, which ultimately causes the aberrant proliferation and survival of malignant myeloid clones. The three major downstream signaling pathways that are activated by JAK2 are JAK2/STATs, MAPK/ERK, and PI3K/AKT (Figure 1). The evidence suggests that each of these pathways plays an important role in MPNs, although the JAK2/STAT pathway appears to be the main one. In fact, dysregulation of JAK2/STAT signaling has been identified in all MPNs regardless of mutational status [104].

2.1. JAK2/STAT Pathway

In MPNs, JAK2 phosphorylates and activates STATs (mainly STAT1, STAT3 and STAT5). It seems that STATs are differentially activated depending on the type of MPN. For example, *MPL* mutations increase STAT3 and STAT5 signaling. In PV patients, JAK2^{V617F} binds to EPOR promoting STAT5 activation. In ET patients, both JAK2^{V617F} and CALR^{Mut} bind to TPOR; JAK2^{V617F} enhances the phosphorylation of STAT1 and STAT3 but CALR^{Mut} promotes STAT3 and STAT5 activation. However, in PMF, phosphorylation of STAT3 is decreased in both JAK2^{V617F} and mutant CALRs. To date, the precise mechanisms that explain differential activation of the STATs remain unclear [78].

Once the STATs are phosphorylated, they form a dimer that enters the nucleus to activate the transcription of target genes (Figure 1). In this way, JAK2/STAT signaling stimulates cell proliferation, differentiation and survival.

2.2. MAPK/ERK Pathway

The activated JAK2 can also lead to the phosphorylation of ERK, a serine threonine kinase that activates multiple proteins in both the cytoplasm and the nucleus. ERK is a key regulator of a wide variety of signaling pathways, so its deregulation could disrupt multiple processes. In the cytoplasm, ERK contributes to ion transport, apoptosis, and regulation of metabolism, among others. In the nucleus, it targets regulators of cell cycle and multiple transcription factors (Figure 1) [105].

2.3. PI3K/AKT Pathway

JAK2 activation also stimulates the PI3K/AKT pathway. AKT is a cell survival kinase which inhibits apoptosis by phosphorylating the proapoptotic protein BAD and the transcription factor FOXO3A. In addition, AKT can activate a wide range of mechanisms such as protein translation through mTOR or the cell cycle machinery (Figure 1) [105].

3. Non-Canonical Signaling Pathways

3.1. JAK2-Related Non-Canonical Signaling

In 2009, activated JAK2 was described to be in the nucleus of hematopoietic cells and to phosphorylate Y41 on histone 3 (H3Y41). This event prevents the binding of heterochromatin protein 1 alpha (HP1α) to H3Y41 [17]. HP1α shows a proliferation-dependent regulation and is involved in gene silencing, genome stability, and chromosome segregation (Figure 2). It has been found overexpressed in some tumors, and it has been proposed as a potential hallmark of cell proliferation that could be relevant in clinical oncology [18].

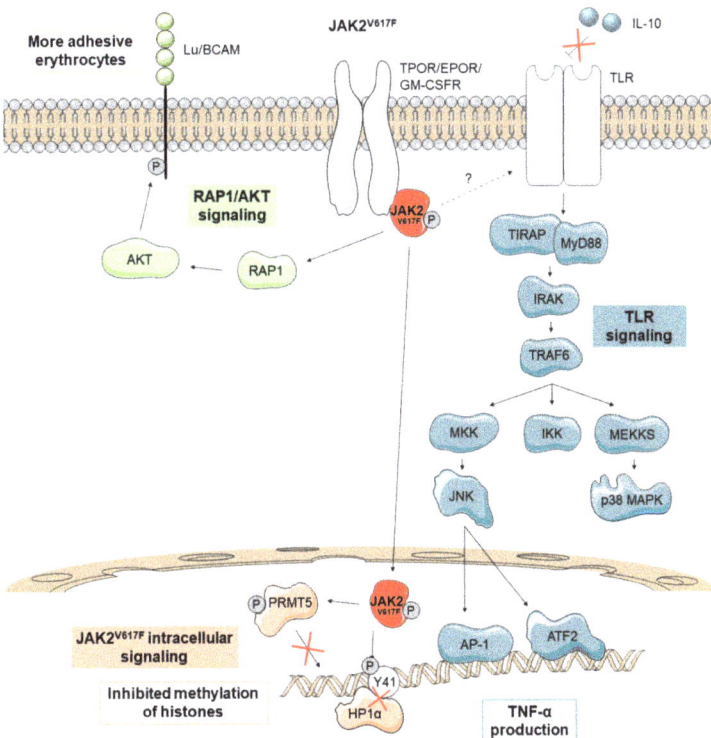

Figure 2. Main non-canonical signaling pathways activated by JAK2^{V617F} in *Ph*-negative MPNs. In PV patients, JAK2^{V617F} (depicted in red) activates the adhesion receptor Lu/BCAM through the RAP1-AKT signaling pathway, making their erythrocytes more adhesive. JAK2^{V617F} has also been described to promote aberrant signaling in the nucleus, where it prevents the binding of heterochromatin protein 1 alpha (HP1α) and inhibits the methylation of histones via protein arginine methyltransferase 5 (PRMT5) impairment. MPN patients with JAK2^{V617F} also seem to be insensitive to the anti-inflammatory cytokine IL-10, increasing TNF-α production through Toll-Like Receptor (TLR) signaling.

JAK2^{V617F} also acquires the ability to phosphorylate the protein arginine methyltransferase 5 (PRMT5) leading to an impairment in its ability to methylate histones (Figure 2). When PRMT5 is knocked down in CD34+ cells, an increased colony formation and erythroid differentiation can be observed [19].

A recent study also suggests that erythrocytes from PV patients are more adhesive since JAK2^{V617F} activates the erythrocyte adhesion receptor Lu/BCAM through an EPOR-independent RAP1/AKT signaling pathway (Figure 2) [20].

Finally, monocytes from MPN patients with JAK2^{V617F} have been found to have a defective negative regulation of toll-like receptor (TLR) signaling leading to increased production of the inflammatory cytokine TNF-α. These monocytes are insensitive to the anti-inflammatory cytokine IL-10, which in turn negatively regulates TNF-α production through TLR (Figure 2) [21]. Studies on TNF-α knockout mice have demonstrated that this cytokine is required for the development of an MPN-like disease [22]. Unrestrained production of TNF-α has been observed in an MPN patient but also in his identical twin, suggesting that it may be a genetic feature rather than a consequence of the disease [21]. In any case, the inflammatory environment can favor the maintenance and expansion of the JAK2^{V617F} mutant clone since these cells are resistant to inflammation whereas non-mutant cells are not [22]. Thus, the JAK2^{V617F} mutant clone seems to induce non-mutant cells to produce inflammatory cytokines, reinforcing the self-perpetuating environment for its continuous selection [23]. Finally, CD34+ progenitors of a PV patient with JAK2^{V617F} have been reported to use dual-specificity phosphatase 1 (DUSP1) to protect themselves against inflammatory stress and DNA damage, promoting their proliferation and survival in this microenvironment (Figure 2) [24].

3.2. CALR-Related Non-Canonical Signaling

Several studies have identified novel mechanisms that collaborate with the activation of TPOR in CALR-mediated cellular transformation (Figure 3). CALR^{Mut} seems to cause reduced activation of the UPR pro-apoptotic pathway and to have an increased sensitivity to oxidative stress by the down-modulation of oxidation resistance 1 (OXR1) in K562 cells. These mechanisms lead to resistance to UPR-induced apoptosis and genomic instability, respectively [25]. Moreover, CALR^{del52} causes increased recruitment of the friend leukemia integration 1 (FLI1) transcription factor to the *MPL* promoter to enhance transcription [26], which suggests a promotion of tumorigenesis by modulating transcription through interactions with transcription factors in the nucleus.

Bioinformatic analyses of CALR^{Mut} revealed the appearance of potential phosphorylation sites for kinases that may have a role in the regulation of multiple cellular activities [27] and recent studies have shown that CALR^{Mut} causes increased binding affinities for proteins involved in the activation of the UPR (HSPA5, HSPA9, and HSPA8) and cytoskeletal (MYL9 and APRC4) and ribosomal proteins (RP17, RSP23, and RPL11), as well as reduced binding to MSI2, a transcriptional regulator that targets genes mainly involved in cell cycle regulation [26].

On the other hand, CALR is an integral part of the peptide loading complex (PLC), which mediates the loading of cellular antigens onto major histocompatibility complex class I (MHC-I) molecules. In addition to CALR, the PLC is composed of PDIA3, TAP-binding protein, TAP1, and TAP2. Specifically, CALR interacts with PDIA3 in a glycan-dependent manner and preserves steady-state levels of TAP-binding protein and MHC-I heavy chains. Besides, it rescues suboptimally assembled MHC-I molecules from post-ER compartments [28]. HEK293T cells lacking CALR expression show a reduction of properly loaded MHC-I on the cell surface, a defect that is not restored by expression of CALR^{Mut} [29]. Consistent with this, cells with CALR^{Mut} show reduced antigen presentation on MHC-I (Figure 3) [54] and decreased binding affinities for PDIA3 [26]. These results suggest that *CALR* mutations have a loss-of-function effect on PLC and, therefore, may contribute to the development of MPN by promoting immunoevasion after loss of tumor antigenicity [28]. Additionally, CALR operates as a key damage-associated molecular pattern (DAMP) when it is translocated to the outer cell membrane of dying cancer cells. CALR-exposing cancer cells deliver pro-phagocytic signals to antigen presenting cells (APCs) and activate dendritic cell efferocytosis. Mutations in *CALR* increase the secretion of the protein both in vitro and in vivo since the ER retention motif (KDEL) is compromised. Soluble CALR binds to CALR receptors in the APCs and limit their ability to phagocytise, leading to immunosuppressive effects (Figure 3) [30].

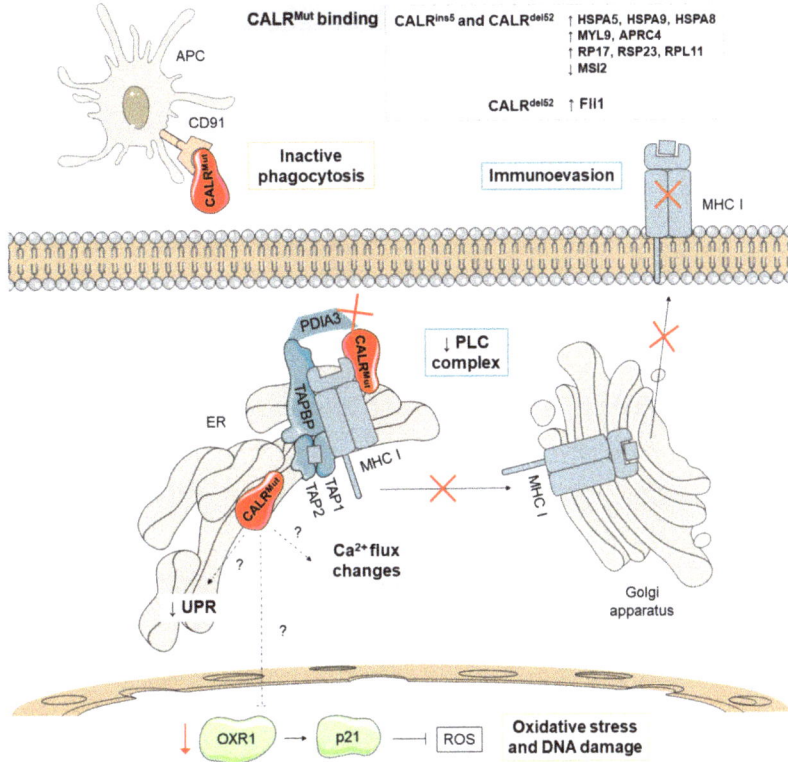

Figure 3. Major non-canonical mechanisms derived from CALR^{Mut}. CALR^{Mut} (depicted in red) shows different binding affinities for proteins implicated in the unfolding protein response (UPR) (HSPA5, HSPA9, and HSPA8), proteins of the cytoskeleton (MYL9 and APRC4), and ribosomal proteins (RP17, RSP23, and RPL11), as well as reduced binding to MSI2, a transcriptional regulator that target genes mainly involved in cell cycle regulation. Additionally, CALR^{Mut} seems to reduce the activation of the pro-apoptotic pathway of the UPR and increases oxidative stress and DNA damage through the downmodulation of oxidation resistance 1 (OXR1). CALR^{Mut} also shows decreased binding affinities for PDIA3 and has a loss-of-function effect on the peptide loading complex (PLC), which mediates the loading of cellular antigens onto major histocompatibility complex class I (MHC-I) molecules, favoring immunoevasion. Mutations in *CALR* increase the secretion of the protein and bind to CALR receptors in antigen presenting cells (APCs), limiting their ability to phagocytize wild-type CALR-exposing cancer cells. The main differences between the phenotypes observed in patients with type 1 (del52) and type 2 (ins5) mutations have been attributed to thrombopoietin receptor (TPOR)-independent cytosolic calcium fluxes and the binding affinity for the transcription factor FLI1.

The wild-type CALR protein also regulates the activation of the stored-operated calcium entry (SOCE) machinery by interacting with PDIA3 and STIM1. Concretely,

STIM1 is a protein of the SOCE machinery that leads to calcium mobilization. $CALR^{Mut}$ has been shown to trigger TPOR-independent cytosolic calcium fluxes in megakaryocytes through defective interactions between $CALR^{Mut}$, PDIA3 and the SOCE machinery. This results in uncontrolled proliferation of megakaryocytes that can be reversed with a SOCE inhibitor [31].

The type of *CALR* mutation has been associated with different disease features. Thus, type 1 mutations are more often associated with PMF (70%) or progression from ET to a myelofibrotic state [32], while type 2 mutations are more often associated with ET [91]. The mechanisms underlying this phenomenon have not been fully elucidated, but it has been demonstrated that type 2 mutants retain longer stretches of the negatively charged amino acids of wild-type CALR than type 2 mutants, which may neutralize the positive electronic charge generated at the C-terminal end. Additionally, type 1 mutant C-terminus generates greater changes in megakaryocyte cytosolic calcium flux than type 2 mutants [33].

3.3. Additional Non-Canonical Signaling

Non-canonical mechanisms affecting inflammatory signaling pathways and the bone marrow microenvironment have been widely observed in all MPNs, regardless of subtype and driver mutation.

3.3.1. Inflammatory Signaling Pathways

As previously noted, chronic inflammation is a characteristic feature of MPNs (Figure 4). In fact, MPN patients typically exhibit increased levels of inflammatory cytokines [34,106]. The impaired JAK2/STAT signaling is not the only contributor to inflammation in these diseases, as the inhibition of JAK2 is not sufficient to normalize the levels of inflammatory cytokines [35]. On the contrary, a significant enrichment of the NF-κB signaling pathway has been observed in both malignant and non-malignant cells in MPNs [36].

NFE2 overexpression has also been reported in most patients and seems to play a role in chronic inflammation [37,38]. NFE2 participates in inflammatory cascades by increasing IL-8 transcription and promotes proliferation by activating the expression of CDK4, CDK6 and cyclin D3 [39,40]. In addition, it produces reactive oxygen species (ROS), a group of highly reactive oxygen-containing molecules which participate in numerous biological processes [41]. This results in lipid and protein oxidation, increased oxidative DNA damage (8-oxo-G), and subsequent double-stranded DNA breaks that induce instability [38]. Excessive ROS production and subsequent oxidative stress confer a proliferative advantage to $JAK2^{V617F}$ clones and activate proinflammatory pathways (NF-κB) that create more ROS. In this way, MPNs have recently been described as "a human inflammation model for cancer development", as they are characterized by a self-perpetuating circle in which inflammation creates ROS which in turn creates more inflammation [42].

Multiple inflammatory signaling pathways such as IFN-α and IL-1β have been also found to be involved in the pathogenesis of MPN. Interferons are key regulators of HSCs. Data from murine PV $JAK2^{V617F}$ models have shown that hematopoietic stem progenitor cells (HSPCs) become more proliferative and lose quiescence when treated with IFN-α, leading to their depletion [43,44]. The ability to deplete previously dormant malignant stem cells together with the enhancement of the immune response have made IFN-α one of the most efficient treatment options in MPNs [107]. On the other hand, IL-1β is a proinflammatory cytokine released by myeloid cells in response to TLR stimulation, that activates multiple downstream pathways such as NF-kB and p38 MAPK [45]. The preleukemic niche of MPNs secretes high levels of IL-1, which drives granulocyte/macrophage differentiation [46]. IL-6 and IL-8 also seem to participate in MPN pathogenesis. IL-6 is a proinflammatory cytokine produced by monocytes, macrophages and T-cells that signals via JAK1/STAT3 [45]. Several mouse models for MPNs have shown a high expression of IL-6 in both mutant and wild-type HSCs [23]. Additionally, elevated IL-6 levels have been observed in $JAK2^{V617F}$ PV and PMF patients [47]. In fact, some studies point that IL-6 may participate in the progression of MPN to AML [45]. IL-8 is also a proinflammatory chemokine released in response to IL-1 or TNF-α that binds to CXCR1 or CXCR2 and activate JAK/STAT, PI3K/AKT, MAPK, PLC/PKC and FAK [45]. Elevated levels of IL-8 have been found in PV and ET patients [48].

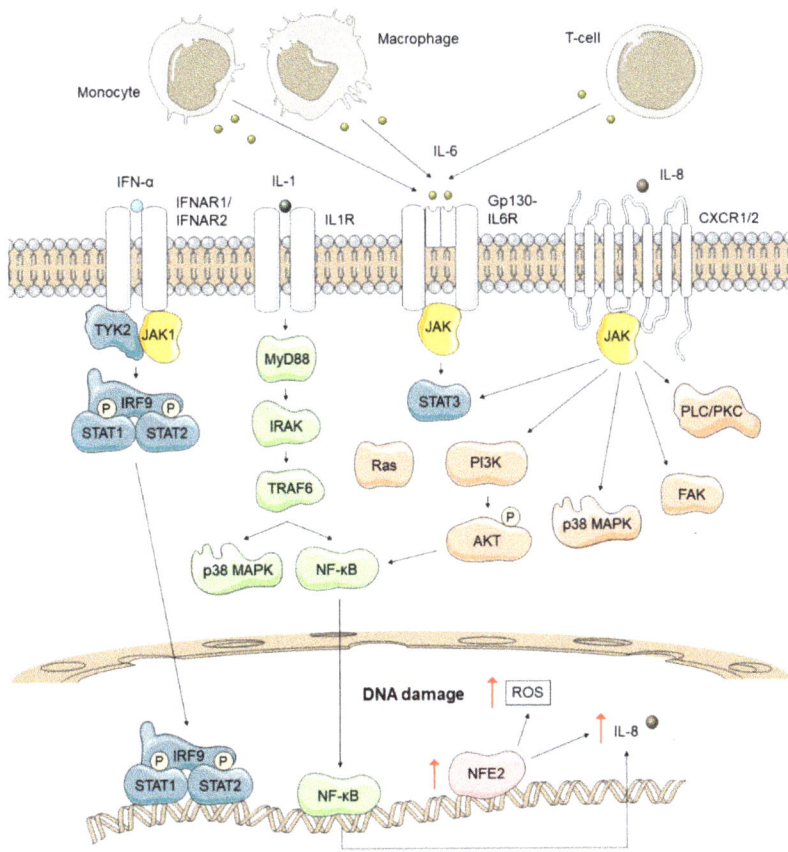

Figure 4. Non-canonical inflammatory signaling pathways affected in *Ph*-negative MPNs, regardless of subtype and driver mutation. The preleukemic niche of MPNs secretes high levels of IL-1, a proinflammatory cytokine that activates multiple downstream pathways, such as p38 MAPK and NF-κB. NF-κB, in turn, generates high levels of IL-8, a proinflammatory cytokine that binds to CXCR1 or CXCR2 and activates STAT3, PI3K/AKT, p38 MAPK, FAK and PLC/PKC. NFE2 overexpression has also been reported in most MPN patients and has been associated with high IL-8 levels and increased ROS and DNA damage. On the other hand, IL-6 is a proinflammatory cytokine produced by monocytes, macrophages and T-cells that signals via JAK1/STAT3, whose levels have been found elevated in JAK2^{V617F} PV and PMF patients. Finally, IFN-α is a key regulator of hematopoietic stem cells (HSCs) that depletes previously dormant hematopoietic stem progenitor cells (HSPCs) and enhances the immune response. A pathogenic role of oncostatin-M, TGF-β1, platelet-derived growth factor (PDGF), basic fibroblast growth factor (BFGF), VEGF, bone morphogenic proteins, inhibitors of matrix metalloproteinases (MMPs) and lipocalin-2 has been suggested in *Ph*-negative MPNs.

Numerous cytokines have been implicated in mediating fibrosis, osteosclerosis and angiogenesis in PMF patients. Thus, several studies have suggested a pathogenic role for oncostatin-M [49], TGF-β1 [50,51], platelet-derived growth factor [51], basic fibroblast growth factor [50], VEGF [52], bone morphogenetic proteins [53], and inhibitors of matrix metalloproteinases [54,55].

Myeloid cells have been reported also to produce elevated levels of lipocalin-2 in PV, ET, and PMF patients. This protein increases the growth of bone marrow cells in PMF patients, but not in healthy donors. On the contrary, it increases reactive oxygen species, DNA damage, and apoptosis in normal cells, but not in PMF patients. Lipocalin-2 also induces the expression of factors that contribute to fibrosis, such as VEGF, TGF-β1, bone morphogenetic protein-2, RUNX2, osteoprotegerin and collagen type I [56,108].

Heat shock proteins (HSPs) are key players during inflammation. HSP90 stabilizes numerous proteins, such as JAK2. The HSP70 family is composed of some proteins (HSPA5, HSPA8, and HSPA8) that have been found to be enriched in fractions bound to CALR^{Mut} [26]. HSP70 also seems to contribute to cell proliferation through regulation of JAK2/STAT signaling. In fact, the inhibition of HSP70 expression in an ex vivo model of PV and ET increased apoptosis of the erythroid lineage and decreased JAK2 signaling [57]. HSP70 also activates TLR2 and TLR4, leading to NF-κB activation, rapid calcium flux, and TNF-α, IL1-β and IL-6 production [58]. Moreover, HSP70 can be secreted as a "danger signal" and bind peptides to form a complex that binds to cell surface receptors, such as CD91 and Lox-1 [59].

Finally, there is also evidence for a link between inflammation and thrombosis. Thrombosis in MPN patients has been associated with an increased platelet-leukocyte interaction. While MPN leukocytes overexpress the surface protein CD11b, its receptor (CD62p) is upregulated on platelets. This results in increased formation of leukocyte-platelet complexes [60–62].

3.3.2. Bone Marrow Microenvironment

The bone marrow microenvironment is a complex and dynamic structure composed of multiple cell types. Clonal HSCs in MPNs interact with other cells in this microenvironment and remodel it allowing further malignant expansion (Figure 5). There is a growing evidence that endothelial cells, mesenchymal stem cells, stromal cells, osteoblasts, and osteoclasts may contribute to the pathogenesis of these diseases in the bone marrow [63].

In a mouse model, endothelial cells expressing JAK2^{V617F} have been shown to be capable of causing the expansion of hematopoietic stem and progenitor cells, which could be caused by increased expression of the cytokines CXCL12 (C-X-C motif chemokine ligand 12) and SCF (stem cell factor) by endothelial cells [64,65].

Mesenchymal stem cells (MSCs) also seem to be important in the pathogenesis of MPNs. In contrast to endothelial cells expressing JAK2^{V617F}, MSCs negative for JAK2^{V617F} have been reported to reduce the expression of CXCL12 and SCF [109,110]. They also support HPSC proliferation [66] and overexpress galectin-1 in all MPN subtypes and galectin-3 in PV patients [67]. Galectins mediate cell adhesion and stimulate cell migration, proliferation and apoptosis through interactions with integrins, laminin and fibronectin. In addition, MSCs promote the expansion of osteoblasts by cell contact and excessive TGF-β1, Notch, IL-6, IL-1β, and TNF-β signaling. Abnormal osteoblasts overproduce inflammatory cytokines, promote fibrogenesis and reduce CXCL12 expression [88]. By contrast, monocytes with JAK2^{V617F} seem to increase osteoclast forming ability in MPN patients, favoring the survival of clonal HSCs [68].

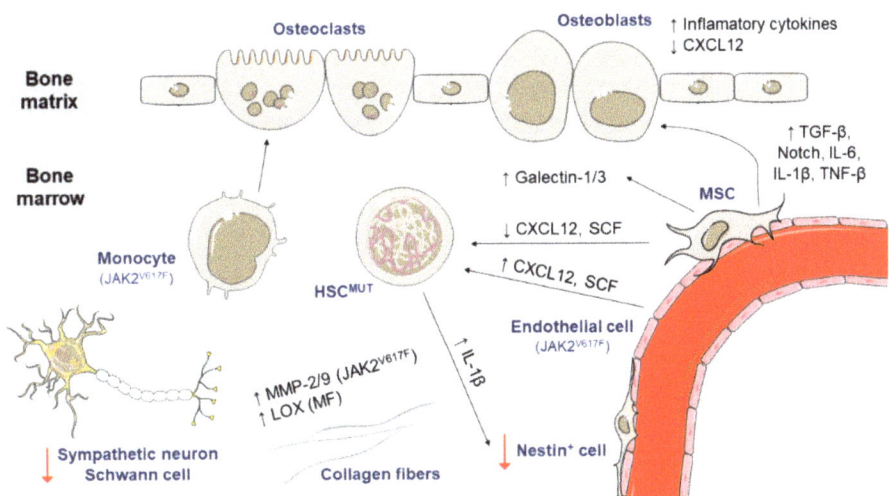

Figure 5. Role of the bone marrow microenvironment in the pathogenesis of *Ph*-negative MPNs. Endothelial cells expressing JAK2^{V617F} increase the expression of CXCL12 and stem cell factor (SCF) and cause the expansion of HSCs and progenitor cells. On the other hand, mesenchymal stem cells (MSCs) negative for JAK2^{V617F} show a reduced expression of CXCL12 and SCF. MSCs also overexpress galectin-1 in all MPN subtypes and galectin-3 in PV patients, and promote the expansion of osteoblasts by cell contact and excessive TGF-1β, Notch, IL-6, IL-1β, and TNF-β signaling. Osteoblasts overproduce inflammatory cytokines and reduce CXCL12 expression. By contrast, monocytes with JAK2^{V617F} seem to increase osteoclast forming ability and favor the survival of clonal HSCs. Meanwhile, clonal HSCs produce high levels of IL-1β, which induces nestin-positive MSCs death. Additionally, the sympathetic nerve fibers supporting Schwann cells are reduced in the bone marrow of MPN patients. Regarding the extracellular matrix, MPN patients with JAK2^{V617F} show increased levels of MMP-2 and MMP-9 and patients with primary myelofibrosis (PMF) have increased levels of all LOX family members.

A recent study has recently found numerous differences between the bone marrow niche of ET and PV patients. In ET, the HSPCs move faster and more frequently towards the endosteal niche and the number of osteoblasts and osteoclasts increases. However, in PV, only the non-endosteal sinusoids are dilated [69]. Other studies have demonstrated that the sympathetic nervous system has a role in the bone marrow niche of MPN patients. Specifically, sympathetic nerve fibers supporting Schwann cells and nestin-positive MSCs are reduced in the bone marrow of MPN patients. In a murine MPN model harboring JAK2^{V617F}, stem cells secreted IL-1β, which induces nestin-positive MSCs death and enables disease expansion [70].

Regarding the extracellular matrix, several studies have also pointed to a role of matrix metalloproteinases (MMPs) and lysyl oxidase (LOX) in the pathogenesis of MPNs. MPN patients with JAK2^{V617F} show increased levels of MMP-2 and MMP-9 [71] and patients with PMF have increased levels of all LOX family members. LOX is involved in collagen cross-linking and promotes fibrogenesis [72].

4. Disease Modifiers

Several non-driver somatic mutations have been identified in MPN patients. According to recent studies, more than 80% of patients with PMF [73] and over 50% of PV/ET patients have at least one additional somatic mutation of this type [74]. These mutations occur in genes affecting a wide variety of processes like epigenetic regulation, tumor suppression, transcription regulation or splicing, but also additional signaling pathways (Figure 6). They often modify the course of the disease and the presence of more than one such aberration has been associated with a worse survival [75].

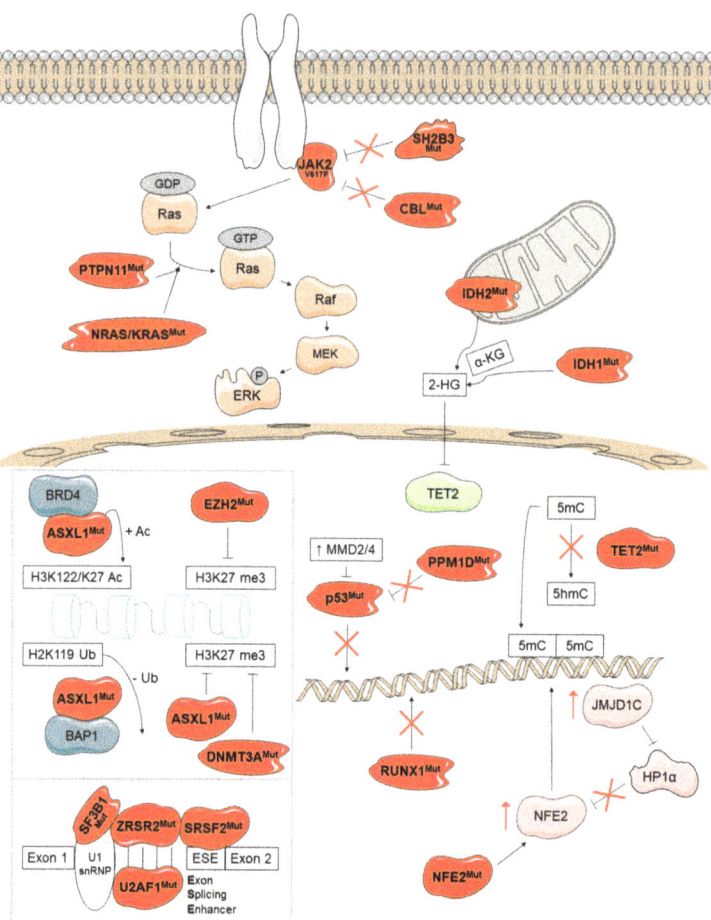

Figure 6. Overview of the disease-modifying genes mutated in *Ph*-negative MPNs and their molecular consequences. These mutations occur in genes affecting epigenetic regulation (*ASXL1*, *EZH2*, *DNMT3A*, *TET2*, *IDH1*, and *IDH2*), tumor suppression (*TP53* and *PPM1D*), transcription regulation (*RUNX1* and *NFE2*), splicing (*SRSF2*, *U2AF1*, *SF3B1*, and *ZRSR2*), and other signaling pathways (*SH2B3*, *CBL*, *NRAS/KRAS*, *PTPN11*). Mutant proteins are depicted in red.

4.1. Epigenetic Regulation

The most common non-driver somatic mutations affect epigenetic regulation and have been identified in *ASXL1* (ASXL transcriptional regulator 1), *EZH2* (enhancer of zeste polycomb repressive complex 2 subunit), *DNMT3A* (DNA methyltransferase 3 alpha), *TET2* (TET methylcitosine dioxygenase 2), *IDH1* and *IDH2* (isocitrate dehydrogenase NADP+, 1 and 2).

The products of *ASXL1* and *EZH2* are involved in chromatin modification (Figure 6, upper box). Normal ASXL1 interacts with the polycomb repressor complex 2 (PRC2) and enhances its function as methylator of H3K27. H3K27 trimethylation results in the silencing of the *HOXA* gene family which participates in chromatin remodeling. Additionally, ASXL1 interacts with BRCA1-associated protein 1 (BAP1), creating the polycomb group repressive deubiquitinase complex, which globally removes monoubiquitin from H2AK119 and locally at *HOXA* and *IRF8* in HSCs [76,111,112]. *ASXL1* mutations are almost exclusively frameshift and nonsense mutations in exon 12, decrease H3K27 trimethylation [111] and enhance the activity of the ASXL1-BAP deubiquitinase complex [113]. This causes the deregulated expression of genes critical for HSC self-renewal and differentiation, as well as more open chromatin in c-Kit+ cells. Mutant ASXL1 also binds to the bromodomain-containing protein 4 (BDR4), resulting in the phosphorylation of RNA polymerase II and the acetylation of H3K27 and H3K122, which lead to the upregulation of genes governing myeloid differentiation [76,114]. Another mechanism reported for mutant ASXL1 consists of the repression of TGF-β pathway through H3K and H4K deacetylation [115]. Although normal ASXL1 activates the retinoic acid receptor [116] and interacts with the peroxisome proliferator activated receptor gamma (PPARγ) to repress lipogenesis [117], the effects of *ASXL1* mutations on these mechanisms are still unknown. In summary, the consequences of *ASXL1* mutations are diverse and are not fully elucidated; the mutant protein shows a loss of function in some mechanisms but a gain of function in others.

EZH2 encodes a histone lysine N-methyltransferase that constitutes the catalytic component of PRC2. The majority of *EZH2* mutations are missense with loss of function effects resulting in the silencing of *HOXA9*. This supports myeloid progenitor self-renewal and leukemic transformation [118,119].

DNMT3A, *TET2*, *IDH1* and *IDH2* encode DNA methylation modifiers (Figure 6). *DNMT3A* encodes a *de novo* DNA methyltransferase responsible for DNA methylation at CpG dinucleotides. The mutation most frequently observed is p.R882H, that impairs the CpG specificity, flanking sequence preference and DNMT3A enzymatic activity [120]. Mechanistic studies in mice indicate that mutant DNMT3A decreases PRC2 recruitment at H3K27 favoring accessibility at enhancer chromatin marks and persistent HSC gene expression. JAK2^{V617F} patients also harboring *DNMT3A* mutations show aberrant self-renewal and altered inflammatory signaling pathways [121].

TET2 encodes an enzyme that catalyzes the oxidation of 5-methylcytosine (5mC) to 5-hydroxymethylcytosine (5-hmC). Mutations in *TET2* are nonsense or missense changes that lead to a loss of function [122] and DNA hypermethylation due to decreased production of 5-hmC. Mutant TET2 increases the expression of HSC self-renewal genes and sensitizes hematopoietic cells to acquire other mutations and leads to significant myeloid lineage skewing [123] and increased IL-6 production [124]. The order of mutation acquisition can influence the MPN phenotype; mutations in *TET2* arising prior to JAK2^{V617F} favors the ET phenotype, but the acquisition of JAK2^{V617F} in a *TET2* non-mutated background is more likely to result in the PV phenotype [125].

IDH1 and *IDH2* encode isocitrate dehydrogenases that catalyze decarboxylation of isocitrate into alpha ketoglutarate (α-KG). While IDH1 acts in the cytosol, IDH2 works in the mitochondria. The most common *IDH1* (p.R132H and p.R132C) and *IDH2* mutations (p.R140Q) increase 2-hydroxyglutarate (2-HG) production. 2-HG prevents histone demethylation and the expression of lineage-specific differentiation genes, leading to a block to cell differentiation [126–128]. This compound can also bind ten-eleven translocation (TET) and Jumonji proteins, inhibiting their functions [129]. IDH mutations have also been associated to enhanced aberrant splicing of mutant SRSF2, leading to genomic instability and risk of leukemic transformation [130].

4.2. Tumor Suppression

TP53 (tumor protein P53) and *PPM1D* (protein phosphatase, Mg^{2+}/Mn^{2+} dependent 1D or P53-induced protein phosphatase 1) are involved in tumor suppression (Figure 6). TP53 is a transcription factor that responds to DNA damage inducing transcriptional programs that result in cell cycle arrest or apoptosis [131]. *TP53* mutations are missense changes with several non-mutually exclusive effects: loss of function, gain of function, and dominant-negative effect on normal TP53 [77]. It has been also demonstrated that mutant TP53 increases HSC self-renewal and resistance to cellular stress [132]. There are several upstream regulators of TP53, which are overexpressed in MPNs, such as MDM2 and

MDM4. Both of them inhibit TP53 function by facilitating nuclear export and by inducing its degradation [133].

PPM1D is a serin-threonine phosphatase which negatively regulates TP53 and is transcriptionally upregulated on TP53 induction [134]. Mutations in *PPM1D* are truncating and frameshift changes in exon 6 that lead to a protein that lacks a carboxyterminal degradation domain. This results in altered cell cycle progression, decreased apoptosis and reduced mitochondrial priming [135].

4.3. Regulation of Transcription

RUNX1 (RUNX family transcription factor 1) and *NFE2* (nuclear factor, erythroid 2) encode transcription factors and have been also found mutated in MPNs (Figure 6). RUNX1 contains a runt homology domain (RHD) responsible for DNA binding and heterodimerization with core binding factor β (CBF-β). Through this interaction, RUNX1 controls key hematopoietic transcriptional programs. Specifically, RUNX1 participates in hematopoietic differentiation, cell cycle regulation, ribosome biogenesis, and p53 and TGF-β pathways [136]. RUNX1 mutations are missense, frameshift, and non-sense changes that inactivate the protein leading to a reduced myeloid differentiation and an increase in HSC self-renewal [77].

Mutations described in *NFE2* are a 4-amino acid in-frame deletion and frameshift changes that lead to a carboxy-terminally truncated protein [40]. Mutant NFE2 promotes myelopoiesis and causes elevated expression of wild-type NFE2 and histone demethylase JMJD1C maybe by a decreased binding of the repressor HP1α [137].

4.4. Splicing

Pre-mRNA splicing is catalyzed by the spliceosome, a complex of five snRNPs and multiple proteins. Mutually exclusive mutations in RNA splicing factors encoded by *SRSF2* (serine and arginine rich splicing factor 2), *U2AF1* (U2 small nuclear RNA auxiliary factor 1), *SF3B1* (splicing factor 3b subunit 1) and *ZRSR2* (zinc finger CCCH-type, RNA binding motif and serine/arginine rich 2) have been reported in MPNs (Figure 6, lower box).

SRSF2 contains a ribonucleoprotein with an RNA binding motif and a carboxyl-terminal serine/arginine rich domain [138], both involved in the recognition and binding to the RNA sequences GGNG and CCNG in exon splicing enhancers (ESEs). The most frequent mutation is p.P95H, that leads to a preferential recognition of CCNG motifs and alters the balance of splicing of multiple pre-mRNAs, which cause downregulation of *EZH2* [139], as well as the mis-splicing of *CASP8*, which activates NF-κB signaling [140]. The expression of mutant SRSF2 has also been demonstrated to cause accumulation of R loops, replication stress and activation of ATR-Chk1 signaling [141,142]. Additionally, mutant SRSF2 seems to predominantly form RUNX1a over RUNX1b and regulate DNA stability [143,144].

U2AF1 recognizes pyrimidine-rich tracts with a conserved terminal AG in 3′ splice sites [145]. The most prevalent somatic mutations affect Q157 and its surroundings; p.Q157 mutants generate mis-splicing of ARID2 and EZH2 [123] and are associated with a worse outcome [146]. Patients can also harbor mutations in serine 34 (p.S34F/Y) that cause different expression and splicing patterns than p.Q157 mutations and have been associated with increased splicing, accumulation of R loops and exon skipping [142,147]. Both types of mutations are located within the CCCH zinc fingers of U2AF1, that are critical for RNA binding [148]. This protein has also been shown to bind to mRNA and repress translation; p.S34F mutation seems to affect the translation of hundreds of mRNAs, but the effect of the other mutations on translation is still unknown [149].

ZRSR2 heterodimerizes with U2AF2 and participates in the recognition of the 3′ splice site. Mutations in this gene are mostly frameshift and nonsense loss-of-function changes that affect splicing and lead to intron retention. Mutant ZRSR2 has been reported to cause increased MAPK and ERBB signaling in myelodysplastic syndromes [150].

SF3B1 forms part of the spliceosome complex. Mutations in *SF3B1* are missense changes (p.K700E and p.H662Q) that cause alternative 3′ splice site selection [151]. These mutations block erythroid maturation [152] and modify the expression of genes involved in RNA processing, cell cycle, heme metabolism and nonsense-mediated RNA decay [77].

4.5. Additional Signaling Pathways

Finally, other mutations have been found in *SH2B3* (SH2B adaptor protein 3, previously known as *LNK*), *CBL* (CBL proto-oncogene), *NRAS* and *KRAS* (NRAS and KRAS proto-oncogene, GTPase) and *PTPN11* (protein tyrosine phosphatase non-receptor type 11), all of them encoding elements involved in signaling (Figure 6).

SH2B3 is an adaptor protein that interacts with and inhibits signaling through cytokine receptors and kinases such JAK2 [153–155] decreasing the proliferation of hematopoietic cells [156–158]. In addition, this protein can recruit the E3-ubiquitin ligase CBL for degradation of receptors and other molecules [157]. Mutations in *SH2B3* are mainly missense changes that disrupt the negative-feedback loops on growth stimulation [155,157].

CBL recognizes and ubiquitinates activated tyrosine kinase receptors and JAK2 leading to their proteasomal degradation. Mutations in *CBL* are mostly missense changes that reduce the E3 ligase activity and the degradation of its substrates [159–161]. However, they are not merely loss-of-function mutations since *CBL* knockout cells show increased cytokine sensitivity [162].

Missense substitutions affecting *NRAS/KRAS* favor the GTP-bound state of RAS, causing a constitutive activation of growth signaling [163].

Finally, *PTPN11* encodes a protein tyrosine phosphatase which dephosphorylates RAS [164]. *PTPN11* mutations increase its phosphatase activity [165], leading to a high dephosphorylation of RAS which increases the activation of RAS-RAF-MEK-ERK pathway [166].

5. Additional Factors Involved in Disease

There are several factors that have been shown to influence heterogeneity in MPN phenotypes, such as the HSC in which the mutation appears first, genetic background, gender, age, and environmental factors.

HSCs are highly heterogeneous and carry a lineage-bias [167]. It has been demonstrated that the acquisition of a driver mutation in a platelet-biased HSC may drive to an ET phenotype, whereas the PV phenotype is more probable when mutation is acquired in balanced/myeloid-biased HSCs [168].

It is well known that there is an association between the *JAK2* haplotype 46/1 or GGCC and MPNs. This haplotype is found in 24% of the population and in the 56% of MPN patients [169] increasing the susceptibility of developing a *JAK2* mutation, but also to *CALR* mutations and weakly to *MPL* mutations [169,170]. Recent studies have identified several SNPs in different loci which have been associated with an increased risk of developing some MPN subtypes [171–173].

Regarding gender, the ET phenotype has been mostly reported in women, while PV/PMF are more prevalent in men [174,175]. Women seem to have a greater symptom burden than men [175], but the male gender has been associated with a higher likelihood of myelofibrotic transformation in ET patients [176].

The incidence of MPNs also increases with age, and this factor is the strongest predictor of death in PV and ET [177,178]. This phenomenon has been related to the influence of aging in hematopoiesis, maybe due to a greater probability of acquiring somatic mutations in HSCs [78] favored by a pro-inflammatory state due to the accumulation of inflammatory cytokines associated with age [45]. This higher probability would also explain the increased risk of disease progression in these patients [78].

Retrospective observational studies have reported that the occupational exposure to benzene and/or petroleum, prior blood donation (specifically for PV) [179], and smoking [180,181] are associated with a higher risk of MPNs.

6. Conclusions

The understanding of the pathogenesis of MPNs has undergone a complete revolution in the last 15 years, especially since the p.V617F mutation in *JAK2* was characterized. Since then, MPNs have basically been considered signaling disorders, especially affecting the JAK2/STAT pathway, but also the MAPK/ERK and PI3K/AKT pathways. Further characterization of mutations in *MPL*, and the mechanism by which *CALR* mutations activate TPOR, reinforced this view. However, although the pathogenic mechanisms of the JAK2, TPOR, and CALR mutants seem quite straightforward and simple, various studies have shown that these alterations can cause more complex disturbances in the cell through non-canonical mechanisms. This, together with the characterization of new somatic genetic alterations that affect genes involved in other processes and signaling pathways, have revealed the complexity of the pathogenesis of MPN, which could partly explain the phenotypic heterogeneity observed among patients.

Author Contributions: Conceptualization: J.L.V. and A.G.-H.; review of the literature: A.G.-H.; writing—original draft preparation: A.G.-H.; writing—review and editing: J.L.V. All authors have read and agreed to the published version of the manuscript.

Funding: J.L.V. and A.G.-H. research are supported by PIUNA 2020 program of the University of Navarra (Code 15058203).

Acknowledgments: The authors acknowledge Cristina Hurtado by her technical support.

Conflicts of Interest: The authors declare no conflict of interest.

References

1. Tefferi, A.; Vardiman, J.W. Classification and diagnosis of myeloproliferative neoplasms: The 2008 World Health Organization criteria and point-of-care diagnostic algorithms. *Leukemia* **2008**, *22*, 14–22. [CrossRef] [PubMed]
2. Druker, B.J.; Sawyers, C.L.; Kantarjian, H.; Resta, D.J.; Reese, S.F.; Ford, J.M.; Capdeville, R.; Talpaz, M. Activity of a specific inhibitor of the bcr-abl tyrosine kinase in the blast crisis of chronic myeloid leukemia and acute lymphoblastic leukemia with the Philadelphia chromosome. *N. Engl. J. Med.* **2001**, *344*, 1038–1042. [CrossRef] [PubMed]
3. Druker, B.J.; Talpaz, M.; Resta, D.J.; Peng, B.; Buchdunger, E.; Ford, J.M.; Lydon, N.B.; Kantarjian, H.; Capdeville, R.; Ohno-Jones, S.; et al. Efficacy and safety of a specific inhibitor of the BCR-ABL tyrosine kinase in chronic myeloid leukemia. *N. Engl. J. Med.* **2001**, *344*, 1031–1037. [CrossRef]
4. Druker, B.J. Inhibition of the Bcr-Abl tyrosine kinase as a therapeutic strategy for CML. *Oncogene* **2002**, *21*, 8541–8546. [CrossRef]
5. Redner, R.L. Why doesn't imatinib cure chronic myeloid leukemia? *Oncologist* **2010**, *15*, 182–186. [CrossRef] [PubMed]
6. Kalmanti, L.; Saussele, S.; Lauseker, M.; Müller, M.C.; Dietz, C.; Heinrich, L.; Hanfstein, B.; Proetel, U.; Fabarius, A.; Krause, S.W.; et al. Safety and efficacy of imatinib in CML over a period of 10 years: Data from the randomized CML-study IV. *Leukemia* **2015**, *29*, 1123–1132. [CrossRef] [PubMed]
7. Hochhaus, A.; Larson, R.A.; Guilhot, F.; Radich, J.P.; Branford, S.; Hughes, T.P.; Baccarani, M.; Deininger, M.W.; Cervantes, F.; Fujihara, S.; et al. Long-Term Outcomes of Imatinib Treatment for Chronic Myeloid Leukemia. *N. Engl. J. Med.* **2017**, *376*, 917–927. [CrossRef]
8. Verstovsek, S.; Mesa, R.A.; Gotlib, J.; Levy, R.S.; Gupta, V.; DiPersio, J.F.; Catalano, J.V.; Deininger, M.; Miller, C.; Silver, R.T.; et al. A double-blind, placebo-controlled trial of ruxolitinib for myelofibrosis. *N. Engl. J. Med.* **2012**, *366*, 799–807. [CrossRef] [PubMed]
9. Brkic, S.; Meyer, S.C. Challenges and perspectives for therapeutic targeting of myeloproliferative neoplasms. *Hemasphere* **2020**, *5*, e516. [CrossRef]
10. Vannucchi, A.M.; Kiladjian, J.J.; Griesshammer, M.; Masszi, T.; Durrant, S.; Passamonti, F.; Harrison, C.N.; Pane, F.; Zachee, P.; Mesa, R.; et al. Ruxolitinib versus standard therapy for the treatment of polycythemia vera. *N. Engl. J. Med.* **2015**, *372*, 426–435. [CrossRef]
11. Deininger, M.; Radich, J.; Burn, T.C.; Huber, R.; Paranagama, D.; Verstovsek, S. The effect of long-term ruxolitinib treatment on JAK2p.V617F allele burden in patients with myelofibrosis. *Blood* **2015**, *126*, 1551–1554. [CrossRef] [PubMed]
12. Greenfield, G.; McPherson, S.; Mills, K.; McMullin, M.F. The ruxolitinib effect: Understanding how molecular pathogenesis and epigenetic dysregulation impact therapeutic efficacy in myeloproliferative neoplasms. *J. Transl. Med.* **2018**, *16*, 1–16. [CrossRef]
13. Martí-Carvajal, A.J.; Anand, V.; Solà, I. Janus kinase-1 and Janus kinase-2 inhibitors for treating myelofibrosis. *Cochrane Database Syst. Rev.* **2015**, CD010298. [CrossRef]
14. Cervantes, F.; Pereira, A. Does ruxolitinib prolong the survival of patients with myelofibrosis? *Blood* **2017**, *129*, 832–838. [CrossRef]
15. Verstovsek, S.; Kantarjian, H.; Mesa, R.A.; Pardanani, A.D.; Cortes-Franco, J.; Thomas, D.A.; Estrov, Z.; Fridman, J.S.; Bradley, E.C.; Erickson-Viitanen, S.; et al. Safety and efficacy of INCB018424, a JAK1 and JAK2 inhibitor, in myelofibrosis. *N. Engl. J. Med.* **2010**, *363*, 1117–1127. [CrossRef]

16. Kaplan, J.B.; Stein, B.L.; McMahon, B.; Giles, F.J.; Platanias, L.C. Evolving therapeutic strategies for the classic philadelphia-negative myeloproliferative neoplasms. *EBioMedicine* **2016**, *3*, 17–25. [CrossRef] [PubMed]
17. Dawson, M.A.; Bannister, A.J.; Göttgens, B.; Foster, S.D.; Bartke, T.; Green, A.R.; Kouzarides, T. JAK2 phosphorylates histone H3Y41 and excludes HP1α from chromatin. *Nature* **2009**, *461*, 819–822. [CrossRef]
18. De Koning, L.; Sauignoni, A.; Boumendil, C.; Rehman, H.; Asselain, B.; Sastre-Garau, X.; Almouzni, G. Heterochromatin protein 1α: A hallmark of cell proliferation relevant to clinical oncology. *EMBO Mol. Med.* **2009**, *1*, 178–191. [CrossRef] [PubMed]
19. Liu, F.; Zhao, X.; Perna, F.; Wang, L.; Koppikar, P.; Abdel-Wahab, O.; Harr, M.W.; Levine, R.L.; Xu, H.; Tefferi, A.; et al. JAK2V617F-mediated phosphorylation of PRMT5 downregulates its methyltransferase activity and promotes myeloproliferation. *Cancer Cell* **2011**, *19*, 283–294. [CrossRef] [PubMed]
20. De Grandis, M.; Cambot, M.; Wautier, M.P.; Cassinat, B.; Chomienne, C.; Colin, Y.; Wautier, J.-L.; Le Van Kim, C.; El Nemer, W. JAK2V617F activates Lu/BCAM-mediated red cell adhesion in polycythemia vera through an EpoR-independent Rap1/Akt pathway. *Blood* **2013**, *121*, 658–665. [CrossRef] [PubMed]
21. Lai, H.Y.; Brooks, S.A.; Craver, B.M.; Morse, S.J.; Nguyen, T.K.; Haghighi, N.; Garbati, M.R.; Fleischman, A.G. Defective negative regulation of Toll-like receptor signaling leads to excessive TNF-α in myeloproliferative neoplasm. *Blood Adv.* **2019**, *3*, 122–131. [CrossRef]
22. Fleischman, A.G.; Aichberger, K.J.; Luty, S.B.; Bumm, T.G.; Petersen, C.L.; Doratotaj, S.; Vasudevan, K.B.; LaTocha, D.H.; Yang, F.; Press, R.D.; et al. TNFα facilitates clonal expansion of JAK2V617F positive cells in myeloproliferative neoplasms. *Blood* **2011**, *118*, 6392–6398. [CrossRef] [PubMed]
23. Kleppe, M.; Kwak, M.; Koppikar, P.; Riester, M.; Keller, M.; Bastian, L.; Hricik, T.; Bhagwat, N.; McKenney, A.S.; Papalexi, E.; et al. JAK-STAT pathway activation in malignant and non-malignant cells contributes to MPN pathogenesis and therapeutic response. *Cancer Discov.* **2015**, *5*, 316–331. [CrossRef]
24. Stetka, J.; Vyhlidalova, P.; Lanikova, L.; Koralkova, P.; Gursky, J.; Hlusi, A.; Flodr, P.; Hubackova, S.; Bartek, J.; Hodny, Z.; et al. Addiction to DUSP1 protects JAK2V617F-driven polycythemia vera progenitors against inflammatory stress and DNA damage, allowing chronic proliferation. *Oncogene* **2019**, *38*, 5627–5642. [CrossRef]
25. Salati, S.; Genovese, E.; Carretta, C.; Zini, R.; Bartalucci, N.; Prudente, Z.; Pennucci, V.; Ruberti, S.; Rossi, C.; Rontauroli, S.; et al. Calreticulin Ins5 and Del52 mutations impair unfolded protein and oxidative stress responses in K562 cells expressing CALR mutants. *Sci. Rep.* **2019**, *9*, 10558. [CrossRef]
26. Pronier, E.; Cifani, P.; Merlinsky, T.R.; Berman, K.B.; Somasundara, A.V.H.; Rampal, R.K.; LaCava, J.; Wei, K.E.; Pastore, F.; Maag, J.L.; et al. Targeting the CALR interactome in myeloproliferative neoplasms. *JCI Insight.* **2018**, *3*, e122703. [CrossRef] [PubMed]
27. Eder-Azanza, L.; Navarro, D.; Aranaz, P.; Novo, F.J.; Cross, N.C.P.; Vizmanos, J.L. Bioinformatic analyses of CALR mutations in myeloproliferative neoplasms support a role in signaling. *Leukemia* **2014**, *28*, 2106–2109. [CrossRef]
28. Fucikova, J.; Spisek, R.; Kroemer, G.; Galluzzi, L. Calreticulin and cancer. *Cell Res.* **2021**, *31*, 5–16. [CrossRef] [PubMed]
29. Arshad, N.; Cresswell, P. Tumor-associated calreticulin variants functionally compromise the peptide loading complex and impair its recruitment of MHC-I. *J. Biol. Chem.* **2018**, *293*, 9555–9569. [CrossRef] [PubMed]
30. Liu, P.; Zhao, L.; Loos, F.; Marty, C.; Xie, W.; Martins, I.; Lachkar, S.; Qu, B.; Waeckel-Énée, E.; Plo, I.; et al. Immunosuppression by mutated calreticulin released from malignant cells. *Mol. Cell.* **2020**, *77*, 748–760.e9. [CrossRef] [PubMed]
31. Di Buduo, C.A.; Abbonante, V.; Marty, C.; Moccia, F.; Rumi, E.; Pietra, D.; Soprano, P.M.; Lim, D.; Cattaneo, D.; Iurlo, A.; et al. Defective interaction of mutant calreticulin and SOCE in megakaryocytes from patients with myeloproliferative neoplasms. *Blood* **2020**, *135*, 133–144. [CrossRef]
32. Cabagnols, X.; Defour, J.P.; Ugo, V.; Ianotto, J.C.; Mossuz, P.; Mondet, J.; Girodon, F.; Alexandre, J.H.; Mansier, O.; Viallard, J.F.; et al. Differential association of calreticulin type 1 and type 2 mutations with myelofibrosis and essential thrombocytemia: Relevance for disease evolution. *Leukemia* **2015**, *29*, 249–252. [CrossRef]
33. Pietra, D.; Rumi, E.; Ferretti, V.V.; Di Buduo, C.A.; Milanesi, C.; Cavalloni, C.; Sant'Antonio, E.; Abbonante, V.; Moccia, F.; Casetti, I.C.; et al. Differential clinical effects of different mutation subtypes in CALR-mutant myeloproliferative neoplasms. *Leukemia* **2016**, *30*, 431–438. [CrossRef]
34. Hoermann, G.; Greiner, G.; Valent, P. Cytokine regulation of microenvironmental cells in myeloproliferative neoplasms. *Mediators Inflamm.* **2015**, *2015*, 869242. [CrossRef] [PubMed]
35. Fisher, D.A.C.; Miner, C.A.; Engle, E.K.; Hu, H.; Collins, T.B.; Zhou, A.; Allen, M.J.; Malkova, O.; Oh, S.T. Cytokine production in myelofibrosis exhibits differential responsiveness to JAK-STAT, MAP Kinase, and NFκB signaling. *Leukemia* **2019**, *33*, 1978–1995. [CrossRef] [PubMed]
36. Kleppe, M.; Koche, R.; Zou, L.; van Galen, P.; Hill, C.E.; Dong, L.; De Groote, S.; Papalexi, E.; Hanasoge Somasundara, A.V.; Cordner, K.; et al. Dual targeting of oncogenic activation and inflammatory signaling increases therapeutic efficacy in myeloproliferative neoplasms. *Cancer Cell* **2018**, *33*, 785–787. [CrossRef]
37. Wang, W.; Schwemmers, S.; Hexner, E.O.; Pahl, H.L. AML1 is overexpressed in patients with myeloproliferative neoplasms and mediates JAK2V617F-independent overexpression of NF-E2. *Blood* **2010**, *116*, 254–266. [CrossRef] [PubMed]
38. Hasselbalch, H.C.; Thomassen, M.; Riley, C.H.; Kjær, L.; Larsen, T.S.; Jensen, M.K.; Bjerrum, O.W.; Kruse, T.A.; Skov, V. Whole blood transcriptional profiling reveals deregulation of oxidative and antioxidative defence genes in myelofibrosis and related neoplasms. Potential implications of downregulation of Nrf2 for genomic instability and disease progression. *PLoS ONE* **2014**, *9*, e112786. [CrossRef] [PubMed]

39. Wehrle, J.; Seeger, T.S.; Schwemmers, S.; Pfeifer, D.; Bulashevska, A.; Pahl, H.L. Transcription factor nuclear factor erythroid-2 mediates expression of the cytokine interleukin 8, a known predictor of inferior outcome in patients with myeloproliferative Neoplasms. *Haematologica* **2013**, *98*, 1073–1080. [CrossRef] [PubMed]
40. Jutzi, J.S.; Bogeska, R.; Nikoloski, G.; Schmid, C.A.; Seeger, T.S.; Stegelmann, F.; Schwemmers, S.; Gründer, A.; Peeken, J.C.; Gothwal, M.; et al. MPN patients harbor recurrent truncating mutations in transcription factor NF-E2. *J. Exp. Med.* **2013**, *210*, 1003–1019. [CrossRef] [PubMed]
41. Motohashi, H.; Kimura, M.; Fujita, R.; Inoue, A.; Pan, X.; Takayama, M.; Katsuoka, F.; Aburatani, H.; Bresnick, E.H.; Yamamoto, M. NF-E2 domination over Nrf2 promotes ROS accumulation and megakaryocytic maturation. *Blood* **2010**, *115*, 677–686. [CrossRef] [PubMed]
42. Hasselbalch, H.C. Chronic inflammation as a promotor of mutagenesis in essential thrombocythemia, polycythemia vera and myelofibrosis. A human inflammation model for cancer development? *Leuk. Res.* **2013**, *37*, 214–220. [CrossRef] [PubMed]
43. Hasan, S.; Lacout, C.; Marty, C.; Cuingnet, M.; Solary, E.; Vainchenker, W.; Villeval, J.-L. JAK2V617F expression in mice amplifies early hematopoietic cells and gives them a competitive advantage that is hampered by IFNα. *Blood* **2013**, *22*, 1464–1477. [CrossRef] [PubMed]
44. Mullally, A.; Bruedigam, C.; Poveromo, L.; Heidel, F.H.; Purdon, A.; Vu, T.; Austin, R.; Heckl, D.; Breyfogle, L.J.; Kuhn, C.P.; et al. Depletion of Jak2V617F myeloproliferative neoplasm-propagating stem cells by interferon-α in a murine model of polycythemia vera. *Blood* **2013**, *121*, 3692–3702. [CrossRef] [PubMed]
45. Hemmati, S.; Haque, T.; Gritsman, K. Inflammatory signaling pathways in preleukemic and leukemic stem cells. *Front. Oncol.* **2017**, *7*, 265. [CrossRef]
46. Hérault, A.; Binnewies, M.; Leong, S.; Calero-Nieto, F.J.; Zhang, Y.; Kang, Y.; Wang, X.; Pietras, E.M.; Chu, S.H.; Barry-Holson, K.; et al. Myeloid progenitor cluster formation drives emergency and leukemic myelopoiesis. *Nature* **2017**, *544*, 53–58. [CrossRef] [PubMed]
47. Geyer, H.L.; Dueck, A.C.; Scherber, R.M.; Mesa, R.A. Impact of inflammation on myeloproliferative neoplasm symptom development. *Mediators Inflamm.* **2015**, *2015*, 284706. [CrossRef]
48. Pourcelot, E.; Trocme, C.; Mondet, J.; Bailly, S.; Toussaint, B.; Mossuz, P. Cytokine profiles in polycythemia vera and essential thrombocythemia patients: Clinical implications. *Exp. Hematol.* **2014**, *42*, 360–368. [CrossRef]
49. Hoermann, G.; Cerny-Reiterer, S.; Herrmann, H.; Blatt, K.; Bilban, M.; Gisslinger, H.; Müllauer, L.; Kralovics, R.; Mannhalter, C.; Valent, P.; et al. Identification of oncostatin M as a JAK2 V617F-dependent amplifier of cytokine production and bone marrow remodeling in myeloproliferative neoplasms. *FASEB J.* **2012**, *26*, 894–906. [CrossRef]
50. Le Bousse-Kerdilès, M.C.; Chevillard, S.; Charpentier, A.; Romquin, N.; Clay, D.; Smadja-Joffe, F.; Praloran, V.; Dupriez, B.; Demory, J.L.; Jasmin, C.; et al. Differential expression of transforming growth factor-beta, basic fibroblast growth factor, and their receptors in CD34+ hematopoietic progenitor cells from patients with myelofibrosis and myeloid metaplasia. *Blood* **1996**, *88*, 4534–4546. [CrossRef] [PubMed]
51. Martyré, M.-C.; Magdelenat, H.; Bryckaert, M.-C.; Laine-Bidron, C.; Calvo, F. Increased intraplatelet levels of platelet-derived growth factor and transforming growth factor-β in patients with myelofibrosis with myeloid metaplasia. *Br. J. Haematol.* **1991**, *77*, 80–86. [CrossRef] [PubMed]
52. Di Raimondo, F.; Azzaro, M.P.; Palumbo, G.A.; Bagnato, S.; Stagno, F.; Giustolisi, G.M.; Cacciola, E.; Sortino, G.; Guglielmo, P.; Giustolisi, R. Elevated vascular endothelial growth factor [VEGF] serum levels in idiopathic myelofibrosis. *Leukemia* **2001**, *15*, 976–980. [CrossRef]
53. Bock, O.; Höftmann, J.; Theophile, K.; Hussein, K.; Wiese, B.; Schlué, J.; Kreipe, H. Bone morphogenetic proteins are overexpressed in the bone marrow of primary myelofibrosis and are apparently induced by fibrogenic cytokines. *Am. J. Pathol.* **2008**, *172*, 951–960. [CrossRef] [PubMed]
54. Wang, J.C.; Novetsky, A.; Chen, C.; Novetsky, A.D. Plasma matrix metalloproteinase and tissue inhibitor of metalloproteinase in patients with agnogenic myeloid metaplasia or idiopathic primary myelofibrosis. *Br. J. Haematol.* **2002**, *119*, 709–712. [CrossRef] [PubMed]
55. Jensen, M.K.; Holten-Andersen, M.N.; Riisbro, R.; De Nully Brown, P.; Larsen, M.B.; Kjeldsen, L.; Heickendorff, L.; Brünner, N.; Hasselbalch, H.C. Elevated plasma levels of TIMP-1 correlate with plasma suPAR/uPA in patients with chronic myeloproliferative disorders. *Eur. J. Haematol.* **2003**, *71*, 377–384. [CrossRef]
56. Lu, M.; Xia, L.; Liu, Y.C.; Hochman, T.; Bizzari, L.; Aruch, D.; Lew, J.; Weinberg, R.; Goldberg, J.D.; Hoffman, R. Lipocalin produced by myelofibrosis cells affects the fate of both hematopoietic and marrow microenvironmental cells. *Blood* **2015**, *126*, 972–982. [CrossRef]
57. Gallardo, M.; Barrio, S.; Fernandez, M.; Paradela, A.; Arenas, A.; Toldos, O.; Ayala, R.; Albizua, E.; Jimenez, A.; Redondo, S.; et al. Proteomic analysis reveals heat shock protein 70 has a key role in polycythemia vera. *Mol. Cancer* **2013**, *12*, 142. [CrossRef] [PubMed]
58. Asea, A.; Kraeft, S.K.; Kurt-Jones, E.A.; Stevenson, M.A.; Chen, L.B.; Finberg, R.W.; Koo, G.C.; Calderwood, S.K. HSP70 stimulates cytokine production through a CD 14-dependant pathway, demonstrating its dual role as a chaperone and cytokine. *Nat. Med.* **2000**, *6*, 435–442. [CrossRef] [PubMed]
59. Sevin, M.; Girodon, F.; Garrido, C.; De Thonel, A. HSP90 and HSP70: Implication in inflammation processes and therapeutic approaches for myeloproliferative neoplasms. *Mediators Inflamm.* **2015**, *2015*, 970242. [CrossRef]

60. Falanga, A.; Marchetti, M.; Evangelista, V.; Vignoli, A.; Licini, M.; Balicco, M.; Manarini, S.; Finazzi, G.; Cerletti, C.; Barbui, T. Polymorphonuclear leukocyte activation and hemostasis in patients with essential thrombocythemia and polycythemia vera. *Blood* **2000**, *96*, 4261–4266. [CrossRef]
61. Villmow, T.; Kemkes-Matthes, B.; Matzdorff, A.C. Markers of platelet activation and platelet-leukocyte interaction in patients with myeloproliferative syndromes. *Thromb. Res.* **2002**, *108*, 139–145. [CrossRef]
62. Falanga, A.; Marchetti, M.; Vignoli, A.; Balducci, D.; Barbui, T. Leukocyte-platelet interaction in patients with essential thrombocythemia and polycythemia vera. *Exp. Hematol.* **2005**, *33*, 523–530. [CrossRef] [PubMed]
63. Curto-Garcia, N.; Harrison, C.; McLornan, D.P. Bone marrow niche dysregulation in myeloproliferative neoplasms. *Haematologica* **2020**, *105*, 1189–1200. [CrossRef] [PubMed]
64. Zhan, H.; Lin, C.H.S.; Segal, Y.; Kaushansky, K. The JAK2V617F-bearing vascular niche promotes clonal expansion in myeloproliferative neoplasms. *Leukemia* **2018**, *32*, 462–469. [CrossRef] [PubMed]
65. Lin, C.H.S.; Zhang, Y.; Kaushansky, K.; Zhan, H. JAK2V617F-bearing vascular niche enhances malignant hematopoietic regeneration following radiation injury. *Haematologica* **2018**, *103*, 1160–1168. [CrossRef]
66. Ramos, T.L.; Sánchez-Abarca, L.I.; Rosón-Burgo, B.; Redondo, A.; Rico, A.; Preciado, S.; Ortega, R.; Rodríguez, C.; Muntión, S.; Hernández-Hernández, A.; et al. Mesenchymal stromal cells [MSC] from JAK2+ myeloproliferative neoplasms differ from normal MSC and contribute to the maintenance of neoplastic hematopoiesis. *PLoS ONE* **2017**, *12*, 1–21. [CrossRef]
67. Koopmans, S.M.; Bot, F.J.; Schouten, H.C.; Janssen, J.; van Marion, A.M. The involvement of Galectins in the modulation of the JAK/STAT pathway in myeloproliferative neoplasia. *Am. J. Blood Res.* **2012**, *2*, 119–127. [PubMed]
68. Spanoudakis, E.; Papoutselis, M.; Bazdiara, I.; Lamprianidi, E.; Kordella, X.; Tilkeridis, C.; Tsatalas, C.; Kotsianidis, I. The JAK2V617F point mutation increases the osteoclast forming ability of monocytes in patients with chronic myeloproliferative neoplasms and makes their osteoclasts more susceptible to JAK2 inhibition. *Mediterr. J. Hematol. Infect. Dis.* **2018**, *10*, e2018058. [CrossRef]
69. Korn, C.; Rak, J.; García-García, A.; Fielding, C.; Khorshed, R.; González-Antón, S.; Li, J.; Norfo, R.; Baxter, E.J.; McKerrell, T.; et al. Niche heterogeneity impacts evolution of myeloproliferative neoplasms driven by the same oncogenic pathway. *Blood* **2018**, *132* (Suppl. 1), 98. [CrossRef]
70. Arranz, L.; Sánchez-Aguilera, A.; Martín-Pérez, D.; Isern, J.; Langa, X.; Tzankov, A.; Lundberg, P.; Muntión, S.; Tzeng, Y.-S.; Lai, D.-M.; et al. Neuropathy of haematopoietic stem cell niche is essential for myeloproliferative neoplasms. *Nature* **2014**, *512*, 78–81. [CrossRef] [PubMed]
71. Liu, G.M.; Zhang, L.J.; Fu, J.Z.; Liang, W.T.; Cheng, Z.Y.; Bai, P.; Bian, Y.S.; Wan, J.S. Regulation of Ruxolitinib on matrix metalloproteinase in JAK2V617F positive myeloroliferative neoplasms cells. *Zhonghua Xue Ye Xue Za Zhi* **2017**, *38*, 140–145. [CrossRef] [PubMed]
72. Tadmor, T.; Bejar, J.; Attias, D.; Mischenko, E.; Sabo, E.; Neufeld, G.; Vadasz, Z. The expression of lysyl-oxidase gene family members in myeloproliferative neoplasms. *Am. J. Hematol.* **2013**, *88*, 355–358. [CrossRef] [PubMed]
73. Tefferi, A.; Lasho, T.L.; Finke, C.M.; Elala, Y.; Hanson, C.A.; Ketterling, R.P.; Gangat, N.; Pardanani, A. Targeted deep sequencing in primary myelofibrosis. *Blood Adv.* **2016**, *1*, 105–111. [CrossRef] [PubMed]
74. Tefferi, A.; Lasho, T.L.; Guglielmelli, P.; Finke, C.M.; Rotunno, G.; Elala, Y.; Pacilli, A.; Hanson, C.A.; Pancrazzi, A.; Ketterling, R.P.; et al. Targeted deep sequencing in polycythemia vera and essential thrombocythemia. *Blood Adv.* **2016**, *1*, 21–30. [CrossRef] [PubMed]
75. Guglielmelli, P.; Lasho, T.L.; Rotunno, G.; Score, J.; Mannarelli, C.; Pancrazzi, A.; Biamonte, F.; Pardanani, A.; Zoi, K.; Reiter, A.; et al. The number of prognostically detrimental mutations and prognosis in primary myelofibrosis: An international study of 797 patients. *Leukemia* **2014**, *28*, 1804–1810. [CrossRef]
76. Grabek, J.; Straube, J.; Bywater, M.; Lane, S.W. MPN: The molecular drivers of disease initiation, progression and transformation and their effect on treatment. *Cells* **2020**, *9*, 1901. [CrossRef] [PubMed]
77. Marneth, A.E.; Mullally, A. The molecular genetics of myeloproliferative neoplasms. *Cold Spring Harb. Perspect. Med.* **2020**, *10*, a034876. [CrossRef] [PubMed]
78. O'Sullivan, J.; Mead, A.J. Heterogeneity in myeloproliferative neoplasms: Causes and consequences. *Adv. Biol. Regul.* **2019**, *71*, 55–68. [CrossRef] [PubMed]
79. Baxter, E.J.; Scott, L.M.; Campbell, P.J.; East, C.; Fourouclas, N.; Swanton, S.; Vassiliou, G.S.; Bench, A.J.; Boyd, E.M.; Curtin, N.; et al. Acquired mutation of the tyrosine kinase JAK2 in human myeloproliferative disorders. *Lancet* **2005**, *365*, 1054–1061. [CrossRef]
80. James, C.; Ugo, V.; Le Couédic, J.P.; Staerk, J.; Delhommeau, F.; Lacout, C.; Garçon, L.; Raslova, H.; Berger, R.; Bennaceur-Griscelli, A.; et al. A unique clonal JAK2 mutation leading to constitutive signalling causes polycythaemia vera. *Nature* **2005**, *434*, 1144–1148. [CrossRef]
81. Kralovics, R.; Teo, S.-S.; Li, S.; Theocharides, A.; Buser, A.S.; Tichelli, A.; Skoda, R.C. Acquisition of the V617F mutation of JAK2 is a late genetic event in a subset of patients with myeloproliferative disorders. *Blood* **2006**, *108*, 1377–1380. [CrossRef] [PubMed]
82. Levine, R.L.; Wadleigh, M.; Cools, J.; Ebert, B.L.; Wernig, G.; Huntly, B.J.P.; Boggon, T.J.; Wlodarska, I.; Clark, J.J.; Moore, S.; et al. Activating mutation in the tyrosine kinase JAK2 in polycythemia vera, essential thrombocythemia, and myeloid metaplasia with myelofibrosis. *Cancer Cell* **2005**, *7*, 387–397. [CrossRef]

83. Zhao, R.; Xing, S.; Li, Z.; Fu, X.; Li, Q.; Krantz, S.B.; Zhao, Z.J. Identification of an acquired JAK2 mutation in polycythemia vera. *J. Biol. Chem.* **2005**, *280*, 22788–22792. [CrossRef]
84. Tefferi, A.; Barbui, T. Polycythemia vera and essential thrombocythemia: 2019 update on diagnosis, risk-stratification and management. *Am. J. Hematol.* **2019**, *94*, 133–143. [CrossRef]
85. Scott, L.M.; Tong, W.; Levine, R.L.; Scott, M.A.; Beer, P.A.; Stratton, M.R.; Futreal, P.A.; Erber, W.N.; McMullin, M.F.; Harrison, C.N.; et al. JAK2 exon 12 mutations in polycythemia vera and idiopathic erythrocytosis. *N. Engl. J. Med.* **2007**, *356*, 459–468. [CrossRef]
86. Passamonti, F.; Elena, C.; Schnittger, S.; Skoda, R.C.; Green, A.R.; Girodon, F.; Kiladjian, J.-J.; McMullin, M.F.; Ruggeri, M.; Besses, C.; et al. Molecular and clinical features of the myeloproliferative neoplasm associated with JAK2 exon 12 mutations. *Blood* **2011**, *117*, 2813–2816. [CrossRef] [PubMed]
87. Pikman, Y.; Lee, B.H.; Mercher, T.; McDowell, E.; Ebert, B.L.; Gozo, M.; Cuker, A.; Wernig, G.; Moore, S.; Galinsky, I.; et al. MPLW515L is a novel somatic activating mutation in myelofibrosis with myeloid metaplasia. *PLoS Med.* **2006**, *3*, e270. [CrossRef]
88. Pardanani, A.D.; Levine, R.L.; Lasho, T.; Pikman, Y.; Mesa, R.A.; Wadleigh, M.; Steensma, D.P.; Elliott, M.A.; Wolanskyj, A.P.; Hogan, W.J.; et al. MPL515 mutations in myeloproliferative and other myeloid disorders: A study of 1182 patients. *Blood* **2006**, *108*, 3472–3476. [CrossRef]
89. Defour, J.P.; Itaya, M.; Gryshkova, V.; Brett, I.C.; Pecquet, C.; Sato, T.; Smith, S.O.; Constantinescu, S.N. Tryptophan at the transmembrane-cytosolic junction modulates thrombopoietin receptor dimerization and activation. *Proc. Natl. Acad. Sci. USA* **2013**, *110*, 2540–2545. [CrossRef] [PubMed]
90. Nangalia, J.; Grinfeld, J.; Green, A.R. Pathogenesis of myeloproliferative disorders. *Annu. Rev. Pathol.* **2016**, *11*, 101–126. [CrossRef] [PubMed]
91. Nangalia, J.; Massie, C.E.; Baxter, E.J.; Nice, F.L.; Gundem, G.; Wedge, D.C.; Avezov, E.; Li, J.; Kollmann, K.; Kent, D.G.; et al. Somatic CALR mutations in myeloproliferative neoplasms with nonmutated JAK2. *N. Engl. J. Med.* **2013**, *369*, 2391–2405. [CrossRef]
92. Klampfl, T.; Gisslinger, H.; Harutyunyan, A.S.; Nivarthi, H.; Rumi, E.; Milosevic, J.D.; Them, N.C.C.; Berg, T.; Gisslinger, B.; Pietra, D.; et al. Somatic mutations of calreticulin in myeloproliferative neoplasms. *N. Engl. J. Med.* **2013**, *369*, 2379–2390. [CrossRef] [PubMed]
93. Michalak, M.; Corbett, E.F.; Mesaeli, N.; Nakamura, K.; Opas, M. Calreticulin: One protein, one gene, many functions. *Biochem. J.* **1999**, *344*, 281–292. [CrossRef] [PubMed]
94. Wang, W.A.; Groenendyk, J.; Michalak, M. Calreticulin signaling in health and disease. *Int. J. Biochem. Cell Biol.* **2012**, *44*, 842–846. [CrossRef] [PubMed]
95. Shivarov, V.; Ivanova, M.; Tiu, R.V. Mutated calreticulin retains structurally disordered C terminus that cannot bind Ca[2+]: Some mechanistic and therapeutic implications. *Blood Cancer J.* **2014**, *4*, e185. [CrossRef]
96. Araki, M.; Yang, Y.; Masubuchi, N.; Hironaka, Y.; Takei, H.; Morishita, S.; Mizukami, Y.; Kan, S.; Shirane, S.; Edahiro, Y.; et al. Activation of the thrombopoietin receptor by mutant calreticulin in CALR-mutant myeloproliferative neoplasms. *Blood* **2016**, *127*, 1307–1316. [CrossRef]
97. Chachoua, I.; Pecquet, C.; El-Khoury, M.; Nivarthi, H.; Albu, R.I.; Marty, C.; Gryshkova, V.; Defour, J.-P.; Vertenoeil, G.; Ngo, A.; et al. Thrombopoietin receptor activation by myeloproliferative neoplasm associated calreticulin mutants. *Blood* **2016**, *127*, 1325–1335. [CrossRef] [PubMed]
98. Elf, S.; Abdelfattah, N.S.; Chen, E.; Perales-Patón, J.; Rosen, E.A.; Ko, A.; Peisker, F.; Florescu, N.; Giannini, S.; Wolach, O.; et al. Mutant calreticulin requires both its mutant C-terminus and the thrombopoietin receptor for oncogenic transformation. *Cancer Discov.* **2016**, *6*, 368–381. [CrossRef] [PubMed]
99. Vainchenker, W.; Kralovics, R. Genetic basis and molecular pathophysiology of classical myeloproliferative neoplasms. *Blood* **2017**, *129*, 667–679. [CrossRef]
100. Elf, S.; Abdelfattah, N.S.; Baral, A.J.; Beeson, D.; Rivera, J.F.; Ko, A.; Florescu, N.; Birrane, G.; Chen, E.; Mullally, A. Defining the requirements for the pathogenic interaction between mutant calreticulin and MPL in MPN. *Blood* **2018**, *131*, 782–786. [CrossRef] [PubMed]
101. Araki, M.; Komatsu, N. The role of calreticulin mutations in myeloproliferative neoplasms. *Int. J. Hematol.* **2020**, *111*, 200–205. [CrossRef]
102. Han, L.; Schubert, C.; Köhler, J.; Schemionek, M.; Isfort, S.; Brümmendorf, T.H.; Koschmieder, S.; Chatain, N. Calreticulin-mutant proteins induce megakaryocytic signaling to transform hematopoietic cells and undergo accelerated degradation and Golgi-mediated secretion. *J. Hematol. Oncol.* **2016**, *9*, 45. [CrossRef]
103. Pecquet, C.; Balligand, T.; Chachoua, I.; Roy, A.; Vertenoeil, G.; Colau, D.; Fertig, E.; Marty, C.; Nivarthi, H.; Defour, J.-P.; et al. Secreted mutant calreticulins as rogue cytokines trigger thrombopoietin receptor activation specifically in CALR mutated cells: Perspectives for MPN therapy. *Blood* **2018**, *132* (Suppl. 1), 4. [CrossRef]
104. Rampal, R.; Al-Shahrour, F.; Abdel-Wahab, O.; Patel, J.; Brunel, J.-P.; Mermel, C.H.; Bass, A.J.; Pretz, J.; Ahn, J.; Hricik, T.; et al. Integrated genomic analysis illustrates the central role of JAK-STAT pathway activation in myeloproliferative neoplasm pathogenesis. *Blood* **2014**, *123*, e123–e133. [CrossRef] [PubMed]
105. Reuther, G.W. Myeloproliferative neoplasms: Molecular drivers and therapeutics. *Prog. Mol. Biol. Transl. Sci.* **2016**, *144*, 437–484. [CrossRef] [PubMed]

106. Tefferi, A.; Vaidya, R.; Caramazza, D.; Finke, C.; Lasho, T.; Pardanani, A. Circulating interleukin (IL)-8, IL-2R, IL-12, and IL-15 levels are independently prognostic in primary myelofibrosis: A comprehensive cytokine profiling study. *J. Clin. Oncol.* **2011**, *29*, 1356–1363. [CrossRef] [PubMed]
107. Kiladjian, J.J.; Giraudier, S.; Cassinat, B. Interferon-alpha for the therapy of myeloproliferative neoplasms: Targeting the malignant clone. *Leukemia* **2016**, *30*, 776–781. [CrossRef] [PubMed]
108. Kagoya, Y.; Yoshimi, A.; Tsuruta-Kishino, T.; Arai, S.; Satoh, T.; Akira, S.; Kurokawa, M. JAK2V617F+ myeloproliferative neoplasm clones evoke paracrine DNA damage to adjacent normal cells through secretion of lipocalin-2. *Blood* **2014**, *124*, 2996–3006. [CrossRef] [PubMed]
109. Decker, M.; Martinez-Morentin, L.; Wang, G.; Lee, Y.; Liu, Q.; Leslie, J.; Ding, L. Leptin-receptor-expressing bone marrow stromal cells are myofibroblasts in primary myelofibrosis. *Nat. Cell Biol.* **2017**, *19*, 677–688. [CrossRef] [PubMed]
110. Schneider, R.K.; Mullally, A.; Dugourd, A.; Peisker, F.; Hoogenboezem, R.; Van Strien, P.M.H.; Bindels, E.M.; Heckl, D.; Büsche, G.; Fleck, D.; et al. Gli1+ mesenchymal stromal cells are a key driver of bone marrow fibrosis and an important cellular therapeutic target. *Cell. Stem Cell.* **2017**, *20*, 785–800. [CrossRef] [PubMed]
111. Abdel-Wahab, O.; Adli, M.; LaFave, L.M.; Gao, J.; Hricik, T.; Shih, A.H.; Pandey, S.; Patel, J.P.; Chung, Y.R.; Koche, R.; et al. ASXL1 mutations promote myeloid transformation through loss of PRC2-mediated gene repression. *Cancer Cell* **2012**, *22*, 180–193. [CrossRef]
112. Asada, S.; Goyama, S.; Inoue, D.; Shikata, S.; Takeda, R.; Fukushima, T.; Yonezawa, T.; Fujino, T.; Hayashi, Y.; Kawabata, K.C.; et al. Mutant ASXL1 cooperates with BAP1 to promote myeloid leukaemogenesis. *Nat. Commun.* **2018**, *9*, 2733. [CrossRef] [PubMed]
113. Balasubramani, A.; Larjo, A.; Bassein, J.A.; Chang, X.; Hastie, R.B.; Togher, S.M.; Lähdesmäki, H.; Rao, A. Cancer-associated ASXL1 mutations may act as gain-of-function mutations of the ASXL1-BAP1 complex. *Nat. Commun.* **2015**, *6*, 7307. [CrossRef] [PubMed]
114. Yang, H.; Kurtenbach, S.; Guo, Y.; Lohse, I.; Durante, M.A.; Li, J.; Li, Z.; Al-Ali, H.; Li, L.; Chen, Z.; et al. Gain of function of ASXL1 truncating protein in the pathogenesis of myeloid malignancies. *Blood* **2018**, *131*, 328–341. [CrossRef] [PubMed]
115. Saika, M.; Inoue, D.; Nagase, R.; Sato, N.; Tsuchiya, A.; Yabushita, T.; Kitamura, T.; Goyama, S. ASXL1 and SETBP1 mutations promote leukaemogenesis by repressing TGFβ pathway genes through histone deacetylation. *Sci. Rep.* **2018**, *8*, 15873. [CrossRef]
116. Cho, Y.-S.; Kim, E.-J.; Park, U.-H.; Sin, H.-S.; Um, S.-J. Additional sex comb-like 1 [ASXL1], in cooperation with SRC-1, acts as a ligand-dependent coactivator for retinoic acid receptor. *J. Biol. Chem.* **2006**, *281*, 17588–17598. [CrossRef] [PubMed]
117. Park, U.-H.; Yoon, S.-K.; Park, T.; Kim, E.-J.; Um, S.-J. Additional sex comb-like [ASXL] proteins 1 and 2 play opposite roles in adipogenesis via reciprocal regulation of peroxisome proliferator-activated receptor γ. *J. Biol. Chem.* **2011**, *286*, 1354–1363. [CrossRef] [PubMed]
118. Khan, S.N.; Jankowska, A.M.; Mahfouz, R.; Dunbar, A.J.; Sugimoto, Y.; Hosono, N.; Hu, Z.; Cheriyath, V.; Vatolin, S.; Przychodzen, B.; et al. Multiple mechanisms deregulate EZH2 and histone H3 lysine 27 epigenetic changes in myeloid malignancies. *Leukemia* **2013**, *27*, 1301–1309. [CrossRef] [PubMed]
119. Rinke, J.; Chase, A.; Cross, N.C.P.; Hochhaus, A.; Ernst, T. EZH2 in myeloid malignancies. *Cells* **2020**, *9*, 1639. [CrossRef]
120. Anteneh, H.; Fang, J.; Song, J. Structural basis for impairment of DNA methylation by the DNMT3A R882H mutation. *Nat. Commun.* **2020**, *11*, 2294. [CrossRef] [PubMed]
121. Jacquelin, S.; Straube, J.; Cooper, L.; Vu, T.; Song, A.; Bywater, M.; Baxter, E.; Heidecker, M.; Wackrow, B.; Porter, A.; et al. Jak2V617F and Dnmt3a loss cooperate to induce myelofibrosis through activated enhancer-driven inflammation. *Blood* **2018**, *132*, 2707–2721. [CrossRef]
122. Abdel-Wahab, O.; Mullally, A.; Hedvat, C.; Garcia-Manero, G.; Patel, J.; Wadleigh, M.; Malinge, S.; Yao, J.; Kilpivaara, O.; Bhat, R.; et al. Genetic characterization of TET1, TET2, and TET3 alterations in myeloid malignancies. *Blood* **2009**, *114*, 144–147. [CrossRef] [PubMed]
123. Ostrander, E.L.; Kramer, A.C.; Mallaney, C.; Celik, H.; Koh, W.K.; Fairchild, J.; Haussler, E.; Zhang, C.R.C.; Challen, G.A. Divergent effects of Dnmt3a and Tet2 mutations on hematopoietic progenitor cell fitness. *Stem Cell Reports* **2020**, *14*, 551–560. [CrossRef] [PubMed]
124. Zhang, Q.; Zhao, K.; Shen, Q.; Han, Y.; Gu, Y.; Li, X.; Zhao, D.; Liu, Y.; Wang, C.; Zhang, X.; et al. Tet2 is required to resolve inflammation by recruiting Hdac2 to specifically repress IL-6. *Nature* **2015**, *525*, 389–393. [CrossRef]
125. Ortmann, C.A.; Kent, D.G.; Nangalia, J.; Silber, Y.; Wedge, D.C.; Grinfeld, J.; Baxter, E.J.; Massie, C.E.; Papaemmanuil, E.; Menon, S.; et al. Effect of mutation order on myeloproliferative neoplasms. *N. Engl. J. Med.* **2015**, *372*, 601–612. [CrossRef]
126. Lu, C.; Ward, P.S.; Kapoor, G.S.; Rohle, D.; Turcan, S.; Abdel-Wahab, O.; Edwards, C.R.; Khanin, R.; Figueroa, M.E.; Melnick, A.; et al. IDH mutation impairs histone demethylation and results in a block to cell differentiation. *Nature* **2012**, *483*, 474–478. [CrossRef] [PubMed]
127. Tefferi, A.; Lasho, T.L.; Abdel-Wahab, O.; Guglielmelli, P.; Patel, J.; Caramazza, D.; Pieri, L.; Finke, C.M.; Kilpivaara, O.; Wadleigh, M.; et al. IDH1 and IDH2 mutation studies in 1473 patients with chronic-, fibrotic- or blast-phase essential thrombocythemia, polycythemia vera or myelofibrosis. *Leukemia* **2010**, *24*, 1302–1309. [CrossRef]
128. Pardanani, A.; Lasho, T.L.; Finke, C.M.; Mai, M.; McClure, R.F.; Tefferi, A. IDH1 and IDH2 mutation analysis in chronic-and blast-phase myeloproliferative neoplasms. *Leukemia* **2010**, *24*, 1146–1151. [CrossRef] [PubMed]
129. Xu, W.; Yang, H.; Liu, Y.; Yang, Y.; Wang, P.; Kim, S.H.; Ito, S.; Yang, C.; Wang, P.; Xiao, M.T.; et al. Oncometabolite 2-hydroxyglutarate is a competitive inhibitor of α-ketoglutarate-dependent dioxygenases. *Cancer Cell* **2011**, *19*, 17–30. [CrossRef]

130. Yoshimi, A.; Lin, K.T.; Wiseman, D.H.; Rahman, M.A.; Pastore, A.; Wang, B.; Lee, S.C.; Micol, J.B.; Zhang, X.J.; de Botton, S.; et al. Coordinated alterations in RNA splicing and epigenetic regulation drive leukaemogenesis. *Nature* **2019**, *574*, 273–277. [CrossRef]
131. Hafner, A.; Bulyk, M.L.; Jambhekar, A.; Lahav, G. The multiple mechanisms that regulate p53 activity and cell fate. *Nat. Rev. Mol. Cell Biol.* **2019**, *20*, 199–210. [CrossRef] [PubMed]
132. Liu, Y.; Elf, S.E.; Miyata, Y.; Sashida, G.; Liu, Y.; Huang, G.; Di Giandomenico, S.; Lee, J.M.; Deblasio, A.; Menendez, S.; et al. p53 regulates hematopoietic stem cell quiescence. *Cell Stem Cell.* **2009**, *4*, 37–48. [CrossRef] [PubMed]
133. Marcellino, B.K.; Hoffman, R.; Tripodi, J.; Lu, M.; Kosiorek, H.; Mascarenhas, J.; Rampal, R.K.; Dueck, A.; Najfeld, V. Advanced forms of MPNs are accompanied by chromosomal abnormalities that lead to dysregulation of TP53. *Blood Adv.* **2018**, *2*, 3581–3589. [CrossRef]
134. Fiscella, M.; Zhang, H.; Fan, S.; Sakaguchi, K.; Shen, S.; Mercer, W.E.; Vande Woude, G.F.; O'Connor, P.M.; Appella, E. Wip1, a novel human protein phosphatase that is induced in response to ionizing radiation in a p53-dependent manner. *Proc. Natl. Acad. Sci. USA* **1997**, *94*, 6048–6053. [CrossRef] [PubMed]
135. Kahn, J.D.; Miller, P.G.; Silver, A.J.; Sellar, R.S.; Bhatt, S.; Gibson, C.; McConkey, M.; Adams, D.; Mar, B.; Mertins, P.; et al. PPM1D-truncating mutations confer resistance to chemotherapy and sensitivity to PPM1D inhibition in hematopoietic cells. *Blood* **2018**, *132*, 1095–1105. [CrossRef]
136. Sood, R.; Kamikubo, Y.; Liu, P. Role of RUNX1 in hematological malignancies. *Blood* **2017**, *129*, 2070–2082. [CrossRef] [PubMed]
137. Peeken, J.C.; Jutzi, J.S.; Wehrle, J.; Koellerer, C.; Staehle, H.F.; Becker, H.; Schoenwandt, E.; Seeger, T.S.; Schanne, D.H.; Gothwal, M.; et al. Epigenetic regulation of NFE2 overexpression in myeloproliferative neoplasms. *Blood* **2018**, *131*, 2065–2073. [CrossRef]
138. Will, C.L.; Lührmann, R. Spliceosome structure and function. *Cold Spring Harb. Perspect. Biol.* **2011**, *3*, a003707. [CrossRef] [PubMed]
139. Kim, E.; Ilagan, J.O.; Liang, Y.; Daubner, G.M.; Lee, S.C.; Ramakrishnan, A.; Li, Y.; Chung, Y.R.; Micol, J.B.; Murphy, M.E.; et al. SRSF2 mutations contribute to myelodysplasia by mutant-specific effects on exon recognition. *Cancer Cell* **2015**, *27*, 617–630. [CrossRef]
140. Lee, S.C.; North, K.; Kim, E.; Jang, E.; Obeng, E.; Lu, S.X.; Liu, B.; Inoue, D.; Yoshimi, A.; Ki, M.; et al. Synthetic lethal and convergent biological effects of cancer-associated spliceosomal gene mutations. *Cancer Cell* **2018**, *34*, 225–241.e8. [CrossRef] [PubMed]
141. Chen, L.; Chen, J.Y.; Huang, Y.J.; Gu, Y.; Qiu, J.; Qian, H.; Shao, C.; Zhang, X.; Hu, J.; Li, H.; et al. The augmented R-loop is a unifying mechanism for myelodysplastic syndromes induced by high-risk splicing factor mutations. *Mol. Cell* **2018**, *69*, 412–425.e6. [CrossRef] [PubMed]
142. Nguyen, H.D.; Leong, W.Y.; Li, W.; Reddy, P.N.G.; Sullivan, J.D.; Walter, M.J.; Zou, L.; Graubert, T.A. Spliceosome mutations induce R loop-associated sensitivity to ATR inhibition in myelodysplastic syndromes. *Cancer Res.* **2018**, *78*, 5363–5374. [CrossRef]
143. Sakurai, H.; Harada, Y.; Ogata, Y.; Kagiyama, Y.; Shingai, N.; Doki, N.; Ohashi, K.; Kitamura, T.; Komatsu, N.; Harada, H. Overexpression of RUNX1 short isoform has an important role in the development of myelodysplastic/myeloproliferative neoplasms. *Blood Adv.* **2017**, *1*, 1382–1386. [CrossRef]
144. Xiao, R.; Sun, Y.; Ding, J.H.; Lin, S.; Rose, D.W.; Rosenfeld, M.G.; Fu, X.D.; Li, X. Splicing regulator SC35 is essential for genomic stability and cell proliferation during mammalian organogenesis. *Mol. Cell Biol.* **2007**, *27*, 5393–5402. [CrossRef]
145. Soares, L.M.; Zanier, K.; Mackereth, C.; Sattler, M.; Valcárcel, J. Intron removal requires proofreading of U2AF/3' splice site recognition by DEK. *Science* **2006**, *312*, 1961–1965. [CrossRef] [PubMed]
146. Tefferi, A.; Finke, C.M.; Lasho, T.L.; Hanson, C.A.; Ketterling, R.P.; Gangat, N.; Pardanani, A. U2AF1 mutation types in primary myelofibrosis: Phenotypic and prognostic distinctions. *Leukemia* **2018**, *32*, 2274–2278. [CrossRef] [PubMed]
147. Graubert, T.A.; Shen, D.; Ding, L.; Okeyo-Owuor, T.; Lunn, C.L.; Shao, J.; Krysiak, K.; Harris, C.C.; Koboldt, D.C.; Larson, D.E.; et al. Recurrent mutations in the U2AF1 splicing factor in myelodysplastic syndromes. *Nat. Genet.* **2011**, *44*, 53–57. [CrossRef] [PubMed]
148. Webb, C.J.; Wise, J.A. The splicing factor U2AF small subunit is functionally conserved between fission yeast and humans. *Mol. Cell Biol.* **2004**, *24*, 4229–4240. [CrossRef] [PubMed]
149. Palangat, M.; Anastasakis, D.G.; Fei, D.L.; Lindblad, K.E.; Bradley, R.; Hourigan, C.S.; Hafner, M.; Larson, D.R. The splicing factor U2AF1 contributes to cancer progression through a noncanonical role in translation regulation. *Genes Dev.* **2019**, *33*, 482–497. [CrossRef] [PubMed]
150. Madan, V.; Kanojia, D.; Li, J.; Okamoto, R.; Sato-Otsubo, A.; Kohlmann, A.; Sanada, M.; Grossmann, V.; Sundaresan, J.; Shiraishi, Y.; et al. Aberrant splicing of U12-type introns is the hallmark of ZRSR2 mutant myelodysplastic syndrome. *Nat. Commun.* **2015**, *6*, 6042. [CrossRef]
151. Cazzola, M.; Rossi, M.; Malcovati, L. Biologic and clinical significance of somatic mutations of SF3B1 in myeloid and lymphoid neoplasms. *Blood* **2013**, *121*, 260–269. [CrossRef]
152. Obeng, E.A.; Chappell, R.J.; Seiler, M.; Chen, M.C.; Campagna, D.R.; Schmidt, P.J.; Schneider, R.K.; Lord, A.M.; Wang, L.; Gambe, R.G.; et al. Physiologic expression of Sf3b1[K700E] causes impaired erythropoiesis, aberrant splicing, and sensitivity to therapeutic spliceosome modulation. *Cancer Cell* **2016**, *30*, 404–417. [CrossRef]
153. Tong, W.; Zhang, J.; Lodish, H.F. Lnk inhibits erythropoiesis and Epo-dependent JAK2 activation and downstream signaling pathways. *Blood* **2005**, *105*, 4604–4612. [CrossRef] [PubMed]

154. Bersenev, A.; Wu, C.; Balcerek, J.; Tong, W. Lnk controls mouse hematopoietic stem cell self-renewal and quiescence through direct interactions with JAK2. *J. Clin. Investig.* **2008**, *118*, 2832–2844. [CrossRef]
155. Simon, C.; Dondi, E.; Chaix, A.; de Sepulveda, P.; Kubiseski, T.J.; Varin-Blank, N.; Velazquez, L. Lnk adaptor protein downregulates specific Kit-induced signaling pathways in primary mast cells. *Blood* **2008**, *112*, 4039–4047. [CrossRef] [PubMed]
156. Takaki, S.; Sauer, K.; Iritani, B.M.; Chien, S.; Ebihara, Y.; Tsuji, K.; Takatsu, K.; Perlmutter, R.M. Control of B cell production by the adaptor protein Lnk: Definition of a conserved family of signal-modulating proteins. *Immunity* **2000**, *13*, 599–609. [CrossRef]
157. Takaki, S.; Morita, H.; Tezuka, Y.; Takatsu, K. Enhanced hematopoiesis by hematopoietic progenitor cells lacking intracellular adaptor protein, Lnk. *J. Exp. Med.* **2002**, *195*, 151–160. [CrossRef] [PubMed]
158. Velazquez, L.; Cheng, A.M.; Fleming, H.E.; Furlonger, C.; Vesely, S.; Bernstein, A.; Paige, C.J.; Pawson, T. Cytokine signaling and hematopoietic homeostasis are disrupted in Lnk-deficient mice. *J. Exp. Med.* **2002**, *195*, 1599–1611. [CrossRef] [PubMed]
159. Thien, C.B.; Langdon, W.Y. Negative regulation of PTK signalling by Cbl proteins. *Growth Factors.* **2005**, *23*, 161–167. [CrossRef] [PubMed]
160. Mohapatra, B.; Ahmad, G.; Nadeau, S.; Zutshi, N.; An, W.; Scheffe, S.; Dong, L.; Feng, D.; Goetz, B.; Arya, P.; et al. Protein tyrosine kinase regulation by ubiquitination: Critical roles of Cbl-family ubiquitin ligases. *Biochim. Biophys. Acta.* **2013**, *1833*, 122–139. [CrossRef] [PubMed]
161. Lv, K.; Jiang, J.; Donaghy, R.; Riling, C.R.; Cheng, Y.; Chandra, V.; Rozenova, K.; An, W.; Mohapatra, B.C.; Goetz, B.T.; et al. CBL family E3 ubiquitin ligases control JAK2 ubiquitination and stability in hematopoietic stem cells and myeloid malignancies. *Genes Dev.* **2017**, *31*, 1007–1023. [CrossRef] [PubMed]
162. Sanada, M.; Suzuki, T.; Shih, L.Y.; Otsu, M.; Kato, M.; Yamazaki, S.; Tamura, A.; Honda, H.; Sakata-Yanagimoto, M.; Kumano, K.; et al. Gain-of-function of mutated C-CBL tumour suppressor in myeloid neoplasms. *Nature* **2009**, *460*, 904–908. [CrossRef] [PubMed]
163. Schubbert, S.; Shannon, K.; Bollag, G. Hyperactive Ras in developmental disorders and cancer. *Nat. Rev. Cancer.* **2007**, *7*, 295–308. [CrossRef] [PubMed]
164. Bunda, S.; Burrell, K.; Heir, P.; Zeng, L.; Alamsahebpour, A.; Kano, Y.; Raught, B.; Zhang, Z.Y.; Zadeh, G.; Ohh, M. Inhibition of SHP2-mediated dephosphorylation of Ras suppresses oncogenesis. *Nat. Commun.* **2015**, *6*, 8859. [CrossRef]
165. Niihori, T.; Aoki, Y.; Ohashi, H.; Kurosawa, K.; Kondoh, T.; Ishikiriyama, S.; Kawame, H.; Kamasaki, H.; Yamanaka, T.; Takada, F.; et al. Functional analysis of PTPN11/SHP-2 mutants identified in Noonan syndrome and childhood leukemia. *J. Hum. Genet.* **2005**, *50*, 192–202. [CrossRef] [PubMed]
166. Shi, Z.Q.; Yu, D.H.; Park, M.; Marshall, M.; Feng, G.S. Molecular mechanism for the Shp-2 tyrosine phosphatase function in promoting growth factor stimulation of Erk activity. *Mol. Cell Biol.* **2000**, *20*, 1526–1536. [CrossRef]
167. Eaves, C.J. Hematopoietic stem cells: Concepts, definitions, and the new reality. *Blood* **2015**, *125*, 2605–2613. [CrossRef]
168. Mead, A.J.; Mullally, A. Myeloproliferative neoplasm stem cells. *Blood* **2017**, *129*, 1607–1616. [CrossRef] [PubMed]
169. Jones, A.V.; Chase, A.; Silver, R.T.; Oscier, D.; Zoi, K.; Wang, Y.L.; Cario, H.; Pahl, H.L.; Collins, A.; Reiter, A.; et al. JAK2 haplotype is a major risk factor for the development of myeloproliferative neoplasms. *Nat. Genet.* **2009**, *41*, 446–449. [CrossRef]
170. Jones, A.V.; Campbell, P.J.; Beer, P.A.; Schnittger, S.; Vannucchi, A.M.; Zoi, K.; Percy, M.J.; McMullin, M.F.; Scott, L.M.; Tapper, W.; et al. The JAK2 46/1 haplotype predisposes to MPL-mutated myeloproliferative neoplasms. *Blood* **2010**, *115*, 4517–4523. [CrossRef]
171. Tapper, W.; Jones, A.V.; Kralovics, R.; Harutyunyan, A.S.; Zoi, K.; Leung, W.; Godfrey, A.L.; Guglielmelli, P.; Callaway, A.; Ward, D.; et al. Genetic variation at MECOM, TERT, JAK2 and HBS1L-MYB predisposes to myeloproliferative neoplasms. *Nat. Commun.* **2015**, *6*, 6691. [CrossRef] [PubMed]
172. Trifa, A.P.; Bănescu, C.; Bojan, A.S.; Voina, C.M.; Popa, Ș.; Vișan, S.; Ciubean, A.D.; Tripon, F.; Dima, D.; Popov, V.M.; et al. MECOM, HBS1L-MYB, THRB-RARB, JAK2, and TERT polymorphisms defining the genetic predisposition to myeloproliferative neoplasms: A study on 939 patients. *Am. J. Hematol.* **2018**, *93*, 100–106. [CrossRef] [PubMed]
173. Hinds, D.A.; Barnholt, K.E.; Mesa, R.A.; Kiefer, A.K.; Do, C.B.; Eriksson, N.; Mountain, J.L.; Francke, U.; Tung, J.Y.; Nguyen, H.M.; et al. Germ line variants predispose to both JAK2 V617F clonal hematopoiesis and myeloproliferative neoplasms. *Blood* **2016**, *128*, 1121–1128. [CrossRef] [PubMed]
174. Godfrey, A.L.; Chen, E.; Pagano, F.; Silber, Y.; Campbell, P.J.; Green, A.R. Clonal analyses reveal associations of JAK2V617F homozygosity with hematologic features, age and gender in polycythemia vera and essential thrombocythemia. *Haematologica* **2013**, *98*, 718–721. [CrossRef] [PubMed]
175. Geyer, H.L.; Kosiorek, H.; Dueck, A.C.; Scherber, R.; Slot, S.; Zweegman, S.; Te Boekhorst, P.A.; Senyak, Z.; Schouten, H.C.; Sackmann, F.; et al. Associations between gender, disease features and symptom burden in patients with myeloproliferative neoplasms: An analysis by the MPN QOL International Working Group. *Haematologica* **2017**, *102*, 85–93. [CrossRef]
176. Alvarez-Larrán, A.; Cervantes, F.; Bellosillo, B.; Giralt, M.; Juliá, A.; Hernández-Boluda, J.C.; Bosch, A.; Hernández-Nieto, L.; Clapés, V.; Burgaleta, C.; et al. Essential thrombocythemia in young individuals: Frequency and risk factors for vascular events and evolution to myelofibrosis in 126 patients. *Leukemia* **2007**, *21*, 1218–2123. [CrossRef] [PubMed]
177. Srour, S.A.; Devesa, S.S.; Morton, L.M.; Check, D.P.; Curtis, R.E.; Linet, M.S.; Dores, G.M. Incidence and patient survival of myeloproliferative neoplasms and myelodysplastic/myeloproliferative neoplasms in the United States, 2001–2012. *Br. J. Haematol.* **2016**, *174*, 382–396. [CrossRef]

178. Grinfeld, J.; Nangalia, J.; Baxter, E.J.; Wedge, D.C.; Angelopoulos, N.; Cantrill, R.; Godfrey, A.L.; Papaemmanuil, E.; Gundem, G.; MacLean, C.; et al. Classification and personalized prognosis in myeloproliferative neoplasms. *N. Engl. J. Med.* **2018**, *379*, 1416–1430. [CrossRef] [PubMed]
179. Anderson, L.A.; Duncombe, A.S.; Hughes, M.; Mills, M.E.; Wilson, J.C.; McMullin, M.F. Environmental, lifestyle, and familial/ethnic factors associated with myeloproliferative neoplasms. *Am. J. Hematol.* **2012**, *87*, 175–182. [CrossRef]
180. Jayasuriya, N.A.; Ellervik, C.; Hasselbalch, H.C.; Sørensen, A. Cigarette smoking, complete blood count, and myeloproliferative neoplasms—A meta-analysis. *Blood* **2017**, *130*, 4199. [CrossRef]
181. Jayasuriya, N.A.; Kjaergaard, A.D.; Pedersen, K.M.; Sørensen, A.L.; Bak, M.; Larsen, M.K.; Nordestgaard, B.G.; Bojesen, S.E.; Çolak, Y.; Skov, V.; et al. Smoking, blood cells and myeloproliferative neoplasms: Meta-analysis and Mendelian randomization of 2·3 million people. *Br. J. Haematol.* **2020**, *189*, 323–334. [CrossRef] [PubMed]

Article

CD99–PTPN12 Axis Suppresses Actin Cytoskeleton-Mediated Dimerization of Epidermal Growth Factor Receptor

Kyoung-Jin Lee [1], Yuri Kim [1], Min Seo Kim [1], Hyun-Mi Ju [1], Boyoung Choi [1], Hansoo Lee [2], Dooil Jeoung [3], Ki-Won Moon [4], Dongmin Kang [5], Jiwon Choi [6,7], Jong In Yook [6,7] and Jang-Hee Hahn [1,*]

[1] Department of Anatomy and Cell Biology, School of Medicine, Kangwon National University, Chuncheon 24341, Korea; jin.lee@supadelixir.com (K.-J.L.); yuri8686@sunmoon.ac.kr (Y.K.); ms.kim@supadelixir.com (M.S.K.); hm.ju@supadelixir.com (H.-M.J.); boyoung630@naver.com (B.C.)
[2] Department of Biological Sciences, College of Natural Sciences, Kangwon National University, Chuncheon 24341, Korea; hslee@kangwon.ac.kr
[3] Department of Biochemistry, College of Natural Sciences, Kangwon National University, Chuncheon 24341, Korea; jeoungd@kangwon.ac.kr
[4] Department of Rheumatology, Kangwon National University Hospital, Chuncheon 24289, Korea; kiwonmoon@kangwon.ac.kr
[5] Department of Life Science, Ewha Womans University, Seoul 03760, Korea; dkang@ewha.ac.kr
[6] Met Life Sciences Co., Ltd., Seoul 03722, Korea; edccjw@gmail.com (J.C.); jiyook@yuhs.ac (J.I.Y.)
[7] Department of Oral Pathology, Oral Cancer Research Institute, College of Dentistry, Yonsei University, Seoul 03722, Korea
* Correspondence: jhahn@kangwon.ac.kr; Tel.: +82-70-4165-5568

Received: 4 September 2020; Accepted: 5 October 2020; Published: 9 October 2020

Simple Summary: The epidermal growth factor receptor (EGFR) is activated through growth factor-dependent dimerization accompanied by functional reorganization of the actin cytoskeleton. Lee et al. demonstrate that CD99 activation by agonist ligands inhibits epidermal growth factor (EGF)-induced EGFR dimerization through impairment of cytoskeletal reorganization by protein tyrosine phosphatase non-receptor type 12 (PTPN12)-dependent c-Src/focal adhesion kinase (FAK) inactivation, thereby suppressing breast cancer growth.

Abstract: The epidermal growth factor receptor (EGFR), a member of ErbB receptor tyrosine kinase (RTK) family, is activated through growth factor-induced reorganization of the actin cytoskeleton and subsequent dimerization. We herein explored the molecular mechanism underlying the suppression of ligand-induced EGFR dimerization by CD99 agonists and its relevance to tumor growth in vivo. Epidermal growth factor (EGF) activated the formation of c-Src/focal adhesion kinase (FAK)-mediated intracellular complex and subsequently induced RhoA-and Rac1-mediated actin remodeling, resulting in EGFR dimerization and endocytosis. In contrast, CD99 agonist facilitated FAK dephosphorylation through the HRAS/ERK/PTPN12 signaling pathway, leading to inhibition of actin cytoskeletal reorganization via inactivation of the RhoA and Rac1 signaling pathways. Moreover, CD99 agonist significantly suppressed tumor growth in a BALB/c mouse model injected with MDA-MB-231 human breast cancer cells. Taken together, these results indicate that CD99-derived agonist ligand inhibits epidermal growth factor (EGF)-induced EGFR dimerization through impairment of cytoskeletal reorganization by PTPN12-dependent c-Src/FAK inactivation, thereby suppressing breast cancer growth.

Keywords: actin cytoskeletal reorganization; breast cancer; CD99 agonist; EGFR dimerization; endocytosis; FAK dephosphorylation; PTPN12; Rac1; RhoA; tripeptide

1. Introduction

Many studies have focused on uncovering the molecular basis of epidermal growth factor receptor (EGFR) activation and its implication in tumor development and progression. EGFR is activated by ligand binding, which induces sequentially their conformational change, auto- and trans-phosphorylation, dimerization, and internalization [1–3]. Structural study demonstrated that EGFR can be multimerized through a specific region of subdomain IV of the extracellular domain [4]. On the other hand, an increasing number of studies have suggested different aspects of EGFR activation. An inactive pre-formed dimer of EGFR without ligand was identified at the cell surface, which undergoes conformational changes during the activation process by stimulated ligand binding [5–7]. In spite of various aspects of the regulation of EGFR activation, dimerization of EGFR is a common feature required for its activation and transmission of downstream signals in tumorigenesis.

Non-receptor type 12 protein tyrosine phosphatase (PTPN12) acts as a core regulator in actin cytoskeleton-mediated modulation of growth factor receptor dynamics [8]. PTPN12 controls Rho GTPase activity by suppressing the interaction of p120 catenin with guanine nucleotide exchange factor VAV2 [9–12]. More recently, it was demonstrated that ephrin receptor (Eph) signaling depends on cytoskeletal reorganization to form polymeric assembly of the receptors and that PTPN12 contrarily downregulates EphA3 activity by inhibiting actin cytoskeletal remodeling. Interestingly, PTPN12 acts as a tumor suppressor which regulates the activities of multiple oncogenic tyrosine kinases, including EGFR, human epidermal growth factor receptor 2 (HER2), and platelet-derived growth factor receptor-β (PDGFRβ), and its deficiency is identified in several carcinomas [13,14]. Loss of PTPN12 promotes in vivo tumor progression of the implanted breast cancer cells, which express a constitutively active form of ErbB2 (CA-ErbB2), and correlates with the impaired feedback regulation of RTKs, thereby resulting in their aberrant activation [15,16]. In this regard, the expression levels of PTPN12 correlate inversely with poor prognosis of hepatocellular carcinoma [17]. Therefore, these results suggest that PTPN12 may play a role in regulation of growth factor receptor dimerization through actin cytoskeleton remodeling.

CD99 is a 32-kDa heavily O-glycosylated type I transmembrane protein [18]. CD99 is expressed on the surface of nearly all normal cell types including thymocytes, peripheral T cells, hematopoietic cells, and also several tumors including Ewing's sarcoma [19,20]. It has been known that CD99 is implicated in various cellular processes including differentiation, apoptosis, homotypic aggregation, and proliferation of lymphocytes, extravasation of leukocytes, transport of several transmembrane proteins, and apoptosis of tumor cells [21–23]. We previously reported that CD99CRIII3, a CD99 agonistic peptide ligand, activated PKA-SHP2-HRAS-ERK1/2 signal transduction pathway, which led to upregulation of PTPN12 expression and interaction with its downstream targets, FAK and PIN1, resulting in dephosphorylation of FAK at Y397 [24]. Consistent with our study, CD99 regulates contact strength and motility of osteosarcoma cells through inhibition of the expression of coiled-coil containing protein kinase 2 (ROCK2), which is a crucial mediator of actin cytoskeleton remodeling [25]. Inhibition of ROCK2 expression leads to a significant decrease in expression and phosphorylation of Ezrin, thereby collapsing the crosslinks between the plasma membrane and cytoskeleton. These results prompted us to hypothesize that CD99 activation can regulate actin cytoskeleton dynamics through the PTPN12/FAK/Rho/Rac axis, thereby suppressing EGFR dimerization and activation.

In this study, we examined the molecular mechanism through which CD99 agonist ligand suppresses ligand-induced dimerization and internalization of EGFR in breast carcinoma cells. Our study suggests that CD99-derived agonist ligands inhibit EGF-induced EGFR dimerization through impairing RhoA-Rac1 signaling-mediated reorganization of the actin cytoskeleton, thereby contributing to the suppression of breast cancer growth.

2. Results

2.1. Epidermal Growth Factor Stimulates Dimerization and Activation of the Epidermal Growth Factor Receptor through c-Src/FAK-Mediated Actin Cytoskeleton Remodeling

Previous studies showed that lovastatin, a statin medication, inhibits EGF-induced EGFR dimerization, activation, and downstream signaling through inhibition of RhoA-mediated actin polymerization and that ligand-induced remodeling of the actin cytoskeleton is required for clustering of transmembrane receptors, thereby resulting in endocytosis and signal transduction [26–28]. We determined whether impairing actin polymerization could disrupt ligand-induced dimerization of receptor tyrosine kinases in two human breast cancer cell lines, low EGFR-expressing MCF-7 and high EGFR-expressing MDA-MB-231. Recombinant human EGF induced EGFR dimerization in a time-dependent manner in MDA-MB-231 cells, but not in actin filament-disrupted cells treated with cytochalasin D (Figure 1A). EGF treatment could induce actin polymerization and stimulate EGFR dimerization and phosphorylation at tyrosine (Y) 1068 residue in a dose-dependent manner (Figure 1B,F and Figure S1A,B,E). In contrast, disruption of actin filaments by cytochalasin D significantly interfered with EGF-induced phosphorylation and dimerization of EGFR. Dose-dependent inhibitory effect of cytochalasin D on EGFR dimerization was confirmed by in situ proximity ligation assay (PLA) (Figure S1B). Furthermore, we confirmed that actin polymerization is critical for not only EGFR/EGFR homo-dimerization but also EGFR/HER2 hetero-dimerization. EGFR/HER2 hetero-dimerization was observed from a very early time point after treatment of MCF-7 cells with EGF and increased in a time-dependent manner, whereas cotreatment with cytochalasin D significantly reduced hetero-dimerization (Figure S1C). These results indicate that actin polymerization is necessarily required for ligand-induced receptor dimerization.

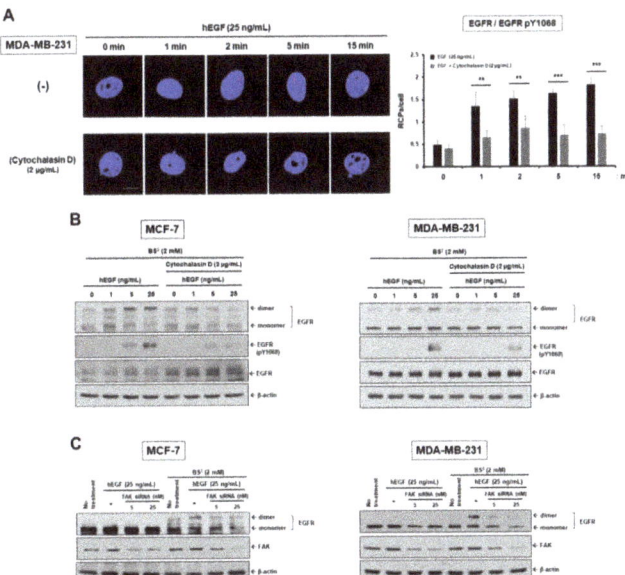

Figure 1. *Cont.*

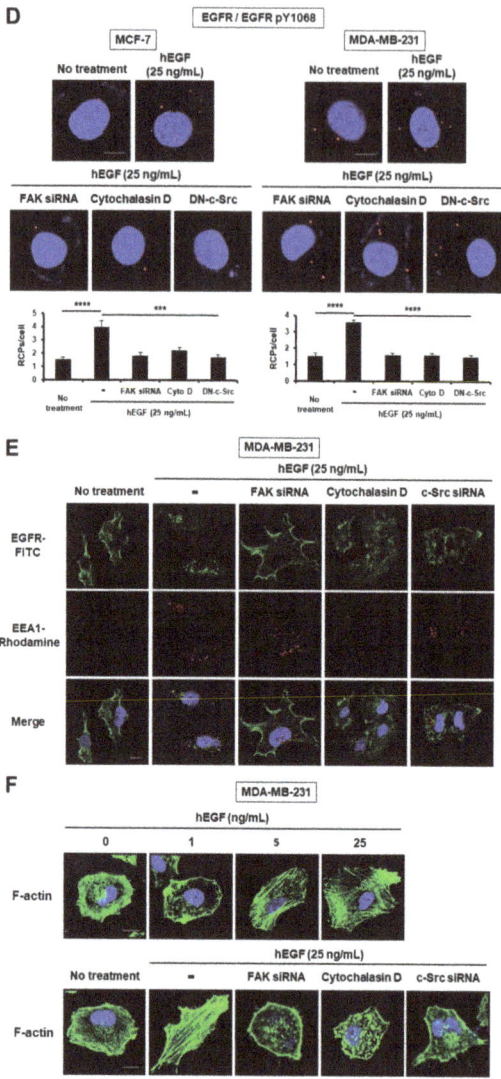

Figure 1. EGF induces EGFR dimerization and endocytosis through c-Src/FAK-mediated cytoskeleton reorganization. (**A,D**) The dimerization level of EGFR was assessed by in situ proximity ligation assay (PLA). (**B,C**) For dimerization assay, human breast carcinoma cells were treated with increasing concentrations of EGF in the presence or absence of cytochalasin D for 1 h on ice, to allow for EGF-induced EGFR dimerization but not endocytosis. Cells were subjected to BS^3 chemical-mediated crosslinking as described in Materials and Methods. To determine the phosphorylation level of EGFR at Y1068, cells were incubated in serum-free medium (SFM) with EGF for 15 min at 37 °C. Cell extracts were assessed by Western blot analysis with the indicated antibodies. β-actin was used as a loading control. ** $p < 0.01$; *** $p < 0.001$; **** $p < 0.0001$. (**E,F**) EGFR endocytosis and actin cytoskeleton organization were determined by immunofluorescent assay (IFA). (**A,D,E,F**) Original magnification of representative images, 600×. Scale bars = 10 μm.

Recruitment and activation of c-Src and FAK have been implicated in cell adhesion and motility by regulating actin cytoskeleton rearrangement and focal adhesion dynamics via activation of RhoA or Rac1/Cdc42 GTPases [29–31]. We determined whether inhibition of FAK function affects EGFR dimerization in the breast carcinoma cells. It was observed that EGF dose-dependently induced FAK phosphorylation at residue Y397 (Figure S1A). FAK knockdown revealed a markedly decreased rate of EGFR dimerization upon EGF binding (Figure 1C). To further investigate the functional relationship between c-Src/FAK-mediated actin rearrangement and EGFR dimerization and endocytosis, we carried out in situ PLA and immunofluorescent assay (IFA) after treatment with FAK small interfering RNA (siRNA), cytochalasin D, and dominant negative c-Src plasmid. Impairing actin polymerization with cytochalasin D or inhibiting c-Src/FAK signaling using dominant negative c-Src (DN-c-Src) or siRNA against FAK or c-Src inhibited EGF-induced EGFR receptor–receptor interaction, endocytosis, as well as actin polymerization (Figure 1D–F and Figure S1D,E). These results suggest that c-Src/FAK-mediated actin cytoskeleton rearrangement plays an important role in ligand-induced EGFR dimerization and activation.

2.2. EGF Induces EGFR Dimerization and Endocytosis through FAK-Mediated RhoA and Rac1 Signaling

Actin cytoskeletal reorganization is regulated by the Rho family of GTPases, including Rho, Rac, and CDC42 [32–35]. We found that although MCF-7 has low expression level of EGFR, EGF treatment dose-dependently stimulates upregulation of the activity of GTPases, Rac1 and RhoA, which is consistent with the results in Figure 1F and Figure S1E showing the pattern of increase in F-actin polymerization (Figure 2A). To determine the role of FAK in activating small GTPase signaling, we transiently transduced constitutively active FAK mutant (CA-FAK), dominant-negative FAK mutant (FAK Y397F) or FAK siRNA. Interaction of FAK with both the GTP-binding proteins and their GTPase activities were upregulated by overexpressing CA-FAK or treating with EGF (Figure 2B,C and Figure S2A). Contrarily, the increased interaction of GTPases with FAK and their upregulated GTPase activities were suppressed by overexpression of kinase-dead FAK Y397 mutant or by knockdown of FAK using siRNA. In addition, knockdown of FAK resulted in inhibition of EGF-induced EGFR endocytosis (Figure 2G). Furthermore, interactions among signaling molecules downstream of GTPases, including Wiskott-Aldrich syndrome protein (WASp) family Verprolin-homologous protein-2 (WAVE2), Actin-related protein-2 (ARP2), ROCK2, and Ezrin, showed patterns similar to those of FAK with RhoA and Rac1 (Figure 2D and Figure S2B). These results show that FAK contributes as a key regulator of RhoA and Rac1, leading to activation of GTPase signaling.

Next, we investigated the effects of activating and inhibiting RhoA and Rac1 GTPases on dimerization and endocytosis of EGFR. Transiently transfected MCF-7 cells expressing CA-Rac1 or CA-RhoA showed significantly enhanced GTPase activity upon EGF treatment (Figure 2E). However, the CA-GTPases influenced neither the dimerization of EGFR nor its endocytosis, even though they induced actin cytoskeleton polymerization (Figure 2F,G, Figure 3F and Figure S2C). On the other hand, DN-Rac1 or DN-RhoA specifically inhibited EGF-stimulated activation of these GTPases (Figure 2E). Contrary to the effect of CA-GTPases, DN-GTPases efficiently suppressed both EGFR dimerization and endocytosis, which were induced by EGF (Figure 2F,G and Figure S2C). We further confirmed the effect of GTPase signaling activity on EGFR dimerization and endocytosis. Consistent with the results in Figure 2E, transfection with DN-Rac1 specifically inhibited the interaction between WAVE2 and ARP2, while transfection with DN-RhoA inhibited only ROCK2–Ezrin interaction, but not WAVE2–ARP2 interaction (Figure 3A). However, EGF-induced dimerization and phosphorylation at Y1068 of EGFR in MDA-MB-231 cells were significantly reduced, even by a single knockdown of ARP2 or Ezrin (Figure 3B). In ARP2 knockdown cells, EGF-induced EGFR endocytosis as well as actin filament branching was significantly inhibited (Figure 3C,D). Knockdown of Ezrin disrupted actin filament polymerization and also suppressed endocytosis of EGFR. In addition, simultaneous knockdown of ARP2 and Ezrin also inhibited actin polymerization. Consistent with the results of DN-GTPases, transfection with CA-Rac1 stimulated the interaction between WAVE2 and ARP2, whereas transfection with CA-RhoA stimulated the interaction of ROCK2 with Ezrin (Figure 3E). Constitutively active forms of Rac1, RhoA, or FAK induced actin filament polymerization in the presence or absence of EGF (Figure 3H). However, although they induced actin filament polymerization as efficiently as EGF, CA-Rac1, CA-RhoA, or CA-FAK failed to stimulate EGFR dimerization and endocytosis without EGF treatment (Figure 3F,G). In addition, EGF binding to EGFR is necessary to initiate the phosphorylation of EGFR, regardless of actin polymerization. These results suggest that GTPase-driven actin polymerization is necessary, but not sufficient for EGFR dimerization and endocytosis.

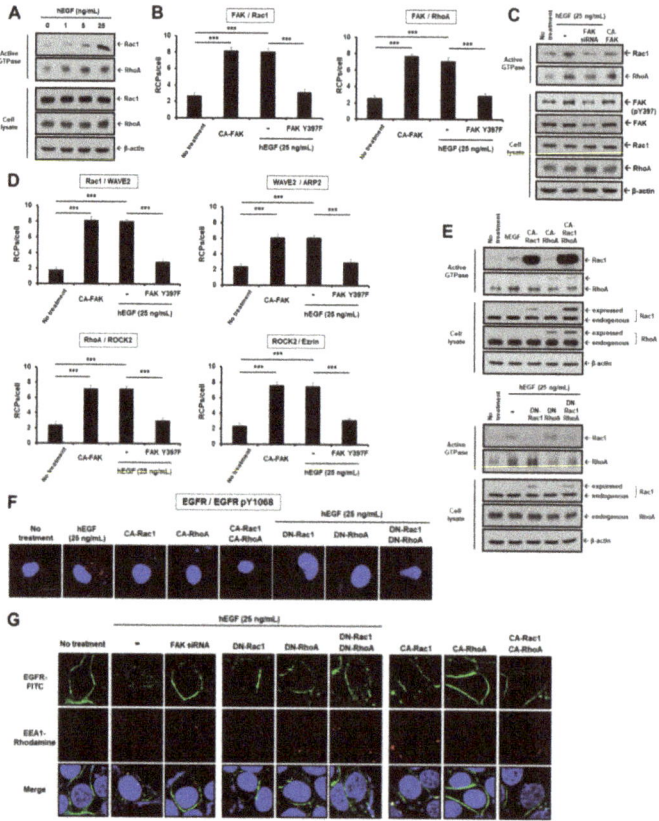

Figure 2. FAK functions as a critical mediator in EGF-induced activation of Rac1 and RhoA GTPases during EGFR signaling. (**A,C**) MCF-7 cells stimulated by binding of ligand to its receptor were analyzed for activation of small GTPases. Activated GTP-bound Rac1 or RhoA in the cell lysates were determined by immunoblotting with anti-Rac1 or anti-RhoA antibodies. β-actin was used as a loading control. (**B,D**) MDA-MB-231 cells were transfected with CA-FAK or FAK Y397F plasmids and incubated in the presence or absence of 25 ng/mL EGF at 37 °C, 5% CO_2 for 15 min. The interactions between the pairs of molecules indicated were assessed by in situ PLA. *** $p < 0.001$. (**E**) Activation of small GTPases in MCF-7 cells was determined by immunoblotting. (**F**) EGFR dimerization in MDA-MB-231 cells was assessed by in situ PLA and the experiments were duplicated. (**G**) EGFR endocytosis in MCF-7 cells was determined by IFA as described above. Original magnification of representative images, 600×. Scale bars = 10 μm.

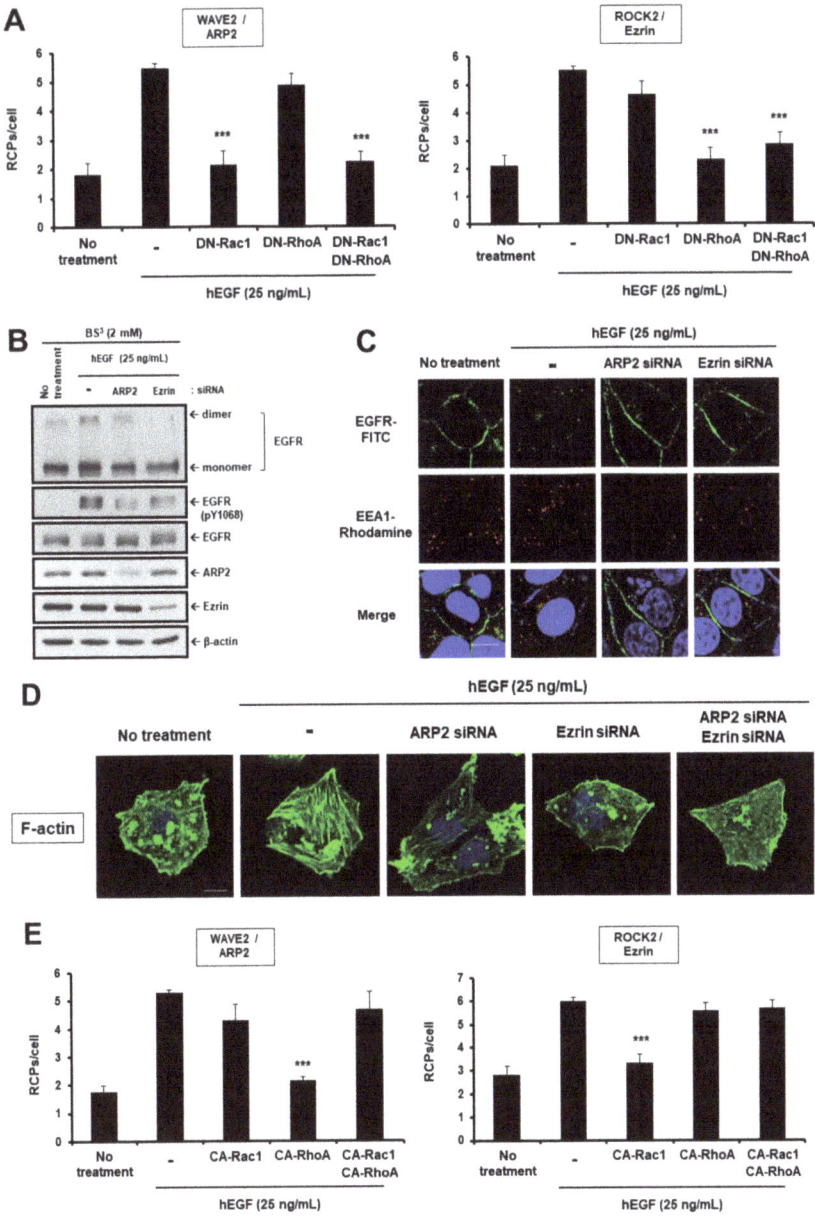

Figure 3. *Cont.*

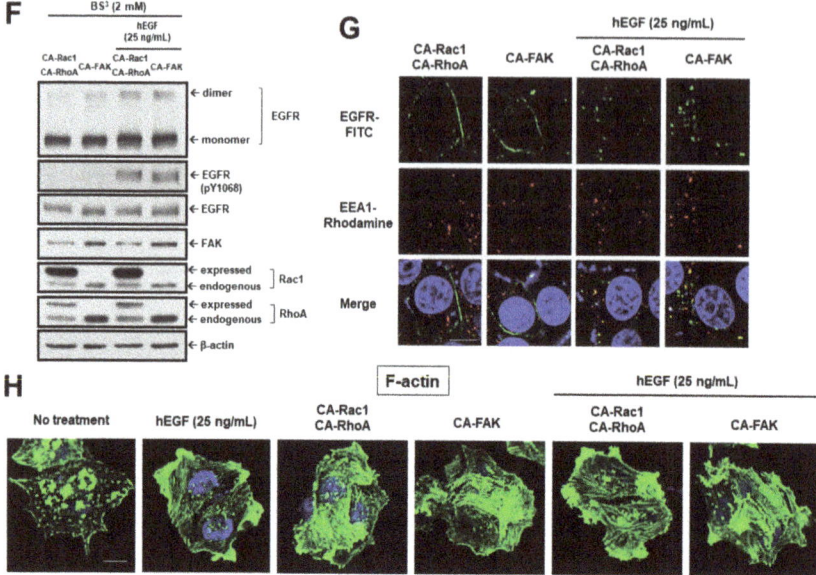

Figure 3. Modulation of actin polymerization by Rac1/RhoA GTPases is essential for EGF-induced dimerization and endocytosis of EGFR. (**A,E**) The changes in the activation of Rac1/RhoA-mediated signaling were observed in MCF-7 cells. The interactions between the pairs of molecules indicated were assessed by in situ PLA. *** $p < 0.001$. (**B,F**) To determine EGFR dimerization, MDA-MB-231 cells were subjected to BS^3 chemical-mediated crosslinking, as described above and in the Materials and Methods. Cell extracts were assessed via Western blotting to determine the dimerization and phosphorylation levels of EGFR and the expression levels of indicated proteins. β-actin was used as a loading control. EGFR endocytosis (**C,G**) and actin cytoskeleton organization (**D,H**) in MCF-7 cells transfected with siRNAs specific for ARP2 and Ezrin or plasmids encoding CA-GTPases or CA-FAK. Original magnification of representative images, 600×. Scale bars = 10 μm.

2.3. CD99 Activation Attenuates EGF-Induced Dimerization and Activation of EGFR via the PKA/SHP2/HRAS/PTPN12/FAK Signaling Pathway

To determine whether CD99 activation can disrupt EGF-induced dimerization and activation of EGFR, two breast cancer cell lines, MDA-MB-231 and MCF-7, were treated with CD99 agonist ligands, CD99CRIII3 or CD99-Fc. We previously demonstrated that CD99CRIII3, a CD99-derived peptide, can function as a CD99 agonist as efficiently as CD99 protein derivatives or anti-CD99 agonist monoclonal antibody [24]. Western blotting and in situ PLA showed that those two CD99 agonists significantly inhibited EGFR dimerization and phosphorylation at Y1068, which were induced by EGF (Figure 4A and Figure S4A). Moreover, neither CD99-Fc nor CD99CRIII3 had any effect on the EGF-induced dimerization and phosphorylation of EGFR at Y1068 in CD99-knockdown cells. EGFR dimerization and phosphorylation at Y1068 were significantly reduced by CD99CRIII3 in a dose-dependent manner (Figure 4B and Figure S4B). CD99CRIII3 inhibited EGF-induced phosphorylation of FAK at Y397. Consistent with this, CD99-Fc and CD99CRIII3 coordinately inhibited EGF-induced interactions of FAK with Rac1 and RhoA in MCF-cells, but not in CD99-knockdown MCF-7 cells (Figure S4C,D). In addition, both molecules suppressed the EGF-induced actin organization in a dose-dependent manner (Figure S4E). These results demonstrate that CD99 agonists inhibited EGF-induced dimerization and activation of EGFR by disrupting FAK-mediated actin organization.

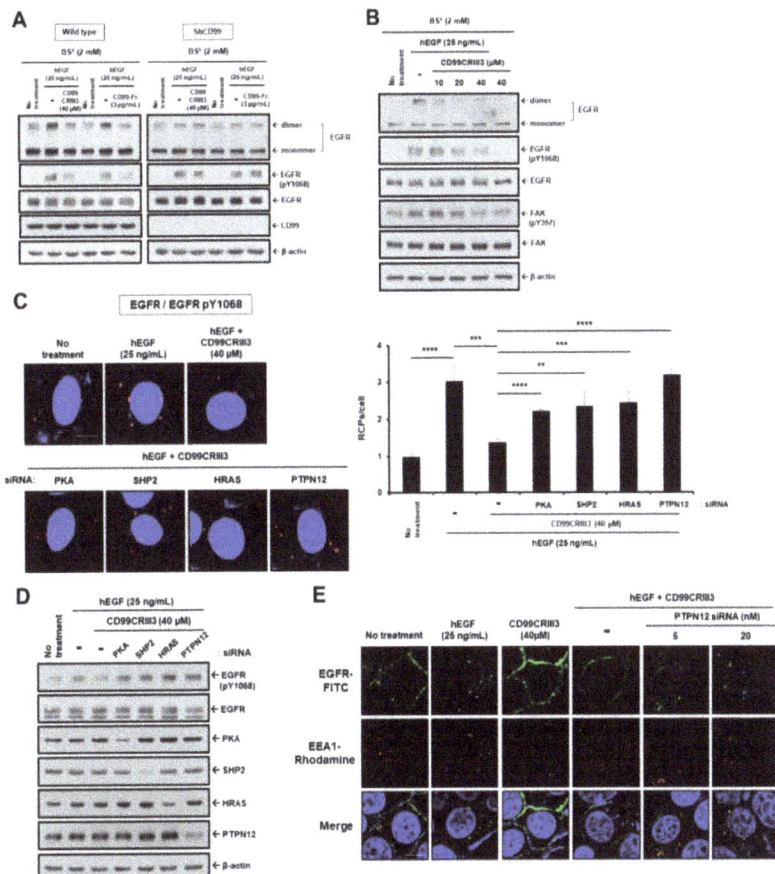

Figure 4. CD99 agonistic ligands inhibit EGFR dimerization and endocytosis via the PKA/SHP2/HRAS/ERK/PTPN12 signaling pathway. (**A,B**) For dimerization assay, wild type or CD99 shRNA stable-expressing MDA-MB-231 cells were treated with CD99CRIII3 or CD99-Fc in the presence of EGF (25 ng/mL) for 1 h on ice. Cells were subjected to BS^3 chemical-mediated crosslinking. Cell extracts were subjected to SDS-PAGE to assess EGFR dimerization and phosphorylation levels of EGFR at Y1068 and FAK at Y397 and the expression levels of indicated proteins. β-actin was used as a loading control. (**C**) In MCF-7 cells, dimerization of EGFR was assessed by in situ PLA. ** $p < 0.01$; *** $p < 0.001$; **** $p < 0.0001$. (**D**) Whole cell lysates extracted from MDA-MB-231 cells treated with EGF with or without CD99CRIII3 were subjected to SDS-PAGE to examine the phosphorylation levels of EGFR and expression levels of each target protein. (**E**) EGFR endocytosis in MCF-7 cells treated with EGF or CD99CRIII3 either alone or combined. (**C,E**) Original magnification of representative images, 600×. Scale bars = 10 μm.

Since our previous results showed that CD99CRIII3 dephosphorylated FAK at Y397 through the PKA/SHP2/HRAS/PTPN12 signaling pathway [24], we next determined whether CD99CRIII3 regulates EGF-induced dimerization and activation of EGFR via the PKA/SHP2/HRAS/PTPN12 signaling pathway. Knockdown of PKA, SHP2, HRAS, or PTPN12 restored EGFR dimerization, which had been inhibited by treatment with CD99CRIII3 (Figure 4C). CD99CRIII3-mediated dephosphorylation of EGFR at Y1068 was also inhibited by knockdown of each of the intracellular signaling molecules (Figure 4D). In particular, knockdown of PTPN12 abrogated the inhibitory effect of CD99CRIII3 on

EGFR endocytosis induced by EGF (Figure 4E). Consistent with our previous results, CD99CRIII3 efficiently inhibited EGF-induced actin rearrangement and EGFR dimerization by dephosphorylating FAK at Y397 via the PKA/SHP2/HRAS/PTPN12 signaling pathway.

To further validate the function of CD99CRIII3 in regulating FAK activity, the cells were treated with a selective FAK inhibitor 14 or transfected with CA-FAK. Inhibition of FAK activity by FAK inhibitor 14 attenuated EGF-induced EGFR dimerization, phosphorylation, and endocytosis by a similar degree to that attenuated by CD99CRIII3 treatment (Figure 5A,B). In contrast, CA-FAK partially recovered the functional activities of EGFR, which had been suppressed by CD99CRIII3, suggesting that persistent activation of FAK partially resists the inhibitory effects of CD99CRIII3 on EGFR dimerization, phosphorylation, and endocytosis. However, CA-FAK alone did not have any effect on dimerization and endocytosis of EGFR. EGFR regulates various cellular signals related to cell growth, proliferation, differentiation, and tumorigenesis [36–38]. As expected, EGF-induced activation of EGFR significantly increased proliferation of MCF-7 cells, whereas CD99CRIII3- or FAK inhibitor 14-induced inhibition of EGFR resulted in a reduced proliferation rate (Figure 5C). The cell proliferation rate, which was suppressed by CD99CRIII3 treatment, was completely restored in both types of cells when transfected with CA-FAK. These results demonstrate that CD99 agonist ligands suppress EGF-induced activation of EGFR through the PKA/SHP2/HRAS/ERK/PTPN12/FAK signaling pathway.

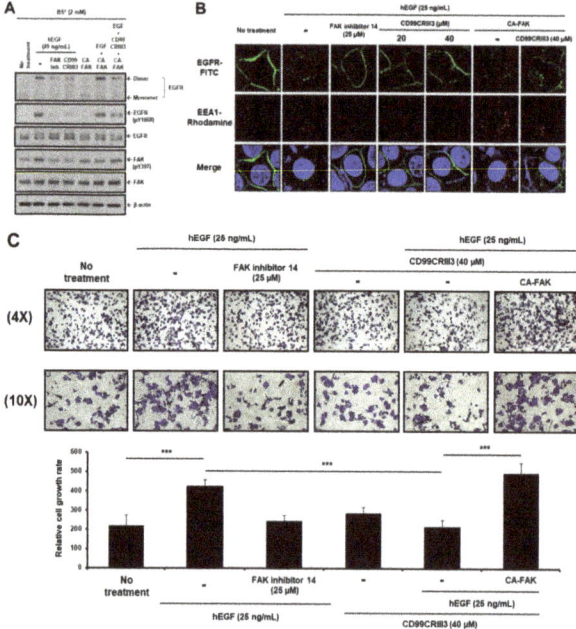

Figure 5. FAK plays an important role in breast cancer cell proliferation induced by EGFR activation. (**A**) MDA-MB-231 cells transfected with CA-FAK plasmid were subjected to BS^3 chemical-mediated crosslinking as described above. Cell extracts were assessed by Western blot analysis to determine the dimerization and phosphorylation levels of EGFR or the expression and phosphorylation levels of FAK. β-actin was used as a loading control. (**B**) EGFR endocytosis in MCF-7 cells was assessed by IFA as described above. Original magnification of representative images, 600×. Scale bars = 10 μm. (**C**) MCF-7 cells were stained with crystal violet. Images were captured using a Nikon Eclipse TE2000-U and the representative images are shown. Lines indicate statistical comparisons, and significant differences between treatments are shown by asterisks as follows: *** $p < 0.001$.

2.4. CD99CRIII3-Activated PTPN12 Regulates the Activation of EGFR Signaling through the PTPN12/FAK/ Rho/Rac Axis

As described above, PTPN12 acts as a negative regulator of multiple RTKs implicated in tumor progression [8,13,15,39]. We hypothesized that PTPN12 may restrain the activation of several cytoplasmic adaptor and kinase proteins that are recruited to EGFR following ligand binding, resulting in attenuation of the activated intracellular signals. Here, using in situ PLA assay, we evaluated the effect of CD99CRIII3-induced PTPN12 on EGFR signaling cascade. Consistent with our hypothesis, EGF treatment facilitated the interactions of EGFR with c-Src, Shc1, Grb2, Gab1, and FAK (Figure 6A). In particular, EGFR showed strongest interaction with c-Src and Shc1 after 5 min of treatment with EGF, whereas the highest degree of interaction between Grb2, Gab1, FAK, and EGFR was observed after 15 min of treatment. Surprisingly, CD99CRIII3 completely attenuated all interactions induced by EGF binding, whereas knockdown of PTPN12 caused a restoration of EGF-induced interactions between EGFR and other intracellular proteins. Consistent with these findings, co-immunoprecipitation revealed that EGF-induced interactions of EGFR with the intracellular molecules were attenuated by co-treating with CD99CRIII3. However, CD99CRIII3 lost its inhibitory effect on EGF-induced EGFR activation by knockdown of PTPN12 (Figure 6B and Figure S5A). To further characterize the kinetics of EGFR-PTPN12 interaction, we evaluated the time-dependent pattern of EGFR-PTPN12 interaction following stimulation with EGF alone or combined stimulation with EGF and CD99CRIII3. PTPN12 was found to co-precipitate with EGFR after treatment with EGF. After 10 min of treatment it showed the highest degree of interaction with EGFR (Figure 6C and Figure S5B). In contrast, the interaction between both molecules in cells treated with EGF plus CD99CRIII3 occurred much earlier than that in cells treated with EGF only and was continued until 10 min after treatment. These results show that PTPN12 activated by CD99CRIII3 plays a critical role in the disruption of the intracellular adapter/kinase complex involved in the EGFR signaling cascade.

It is certain that PTPN12 is involved in regulating cellular motility and morphology, since the phosphatase acts as a central regulator of actin cytoskeleton reorganization [8,9,40]. We performed co-immunoprecipitation to further verify the effects of CD99CRIII3-activated PTPN12 on Rac1/RhoA GTPase signaling pathways. CD99CRIII3 strongly inhibited WAVE2–ARP2 and ROCK2–Ezrin interactions, which were stimulated by EGF treatment in MDA-MB-231 cells (Figure 6D). Contrarily, knockdown of PTPN12 was able to neutralize the effects of CD99CRIII3 and maintain EGF-induced interactions between WAVE2 and ARP2 as well as ROCK2 and Ezrin. Consistent with these observations, while CD99CRIII3 suppressed the EGF-induced activation of Rac1 and RhoA GTPases, its inhibitory effect was neutralized by siRNA-mediated knockdown of PTPN12 in MCF-7 cells (Figure 6E). In addition, transfection with plasmids encoding CA-Rac1, wt-WAVE2, or wt-ARP2 reinstated the Rac1-mediated interaction of WAVE2 with ARP2, which had been inhibited by CD99CRIII3. Similar results were obtained in RhoA-mediated signaling cascade by expression of CA-RhoA, wt-ROCK2, or Ezrin. These results were demonstrated by in situ PLA and immunocytochemical assay for monitoring the localization of each of the Rac1/RhoA GTPase signaling-related proteins and the interactions between them (Figure S6A,B). CD99CRIII3 inhibited colocalization and physical proximity of WAVE2 and ARP2, ROCK2 and Ezrin at the cell membrane region, which were induced by treatment with EGF. Consistent with the above results, knockdown of PTPN12 abrogated the inhibitory effect of CD99CRIII3 on the interactions of actin polymerization-regulating proteins. Moreover, transfection with CA-Rac1 or overexpression of either of WAVE2 or ARP2 maintained the interaction between WAVE2 and ARP2. We also identified similar patterns of results showing RhoA-dependent localization of ROCK2 and Ezrin. Taken together, we found that CD99CRIII3 inhibits EGF-induced dimerization and endocytosis of EGFR, as well as actin polymerization in a PTPN12-dependent manner at a level equivalent to that exhibited by cytochalasin D treatment (Figure 6F–H and Figure S6C). These observations suggest that PTPN12 functions as a key regulator in CD99CRIII3-induced inhibition of EGFR dimerization and endocytosis via suppression of actin polymerization.

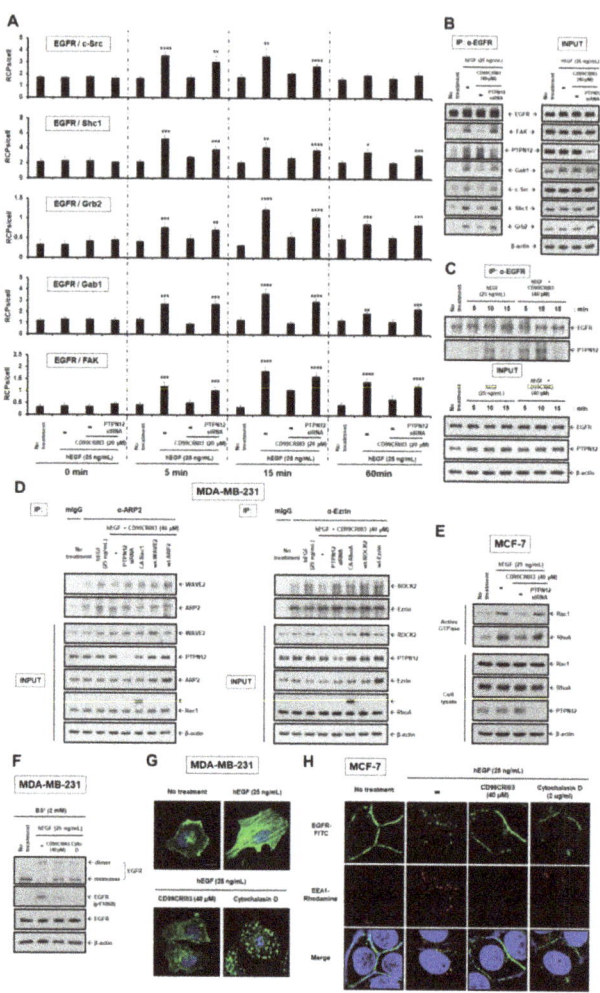

Figure 6. CD99CRIII3 activates PTPN12 to facilitate inhibition of EGFR signaling. (A) In situ PLA performed to assess the interactions between the pairs of molecules indicated in MCF-7 cells. * $p < 0.05$; ** $p < 0.01$; *** $p < 0.001$; **** $p < 0.0001$. (B) MDA-MB-231 cells were transfected with PTPN12 siRNA, followed by treatment with EGF (25 ng/mL) with or without CD99CRIII3 (40 µM) for 15 min. (C) MDA-MB-231 cells were treated with EGF and/or CD99CRIII3 in a time-dependent manner. (D) MDA-MB-231 cells were transiently transfected with PTPN12 siRNA or expression plasmids encoding CA-GTPases or WAVE2, ARP2, ROCK2, and Ezrin. Cell lysates were immunoprecipitated with the antibodies indicated. The immunoprecipitates were analyzed by Western blot with the antibodies indicated. (E) The cells stimulated by binding of ligand to its receptor were assayed for activation of small GTPases. β-actin was used as a loading control. (F) For dimerization assay, MDA-MB-231 cells were subjected to BS^3 chemical-mediated crosslinking as described above. Cell extracts were assessed by Western blot analysis to determine the dimerization and phosphorylation levels of EGFR. β-actin was used as a loading control. Actin cytoskeleton organization in MDA-MB-231 cells (G) and EGFR endocytosis in MCF-7 cells (H) were determined by IFA as described above. Original magnification of representative images, 600×. Scale bars = 10 µm.

2.5. CD99CRIII3 Dose-Dependently Inhibited TNBC Progression In Vivo through PTPN12-Mediated Suppression of Breast Cancer Cell Proliferation

To determine the anti-tumorigenic effect of CD99CRIII3 and the importance of PTPN12 in suppressing tumor progression, we generated a stable MDA-MB-231 cell line (shPTPN12-MDA-MB-231) with 75% reduction in PTPN12 protein using the shRNA system (Figure S7A). shPTPN12-MDA-MB-231 cells exhibited no changes in the expression level of EGFR and CD99. In addition, the dimerization and phosphorylation on Y1068 of EGFR and Y397 of FAK, which had been suppressed by CD99CRIII3 in wt-MDA-MB-231 cells, were not affected in shPTPN12-MDA-MB-231 cells (Figure 7A and Figure S7B). CD99CRIII3 inhibited the proliferation of wt-MDA-MB-231 cells, which was increased by treatment with EGF. Contrarily, the cell proliferation rate, which was enhanced by EGF, was not suppressed by CD99CRIII3 in the PTPN12 knockdown cell line (Figure 7B and Figure S7C). We confirmed the physiological characteristics of shPTPN12-MDA-MB-231 using in situ PLA (Figure S7D). EGF treatment induced the interactions of EGFR with Grb2, c-Src, Shc1, FAK, Gab1, and itself. However, the shPTPN12-MDA-MB-231 cells did not inhibit these interactions by treatment with CD99CRIII3. These results suggest that CD99CRIII3 inhibits EGF-induced EGFR activation via PTPN12-mediated signaling.

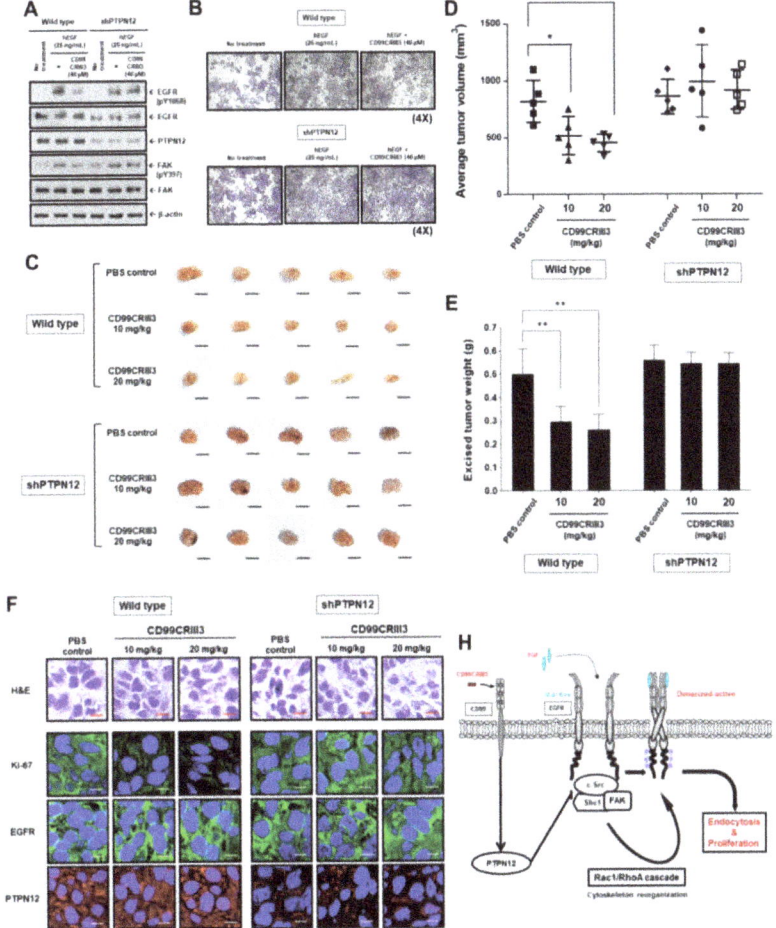

Figure 7. Cont.

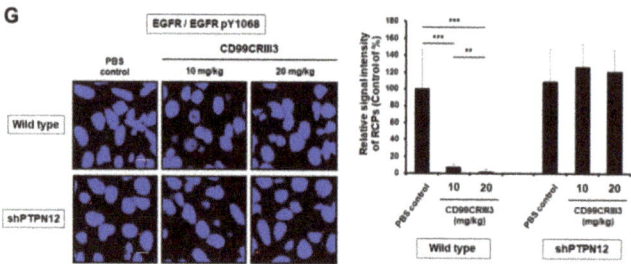

Figure 7. Evaluation of the in vivo efficacy of CD99CRIII3 in the xenograft model of human breast cancer. (**A**) MDA-MB-231 cells were transiently transfected with PTPN12 shRNA plasmid. Cell extracts were assessed by Western blot analysis to determine the phosphorylation levels of EGFR at Y1068 or FAK at Y397. β-actin was used as a loading control. The uncropped Western blots have been shown in Figure S8. (**B**) Comparison of cell growth rate between wt-MDA-MB-231 and shPTPN12-MDA-MB-231 cells. (**C**) Images of tumor xenografts. Scale bar represents 10 mm. (**D,E**) Graph shows the mean difference in tumor volume and weight between wild-type and PTPN12 knockdown cells. Lines indicate statistical comparisons, and significant differences between treatments are shown by asterisks as follows: * $p < 0.05$; ** $p < 0.01$. (**F**) Hematoxylin and Eosin (H&E) staining of tumor xenografts. Scale bar represents 10 μm for 400× magnification. The expression levels of EGFR, PTPN12, and Ki67 by IHC in xenografts. (**G**) In situ PLA analysis was performed to determine the dimerization pattern of EGFR within xenograft tumor tissues. Confocal images were taken from four tumors of each treatment group and displayed in compressed z-stack form. Numerical values are the mean intensities (±SD) of red spots in three randomly selected fields per tumor section. Significant differences between treatments are shown by asterisks as follows: ** $p < 0.01$; *** $p < 0.001$. Scale bar, 10 μm (600×). wt, wild type; sh, short hairpin. (**H**) Schematic model for the inhibitory effect of CD99 agonistic ligand on EGF-induced activation of EGFR.

Finally, we carried out a tumor xenograft assay in the BALB/c nude mouse model with wt- and shPTPN12-MDA-MB-231 human breast carcinoma cells. The daily injection of CD99CRIII3 led to significantly decreased tumor volume and weight in the wt-MDA-MB-231-inoculated mice, compared with PBS-treated mice (Figure 7C–E). However, there were no differences in tumor size and weight in the CD99CRIII3-treated mice injected with shPTPN12-MDA-MB-231 cells, indicating that CD99CRIII3 exerts its anti-tumorigenic activity via the CD99–PTPN12 axis. After 15 days of CD99CRIII3 administration, tumors were collected and sliced into small pieces. Serial sections of the tumor specimens were stained with hematoxylin and eosin (H&E) and antibodies to measure the expression of Ki67, EGFR, and PTPN12 (Figure 7F). Histological analysis of the specimens revealed that CD99CRIII3 led to reduced Ki-67 expression in a group of wt-MDA-MB-231-inoculated mice, but not in the shPTPN12-MDA-MB-231-inoculated mice group. The majority of tumor mass was identified to be positive for EGFR and Ki-67. The number of Ki-67-positive cells was reduced in the CD99CRIII3-treated mice, showing correlation with the reduced tumor size (Figure S7E). In addition, CD99CRIII3 dose-dependently inhibited EGFR dimerization only in wt-MDA-MB-231-originated tumor tissues (Figure 7G). These results indicate that CD99 agonist ligand could significantly suppress the proliferation of MDA-MB-231 human breast cancer cells through PTPN12-mediated inactivation of EGFR.

3. Discussion

In this study, we clearly showed that actin polymerization plays an important role in EGFR receptor dimerization and activation, which was inhibited by the CD99/PTPN12/FAK/Rho/Rac axis. Our novel findings provide an insight into the role of CD99 in the inactivation of several oncogenic tyrosine kinases including EGFR [13,14].

As the actin cytoskeleton plays an important role in controlling the movement of intracellular organelles as well as cell surface receptors [41–43], we elucidated the importance of cytoskeleton reorganization in ligand-induced dimerization and subsequent activation of EGFR. EGFR directly associates with the actin filament via its C-terminal actin-binding domain [44,45]. We found that impairment of actin cytoskeleton organization by cytochalasin D inhibits the phosphorylation, dimerization, and internalization of EGFR, consistent with previous results showing that disruption of actin polymerization inhibits ligand-induced EGFR dimerization, activation, and downstream signaling [26,28]. Besides the role for EGFR dimerization, the blocking of F-actin polymerization inhibits the CXCL12-mediated dimerization of CXCR4 [46]. The actin cytoskeleton intimately interacts with plasma membrane integral proteins and regulates intricate membrane events, such as the formation of focal adhesions as well as the internalization, recycling, compartmentalization, dynamics, clustering, and diffusion of membrane receptor proteins [27,41,47]. The assembly and disassembly of cytoskeletal actin filaments (F-actin) are regulated by c-Src and FAK [31,48,49]. Functional impairment of c-Src or FAK inhibited actin polymerization, leading to the suppression of dimerization and internalization of EGFR. In contrast, transduction with CA-FAK facilitated the FAK-mediated activation of Rac1/RhoA signaling pathways and actin polymerization. Importantly, it looks like dimerization of EGFR is not sufficient to activate its kinase activity. Although CA-FAK could induce the formation of actin filaments without EGF ligand, it failed to proceed to the next step, EGFR dimerization and endocytosis. CA-Rac1 and CA-RhoA also showed similar results. The binding of growth factor ligands to EGFR may be critical for conformational changes of the receptor or its dynamics, leading to dimerization or oligomerization of EGFR and subsequent activation of the downstream signaling pathway. In other words, EGFR activation may require both ligand binding to EGFR and subsequent dimerization. Therefore, disruption of ligand-induced EGFR dimerization as well as ligand binding would be a promising therapeutic strategy for the treatment of breast cancer patients with aberrant expression or activation of EGFR.

Breast cancer can be classified into several subtypes according to the expression level of various surface marker proteins, including estrogen receptor (ER), progesterone (PR), and HER2. On the other hand, EGFR is expressed in a wide range of breast cancer cell lines at different levels. EGFR has long been in spotlight as a reasonable target molecule for developing antitumor strategies, since its aberrant activation by increased expression of a constitutively activated truncated variant EGFRvIII or itself is implicated in the development and progression of a broad range of solid cancer diseases including breast cancer [50]. We adopted two breast cancer cell lines, MDA-MB-231 and MCF-7. MDA-MB-231 cells lack the expression of ER, PR, and HER2, while they show high expression of multiple RTKs. On the other hand, adenocarcinoma MCF-7 cells express ER, PR, and glucocorticoid receptors. We found that MDA-MB-231 cells express EGFR at high levels, whereas MCF-7 cells express very low levels of this receptor. The expression levels of CD99, in contrast, are similar in both cell lines. Despite different levels of EGFR expression, these two breast carcinomas were similarly affected by EGFR ligands and CD99 agonists. These results suggest that EGFR might play a dominant role in cellular and physiological systems of breast cancer cells, so that it can be a valuable target for the development of a broadly applicable anti-cancer drug.

PTPN12 is a tumor suppressor which regulates cellular transformation from normal to malignant cells via the inhibition of multiple oncogenic tyrosine kinases [13,14]. Consistent with this, our data showed that stable knockdown of PTPN12 increased tumor progression in vivo. Although several studies imply the functional significance of PTPN12 in controlling tumor progression, the activator of PTPN12 has not been identified yet. One novel finding of this study is that the CD99–PTPN12 axis participates in the regulation of ligand-induced activation of EGFR by suppressing the reorganization of the actin cytoskeleton. This observation is consistent with a previous study, which demonstrated that PTPN12 controls EphA3 activation by regulating actin cytoskeletal organization during Eph clustering [8]. Furthermore, we previously reported the molecular mechanism by which CD99 induces β1 integrin inactivation via PTPN12 activation [24]. Likewise, CD99CRIII3 showed significant inhibitory effects on EGF-induced EGFR dimerization and internalization via activation of PTPN12. When EGFR is activated with its ligand, PTPN12 is recruited to the activated EGFR to return to an inactive state within 15 min [39]. On the other hand, CD99CRIII3 induced very early recruitment of PTPN12 to the EGF-induced EGFR signaling complex, which led to the inhibition of EGFR dimerization and activation. The remarkable inhibitory effect of CD99CRIII3 on EGFR activation was suppressed when CD99 or PTPN12 expression was downregulated, indicating that CD99 activation by CD99CRIII3 stimulated PTPN12 to inhibit the early stage of the EGFR signaling pathway.

PTPN12 exhibited relatively low expression levels in triple-negative breast cancer (TNBC) cells [13]. However, ectopic restoration of PTPN12 in TNBC resulted in the suppression of anchorage-independent proliferation and metastatic ability. Consistent with this finding, we observed that CD99CRIII3 significantly suppressed the EGF-induced proliferation of MDA-MB-231 and MCF-7 breast cancer cells, which was not observed in PTPN12-knockdown cells. Furthermore, shPTPN12-MDA-MB-231 cells allowed us to examine whether CD99CRIII3 affects in vivo tumorigenesis via the PTPN12-dependent negative feedback loop. CD99CRIII3 dose-dependently suppressed the growth of MDA-MB-231 human breast cancer cells implanted in nude mice, while it failed to suppress the growth of shPTPN12-MDA-MB-231 cells implanted in nude mice, suggesting that PTPN12 serves as a key executor of the CD99 signaling pathway. Consistently, CD99CRIII3 inhibited EGFR dimerization in wt-MDA-MB-231-originated tumor tissues, but not in shPTPN12-MDA-MB-231-originated tumor tissues. Here we pay attention to recent reports showing that CD99 activates p53 tumor suppressor by inducing degradation of Mdm2, an E3 ubiquitin ligase, resulting in the death of Ewing sarcoma (EWS) [20,51]. Collectively, these results suggest that CD99 might play a key role in modulating the activities of intracellular tumor suppressors, PTPN12 and p53, whose interrelationship still remains elusive.

The growth of various tumors is promoted by tumorigenic growth factor receptors, such as FGFR, TGF-βR, IGF-1R, InsR, and PDGF [52–56]. Given that their kinase activity is induced via dimerization and activation according to ligand binding, and actin cytoskeleton is implicated in controlling receptor compartmentalization [27,57,58], it is important to determine whether CD99CRIII3 can regulate the activity of those RTKs. Additionally, protein tyrosine phosphatases (PTPs) act as inhibitors, regulating tumor-inducing activity [53]. Thus, our results suggest that PTPN12 activated by CD99CRIII3 may suppress the activity of other abnormal RTKs as well as EGFR and that their dimerization and activation processes are regulated by actin cytoskeleton-controlled clustering. However, the underlying mechanism by which CD99CRIII3 inhibits the dimerization and activation of other tumorigenic RTKs needs further investigation in a broad range of tumors.

4. Materials and Methods

4.1. Reagents and Antibodies

All cultureware and reagents were purchased from Invitrogen (Carlsbad, CA, USA). Immun-Blot polyvinylidene fluoride (PVDF) membranes for protein blotting were purchased from Bio-Rad Laboratories (Hercules, CA, USA). The WEST-ZOL plus Western blot detection kit was obtained from iNtRON Biotechnology, Inc. (Seongnam, Korea). Lipofectamine LTX/PLUS and RNAiMAX reagents were purchased from Invitrogen (Life Technologies, Grand Island, NY, USA). Protein A/G agarose beads were purchased from Santa Cruz Biotechnology, Inc. (Santa Cruz, CA, USA). Cytochalasin D, FAK inhibitor 14, recombinant human epidermal growth factor (EGF), FITC (Fluorescein isothiocyanate)-conjugated Phalloidin (1:200 for IFA), and purified mouse IgG (1:200 for IFA) were purchased from Sigma-Aldrich Co. (St. Louis, MO, USA). Rhodamine-conjugated anti-mouse IgG antibody, rhodamine-conjugated anti-rabbit IgG antibody, FITC-conjugated anti-mouse IgG antibody, FITC-conjugated anti-rabbit IgG antibody (1:200 for IFA), and Horseradish peroxidase (HRP)-conjugated anti-mouse IgG antibody (1:10,000 for Western blot) were purchased from DiNonA (Seoul, Korea). HRP-conjugated goat anti-rabbit IgG antibody (1:10,000 for Western blot) was purchased from Chemicon (Temecula, CA, USA). Mouse monoclonal anti-human epidermal growth factor receptor (EGFR) antibody (1:150 for IFA), rabbit polyclonal anti-human EGFR antibody (1:150 for IFA), and rabbit polyclonal or mouse monoclonal anti-EEA1 antibody (1:150 for IFA) were purchased from Abcam (Cambridge, UK). Antibodies against HRAS, SHP2, PKA, Ezrin, WAVE2, Arp2, ROCK2, Grb2, Shc1, Rac1, RhoA, EGFR, β-actin, and HRP-conjugated donkey anti-goat IgG antibody (1:10,000 for Western blot) were obtained from Santa Cruz Biotechnology, Inc. (Santa Cruz, CA, USA). Antibodies against phospho-FAK (Tyr397), FAK, phospho-EGFR (Tyr1068), PTPN12, c-Src, HER2, and Gab1 were purchased from Cell Signaling Technology (Danvers, MA, USA).

4.2. Cell Culture

Human breast adenocarcinoma cell line MCF-7 was obtained from American Type Culture Collection (ATCC). Triple-negative breast carcinoma cell line MDA-MB-231 was kindly provided by Dr. Hyung Geun Song (DiNonA Inc., Seoul, Korea). MCF-7 cells were cultured in Dulbecco's modified Eagle's medium (DMEM) containing 10% (*v/v*) fetal bovine serum (FBS), 100 unit/mL penicillin, and 100 μg/mL streptomycin (Gibco-BRL, Grand Island, NY, USA). MDA-MB-231 cells were cultured in Roswell Park memorial Institute (RPMI) 1640 (10% FBS, 100 unit/mL penicillin, 100 μg/mL streptomycin, and 25 mM HEPES). All cells were maintained at 37 °C in a humidified 5% CO_2 incubator.

4.3. Synthesis of Polypeptides

CD99 agonist polypeptide CD99CRIII3 was synthesized using an automatic peptide synthesizer (PeptrEx-R48, Peptron, Daejeon, Korea) according to the 9-fluorenylmethoxycarbonyl (Fmoc) solid-phase method. The synthesized polypeptides were purified and analyzed using reverse-phase high-performance liquid chromatography (Prominence LC-20AB, Shimadzu, Japan) equipped with a C18 analytical RP column (Capcell Pak column, Shiseido Co., Ltd., Japan). The mass was analyzed using a mass spectrometer (HP1100 Series LC/MSD, Hewlett-Packard, Roseville, CA, USA). The analytical results are described in Figure S3.

4.4. Plasmids and RNA Interference

The coding sequences of human WAVE2 and Arp2 were obtained by PCR with respective pairs of primers. Sense primer 5′-GGGGTACCGCCACCATGCCGTTAGTAACGAGGAAC-3′ and antisense primer 5′-GCTCTAGAGAGTTAATCGGACCAGTCGTC-3′ for the cDNA of WAVE2, sense primer 5′-GGGGTACCGCCACCATGGACAGCCAGGGCAGG-3′ and antisense primer 5′-GCTCTAGATTATCGAACAGTCACACCAAG-3′ for the cDNA of Arp2. Full length human WAVE2 and Arp2 cDNAs were subcloned into KpnI and XbaI sites of the pcDNA3 vector. The sequences of the constructs were confirmed by DNA sequencing. The expression vectors pEXV/constitutively active Rac1, pEXV/dominant negative Rac1, pEXV/constitutively active RhoA, pEXV/dominant negative RhoA, and pcDNA3.1/dominant negative c-Src were kindly donated by Dr. Hansoo Lee. The expression vector kinase-dead, non-phosphorylatable dominant negative FAK Y397F (pcDNA3/FAK Y397F) was kindly provided by Dr. Soo-Chul Park (Sookmyung Women's University, Seoul, S. Korea). Constitutively active FAK plasmid (pCDM8/CD2-FAK) was kindly provided by Dr. Andrey V. Cybulsky (McGill University, Montreal, QC, Canada). The pCS2/ROCK2 vector was kindly provided by Dr. Anming Meng (Tsinghua University, Beijing, China). The pCB6/rsr-G-Tag/Ezrin vector was kindly provided by Dr. Janet Allopenna (Stony Brook Medicine, NY, USA). For gene knockdown experiments, the small interfering RNAs (siRNAs) against FAK, Shc1, c-Src, Arp2, Ezrin, PKA-α, SHP2, HRAS, PTPN12, and shRNA targeting PTPN12 were purchased from Santa Cruz Biotechnology, Inc. (Santa Cruz, CA, USA). Plasmids or siRNA duplexes were transfected into cells using Lipofectamine LTX/PLUS or RNAiMAX (Invitrogen Life Technologies, Grand Island, NY, USA). The PTPN12 knockdown MDA-MB-231 resistant clone was established by selecting with 0.4 mg/mL puromycin. After transfection, knockdown of each of the target molecules or expression of dominant negative or constitutively active DNA was confirmed by Western blotting.

4.5. In Situ Proximity Ligation Assay (PLA)

The in situ PLA analysis was performed using Duolink® in situ reagents (O-LINK® Bioscience, Uppsala, Sweden) according to the manufacturer's instructions. Cells were transfected with plasmids or siRNAs and then seeded on glass coverslips in 24-well cell culture plates (1×10^5 cells/well). After 24 h growth under standard conditions, cells were treated with EGF (25 ng/mL) in the presence or absence of peptides and each reagent for 15 min in a CO_2 incubator at 37 °C, and then washed twice with 1X PBS. Cells were fixed with 2% formaldehyde in PBS for 10 min at room temperature (RT), and subsequently washed twice with 1X PBS, permeabilized with 0.1% Triton X-100 in PBS, and then washed twice with wash buffer A. Cells were incubated with blocking solution at 37 °C for 30 min, and then washed twice with wash buffer A. Cells were stained with specific antibodies (1:100 for in situ PLA) as indicated. Protein–protein interactions were analyzed using a confocal laser scanning microscope Olympus FluoView FV1000 (Olympus, Tokyo, Japan). PLA signals in cell populations ($n = 4$) were quantified by NIS-Elements analysis, and four or two independent experiments were performed. The average number of rolling-circle products (RCPs) per cell ± standard error is shown.

4.6. Dimerization Assay

BS^3 [bis(sulfosuccinimidyl) suberate] was obtained from Thermo Scientific (Waltham, MA, USA) and used according to the manufacturer's instruction and reference [59]. Cells were serum-starved in DMEM or RPMI containing 0.1% bovine serum albumin (BSA) and incubated in serum-free medium supplemented with human EGF in the presence or absence of CD99CRIII3 for 1 h at 4 °C (incubation on ice during ligand stimulation allows for ligand-induced receptor dimerization but inhibits receptor endocytosis). Cells were washed three times with ice-cold 1X Ca^{2+}-, Mg^{2+}-free PBS, then incubated with BS^3 (2 mM) at 4 °C for 30 min and an additional 20 min at RT, followed by quenching with 1M of Tris (pH 7.5). Cells were lysed with 1% NP40 buffer containing 10 mM of β-mercaptoethanol. Cell lysates were subjected to SDS-PAGE and analyzed by Western blotting.

4.7. Active GTPase Detection

Active GTPase assay was performed using an active Rac1 or RhoA detection kit (Cell Signaling Technology, Danvers, MA, USA) according to the manufacturer's instructions. Cells were rinsed with 1× ice-cold PBS, then lysed with 1× lysis/binding/wash buffer plus 1 mM PMSF. Whole cell lysate was harvested and incubated on ice for 5 min, and then centrifuged at $16,000 \times g$ at 4 °C for 15 min. The clear supernatant was transferred to a new tube and subjected to active GTPase assay. Glutathione resin slurry (50%, 100 µL) was added to a spin cup with a collection tube and the tube was centrifuged at $6000 \times g$ for 1 min. After washing the resin with 400 µL of 1× lysis/binding/wash buffer, 20 µg of GST-PAK1-p21 binding domain (PBD) (for GTP-bound Rac1) or GST-Rhotekin-Rho binding domain (RBD) (for GTP-bound RhoA) was added to the spin cup containing glutathione resin. The cell lysate was immediately transferred to the spin cup and vortexed. The reaction mixture was incubated at 4 °C for 1 h with gentle rocking. The active GTPase-bound GST resin was washed with 1X lysis/binding/wash buffer containing 1 mM PMSF. GTP-bound Rac1 or RhoA was eluted with 2X SDS reducing buffer containing 200 mM 1,4-dithiothreitol (DTT), followed by Western blotting with mouse anti-Rac1 mAb or rabbit anti-RhoA pAb.

4.8. Western Blot Analysis and Immunoprecipitation

Western blotting and immunoprecipitation were carried out as described previously [24]. Serum-starved breast carcinoma cells were treated with the appropriate reagents for 15 min at 37 °C, 5% CO_2. Cells were harvested and lysed with 1% NP40 lysis buffer (1% Nonidet P40, 150 mM NaCl, 50 mM Tris-HCl (pH 8.0), 5 mM EDTA) containing 10 mM phenylmethylsulfonyl fluoride, 1 µg/mL pepstatin A, 10 µg/mL leupeptin, 1 µg/mL aprotinin, and 1 mM sodium orthovanadate. Cell extracts were subjected to SDS-PAGE and subsequently transferred to PVDF membranes. Immunoblotting was carried out with the indicated antibodies (1:1000 for Western blot) to detect the target proteins.

For immunoprecipitation, cells were treated for the indicated time with each set of reagents at 37 °C, 5% CO_2. Cells were harvested and lysed with PRO-PREP^{TM} protein extraction solution (iNtRON Biotechnology, Inc., Seongnam, Korea). After centrifugation at 13,000 rpm and 4 °C for 15 min, supernatants were collected, and then incubated overnight with the appropriate antibodies at 4 °C on a nutator. The immunoprecipitates were incubated with Protein A/G PLUS-Agarose (Santa Cruz Biotechnology, Inc., Santa Cruz, CA, USA) beads for 3 h at 4 °C on a rotator and washed with PRO-PREP^{TM} solution. The precipitates were eluted with 1× sample buffer (50 mM Tris-HCl (pH 6.8), 100 mM DTT, 2% SDS, 0.1% bromophenol blue, and 10% glycerol). Western blot analysis was carried out with the indicated antibodies to detect the target proteins.

4.9. Immunofluorescence Assay (IFA)

The EGFR distribution, cytoskeletal organization, and localization of the related proteins were detected by immunofluorescence assay. To determine the changes in RTK distribution, cytoskeletal organization, and localization of the related proteins, cells were seeded on round-shaped glass coverslips as described above. The following day, cells were treated with the appropriate reagents, then washed with ice-cold PBS and fixed with 4% paraformaldehyde (PFA) in 1× PBS for 10 min at RT. Subsequently, cells were washed twice with PBS, permeabilized for 5 min with 0.1% Triton X-100 in PBS. After washing with PBS, the cells were incubated with appropriate primary and secondary antibodies to detect the target proteins. Alternatively, cells were stained with 0.2 µM of FITC-conjugated phalloidin to detect the fibrous actin filaments. The stained cells were mounted onto slides with an aqueous mounting medium. Fluorescence images were acquired using a confocal microscope Olympus FluoView FV1000 (Olympus, Tokyo, Japan).

4.10. Proliferation Assay

Cell proliferation was assessed by the Cell Counting Kit-8 (CCK-8) assay or crystal violet staining method. Wild-type or CA-FAK-transfected cells were seeded at a density of 5×10^3 cells per well in 96-well culture plates. After 24 h incubation, cells were treated with EGF (25 ng/mL) in the presence or absence of CD99CRIII3 (40 µM) or FAK inhibitor (25 µM) in 100 µL of serum-free medium (SFM) for 24 h, 48 h, and 72 h. At the indicated time points, cell proliferation was assessed using Cell Counting Kit-8 (CCK8, Dojindo Molecular Technologies, Inc., Rockville, MD, USA)-based assay or crystal violet staining method. CCK-8 colorimetric reactions were assessed by measuring the absorbance at 450 nm using a microplate reader (Versa Max, NY, USA). The images of crystal violet-stained cells were captured with a Nikon Eclipse TE2000-U (Nikon Instruments Inc., Melville, NY, USA).

4.11. Tumor Xenograft and Immunohistochemistry (IHC)

All animal experiments were performed in accordance with the Institutional Guidelines of the Animal Care and Use Committees (IACUC) of Kangwon National University. This research has been approved by IACUC of Kangwon National University on 26 October 2016 (KW-161020-1). MDA-MB-231 cells were cultured in complete Roswell Park Memorial Institute (RPMI) 1640 (10% FBS, 25 mM HEPES, 100 units/mL penicillin, and 100 µg/mL streptomycin) medium. Wild-type or PTPN12 shRNA-transfected MDA-MB-231 cells (5×10^6 cells in 50 µL SFM/mouse) were mixed 1:1 (v/v) with Matrigel and subcutaneously injected into the right flanks of 6-week-old female BALB/c nude mice. One week after tumor cell inoculation, mice were divided into three groups of five mice each when the tumor size exceeded 5 mm in diameter (10 mg/kg or 20 mg/kg of body weight of CD99CRIII3 and PBS control). CD99CRIII3 was intraperitoneally administered to mice every day for 14 days. The tumor size was measured using a caliper every other day for 15 days. After 21 days of tumor cell inoculation, mice were sacrificed and the tumor masses were removed and weighed. After measuring the volume and weight, four tumor masses from each treatment group were paraffinized, sectioned with a microtome and stained with hematoxylin and eosin (H&E) following internal procedures. The effect of CD99CRIII3 on EGFR dimerization in tumor xenograft was assessed by in situ PLA assay according to the manufacturer's instructions. Tumor sections were stained with anti-human EGFR and anti-phospho-EGFR (Tyr1068) antibodies. The z-stacks were generated from images taken at 0.2–0.4 μm intervals. Z-stack images were collected from three randomly selected fields per tumor. EGFR–EGFR interaction was quantified and analyzed by mean red intensity of automated measurements. Six tumors, one of each treatment, were frozen using liquid nitrogen, subjected to cryosectioning and stained with primary antibodies specific for EGFR, PTPN12, and ki67, followed by incubation with respective fluorescent secondary antibodies. Fluorescence images were analyzed using a confocal laser scanning microscope Olympus FluoView FV1000 and H&E staining images were captured using an Olympus BX50 microscope (Olympus, Tokyo, Japan).

4.12. Statistical Analysis

Values are given as mean ± standard deviation (SD). Statistical significance was determined by the Student's *t*-test using the statistical analysis software GraphPad Prism (version 8.0; San Diego, CA, USA) and $p < 0.05$ was considered statistically significant. All experiments were conducted twice or more to minimize experimental error. The representative data are shown in the figures.

5. Conclusions

We demonstrated that CD99 activation regulates actin cytoskeleton dynamics through PTPN12/FAK/Rho/Rac axis, thereby suppressing EGFR activation and relevant tumor growth. We propose a schematic model illustrating the possible mechanism for the CD99 agonist ligand-induced suppression of EGFR activation (Figure 7H). CD99 acts as an upstream regulator of the PTPN12-mediated negative feedback loop for regulating ligand-induced dimerization or oligomerization of plasma membrane protein kinases, which are involved in tumor development and progression. Taken together, we propose that CD99 agonist ligands have potential as novel therapeutic drug candidates to suppress human breast carcinoma via inhibition of EGF-mediated EGFR signaling.

Supplementary Materials: The following are available online at http://www.mdpi.com/2072-6694/12/10/2895/s1, Figure S1: c-Src/FAK plays an important role in actin cytoskeleton reorganization, resulting in EGFR dimerization and internalization, Figure S2: Binding of ligand to its receptor is essential to induce Rac1/RhoA-mediated EGFR dimerization, Figure S3: HPLC/MS chromatogram of CD99-derived agonistic peptide (CD99CRIII3), Figure S4: Functional validation of the equivalence of CD99 agonist ligands, Figure S5: PTPN12 plays a critical role in the dissociation of the EGFR-associated signaling complex induced by CD99CRIII3, Figure S6: CD99CRIII3 suppresses EGF-induced Rac1/RhoA GTPase signaling cascades via PTPN12, Figure S7: The physiological characteristics of shPTPN12-MDA-MB-231 cells, Figure S8: Uncropped western blot figures.

Author Contributions: J.-H.H. and K.-J.L. proposed the concept, conceived the entire study, and wrote the paper; K.-J.L., Y.K., M.S.K., B.C., and H.-M.J. performed most of the experiments; H.L., D.J., D.K., K.-W.M., J.C., and J.I.Y. provided discussion and advice. All authors have read and agreed to the published version of the manuscript.

Funding: This work was supported by the Basic science Research Program through the National Research Foundation of Korea (NRF) funded by the Ministry of Education (2018R1D1A3B07043170) and by the 2017 Research Grant from Kangwon National University (No. 520170543).

Acknowledgments: We highly appreciate Andrey V. Cybulsky (Department of Medicine, McGill University, Montreal, Canada) for providing pCDM8/CD2-FAK plasmid; Hyung Geun Song (DiNonA Inc., Seoul, S. Korea) for the triple-negative breast cancer MDA-MB-231 cell line.

Conflicts of Interest: The authors declare no conflict of interest.

References

1. Freed, D.M.; Alvarado, D.; Lemmon, M.A. Ligand regulation of a constitutively dimeric EGF receptor. *Nat. Commun* **2015**, *6*, 7380. [CrossRef] [PubMed]
2. Wang, Q.; Villeneuve, G.; Wang, Z. Control of epidermal growth factor receptor endocytosis by receptor dimerization, rather than receptor kinase activation. *EMBO Rep.* **2005**, *6*, 942–948. [CrossRef] [PubMed]

3. Schlessinger, J. Ligand-induced, receptor-mediated dimerization and activation of EGF receptor. *Cell* **2002**, *110*, 669–672. [CrossRef]
4. Huang, Y.; Bharill, S.; Karandur, D.; Peterson, S.M.; Marita, M.; Shi, X.; Kaliszewski, M.J.; Smith, A.W.; Isacoff, E.Y.; Kuriyan, J. Molecular basis for multimerization in the activation of the epidermal growth factor receptor. *Elife* **2016**, *5*. [CrossRef]
5. Purba, E.R.; Saita, E.I.; Maruyama, I.N. Activation of the EGF Receptor by Ligand Binding and Oncogenic Mutations: The "Rotation Model". *Cells* **2017**, *6*. [CrossRef] [PubMed]
6. Maruyama, I.N. Mechanisms of activation of receptor tyrosine kinases: Monomers or dimers. *Cells* **2014**, *3*, 304–330. [CrossRef]
7. Maruyama, I.N. Activation of transmembrane cell-surface receptors via a common mechanism? The "rotation model". *Bioessays* **2015**, *37*, 959–967. [CrossRef] [PubMed]
8. Mansour, M.; Nievergall, E.; Gegenbauer, K.; Llerena, C.; Atapattu, L.; Halle, M.; Tremblay, M.L.; Janes, P.W.; Lackmann, M. PTP-PEST controls EphA3 activation and ephrin-induced cytoskeletal remodelling. *J. Cell Sci.* **2016**, *129*, 277–289. [CrossRef]
9. Espejo, R.; Jeng, Y.; Paulucci-Holthauzen, A.; Rengifo-Cam, W.; Honkus, K.; Anastasiadis, P.Z.; Sastry, S.K. PTP-PEST targets a novel tyrosine site in p120 catenin to control epithelial cell motility and Rho GTPase activity. *J. Cell Sci.* **2014**, *127*, 497–508. [CrossRef]
10. Noren, N.K.; Liu, B.P.; Burridge, K.; Kreft, B. p120 catenin regulates the actin cytoskeleton via Rho family GTPases. *J. Cell Biol.* **2000**, *150*, 567–580. [CrossRef]
11. Anastasiadis, P.Z.; Moon, S.Y.; Thoreson, M.A.; Mariner, D.J.; Crawford, H.C.; Zheng, Y.; Reynolds, A.B. Inhibition of RhoA by p120 catenin. *Nat. Cell Biol.* **2000**, *2*, 637–644. [CrossRef] [PubMed]
12. Grosheva, I.; Shtutman, M.; Elbaum, M.; Bershadsky, A.D. p120 catenin affects cell motility via modulation of activity of Rho-family GTPases: A link between cell-cell contact formation and regulation of cell locomotion. *J. Cell Sci.* **2001**, *114*, 695–707. [PubMed]
13. Sun, T.; Aceto, N.; Meerbrey, K.L.; Kessler, J.D.; Zhou, C.; Migliaccio, I.; Nguyen, D.X.; Pavlova, N.N.; Botero, M.; Huang, J.; et al. Activation of multiple proto-oncogenic tyrosine kinases in breast cancer via loss of the PTPN12 phosphatase. *Cell* **2011**, *144*, 703–718. [CrossRef] [PubMed]
14. Lee, C.; Rhee, I. Important roles of protein tyrosine phosphatase PTPN12 in tumor progression. *Pharm. Res.* **2019**, *144*, 73–78. [CrossRef] [PubMed]
15. Nair, A.; Chung, H.C.; Sun, T.; Tyagi, S.; Dobrolecki, L.E.; Dominguez-Vidana, R.; Kurley, S.J.; Orellana, M.; Renwick, A.; Henke, D.M.; et al. Combinatorial inhibition of PTPN12-regulated receptors leads to a broadly effective therapeutic strategy in triple-negative breast cancer. *Nat. Med.* **2018**, *24*, 505–511. [CrossRef] [PubMed]
16. Li, J.; Davidson, D.; Martins Souza, C.; Zhong, M.C.; Wu, N.; Park, M.; Muller, W.J.; Veillette, A. Loss of PTPN12 Stimulates Progression of ErbB2-Dependent Breast Cancer by Enhancing Cell Survival, Migration, and Epithelial-to-Mesenchymal Transition. *Mol. Cell Biol.* **2015**, *35*, 4069–4082. [CrossRef]
17. Luo, R.Z.; Cai, P.Q.; Li, M.; Fu, J.; Zhang, Z.Y.; Chen, J.W.; Cao, Y.; Yun, J.P.; Xie, D.; Cai, M.Y. Decreased expression of PTPN12 correlates with tumor recurrence and poor survival of patients with hepatocellular carcinoma. *PLoS ONE* **2014**, *9*, e85592. [CrossRef]
18. Lee, K.J.; Yoo, Y.H.; Kim, M.S.; Yadav, B.K.; Kim, Y.; Lim, D.; Hwangbo, C.; Moon, K.W.; Kim, D.; Jeoung, D.; et al. CD99 inhibits CD98-mediated beta1 integrin signaling through SHP2-mediated FAK dephosphorylation. *Exp. Cell Res.* **2015**, *336*, 211–222. [CrossRef]
19. Lee, K.J.; Lee, S.H.; Yadav, B.K.; Ju, H.M.; Kim, M.S.; Park, J.H.; Jeoung, D.; Lee, H.; Hahn, J.H. The activation of CD99 inhibits cell-extracellular matrix adhesion by suppressing beta(1) integrin affinity. *BMB Rep.* **2012**, *45*, 159–164. [CrossRef]
20. Guerzoni, C.; Fiori, V.; Terracciano, M.; Manara, M.C.; Moricoli, D.; Pasello, M.; Sciandra, M.; Nicoletti, G.; Gellini, M.; Dominici, S.; et al. CD99 triggering in Ewing sarcoma delivers a lethal signal through p53 pathway reactivation and cooperates with doxorubicin. *Clin. Cancer Res.* **2015**, *21*, 146–156. [CrossRef]
21. Waclavicek, M.; Majdic, O.; Stulnig, T.; Berger, M.; Sunder-Plassmann, R.; Zlabinger, G.J.; Baumruker, T.; Stockl, J.; Ebner, C.; Knapp, W.; et al. CD99 engagement on human peripheral blood T cells results in TCR/CD3-dependent cellular activation and allows for Th1-restricted cytokine production. *J. Immunol.* **1998**, *161*, 4671–4678. [PubMed]

22. Sohn, H.W.; Shin, Y.K.; Lee, I.S.; Bae, Y.M.; Suh, Y.H.; Kim, M.K.; Kim, T.J.; Jung, K.C.; Park, W.S.; Park, C.S.; et al. CD99 regulates the transport of MHC class I molecules from the Golgi complex to the cell surface. *J. Immunol.* **2001**, *166*, 787–794. [CrossRef] [PubMed]
23. Sohn, H.W.; Choi, E.Y.; Kim, S.H.; Lee, I.S.; Chung, D.H.; Sung, U.A.; Hwang, D.H.; Cho, S.S.; Jun, B.H.; Jang, J.J.; et al. Engagement of CD99 induces apoptosis through a calcineurin-independent pathway in Ewing's sarcoma cells. *Am. J. Pathol.* **1998**, *153*, 1937–1945. [CrossRef]
24. Lee, K.J.; Kim, Y.; Yoo, Y.H.; Kim, M.S.; Lee, S.H.; Kim, C.G.; Park, K.; Jeoung, D.; Lee, H.; Ko, I.Y.; et al. CD99-Derived Agonist Ligands Inhibit Fibronectin-Induced Activation of beta1 Integrin through the Protein Kinase A/SHP2/Extracellular Signal-Regulated Kinase/PTPN12/Focal Adhesion Kinase Signaling Pathway. *Mol. Cell Biol.* **2017**, *37*. [CrossRef]
25. Zucchini, C.; Manara, M.C.; Pinca, R.S.; De Sanctis, P.; Guerzoni, C.; Sciandra, M.; Lollini, P.L.; Cenacchi, G.; Picci, P.; Valvassori, L.; et al. CD99 suppresses osteosarcoma cell migration through inhibition of ROCK2 activity. *Oncogene* **2014**, *33*, 1912–1921. [CrossRef] [PubMed]
26. Zhao, T.T.; Le Francois, B.G.; Goss, G.; Ding, K.; Bradbury, P.A.; Dimitroulakos, J. Lovastatin inhibits EGFR dimerization and AKT activation in squamous cell carcinoma cells: Potential regulation by targeting rho proteins. *Oncogene* **2010**, *29*, 4682–4692. [CrossRef]
27. Mattila, P.K.; Batista, F.D.; Treanor, B. Dynamics of the actin cytoskeleton mediates receptor cross talk: An emerging concept in tuning receptor signaling. *J. Cell Biol.* **2016**, *212*, 267–280. [CrossRef]
28. Low-Nam, S.T.; Lidke, K.A.; Cutler, P.J.; Roovers, R.C.; van Bergen en Henegouwen, P.M.; Wilson, B.S.; Lidke, D.S. ErbB1 dimerization is promoted by domain co-confinement and stabilized by ligand binding. *Nat. Struct Mol. Biol.* **2011**, *18*, 1244–1249. [CrossRef]
29. Ren, X.D.; Kiosses, W.B.; Sieg, D.J.; Otey, C.A.; Schlaepfer, D.D.; Schwartz, M.A. Focal adhesion kinase suppresses Rho activity to promote focal adhesion turnover. *J. Cell Sci.* **2000**, *113*, 3673–3678.
30. Zhai, J.; Lin, H.; Nie, Z.; Wu, J.; Canete-Soler, R.; Schlaepfer, W.W.; Schlaepfer, D.D. Direct interaction of focal adhesion kinase with p190RhoGEF. *J. Biol. Chem.* **2003**, *278*, 24865–24873. [CrossRef]
31. Westhoff, M.A.; Serrels, B.; Fincham, V.J.; Frame, M.C.; Carragher, N.O. SRC-mediated phosphorylation of focal adhesion kinase couples actin and adhesion dynamics to survival signaling. *Mol. Cell Biol.* **2004**, *24*, 8113–8133. [CrossRef] [PubMed]
32. Suetsugu, S.; Takenawa, T. Regulation of cortical actin networks in cell migration. *Int. Rev. Cytol.* **2003**, *229*, 245–286. [CrossRef] [PubMed]
33. Yamazaki, D.; Kurisu, S.; Takenawa, T. Regulation of cancer cell motility through actin reorganization. *Cancer Sci.* **2005**, *96*, 379–386. [CrossRef] [PubMed]
34. Spiering, D.; Hodgson, L. Dynamics of the Rho-family small GTPases in actin regulation and motility. *Cell Adh. Migr.* **2011**, *5*, 170–180. [CrossRef] [PubMed]
35. Bai, C.Y.; Ohsugi, M.; Abe, Y.; Yamamoto, T. ZRP-1 controls Rho GTPase-mediated actin reorganization by localizing at cell-matrix and cell-cell adhesions. *J. Cell Sci.* **2007**, *120*, 2828–2837. [CrossRef]
36. Fraguas, S.; Barberan, S.; Cebria, F. EGFR signaling regulates cell proliferation, differentiation and morphogenesis during planarian regeneration and homeostasis. *Dev. Biol.* **2011**, *354*, 87–101. [CrossRef]
37. Song, Z.; Fusco, J.; Zimmerman, R.; Fischbach, S.; Chen, C.; Ricks, D.M.; Prasadan, K.; Shiota, C.; Xiao, X.; Gittes, G.K. Epidermal Growth Factor Receptor Signaling Regulates beta Cell Proliferation in Adult Mice. *J. Biol. Chem.* **2016**, *291*, 22630–22637. [CrossRef]
38. Pennock, S.; Wang, Z. Stimulation of cell proliferation by endosomal epidermal growth factor receptor as revealed through two distinct phases of signaling. *Mol. Cell Biol.* **2003**, *23*, 5803–5815. [CrossRef]
39. Zheng, Y.; Zhang, C.; Croucher, D.R.; Soliman, M.A.; St-Denis, N.; Pasculescu, A.; Taylor, L.; Tate, S.A.; Hardy, W.R.; Colwill, K.; et al. Temporal regulation of EGF signalling networks by the scaffold protein Shc1. *Nature* **2013**, *499*, 166–171. [CrossRef]
40. Ayoub, E.; Hall, A.; Scott, A.M.; Chagnon, M.J.; Miquel, G.; Halle, M.; Noda, M.; Bikfalvi, A.; Tremblay, M.L. Regulation of the Src kinase-associated phosphoprotein 55 homologue by the protein tyrosine phosphatase PTP-PEST in the control of cell motility. *J. Biol. Chem.* **2013**, *288*, 25739–25748. [CrossRef]
41. Trimble, W.S.; Grinstein, S. Barriers to the free diffusion of proteins and lipids in the plasma membrane. *J. Cell Biol.* **2015**, *208*, 259–271. [CrossRef]
42. Jung, S.R.; Seo, J.B.; Shim, D.; Hille, B.; Koh, D.S. Actin cytoskeleton controls movement of intracellular organelles in pancreatic duct epithelial cells. *Cell Calcium* **2012**, *51*, 459–469. [CrossRef] [PubMed]

43. Manneville, J.B.; Etienne-Manneville, S.; Skehel, P.; Carter, T.; Ogden, D.; Ferenczi, M. Interaction of the actin cytoskeleton with microtubules regulates secretory organelle movement near the plasma membrane in human endothelial cells. *J. Cell Sci.* **2003**, *116*, 3927–3938. [CrossRef] [PubMed]
44. Tang, J.; Gross, D.J. Regulated EGF receptor binding to F-actin modulates receptor phosphorylation. *Biochem. Biophys. Res. Commun.* **2003**, *312*, 930–936. [CrossRef] [PubMed]
45. Den Hartigh, J.C.; van Bergen en Henegouwen, P.M.; Verkleij, A.J.; Boonstra, J. The EGF receptor is an actin-binding protein. *J. Cell Biol.* **1992**, *119*, 349–355. [CrossRef]
46. Martinez-Munoz, L.; Rodriguez-Frade, J.M.; Barroso, R.; Sorzano, C.O.S.; Torreno-Pina, J.A.; Santiago, C.A.; Manzo, C.; Lucas, P.; Garcia-Cuesta, E.M.; Gutierrez, E.; et al. Separating Actin-Dependent Chemokine Receptor Nanoclustering from Dimerization Indicates a Role for Clustering in CXCR4 Signaling and Function. *Mol. Cell* **2018**, *71*, 873. [CrossRef]
47. Carragher, N.O.; Frame, M.C. Focal adhesion and actin dynamics: A place where kinases and proteases meet to promote invasion. *Trends Cell Biol.* **2004**, *14*, 241–249. [CrossRef]
48. Wehrle-Haller, B. Assembly and disassembly of cell matrix adhesions. *Curr. Opin. Cell Biol.* **2012**, *24*, 569–581. [CrossRef]
49. Li, S.Y.; Mruk, D.D.; Cheng, C.Y. Focal adhesion kinase is a regulator of F-actin dynamics: New insights from studies in the testis. *Spermatogenesis* **2013**, *3*, e25385. [CrossRef]
50. Rae, J.M.; Scheys, J.O.; Clark, K.M.; Chadwick, R.B.; Kiefer, M.C.; Lippman, M.E. EGFR and EGFRvIII expression in primary breast cancer and cell lines. *Breast Cancer Res. Treat.* **2004**, *87*, 87–95. [CrossRef]
51. Manara, M.C.; Terracciano, M.; Mancarella, C.; Sciandra, M.; Guerzoni, C.; Pasello, M.; Grilli, A.; Zini, N.; Picci, P.; Colombo, M.P.; et al. CD99 triggering induces methuosis of Ewing sarcoma cells through IGF-1R/RAS/Rac1 signaling. *Oncotarget* **2016**, *7*, 79925–79942. [CrossRef] [PubMed]
52. Stock, J. Receptor signaling: Dimerization and beyond. *Curr. Biol.* **1996**, *6*, 825–827. [CrossRef]
53. Weiss, A.; Schlessinger, J. Switching signals on or off by receptor dimerization. *Cell* **1998**, *94*, 277–280. [CrossRef]
54. Rowland-Goldsmith, M.A.; Maruyama, H.; Kusama, T.; Ralli, S.; Korc, M. Soluble type II transforming growth factor-beta (TGF-beta) receptor inhibits TGF-beta signaling in COLO-357 pancreatic cancer cells in vitro and attenuates tumor formation. *Clin. Cancer Res.* **2001**, *7*, 2931–2940. [PubMed]
55. Farooqi, A.A.; Siddik, Z.H. Platelet-derived growth factor (PDGF) signalling in cancer: Rapidly emerging signalling landscape. *Cell Biochem. Funct.* **2015**, *33*, 257–265. [CrossRef]
56. Helsten, T.; Elkin, S.; Arthur, E.; Tomson, B.N.; Carter, J.; Kurzrock, R. The FGFR Landscape in Cancer: Analysis of 4,853 Tumors by Next-Generation Sequencing. *Clin. Cancer Res.* **2016**, *22*, 259–267. [CrossRef] [PubMed]
57. Zou, L.; Cao, S.; Kang, N.; Huebert, R.C.; Shah, V.H. Fibronectin induces endothelial cell migration through beta1 integrin and Src-dependent phosphorylation of fibroblast growth factor receptor-1 at tyrosines 653/654 and 766. *J. Biol Chem.* **2012**, *287*, 7190–7202. [CrossRef]
58. Chen, M.; She, H.; Kim, A.; Woodley, D.T.; Li, W. Nckbeta adapter regulates actin polymerization in NIH 3T3 fibroblasts in response to platelet-derived growth factor bb. *Mol. Cell Biol.* **2000**, *20*, 7867–7880. [CrossRef]
59. Turk, H.F.; Chapkin, R.S. Analysis of epidermal growth factor receptor dimerization by BS(3) cross-linking. *Methods Mol. Biol.* **2015**, *1233*, 25–34. [CrossRef]

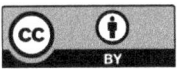

© 2020 by the authors. Licensee MDPI, Basel, Switzerland. This article is an open access article distributed under the terms and conditions of the Creative Commons Attribution (CC BY) license (http://creativecommons.org/licenses/by/4.0/).

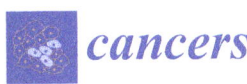

Article

Genomic Mapping of Splicing-Related Genes Identify Amplifications in *LSM1*, *CLNS1A*, and *ILF2* in Luminal Breast Cancer

María del Mar Noblejas-López [1,2,†], Igor López-Cade [3,†], Jesús Fuentes-Antrás [4,5], Gonzalo Fernández-Hinojal [4,5], Ada Esteban-Sánchez [3], Aránzazu Manzano [4,5], José Ángel García-Sáenz [6], Pedro Pérez-Segura [6], Miguel De La Hoya [3], Atanasio Pandiella [7], Balázs Győrffy [8,9,10], Vanesa García-Barberán [3,*] and Alberto Ocaña [1,2,4,5,*]

1 Translational Oncology Laboratory, Translational Research Unit, Albacete University Hospital, 02008 Albacete, Spain; mariadelmar.noblejas@uclm.es
2 Centro Regional de Investigaciones Biomédicas, Castilla-La Mancha University (CRIB-UCLM), 02008 Albacete, Spain
3 Molecular Oncology Laboratory, Hospital Clínico San Carlos (HCSC), Instituto de Investigación Sanitaria San Carlos (IdISSC), 28040 Madrid, Spain; ilopez.7@alumni.unav.es (I.L.-C.); ada.esteban@salud.madrid.org (A.E.-S.); miguel.hoya@salud.madrid.org (M.D.L.H.)
4 Experimental Therapeutics Unit, Hospital Clínico San Carlos (HCSC), Instituto de Investigación Sanitaria San Carlos (IdISSC), 28040 Madrid, Spain; jfuentesa@salud.madrid.org (J.F.-A.); gfernandezh@salud.madrid.org (G.F.-H.); aranzazu.manzano@salud.madrid.org (A.M.)
5 Centro de Investigación Biomédica en Red en Oncología (CIBERONC), 28029 Madrid, Spain
6 Medical Oncology Department, Hospital Clínico San Carlos (HCSC), Instituto de Investigación Sanitaria San Carlos (IdISSC), 28040 Madrid, Spain; jagarcia.hcsc@salud.madrid.org (J.Á.G.-S.); pedro.perez@salud.madrid.org (P.P.-S.)
7 Instituto de Biología Molecular y Celular del Cáncer (IBMCC-CIC), Instituto de Investigación Biomédica de Salamanca (IBSAL), Consejo Superior de Investigaciones Científicas (CSIC) and CIBERONC, 37007 Salamanca, Spain; atanasio@usal.es
8 Department of Bioinformatics, Semmelweis University, H-1094 Budapest, Hungary; gyorffy.balazs@ttk.mta.hu
9 2nd Department of Pediatrics, Semmelweis University, H-1094 Budapest, Hungary
10 TTK Lendület Cancer Biomarker Research Group, Institute of Enzymology, H-1117 Budapest, Hungary
* Correspondence: vanesa.garciabar@salud.madrid.org (V.G.-B.); alberto.ocana@salud.madrid.org (A.O.)
† Equal contributors.

Simple Summary: The alternative splicing (AS) process is highly relevant, affecting most of the hallmarks of cancer, such as proliferation, angiogenesis, and metastasis. Our study evaluated alterations in 304 splicing-related genes and their prognosis value in breast cancer patients. Amplifications in *CLNS1A*, *LSM1*, and *ILF2* genes in luminal patients were significantly associated with poor outcome. Downregulation of these genes in luminal cell lines showed an antiproliferative effect. Pharmacological modulation of transcription and RNA regulation is key for the optimal development of therapeutic strategies against key proteins. Administration of a BET inhibitor and BET-PROTAC reduced the expression of these identified genes and displayed a significant antiproliferative effect on these cell models. In conclusion, we describe novel splicing genes amplified in luminal breast tumors that are associated with detrimental prognosis and can be modulated pharmacologically. It opens the door for further studies confirming the effect of these genes in patients treated with BET inhibitors.

Abstract: Alternative splicing is an essential biological process, which increases the diversity and complexity of the human transcriptome. In our study, 304 splicing pathway-related genes were evaluated in tumors from breast cancer patients (TCGA dataset). A high number of alterations were detected, including mutations and copy number alterations (CNAs), although mutations were less frequently present compared with CNAs. In the four molecular subtypes, 14 common splice genes showed high level amplification in >5% of patients. Certain genes were only amplified in specific breast cancer subtypes. Most altered genes in each molecular subtype clustered to a few chromosomal regions. In the Luminal subtype, amplifications of *LSM1*, *CLNS1A*, and *ILF2* showed a strong significant association with prognosis. An even more robust association with OS and RFS was observed when expression of these three genes was combined. Inhibition of LSM1, CLNS1A, and ILF2, using siRNA in MCF7 and T47D cells, showed a decrease in cell proliferation. The mRNA expression of these genes was reduced by treatment with BET inhibitors, a family of epigenetic modulators. We map the presence of splicing-related genes in breast cancer, describing three novel genes, LSM1, CLNS1A, and ILF2, that have an oncogenic role and can be modulated with BET inhibitors.

Keywords: splicing pathway; luminal breast cancer; BET inhibitors

1. Introduction

The RNA splicing process regulates gene expression in eukaryotic cells through a complex process in which introns are removed from precursor RNAs (pre-mRNAs) and consecutive exons are precisely joined together to produce mature mRNAs, with the final goal of maintaining mature transcripts to guarantee a successful translation process [1]. The alternative splicing process (AS) is the way in which exons or portions of exons or non-coding regions within a pre-mRNA transcript are differentially joined or skipped, resulting in multiple protein isoforms being encoded by a single gene [1]. Alternative splicing (AS) contributes to transcriptome (and proteome) diversity in development- and tissue-regulated pathways, as well as in response to multiple physiological signals [2]. Remarkably, large-scale proteomic studies suggest that many predicted alternative transcripts are not translated into proteins, so the exact contribution of AS to protein diversity is currently under dispute [3,4]. On top of that, some authors have suggested a role for AS in buffering mutational consequences [5], and mounting evidence indicates that AS coupled to nonsense-mediated decay is a major post-transcriptional regulator of gene expression [6,7]. Five major types of AS have been described: exon skipping, mutually exclusive exons, intron retention, and alternative 5' or 3' splice site [8]. The AS process is carried out by the spliceosome and consists of four stages: assembly, activation, catalysis or splicing, and disassembly. In each specific stage of a splicing cycle, different spliceosome subcomplexes are involved (pre-B, B, Bact, B*, C, C*, P, and ILS complexes), which are composed of small nuclear ribonucleoproteins (snRNPs) and non-snRNPs splicing factors [9]. AS is a highly regulated process, with five snRNPs and over 300 non-snRNP proteins identified as recruited to the spliceosome at these specific stages [10].

Changes due to AS can affect the translation rate and the functional role of the mRNA. AS can act on different cellular and biological processes or be involved in tissue specificity, developmental states, or disease conditions, such as cancer [11]. It has a relevant role in cancer development and maintenance, affecting most of the hallmarks of cancer [12,13]. In addition, it can be involved in cancer relapse or resistance to different treatment modalities [12]. Thus, specific isoforms have been identified promoting and supporting neoplastic transformation and tumor development. In a variety of tumor types, AS has been linked to up-regulation of oncogenes, participating in different processes of tumor development, including angiogenesis, cell division, altered metabolism, proliferation, or metastasis [10,14]. In addition, they can also contribute to the deregulation of several non-oncogenic vulnerabilities that are also relevant in the initiation and maintenance of the oncogenic transformation [12].

Alterations in the AS machinery have been identified in different human tumors, and they can affect a network of downstream splicing targets. Using high throughput methodologies, Seiler et al. have described somatic mutations in 119 splicing factors in 33 tumor types, bladder carcinoma and uveal melanoma being those with higher frequencies [15]. Moreover, mutations in splicing factors appear to be mutually exclusive within a tumor, which might indicate that co-occurrence of these mutations may be lethal [15].

Specifically in breast cancer, AS affects major breast cancer-related proteins, such as the estrogen receptor (ER), BRCA1, and BRCA2, among others [16]. Thus, disequilibrium between ERα66 and ERα36 induce abnormal proliferation, and high levels of ERα36 can cause resistance to Tamoxifen [16]. Alterations in components of the regulatory splicing machinery have been described in breast cancer. For example, SF3B1 is involved in the 3′-SS recognition and is one of the most commonly mutated genes with a higher frequency in the metastatic setting [17]. Mutant SF3B1 produces aberrant splicing, inducing metabolic reprogramming [18]. In addition, AS has been described to have a role in drug resistance. For instance, it has been described that, in carriers of BRCA1 exon 11 premature termination codon variants, tumors upregulate exon 11 skipping to produce isoforms that retain residual activity, contributing to PARPi resistance [19]. Overexpression of SF3B1 and SF3B3 are associated with tamoxifen and fulvestrant resistance, and inhibition of another splicing factors, such as ZRANB2 and SYF2, reduces resistance to doxorubicin in breast cancer cells [20,21]. On the other hand, SRSF4 induces apoptosis in cancer cells, in combination with platinum agents [22].

In our study, alterations in 304 splicing factors were evaluated in breast cancer patients using several large datasets. We found high frequency of amplification in *CLNS1A*, *LSM1*, and *ILF2* in Luminal tumors, with a significant association with poor prognosis. Despite the limited information about these genes, they have been associated with oncogenic processes and resistance to treatments. IFL2 deregulation has been related to an aberrant RNA splicing pattern, mainly deregulated skipped exons in genes involved in DNA repair [23]. LSM1 is included in the heteroheptameric complex LSM1-7, which initiates mRNA decay [24]. CLNS1A acts as a Sm chaperone, recruiting Sm proteins to the PRMT5 complex [25]. In our study, genomic regulation of these genes, with a reduction of their expression, decreased proliferation of luminal tumor cells. In addition, treatment with epigenetic modulators, such as the Bromodomain and extraterminal (BET) family of inhibitors, reduced the expression level of these genes, leading to cell growth reduction.

2. Materials and Methods

2.1. Data Collection and Processing

Processed TCGA (The Cancer Genome Atlas) PanCancer dataset was downloaded through cBioportal (www.cbioportal.org; accessed on 4 December 2019). This dataset contains whole exome sequencing and RNA-Seq data from patients with breast invasive carcinoma, consisting of 696 Luminal, 78 HER2 positive, and 171 Basal tumors and their matched normal tissues. WES data was used to explore CNAs and mutations in 304 splicing factor genes. Splicing related genes were collected from four sources: HUGO Gene Nomenclature Committee and the studies of Hegele et al. [26], Wan et al. [9], and Koedoot et al. [20]. Only somatic non-silent mutations in splicing factor genes were considered (missense, premature termination codon, and IVS+-1,2). Somatic non-silent mutations in splicing factor genes were only considered. In the PanCancer dataset, identification of somatic single nucleotide variations was performed using Mutect. CNAs were assessed as deviations in the tumor sample from the paired normal tissue sample using GISTIC 2.0. GISTIC 2.0 identifies regions significantly amplified or deleted and lists genes found in each "wide peak" region [27]. Value +/− 2 indicates high-level thresholds for amplifications/deletions, respectively, and those with +/− 1 exceed the low-level thresholds but not the high-level thresholds. In addition, the Metabric dataset (www.cbioportal.org; accessed on 4 December 2019) was used to validate results of identified genes with a high level of amplification in >5% of tumors.

2.2. Outcome Analysis

The relationship between gene expression levels and patient clinical prognosis in terms of relapse-free survival (RFS) and overall survival (OS) was evaluated using the Kaplan–Meier Plotter platform, as described previously [28,29] (accessed on 6 June 2020). This tool used gene expression and survival data from 7830 breast tumors (sources include GEO, EGA and TCGA). Samples were split into two groups using the best threshold as the cutoff (auto select best cutoff). When testing multiple genes, the analysis was performed using the mean expression. Patients above the threshold were labelled as "high" expressing, while patients below the threshold were labelled as "low" expressing. The two groups were compared using Cox survival analysis. The prognostic value of the identified signature (containing *LSM1*, *CLSN1A*, and *ILF2*) was validated using the TCGA project.

The correlation between CNAs and patient clinical outcome was analyzed using the Genotype-2-Outcome platform (accessed on 8 January 2021) [30]. This tool links genotype to clinical outcome by utilizing next generation sequencing and gene chip data of 6697 breast cancer patients. It allows the association with prognosis of a specific transcriptomic signature linked to an altered gene, by classifying patients according to the average expression of significant genes designated as a surrogate metagene of its alteration status. The median expression values for different transcripts are used as a cut-off to discriminate "high" and "low" expression cohorts, which are compared using a Cox survival analysis. To identify factors independently associated with OS and RFS, a multivariate analysis (Cox proportional risk regression model) was performed.

2.3. Cell Culture and Compounds

MCF7 and T47D cells (American Type Culture Collection, Manassas, VA, USA) were cultured in DMEM (Sigma-Aldrich, Saint Louis, MO, USA) containing 10% fetal bovine serum with 100 U/mL penicillin, 100 μg/mL streptomycin, and 2 mM L-glutamine, and cells were maintained at 37 °C in a 5% CO_2 atmosphere. The BET inhibitor JQ1 was purchased from Tocris Bioscience, and BET-PROTAC MZ1 was purchased from Selleckchem (Houston, TX, USA).

2.4. Small Interfering RNA

siRNA oligonucleotides (Sigma-Aldrich, Saint Louis, MO, USA) were transfected into cells using Lipofectamine RNAiMax protocol (Thermo Fisher Scientific, Rockford, IL, USA) at a final concentration of 20 nM. References: siLSM1(EHU121391), siCLNS1A (EHU147241), and siILF2 (EHU084311). siGFP (EHUEGFP) was used as the negative control of transfection. Briefly, cells were transfected (~80% of confluency), and after 24 h, cells were reseeded for validation experiments.

2.5. Quantitative Reverse-Transcription PCR

Total RNA was collected from cells using the RNeasy Mini Kit (Qiagen, Hilden, Germany) according to the manufacturer's instructions. Determination of concentration and purity were measured using a NanoDrop ND-1000 spectrophotometer (Thermo Fisher Scientific, Rockford, IL, USA), and then 1 μg of total RNA was reverse transcribed using the RevertAid H Minus first-strand cDNA synthesis kit (Thermo Fisher Scientific) in a thermal cycler (Bio-Rad, Hercules, CA, USA) under the following reaction conditions: 65 °C for 5 min, 42 °C for 60 min, and 70 °C for 10 min. cDNAs were then subjected to real-time PCR analysis using Fast SYBR Green master mix on the StepOnePlus Real-Time PCR system (Applied Biosystems) according to the manufacturer's instructions. Primer sequences used were as follows: h-LSM1 F: TTCCTCGAGGGATTTTTGTG, h-LSM1 R: TTCTCTGCTTCCAGCTTGGT, h-CLNS1A F: TCGGCACTGGTACCCTTTAC, h-CLNS1A R: AATGGTGGGTATTCCAGTG, h-ILF2 F: GCTCCAGGGACATTTGAAGT, h-ILF2 R: CAGCCACATTGTGTCCTGTAG, h-18S F: GAGGATGAGGTGGAACGTGT, h-18S R: TCTTCAGTCGCTCCAGGTCT. An initial step was performed at 95 °C for 5 min, followed by 40 cycles of 95 °C for 15 s, and finished at 60 °C for 1 min. Each sample was analyzed in triplicates, and cycle threshold (Ct) values of transcripts were determined using StepOne Software v.2.1. Ct values were calculated using the 18Sas reference. Untreated control cells were used as the control to calculate the Ct value and determine the X-fold mRNA expression.

2.6. Proliferation MTT Assays

Cell proliferation was measured using MTT reagent (3-(4, 5-dimethylthiazol-2-yl)-2, 5 diphenyltetrazolium bromide) (Sigma-Aldrich). MTT reduction by mitochondria of living cells generate formazan accumulates.

For evaluated siRNAs antiproliferative effect, MCF7 and T47D cells (5000/well, 48-multiwell plates) were seeded after siRNAs transfection during 24, 48, and 120 h.

For antiproliferative drugs validation, MCF7 and T47D cells (5000/well, 48-multiwell plates) were seeded. After, they were treated with increased doses of JQ1 and MZ1 for 72 h. Later medium was replaced with red-phenol free DMEM containing MTT (0.5 mg/mL) and incubated for 45 min at 37 °C. After, medium was removed and dimethylsulfoxide (DMSO) (Thermo Fisher Scientific) was used for dissolved formazan accumulates. Absorbance (A555 nm–A690 nm) was recorded in a multiwell plate reader (BMG labtech, Ortenberg, Germany).

2.7. Growth Studies

To compare the growth between siRNAs-transfected cells and siGFP-transfected cells (control), proliferation rate was studied by cell count. Cell lines were cultured at a density of 50,000 cells in 6-well. At the times of 24 and 48 h, cells were trypsinized and counted. Images was performed at 48 h using inverted microscope (10×).

2.8. Cell Cycle Assay

siRNAs-transfected cells (MCF7 and T47D) were collected and fixed in ethanol (70%, cold) for 30 min. Cell pellets were washed in PBS+2% BSA and incubated in the dark for 1 h at 4 °C with Propidium iodide/RNAse staining solution (Immunostep).

2.9. Statistical Analysis

We used the student's t-test unpaired for independent samples. The level of significance was considered 95%; therefore, p values lower than 0.05 were considered statistically significant: * $p < 0.05$; ** $p < 0.01$, and *** $p < 0.001$. Statistics and representations were made with statistical software GraphPad Prism 7.0. All results (unless indicated) are presented as the mean ± SEM of three independent experiments, each of them performed in triplicate.

3. Results

3.1. Mutations in Splicing-Related Genes

Alterations in 304 splicing-related genes (Supplementary Table S1) were analyzed in 945 breast cancer patients (499 Luminal A, 197 Luminal B, 171 Basal, and 78 HER2+ samples) using the Breast Invasive PanCancer Atlas Dataset, as described in the materials and methods section. Non-synonymous mutations were detected in 278 genes, with 525 tumors showing at least one altered splicing-related gene (Supplementary Table S2, Supplementary Figure S1). When patients were classified based on molecular subtypes, several differences were observed in the distribution of the identified genes. Regarding the 278 genes with presence of mutations, the number of altered genes were 231 (83.1%) for Luminal A, 157 (56.5%) for Luminal B, 175 (62.9%) for Basal, and 150 (54%) for HER2+ subtype (Figure 1A). Tumors with modifications in any of these genes were observed in a higher percentage in HER2+ (70.5%) and Basal (66.1%) compared with the Luminal A and B subtypes (47.1% and 61.9%, respectively) (Figure 1B). When the frequency of tumors with alterations in each gene were evaluated, HER2+ and the basal subtype population showed splicing-related genes with a higher percentage of alterations (Figure 1C; Supplementary Table S2). In the four molecular subtypes, no gene was detected to be mutated in more than 6% of tumors. Splicing genes with mutations in >3% of tumors are displayed in Figure 1C and mainly belonged to the HER2+ and Basal subgroups (Figure 1D).

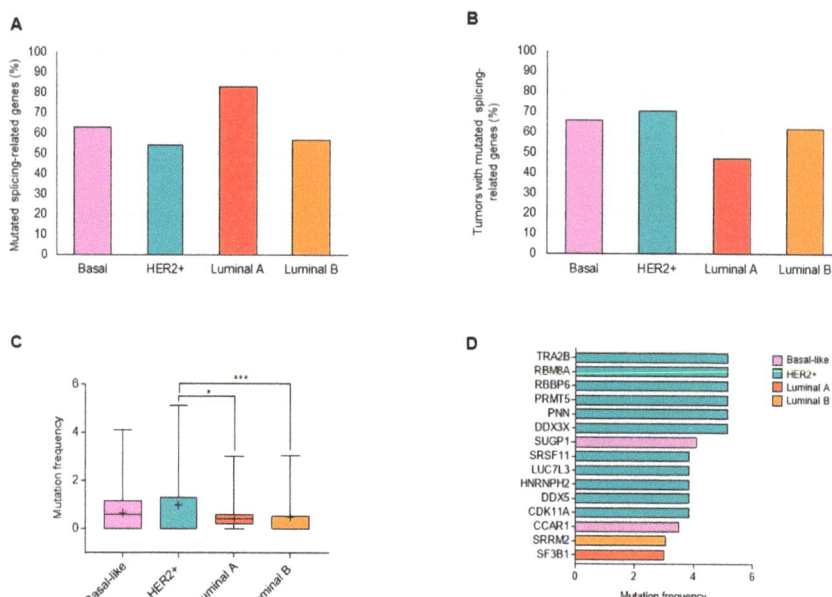

Figure 1. Percentage of splicing-related genes showing mutations in each molecular subtype (**A**). Percentage of tumors with at least one mutated splicing-related gene (**B**). Frequency of non-synonymous mutations in splicing-related genes in each molecular subtype (**C**). List of splicing-related genes mutated in >3% of tumors (**D**). *: $p < 0.05$; ***: $p < 0.001$.

3.2. Copy Number Alterations (CNAs) in Splicing-Related Genes

The TCGA PanCancer series also includes putative copy-number data [31]. Thus, we evaluated the following changes in splicing-related genes: homozygous or hemizygous deletions, no change, gain, and high level of amplification. In this large series of breast cancer patients, we found information about 301 genes from those identified. High level of amplification (GISTIC thresholded CN value of +2) in any of these genes were detected in a high percentage of tumors (HER2+: 87.2%; Basal: 81.3%; Luminal A: 51.1%; and Luminal B: 67.5%). Considering only those genes in regions with homozygous deletion or a high level of amplification in >5% of patients, we found 61 altered splicing-related genes (58 amplified and 3 loss). Regarding the molecular subtypes, 33 (10.9%) splicing-related genes were altered in the Basal subtype (30 amplified and 3 loss), 41 (13.6%) amplified in HER2+, 30 (9.9%) amplified in Luminal A, and 28 (9.3%) altered in Luminal B (26 amplified and 2 loss) (Figure 2A–D, respectively). Therefore, a large number of genes showed higher frequencies of CNAs versus mutations (only 6 genes with mutations in >5% of patients, Figure 1D). In the four molecular subtypes, 14 common splicing-related genes showed a high level of amplification in >5% of tumors (Figure 2E). On the other hand, certain genes were amplified only in specific subtypes (Figure 2F). A complete list of genes is displayed in the Supplementary Table S3.

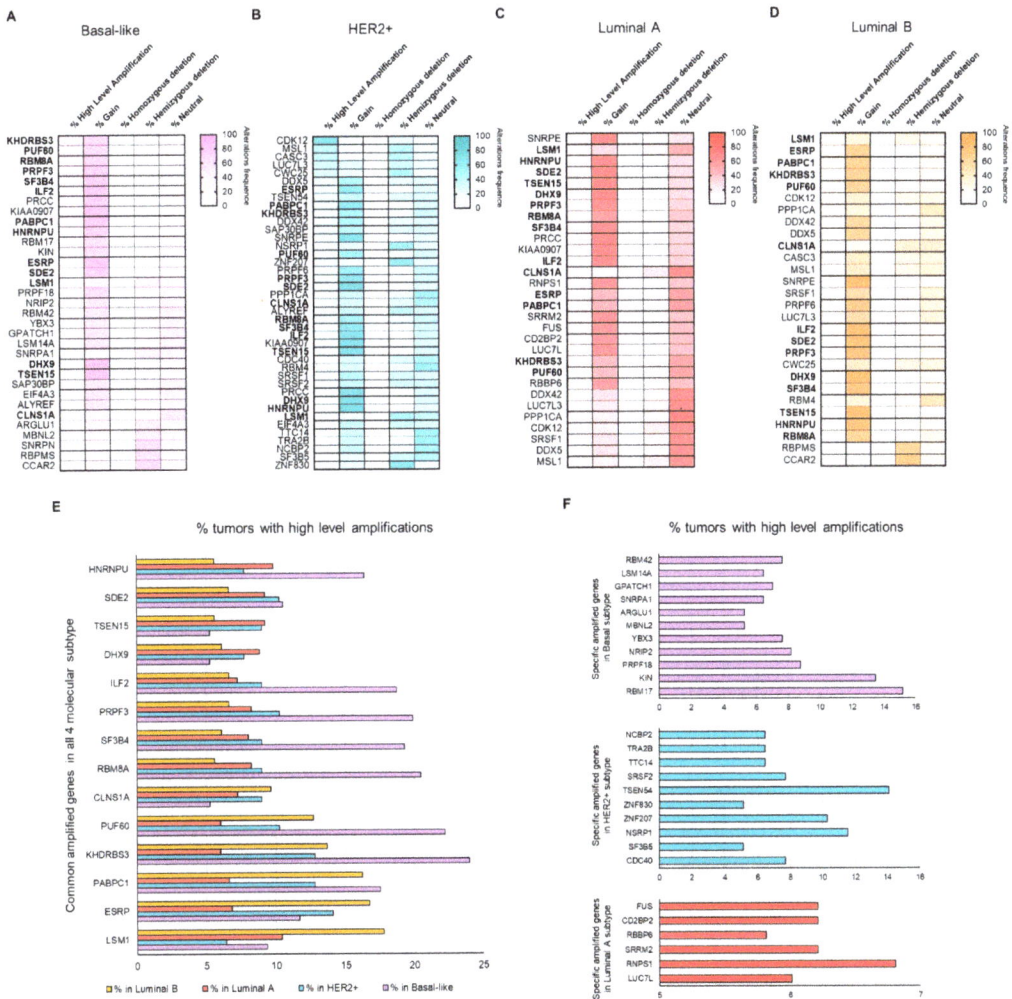

Figure 2. Copy number alteration frequencies in splicing-related genes: list of genes with high amplification in >5% of tumors for Basal (**A**), HER2+ (**B**), Luminal A (**C**), and Luminal B (**D**) molecular subtypes. In total, 14 common splicing-related genes showed high level amplification in >5% of tumors, shown in bold font. Percentage of tumors with presence of amplifications in >5% of tumors in splicing-related genes both common in all molecular subtypes (**E**) and specific in each subtype (**F**).

With this information, we next aimed to explore the chromosome location of splicing-related genes with a high level of amplification or homozygous deletion. Interestingly, most altered splicing-related genes in each molecular subtype were distributed in a few chromosome regions: 1q, 8q, and 17q, as shown in Figure 3A. In total, 12 out of 14 common amplified genes were located in 1q and 8q. Different altered regions were specific for each subtype: (a) 10p, 12p 13q, 15q, and 19q for Basal; (b) 6q, 17q, and 3q for HER2+; (c) all genes in the 16p region for Luminal A; and (d) no one for Luminal B (Figure 3A; Supplementary Table S3). Copy-number gain in these regions is represented in Figure 3B.

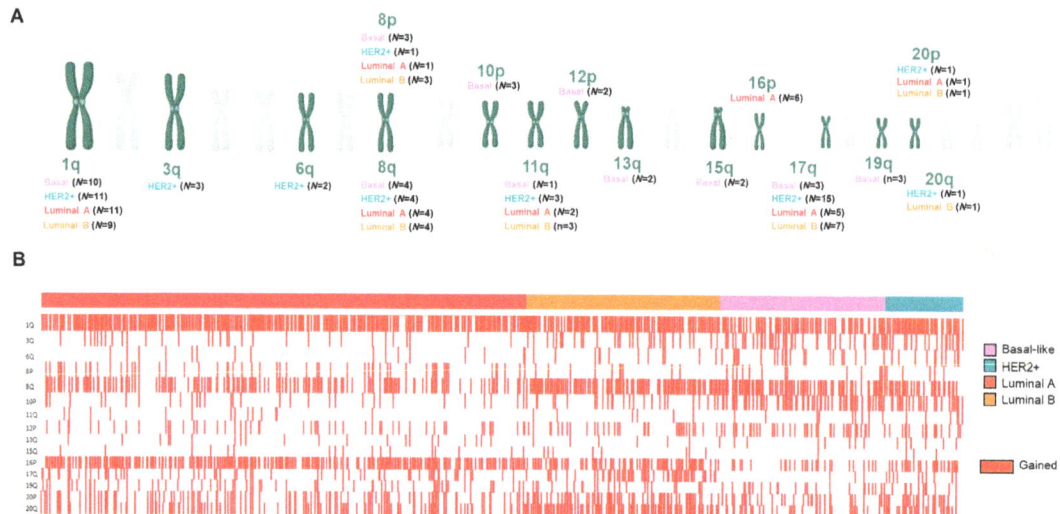

Figure 3. Number of splicing-related genes with high amplification in >5% of patients by chromosome location (**A**) (Created with BioRender.com (accessed on 4 December 2019)). Tumors with chromosomal gain (red) in each molecular subtype (**B**).

3.3. Associations of Splicing-Related Genes with Clinical Outcome in Patients

To identify which of the identified genes could have a role in cancer progression, we intended to link the described data with patient clinical outcome. To do so, we used published transcriptomic microarray data, as described elsewhere [32]. The prognostic value of the high amplified genes (with a cutoff of >5% of tumors) were analyzed in a dataset of 6234 breast cancer patients (Figure 4A). CNA frequencies in identified genes were validated in an additional dataset (Supplementary Figure S2). Frequencies of high level of amplified genes were correlated between both datasets. Alterations in splicing-related genes were most frequently observed in the HER2+ and Basal-like subtypes. However, as there were few patients in these subtypes, it was not possible to establish the prognostic value for most amplified genes. Despite the low number of patients in this subgroup, several genes showed association with RFS and OS (Figure 4B and Supplementary Table S4). We focused on those genes, with a clear impact on survival by using an arbitrary selection based on statistical outcome relevance and low false discovery rate (FDR) ($p < 0.002$, Hazard Ratio (HR) > 1.5; FDR < 5). For Luminal A, high expression of *ESRP1*, *LSM1*, *CLNS1A*, *ILF2*, and *PPP1CA* showed a clear association with detrimental OS and RFS (Figure 4B). In the same way, high levels of these first four genes were associated with a poor prognostic in the Luminal B subtype. In the Luminal series, CNAs were significant associated with expression levels in these genes (Supplementary Figure S3).

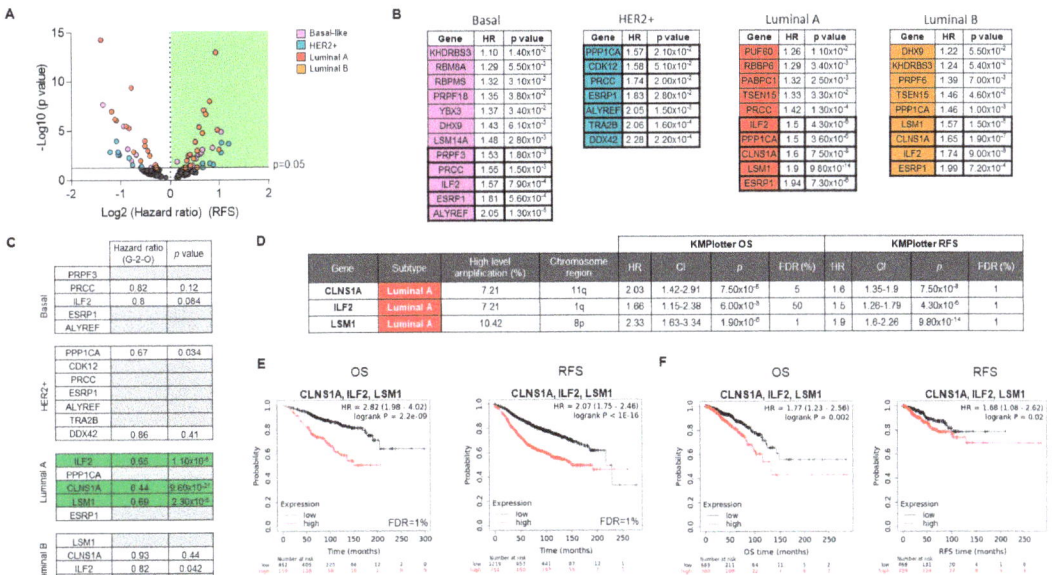

Figure 4. Prognosis value for splicing-related genes with CNAs. Splicing-related genes (only showed those genes with high amplification in >5% of patients) with higher prognostic value based on hazard ratio and *p* values (**A**). List of genes showing significant association between expression levels and detrimental prognosis in RFS (KM Plotter software was used) (**B**). Prognostic value (OS) of selected genes (based on: $p < 0.002$, HR > 1.5; FDR < 5 from KM Plotter) was confirmed using genotype-2-outcome web-server (**C**). Summary of outcome results obtained to *LSM1*, *CLNS1A*, and *ILF2* in the Luminal A subtype (**D**). Kaplan-Meier plots (OS and RFS) for the combination of these three genes using KM Plotter software (**E**) and their validation in another Luminal A cohort (TCGA project) (**F**).

Next, to confirm the prognostic role of the alterations described before, we used a transcriptomic fingerprint of the amplified splicing-related genes by using the genotype-2-outcome (Figure 4C). With this approach, we can obtain the clinical outcome of a gene signature associated with a specific genomic alteration, including gene amplification, as described in the materials and methods section. Thus, the transcriptomic fingerprint associated with the amplification of *LSM1*, *CLNS1A*, and *ILF2* showed a strong association with survival (Supplementary Figure S4). The transcripts included in the signatures associated with the CNA gain of *LSM1*, *CLNS1A*, and *ILF2* are displayed in Supplementary Table S5.

In Figure 4D, we summarized the prognostic value (RFS and OS), percentage of amplification, subtype, and chromosome location of the identified genes. In addition, a more robust association with OS and RFS was observed when expression of these three genes was combined together (Figure 4E). Finally, the prognostic role of the identified signature in the Luminal A subtype was confirmed in a validation cohort, confirming the reproducibility of the findings described before (TCGA dataset; Figure 4F). Univariate and multivariate COX regression analysis showed that the combination of LSM1, CLNS1A, and ILF2 was a clear, independent prognostic factor, mainly with OS (Supplementary Table S6).

3.4. Genomic Down-Regulation of LSM1, CLNS1A, and ILF2 Reduces Cell Proliferation

To validate *LSM1*, *CLNS1A*, and *ILF2* dependency in Luminal breast cancer cells lines, mRNA expression of these genes was downregulated by using small interfering RNA (siRNA). *LSM1*, *CLNS1A*, and *ILF2* downregulation in MCF7 and T47D efficiently reduced gene expression, as shown in Figure 5A. Cell growth (Figure 5B,C) and cell proliferation, evaluated as MTT metabolization (Figure 5D), was reduced after siRNA knockdown of the mentioned splicing genes. Growth reduction was observed clearer with gene interfering of *LSM1* in MCF7 cells and *CLNS1A* in T47D. The antiproliferative effect produced after gene inhibition evaluated as a metabolization of MTT was significantly observed after 120 h, with no differences at a shorter time. To explore how the mechanism for genomic down-regulation of *LSM1*, *CLNS1A*, and *ILF2* inhibits cell proliferation, we performed cell cycle analysis using propidium iodure. No major changes were observed in cell cycle phases, only *CLNS1A* down-regulation showed a G0/G1 arrest in T47D cells in accordance with previous findings (Figure 5E).

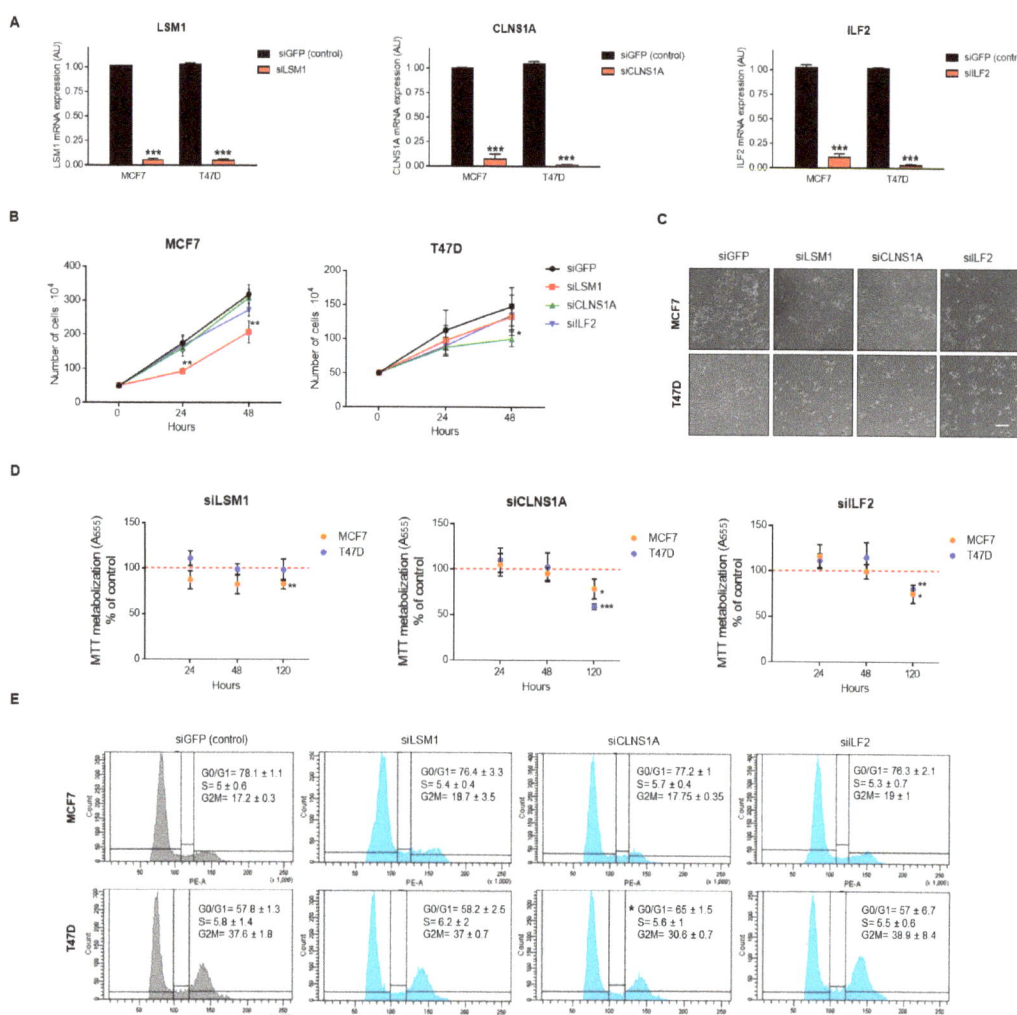

Figure 5. Splicing-related genes genomic inhibition by siRNA and pharmacological inhibition by BET inhibitor and PROTAC. (**A**). *LSM1*, *CLNS1A*, and *ILF2* mRNA expression in MCF7 and T47D luminal A breasts cancer cells after transfection with siRNAs. Cells were transfected using lipofectamine reagent and 24 h later were reseeded. After 24 h, (48 h post-transfection), cells were collected, RNA was extracted, and qPCR was performed. siGFP was used as the control of transfection. (**B**). Transfected cells were seeded (50,000 cells 6-well plate and were counted after 24, 48 and 120 h). (**C**). Images obtained by inverted microscope of transfected cells after 48 h. (**D**). Antiproliferative effect of siRNA evaluated by MTT assays after 24, 48, and 120 h. (**E**). Changes in cell cycle phases after genomic inhibition (representative plot of two independent experiments is shown). Scale bar = 100 µm. * $p < 0.05$; ** $p < 0.01$; *** $p < 0.001$.

3.5. BET Inhibitors Reduce the Expression of LSM1, CLNS1A, and ILF2

Epigenetic agents can modulate the expression of genes that have a role in transcription and maturation [33]. With this in mind, we explored the effect of Bromo and Extra terminal domain (BET) inhibitors and BET derivatives, such as BET-Proteolysis targeting chimeras (PROTAC), on the expression of the identified genes. Administration of the BET inhibitor (JQ1) and BET-PROTAC (MZ1) produced a reduction of the gene expressions of *LSM1*, *CLNS1A*, and *ILF2*. In MCF7 cells, *ILF2* was downregulated with MZ1 treatment after 12 and 24 h of administration. Moreover, *LSM1* was downregulated with MZ1 after 12 h (Figure 6A). In T47D cells, after 12 h of treatment, these three genes were downregulated by both JQ1 and MZ1. This effect was maintained at 24 h of treatment for MZ1, but not for JQ1, suggesting that the PROTAC had a more prolonged effect (Figure 6B). Following these findings, we explored their effect on cell growth. We observed that JQ1 and MZ1 displayed an antiproliferative effect in Luminal cells lines (Figure 6C). EC50 values showed that MZ1 PROTAC was more potent than the inhibitor JQ1 (Figure 6D). In summary, these findings confirm the modulation of the expression of these three genes by JQ1 and MZ1 and the pharmacological effect of these agents on cell proliferation.

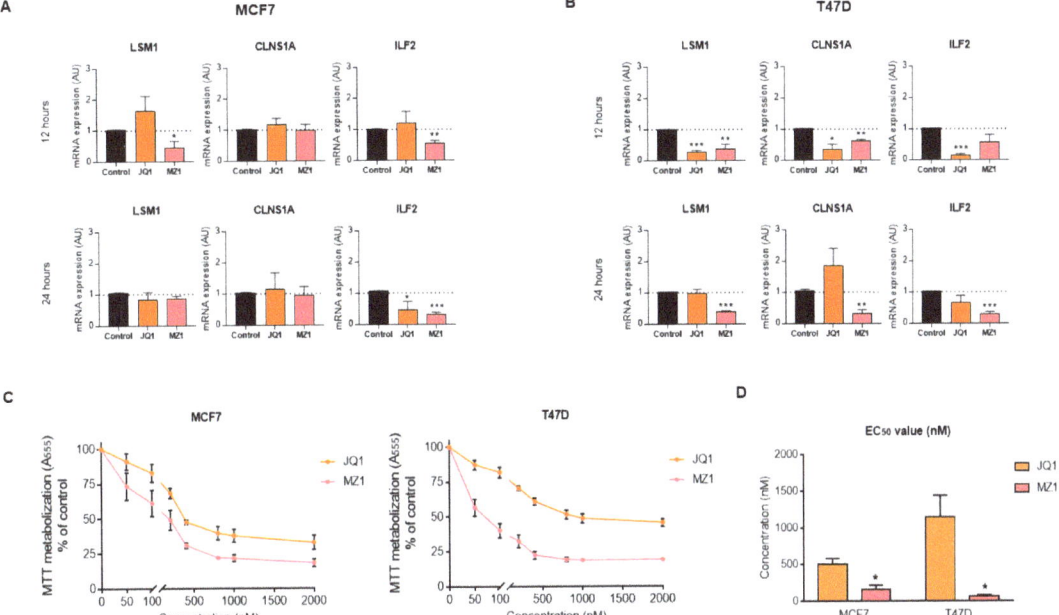

Figure 6. Pharmacological inhibition of splicing-related genes by BET inhibitor and PROTAC. *LSM1*, *CLNS1A*, and *ILF2* mRNA expression in MCF7 (**A**) and T47D (**B**) luminal A breast cancer cell lines after 12 h and 24 h JQ1 and MZ1 exposure. Cell viability evaluated by MTT assays for MCF7 (left) and T47D (right) cells treated with increasing doses of JQ1 and MZ1 (**C**). JQ1, MZ1, and EC50 doses in luminal A cell lines (**D**). * $p < 0.05$; ** $p < 0.01$; *** $p < 0.001$.

4. Discussion

In the present article, we characterize the presence and role of genomic alterations in splicing genes in breast cancer. Splicing is a biological process that permits transcriptional diversity and redundancy of molecular functions, allowing the integrity of key cellular activities [34]. Transcriptional regulation by splicing has been involved in the control of different biological tasks from DNA damage, to cell survival, or stemness, among others [13]. In this context, several genes implicated in splicing have been described in cancer, leading to the promotion of different oncogenic properties. For instance, some known factors, such as SRSF1, have been described as overexpressed in cancer, leading to malignant transformation by an alternative splicing of genes involved in proliferation and apoptosis [35]. Other examples include RBM39 in Acute Myeloid Leukemia or RBM11 in glioblastoma cells, among others [36,37]. In breast cancer, mutations in *SF3B1* are more frequently observed in the metastatic setting, and its potential role in the regulation of protein degradation or metabolism is known [17,18]. In addition, overexpression of *SF3B1* and *SF3B3* has been associated with resistance to hormone therapy, and others, such as *ZRANB2* and *SYF2*, to chemotherapy, particularly for doxorubicin [20,21]. Taking this background into consideration, the identification of deregulated genes involved in splicing and the understanding of their role in cancer is a main objective, with the final goal of designing or implementing therapeutic strategies to reduce their presence.

In our study, we analyzed a set of genes involved in splicing in breast cancer. Genomic modifications of splicing proteins were highly presented in breast cancer, the HER2 subtype being the most common tumor (70.5%), with the less frequency presence observed in the Luminal A subtype (47.1%). Although mutations in splicing genes have been widely reported [15], in our study, no specific gene was mutated in more than 6% of the tumors. On the other hand, when CNAs in our splicing-related gene lists were evaluated, 61 of them were altered in >5% of patients. In a similar way to mutations, the HER2 subtype showed a higher number of altered genes compared with the other groups. This really demonstrates that mutations are less frequently observed than other structural alterations, and the splicing pathway is mainly altered in the HER2 subtype compared with the other breast subtypes. Nevertheless, 14 common splicing-related genes showed high-level amplification in >5% of patients in the four molecular groups, most of them located in 1q and 8q chromosome regions.

The next step in our study was to select those altered splicing-related genes with a role in patient clinical outcome. The results were not conclusive for the HER2 subtype due to the small number of patients. Regarding the Luminal subtype, we identified three genes with clear association with poor prognosis: *ILF2*, *LSM1*, and *CLNS1A*. Although prognosis value cannot be evaluated in HER2 and Basal subtypes, these three genes were also detected as amplified in tumors of these molecular subtypes. Moreover, when the presence of CNAs in our selected genes was analyzed in different tumor types (GDC Data Portal; 67 primary sites), breast cancer was one of most frequently amplified for *LSM1*, *CLNS1A*, and *ILF2* (Supplementary Figure S5). IFL2 has been described as implicated in the RNA splicing regulation of crucial effectors involved in DNA damage response [23]. In addition, overexpression of this gene mediated resistance to DNA damaging agents [23]. Of note, *IFL2* is located at the 8p chromosome, where other genes with a particular oncogenic role in breast cancer, such as FGFR1, has been described as amplified [38]. LSM1 is involved in pre-RNA splicing by acting on the removal of the $5'$ cap structure [24,39,40]. *LSM1* has been studied in other tumor types, such as pancreatic cancer, observing a role in cancer progression, metastasis, and resistance to chemotherapies [41]. CLNS1A is involved in both the assembly of spliceosomal snRNPs and the methylation of Sm proteins [25,42]. CLNS1A cooperates with the protein PRMT5 and functions as an epigenetic activator of AR transcription in castration resistance prostate cancer [43]. *CLNS1A* has also been described in malignant gliomas [44], but data for breast cancer is very limited.

An interesting observation is the fact that the overexpression and amplification of these three genes was associated with detrimental prognosis in two large datasets, particularly in the luminal breast cancer subtype. Furthermore, the genomic knockdown of these transcripts reduced cell proliferation, suggesting an effect on cell growth.

Pharmacological modulation of transcription and RNA regulation is key for the optimal development of therapeutic strategies against key proteins. Spliceosome inhibitors have been developed, particularly those that bind to the HEAT repeats domain of some proteins, such as SF3B1 [45]. A comprehensive description has been recently reviewed elsewhere and beyond the scope of this article [12]. However, another approach to target this family of genes is the use of epigenetic modulators, such as BET inhibitors, to modulate transcriptional regulators or genes involved in RNA maturation. Examples have been provided with BET inhibitors, such as MK-8628 or ZEN003694 [12]. In this context, we observed that administration of the BET inhibitor JQ1 and the BET-PROTAC MZ1 reduced the expression of the three identified genes at different levels in two characteristic estrogen receptor breast cancer cell lines, MCF7 and T47D. In addition, these agents displayed a significant antiproliferative effect on these cell models. Although we agree that the antiproliferative effect of the compound could be multifactorial and the participation of these genes is a part and not a whole, we demonstrate in breast cancer that BETi can modulate the expression of splicing-related agents.

5. Conclusions

In conclusion, we describe novel splicing genes amplified in luminal breast tumors that are associated with detrimental prognosis and can be modulated pharmacologically. This data opens the door for further studies, confirming the effect of these genes in patients treated with BET inhibitors.

Supplementary Materials: The following are available online at https://www.mdpi.com/article/10.3390/cancers13164118/s1, Figure S1: Percentage of tumors with non-silent mutations for each splicing-related gene; Figure S2: Relation between expression level and CNAs for *ILF2*, *CLNS1A*, *LSM1*, and *ESRP1* genes; Figure S3: Associations of the transcriptomic fingerprint associated with amplification of *LSM1*, *CLNS1A*, and *ILF2* genes (genotype-2-outcome) and clinical outcome (OS and RFS); Figure S4: Presence of CNAs in our selected genes (*LSM1*, *CLNS1A*, and *ILF2*) in different tumor types (GDC Data Portal; 67 primary sites; Gain: red and Loss: blue); Table S1: List of splicing related genes evaluated in our study; Table S2: Percentage of tumors with mutation for each gene; Table S3: Common and specific splicing-related genes depending on molecular subtypes. Table shows the percentage of tumors with a high level of amplification for each gene (only included those with high amplification in >5%); Table S4: Prognostic value (RFS and OS) of the amplified genes (with a cutoff of >5% of tumors) in the HER2+ and Basal-like subtypes; Table S5: List of the transcripts included in the signatures associated with the CNA gain of *LSM1*, *CLNS1A*, and *ILF2*. Table S6: Univariate and Multivariate COX regression analysis to assess the potential prognostic value of CLNS1A, ILF2, and LSM1 expression in Luminal breast cancer patients.

Author Contributions: Conceptualization, M.D.L.H., A.P., V.G.-B. and A.O.; data curation, G.F.-H. and B.G.; formal analysis, M.d.M.N.-L., I.L.-C., G.F.-H., A.P., B.G., V.G.-B. and A.O.; funding acquisition, V.G.-B. and A.O.; investigation, A.M., J.Á.G.-S., P.P.-S. and M.D.L.H.; methodology, M.d.M.N.-L., I.L.-C., J.F.-A. and A.E.-S.; project administration, V.G.-B. and A.O.; resources, A.M., J.Á.G.-S., P.P.-S., M.D.L.H. and V.G.-B.; software, M.d.M.N.-L., I.L.-C., G.F.-H. and B.G.; supervision, V.G.-B. and A.O.; validation, I.L.-C., J.F.-A. and A.E.-S.; visualization, M.d.M.N.-L.; writing—original draft, M.d.M.N.-L., I.L.-C., V.G.-B. and A.O.; writing—review and editing, A.M., J.Á.G.-S., P.P.-S., M.D.L.H., A.P. and B.G. All authors have read and agreed to the published version of the manuscript.

Funding: A.O.'s lab is supported by the Instituto de Salud Carlos III (ISCIII, PI19/00808); ACEPAIN; CRIS Cancer Foundation and Diputación de Albacete. This research is also supported by PI18/01020 from the Instituto de Salud Carlos III and co-financed by the European Development Regional Fund (FEDER) "A way to achieve Europe" (ERDF); N.L. MDM was supported by the Spanish Ministry of Education (FPU grant; Ref.: FPU18/01319). B.G. was financed by the 2018-2.1.17-TET-KR-00001, 2020-1.1.6-JÖVŐ-2021-00013, and 2018-1.3.1-VKE-2018-00032 grants and by the Higher Education Institutional Excellence Programme (2020-4.1.1.-TKP2020) of the Ministry for Innovation and Technology in Hungary.

Institutional Review Board Statement: Not applicable. All the data corresponding to the breast cancer patient series used in this study are available in the public functional genomics data repository.

Informed Consent Statement: Not applicable. All the data corresponding to the breast cancer patient series used in this study are available in the public functional genomics data repository.

Data Availability Statement: All the data used in this study are available in public functional genomics data repositories (GEO, EGA, cBioportal, and TCGA).

Acknowledgments: We are grateful to Francisco J. Cimas for support in platforms about mechanism of action of drugs, and to Miguel Burgos for support in cell cycle experiments.

Conflicts of Interest: The authors declare no conflict of interest.

References

1. Dvinge, H.; Kim, E.; Abdel-Wahab, O.; Bradley, R.K. RNA splicing factors as oncoproteins and tumour suppressors. *Nat. Rev. Cancer* **2016**, *16*, 413–430. [CrossRef]
2. Xu, Y.; Zhao, W.; Olson, S.D.; Prabhkara, K.S.; Zhou, X. Alternative splicing links histone modifications to stem cell fate decision. *Genome Biol.* **2018**, *19*, 133. [CrossRef]
3. Djebali, S.; Davis, C.A.; Merkel, A.; Dobin, A.; Lassmann, T.; Mortazavi, A.; Tanzer, A.; Lagarde, J.; Lin, W.; Schlesinger, F.; et al. Landscape of transcription in human cells. *Nature* **2012**, *489*, 101–108. [CrossRef] [PubMed]
4. Kim, E.; Magen, A.; Ast, G. Different levels of alternative splicing among eukaryotes. *Nucleic Acids Res.* **2007**, *35*, 125–131. [CrossRef] [PubMed]
5. Niklas, K.J.; Bondos, S.E.; Dunker, A.K.; Newman, S.A. Rethinking gene regulatory networks in light of alternative splicing, intrinsically disordered protein domains, and post-translational modifications. *Front. Cell Dev. Biol.* **2015**, *3*, 8. [CrossRef] [PubMed]
6. Vohhodina, J.; Barros, E.M.; Savage, A.L.; Liberante, F.G.; Manti, L.; Bankhead, P.; Cosgrove, N.; Madden, A.F.; Harkin, D.P.; Savage, K.I. The RNA processing factors THRAP3 and BCLAF1 promote the DNA damage response through selective mRNA splicing and nuclear export. *Nucleic Acids Res.* **2017**, *45*, 12816–12833. [CrossRef] [PubMed]
7. Mauger, O.; Scheiffele, P. Beyond proteome diversity: Alternative splicing as a regulator of neuronal transcript dynamics. *Curr. Opin. Neurobiol.* **2017**, *45*, 162–168. [CrossRef]
8. Wang, E.; Aifantis, I. RNA Splicing and Cancer. *Trends Cancer* **2020**, *6*, 631–644. [CrossRef]
9. Wan, R.; Bai, R.; Shi, Y. Molecular choreography of pre-mRNA splicing by the spliceosome. *Curr. Opin. Struct. Biol.* **2019**, *59*, 124–133. [CrossRef]
10. Urbanski, L.; Leclair, N.; Anczuków, O. Alternative-splicing defects in cancer: Splicing regulators and their downstream targets, guiding the way to novel cancer therapeutics. *WIREs RNA* **2018**, *9*, e1476. [CrossRef]
11. El Marabti, E.; Younis, I. The Cancer Spliceome: Reprograming of Alternative Splicing in Cancer. *Front. Mol. Biosci.* **2018**, *5*, 80. [CrossRef]
12. Bonnal, S.C.; López-Oreja, I.; Valcárcel, J. Roles and mechanisms of alternative splicing in cancer—Implications for care. *Nat. Rev. Clin. Oncol.* **2020**, *17*, 457–474. [CrossRef]
13. Goodall, G.J.; Wickramasinghe, V.O. RNA in cancer. *Nat. Rev. Cancer* **2021**, *21*, 22–36. [CrossRef]
14. Fish, L.; Khoroshkin, M.; Navickas, A.; Garcia, K.; Culbertson, B.; Hänisch, B.; Zhang, S.; Nguyen, H.C.B.; Soto, L.M.; Dermit, M.; et al. A prometastatic splicing program regulated by SNRPA1 interactions with structured RNA elements. *Science* **2021**, *372*, eabc7531. [CrossRef]
15. Seiler, M.; Peng, S.; Agrawal, A.A.; Palacino, J.; Teng, T.; Zhu, P.; Smith, P.G.; Cancer Genome Atlas Research Network; Buonamici, S.; Yu, L. Somatic Mutational Landscape of Splicing Factor Genes and Their Functional Consequences across 33 Cancer Types. *Cell Rep.* **2018**, *23*, 282–296. [CrossRef]
16. Xiping, Z.; Qingshan, W.; Shuai, Z.; Hongjian, Y.; Xiaowen, D. A summary of relationships between alternative splicing and breast cancer. *Oncotarget* **2017**, *8*, 51986–51993. [CrossRef] [PubMed]
17. Pereira, B.; Chin, S.F.; Rueda, O.M.; Vollan, H.K.; Provenzano, E.; Bardwell, H.A.; Pugh, M.; Jones, L.; Russell, R.; Sammut, S.J.; et al. The somatic mutation profiles of 2433 breast cancers refines their genomic and transcriptomic landscapes. *Nat. Commun.* **2016**, *7*, 11479. [CrossRef]
18. Brian, W.D.; Helmenstine, E.; Walsh, N.; Gondek, L.P.; Kelkar, D.S.; Read, A.; Natrajan, R.; Christenson, E.S.; Roman, B.; Das, S.; et al. Hotspot SF3B1 mutations induce metabolic reprogramming and vulnerability to serine deprivation. *J. Clin. Investig.* **2019**, *129*, 4708–4723. [CrossRef]
19. Wang, Y.; Bernhardy, A.J.; Cruz, C.; Krais, J.J.; Nacson, J.; Nicolas, E.; Peri, S.; van der Gulden, H.; van der Heijden, I.; O'Brien, S.W.; et al. The BRCA1-delta11q Alternative Splice Isoform Bypasses Germline Mutations and Promotes Therapeutic Resistance to PARP Inhibition and Cisplatin. *Cancer Res.* **2016**, *76*, 2778–2790. [CrossRef] [PubMed]
20. Koedoot, E.; Wolters, L.; van de Water, B.; Le Dévédec, S.E. Splicing regulatory factors in breast cancer hallmarks and disease progression. *Oncotarget* **2019**, *10*, 6021–6037. [CrossRef]
21. Tanaka, I.; Chakraborty, A.; Saulnier, O.; Benoit-Pilven, C.; Vacher, S.; Labiod, D.; Lam, E.W.F.; Bièche, I.; Delattre, O.; Pouzoulet, F.; et al. ZRANB2 and SYF2-mediated splicing programs converging on ECT2 are involved in breast cancer cell resistance to doxorubicin. *Nucleic Acids Res.* **2020**, *48*, 2676–2693. [CrossRef]
22. Gabriel, M.; Delforge, Y.; Deward, A.; Habraken, Y.; Hennuy, B.; Piette, J.; Klinck, R.; Chabot, B.; Colige, A.; Lambert, C.; et al. Role of the splicing factor SRSF4 in cisplatin-induced modifications of pre-mRNA splicing and apoptosis. *BMC Cancer* **2015**, *15*, 227. [CrossRef]
23. Marchesini, M.; Ogoti, Y.; Fiorini, E.; Aktas Samur, A.; Nezi, L.; D'Anca, M.; Storti, P.; Samur, M.K.; Ganan-Gomez, I.; Fulciniti, M.T.; et al. ILF2 Is a Regulator of RNA Splicing and DNA Damage Response in 1q21-Amplified Multiple Myeloma. *Cancer Cell* **2017**, *32*, 88–100. [CrossRef]

24. Lobel, J.H.; Tibble, R.W.; Gross, J.D. Pat1 activates late steps in mRNA decay by multiple mechanisms. *Proc. Natl. Acad. Sci. USA* **2019**, *116*, 23512–23517. [CrossRef] [PubMed]
25. Guderian, G.; Peter, C.; Wiesner, J.; Sickmann, A.; Schulze-Osthoff, K.; Fischer, U.; Grimmler, M. RioK1, a new interactor of protein arginine methyltransferase 5 (PRMT5), competes with pICln for binding and modulates PRMT5 complex composition and substrate specificity. *J. Biol. Chem.* **2011**, *286*, 1976–1986. [CrossRef]
26. Hegele, A.; Kamburov, A.; Grossmann, A.; Sourlis, C.; Wowro, S.; Weimann, M.; Will, C.L.; Pena, V.; Lührmann, R.; Stelzlet, U. Dynamic protein-protein interaction wiring of the human spliceosome. *Mol. Cell* **2012**, *45*, 567–580. [CrossRef]
27. Mermel, C.; Schumacher, S.; Hill, B.; Meyerson, M.L.; Beroukhim, R.; Getz, G. GISTIC2.0 facilitates sensitive and confident localization of the targets of focal somatic copy-number alteration in human cancers. *Genome Biol.* **2011**, *12*, R41. [CrossRef] [PubMed]
28. Fuentes-Antrás, J.; Alcaraz-Sanabria, A.L.; Morafraile, E.C.; Noblejas-López, M.D.M.; Galán-Moya, E.M.; Baliu-Pique, M.; López-Cade, I.; García-Barberán, V.; Pérez-Segura, P.; Manzano, A.; et al. Mapping of Genomic Vulnerabilities in the Post-Translational Ubiquitination, SUMOylation and Neddylation Machinery in Breast Cancer. *Cancers* **2021**, *13*, 833. [CrossRef] [PubMed]
29. Nagy, A.; Munkacsy, G.; Győrffy, B. Pancancer survival analysis of cancer hallmark genes. *Sci. Rep.* **2021**, *11*, 6047. [CrossRef] [PubMed]
30. Pongor, L.; Kormos, M.; Hatzis, C.; Pusztai, L.; Szabó, A.; Győrffy, B. A genome-wide approach to link genotype to OS by utilizing next generation sequencing and gene chip data of 6697 breast cancer patients. *Genome Med.* **2015**, *7*, 104. [CrossRef]
31. Ciriello, G.; Gatza, M.L.; Beck, A.H.; Wilkerson, M.D.; Rhie, S.K.; Pastore, A.; Zhang, H.; McLellan, M.; Yau, C.; Kandoth, C.; et al. Comprehensive Molecular Portraits of Invasive Lobular Breast Cancer. *Cell* **2015**, *163*, 506–519. [CrossRef] [PubMed]
32. Győrffy, B.; Lanczky, A.; Eklund, A.C.; Denkert, C.; Budczies, J.; Li, Q.; Szallasi, Z. An online survival analysis tool to rapidly assess the effect of 22,277 genes on breast cancer prognosis using microarray data of 1809 patients. *Breast Cancer Res. Treat.* **2010**, *123*, 725–731. [CrossRef] [PubMed]
33. Ocaña, A.; Pandiella, A. Proteolysis targeting chimeras (PROTACs) in cancer therapy. *J. Exp. Clin. Cancer Res.* **2020**, *39*, 189. [CrossRef] [PubMed]
34. Ken-Ichi, F.; Takaki, I.; Mizuki, M.; Masashi, K.; Seiji, M. Regulating Divergent Transcriptomes through mRNA Splicing and Its Modulation Using Various Small Compounds. *Int. J. Mol. Sci.* **2020**, *21*, 2026. [CrossRef]
35. Denichenko, P.; Mogilevsky, M.; Cléry, A.; Welte, T.; Biran, J.; Shimshon, O.; Barnabas, G.D.; Danan-Gotthold, M.; Kumar, S.; Yavin, E.; et al. Specific inhibition of splicing factor activity by decoy RNA oligonucleotides. *Nat. Commun.* **2019**, *10*, 1590. [CrossRef]
36. Wang, E.; Lu, S.X.; Pastore, A.; Chen, X.; Imig, J.; Chun-Wei Lee, S.; Hockemeyer, K.; Ghebrechristos, Y.E.; Yoshimi, A.; Inoue, D.; et al. Targeting an RNA-Binding Protein Network in Acute Myeloid Leukemia. *Cancer Cell* **2019**, *35*, 369–384.e7. [CrossRef] [PubMed]
37. Pavlyukov, M.S.; Yu, H.; Bastola, S.; Minata, M.; Shender, V.O.; Lee, Y.; Zhang, S.; Wang, J.; Komarova, S.; Wang, J.; et al. Apoptotic Cell-Derived Extracellular Vesicles Promote Malignancy of Glioblastoma Via Intercellular Transfer of Splicing Factors. *Cancer Cell* **2018**, *34*, 119–135. [CrossRef]
38. Voutsadakis, I.A. 8p11.23 Amplification in Breast Cancer: Molecular Characteristics, Prognosis and Targeted Therapy. *J. Clin. Med.* **2020**, *9*, 3079. [CrossRef]
39. Kufel, J.; Bousquet-Antonelli, C.; Beggs, J.D.; Tollervey, D. Nuclear Pre-mRNA Decapping and 5′ Degradation in Yeast Require the Lsm2-8p Complex. *Mol. Cell Biol.* **2004**, *24*, 9646–9657. [CrossRef] [PubMed]
40. Tharun, S.; He, W.; Mayes, A.E.; Lennertz, P.; Beggs, J.D.; Parker, R. Yeast Sm-like proteins function in mRNA decapping and decay. *Nature* **2000**, *404*, 515–518. [CrossRef]
41. Little, E.C.; Camp, E.R.; Wang, C.; Watson, P.M.; Watson, D.K.; Cole, D.J. The CaSm (LSm1) oncogene promotes transformation, chemoresistance and metastasis of pancreatic cancer cells. *Oncogenesis* **2016**, *5*, e182. [CrossRef] [PubMed]
42. Chari, A.; Golas, M.M.; Klingenhäger, M.; Neuenkirchen, N.; Sander, B.; Englbrecht, C.; Sickmann, A.; Stark, H.; Fischer, U. An assembly chaperone collaborates with the SMN complex to generate spliceosomal SnRNPs. *Cell* **2008**, *135*, 497–509. [CrossRef]
43. Beketova, E.; Fang, S.; Owens, J.L.; Liu, S.; Chen, X.; Zhang, Q.; Asberry, A.M.; Deng, X.; Malola, J.; Huang, J.; et al. Protein Arginine Methyltransferase 5 Promotes pICln-Dependent Androgen Receptor Transcription in Castration-Resistant Prostate Cancer. *Cancer Res.* **2020**, *80*, 4904–4917. [CrossRef] [PubMed]
44. Braun, C.J.; Stanciu, M.; Boutz, P.L.; Patterson, J.C.; Calligaris, D.; Higuchi, F.; Neupane, R.; Fenoglio, S.; Cahill, D.P.; Wakimoto, H.; et al. Coordinated Splicing of Regulatory Detained Introns within Oncogenic Transcripts Creates an Exploitable Vulnerability in Malignant Glioma. *Cancer Cell* **2017**, *32*, 411–426. [CrossRef] [PubMed]
45. Read, A.; Natrajan, R. Splicing dysregulation as a driver of breast cancer. *Endocr. Relat. Cancer* **2018**, *25*, R467–R478. [CrossRef]

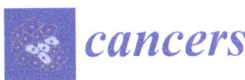

Article

Expression of Phosphorylated BRD4 Is Markedly Associated with the Activation Status of the PP2A Pathway and Shows AStrong Prognostic Value in Triple Negative Breast Cancer Patients

Marta Sanz-Álvarez [1,†], Ion Cristóbal [2,*,†], Melani Luque [1], Andrea Santos [2], Sandra Zazo [1], Juan Madoz-Gúrpide [1], Cristina Caramés [2], Cheng-Ming Chiang [3], Jesús García-Foncillas [4], Pilar Eroles [5], Joan Albanell [6] and Federico Rojo [1,*]

1. Pathology Department, Fundación Jiménez Díaz University Hospital Health Research Institute (IIS—FJD, UAM)-CIBERONC, E-28040 Madrid, Spain; marta.sanza@quironsalud.es (M.S.-Á.); melani.luque@quironsalud.es (M.L.); szazo@fjd.es (S.Z.); JMadoz@fjd.es (J.M.-G.)
2. Cancer Unit for Research on Novel Therapeutic Targets, Oncohealth Institute, IIS-Fundación Jiménez Díaz-UAM, E-28040 Madrid, Spain; andrea.santos@quironsalud.es (A.S.); ccarames@fjd.es (C.C.)
3. Departments of Biochemistry and Pharmacology, Simmons Comprehensive Cancer Center, University of Texas Southwestern Medical Center, Dallas, TX 75390, USA; chen-ming.chiang@UTSouthwestern.edu
4. Medical Oncology Department, University Hospital "Fundación Jiménez Díaz", UAM, E-28040 Madrid, Spain; jesus.garciafoncillas@oncohealth.eu
5. Institute of Health Research INCLIVA-CIBERONC, E-46010 Valencia, Spain; pilar.eroles@uv.es
6. Medical Oncology Department, Hospital del Mar-CIBERONC, E-08003 Barcelona, Spain; 96087@parcdesalutmar.cat
* Correspondence: ion.cristobal@fjd.es (I.C.); frojo@fjd.es (F.R.); Tel.: +34-915504800 (I.C. & F.R.)
† These authors have contributed equally to this work.

Simple Summary: The use of BRD4 inhibitors has emerged as a novel therapeutic approach in a wide variety of tumors including the triple negative breast cancer. Moreover, PP2A has been proposed as the phosphatase involved in regulating BRD4 phosphorylation and stabilization. Our aim was to evaluate for the first time the clinical impact of BRD4 phosphorylation in triple negative breast cancer patients and as well as its potential linking with the PP2A activation status in this disease. Our findings are special relevant since they suggest the prognostic value of BRD4 phosphorylation levels, and the potential clinical usefulness of PP2A inhibition markers to anticipate response to BRD4 inhibitors.

Abstract: The bromodomain-containing protein 4 (BRD4), a member of the bromodomain and extra-terminal domain (BET) protein family, has emerged in the last years as a promising molecular target in many tumors including breast cancer. The triple negative breast cancer (TNBC) represents the molecular subtype with the worst prognosis and a current therapeutic challenge, and TNBC cells have been reported to show a preferential sensitivity to BET inhibitors. Interestingly, BRD4 phosphorylation (pBRD4) was found as an alteration that confers resistance to BET inhibition and PP2A proposed as the phosphatase responsible to regulate pBRD4 levels. However, the potential clinical significance of pBRD4, as well as its potential correlation with the PP2A pathway in TNBC, remains to be investigated. Here, we evaluated the expression levels of pBRD4 in a series of 132 TNBC patients. We found high pBRD4 levels in 34.1% of cases (45/132), and this alteration was found to be associated with the development of patient recurrences ($p = 0.007$). Interestingly, BRD4 hyperphosphorylation predicted significantly shorter overall ($p < 0.001$) and event-free survival ($p < 0.001$). Moreover, multivariate analyses were performed to confirm its independent prognostic impact in our cohort. In conclusion, our findings show that BRD4 hyperphosphorylation is an alteration associated with PP2A inhibition that defines a subgroup of TNBC patients with unfavorable prognosis, suggesting the potential clinical and therapeutic usefulness of the PP2A/BRD4 axis as a novel molecular target to overcome resistance to treatments based on BRD4 inhibition.

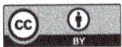

Keywords: pBRD4; SET; PP2A; prognosis; triple negative breast cancer

1. Introduction

Breast cancer has the highest prevalence in cancer diagnosis and represents the second leading cause of female cancer-related deaths [1]. Breast cancer is a very heterogeneous disease, with different molecular subtypes including luminal A, luminal B, HER2+, basal and normal-like tumors [2,3]. The triple negative breast cancer (TNBC) is molecularly characterized by the lack of hormonal receptors expression (estrogen (ER) and progesterone receptors (PR)), and by an absence of expression of the HER2 receptor [3]. TNBC represents 15–20% of all breast carcinomas [4] and shows more aggressive features such as emergence at a younger age, higher tumor size and grade, and greater proportion of positive lymph node metastases. TNBC has been largely described as the breast cancer subtype with the worst overall and progression-free survival rates, and represents a major challenge for current clinical management due to the lack of established and effective therapeutic strategies [5,6]. TNBC cells have very aggressive behavior that leads to a shorter time of disease progression. In fact, TNBCs show the highest recurrence rates, with brain and visceral organs as the main metastatic niches [7]. Triple negative tumors are heterogeneous at the molecular level, and *TP53*, *PIK3CA*, *PTEN*, *RB1*, *EGFR* and *MYC* have been reported as the most commonly mutated genes [8,9]. However, it remains urgent to improve our understanding about the molecular alterations that govern TNBC progression in order to develop novel therapeutic strategies for this disease.

Bromodomain-containing protein 4 (BRD4) is a member of the bromodomain and extra-terminal domain (BET) protein family, along with BRD2, BRD3, and BRDT. BRD4 is structurally composed of two N-terminal bromodomain domains (BD1 and BD2), and a C-terminal extra-terminal domain. BD1 and BD2 allow for the formation of a hydrophobic pocket that binds to acetylated lysine residues of histones or transcription factors [10,11], ultimately regulating a wide variety of cell functions. Specifically, BRD4 is involved in chromatin decompaction, the recruitment of components of the transcriptional complex, as well as in the stages of initiation, release pause and elongation of transcription due to its interaction with PTEF-b that phosphorylates RNA Pol II [10]. Due to its role in important cellular processes, BRD4 dysfunction can lead to the appearance of various human diseases, including inflammation, cardiovascular diseases and cancer [10–12]. BRD4 has been found to play oncogenic roles in many hematological and solid tumors, including melanoma, prostate and breast cancer among others, and has been proposed as a druggable promising target in human cancer [12–16]. BRD4 has been shown to regulate the expression of different set of oncogenic drivers, such as c-MYC [13], NF-κB [16] or Jagged1 [17]. In breast cancer, several BRD4 alterations involved in the different molecular subtypes have been reported to date. Thus, BRD4 activity has been found to be required for proliferation and ERα function in ER+ breast cancer cells [18], and promotes the migration and invasion of triple negative tumors through controlling Jagged1 expression [17]. Regarding its post-translational modifications, CK2-mediated BRD4 hyperphosphorylation has been associated with greater stability and nuclear localization of the BRD4 protein [19], with important functional and therapeutic implications in TNBC [20,21]. In fact, the therapeutic value of BRD4 inhibition in TNBC has been previously reported by Shu and co-workers [21], analyzing a set of BRD4 inhibitors across a panel of cell lines with different breast cancer subtypes, observing that these drugs showed the strongest antitumor effects in the triple negative subtype. These results were confirmed in vivo using primary human TNBC xenografts. After an exhaustive analysis of potential mechanisms of drug resistance, BRD4 was identified as a novel PP2A target and its hyperphosphorylation as an alteration that promotes resistance to BRD4 inhibition in TNBC cells.

In the last years, several studies have evaluated distinct therapeutic approaches related to targeting BRD4 in TNBC. It has been reported promising antitumor properties using cell-penetrating peptides including EGFR and BRD4 siRNAs in TNBC cells [22], or a dual-target small-molecule inhibitor co-targeting PARP1 and BRD4 [23]. Moreover, it has been described that BRD4 regulates PD-L1 expression in TNBC cells, which could have interesting implication for immunotherapy-based treatments [24], or the therapeutic usefulness of strategies based on BRD4 inhibition, due to its role as regulator of the oncogenic c-MYC pathway in this disease [25,26].

Altogether, the different studies in the literature regarding BRD4 in TNBC highlight its promising therapeutic value. However, little is known about its clinical impact as well as the functional and therapeutic significance of pBRD4 in this disease. Moreover, the relevance of the PP2A pathway as a potential regulator of pBRD4 remains to be investigated and confirmed in TNBC patient cohorts.

2. Experimental Section

2.1. Patient Samples

A total number of 132 surgical resection specimens from patients diagnosed with primary breast cancer were included in this study. Formalin-fixed paraffin-embedded breast tumor specimens from this patient cohort were retrospectively selected from Fundación Jiménez Díaz Biobank (Madrid, Spain) following these criteria: infiltrating carcinomas, operable, enough available tissue, molecular and/or clinical follow-up data and triple negative subtype. Clinical data were collected from medical clinical records by oncologists. Samples were taken anonymously. TNM (tumor–node–metastasis) staging classification was performed using the American Joint Committee on Cancer (AJCC) staging system. The Scarff–Bloom–Richardson modified by Elston criteria [27] was used to define the histological grade. Two independent pathologists who were blinded to patient outcomes evaluated tumor tissue staining.

2.2. Determination of the Molecular Subtype

We evaluated the expression of hormonal receptors as well as HER2 to define the molecular subtype and confirm that all patients included in this study have triple negative breast tumors. The expression of both estrogen receptor (ER) and progesterone receptor (PR) were determined by immunohistochemistry (IHC) (SP1 and PgR636 clones, respectively; Dako, Carpinteria, CA, USA), establishing positivity criteria in >1% of nuclear tumor staining [28]. Determination of HER2 amplification was carried out by FISH (Pathvysion; Abbott Laboratories, Green Oaks, IL, USA) [29].

2.3. Ethics Approval and Consent to Participate

This study was conducted in full accordance with the guidelines for Good Clinical Practice and the Declaration of Helsinki. All participants gave written informed consent for tissue storage and analysis at Fundación Jiménez Díaz biobank, Madrid (Spain). The ethical committee institutional review board of Fundación Jiménez Díaz University Hospital reviewed and approved the project (ref. PIC 13-2016).

2.4. Immunohistochemistry

Representative areas of each tumor were carefully selected, and three tissue cores (1mm diameter) were obtained using a tissue microarray (TMA) workstation (T1000 Chemicon). Immunostainings were performed on tissue sections (3 μM) obtained from FFPE tumors, as previously described [30]. Expression levels of Ki-67 were studied by IHC using the MIB1 clone (Dako, Carpinteria, CA, USA) [31]. High proliferation in our breast cancer patient cohort based on Ki-67 labelling by IHC has been defined following the 13th St Gallen International Breast Cancer Conference (2013) criteria based on a threshold $\geq 20\%$ of proliferation [32]. Other antibodies used were: pBRD4 (developed and kindly provided by Prof. Chiang's laboratory) [19,21], rabbit polyclonal anti-SET (ab1183) (Abcam, Cambridge, UK) and rabbit monoclonal anti-PP2AY307 (1155-1) (Abcam, Cambridge, UK). Antibody dilutions were as follows: pBRD4 (1:100), SET (1:5000), and phospho-

PPP2CA (pPPP2CA) (1:2000). pBRD4, SET and pPPP2CA expression blinded to clinical data was evaluated by two pathologists (F.R. and S.Z.). The specific phosphorylation sites recognized by the antibodies were Y307 for PPP2CA and S484/488 for BRD4. A semiquantitative histoscore (Hscore) was calculated by estimation of the percentage of tumor cells positively stained with low, medium, or high staining intensity. The final score was determined after applying a weighting factor to each estimate. The formula used was Hscore = (low%) × 1 + (medium%) × 2 + (high%) × 3, and the results ranged from 0 to 300.

2.5. Statistical Analysis

Statistical analyses were performed using SPSS20 for windows (SPSS Inc, Chicago IL, USA). We applied the χ^2 test (Fisher exact test) based on bimodal distribution of data to evaluate the significance of potential associations between BRD4 phosphorylation and the molecular and clinical characteristics of the tumor specimens included in this study.

Overall survival (OS) was defined as the time from diagnosis to the date of death from any cause or last follow-up. Event-free survival(EFS) was defined as the time from the date of diagnosis until relapse at any location, death or last follow-up. Kaplan–Meier plots and survival comparisons were carried out using the log-rank test if the proportional hazard assumption was fulfilled, and Breslow otherwise. The Cox proportional hazards model was adjusted taking into consideration significant parameters in the univariate analysis. A receiver operating characteristic (ROC) curve was used to determine the optimal cutoff point based on progression end point for pBRD4 as previously described [33,34]. p-Value less than 0.05 was considered statistically significant. This work was carried out in accordance with Reporting Recommendations for Tumor Marker Prognostic Studies(REMARK) guidelines [35].

3. Results

3.1. Prevalence of BRD4 Hyperphosphorylation in Triple Negative Breast Cancer Patients and Its Association with Molecular and Clinical Parameters

To investigate the prevalence and potential clinical impact of pBRD4 in TNBC, we analyzed the expression of pBRD4 by immunohistochemistry in a cohort of 132 patients with early breast cancer and triple negative subtype, observing high pBRD4 levels in 45 of 132 of cases (34.1%). Patient characteristics are presented in Table S1. We next correlated pBRD4 expression with molecular and clinical features of our patient cohort. Interestingly, high pBRD4 levels were found to be strongly associated with the subgroup of patients who relapsed ($p = 0.007$). Associations between pBRD4 status and clinical and molecular characteristics are shown in Table 1.

3.2. Clinical Impact of pBRD4 in Triple Negative Breast Cancer

We analyzed the clinical significance of pBRD4 in the same cohort of 132 TNBC patients. Clinical follow-up data were available in all cases. The median of age was 57 years (with an age range of 31 to 90 years). Interestingly, we found that the subgroup of high pBRD4 expressing patients had a markedly shorter OS ($p < 0.001$) (Figure 1A). Moreover, we observed that pBRD4 also had predictive value for EFS in our patient cohort ($p < 0.001$) (Figure 1B).

Interestingly, multivariate Cox analysis showed that high pBRD4 expression is an unfavorable independent factor associated with patient outcome in our cohort (Hazard ratio (HR) = 5.342; 95% confidence interval (CI), 2.286–12.482; $p < 0.001$) (Table 2).

Table 1. Association of bromodomain-containing protein 4 (BRD4) phosphorylation levels with molecular and clinical parameters in a cohort of 132 triple negative breast cancer (TNBC) patients.

Parameters	No. Cases	No. Low pBRD4	(%)	No. High pBRD4	(%)	p
pBRD4	132	87	(65.9)	45	(34.1)	
Hormonal status	132	87		45		0.261
Premenopausal	36	21	(24.1)	15	(33.3)	
Postmenopausal	96	66	(75.9)	30	(66.7)	
Morphological type	131	86		45		0.427
IDC [1]	122	79	(91.9)	43	(95.6)	
ILC [2]	9	7	(8.1)	2	(4.4)	
T [3]	132	87		45		0.377
1	54	32	(36.8)	22	(48.9)	
2	60	43	(49.4)	17	(37.8)	
3–4	18	12	(13.8)	6	(13.3)	
N [4]	132	87		45		0.457
0	77	52	(59.8)	25	(55.6)	
1	33	19	(21.8)	14	(31.1)	
2–3	22	16	(18.4)	6	(13.3)	
Stage	132	87		45		0.865
I	39	25	(28.7)	14	(31.1)	
II	60	41	(47.1)	19	(42.2)	
III	33	21	(24.2)	12	(27.7)	
Grade	132	87		45		0.448
Low/Moderate	47	29	(33.3)	18	(40)	
High	85	58	(66.7)	27	(60)	
Relapse	132	87		45		0.007
No	98	8	(81.6)	6	(60)	
Yes	34	4	(18.4)	0	(40)	
Ki-67	66	37		29		0.307
Low	34	17	(45.9)	17	(58.6)	
High	32	20	(54.1)	12	(41.4)	

IDC [1] = invasive ductal carcinoma; ILC [2] = invasive lobular carcinoma; T [3] = tumor size; N [4] = lymph node metastases.

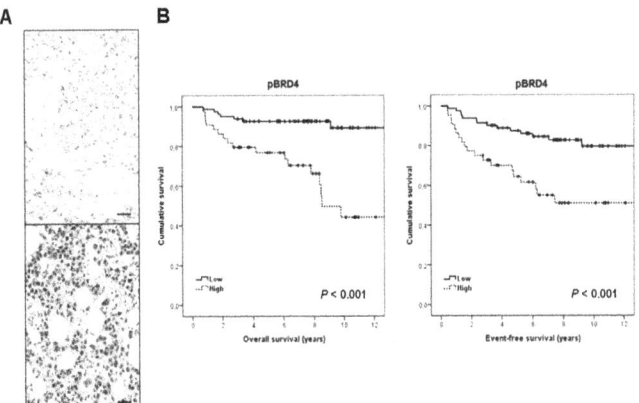

Figure 1. Clinical significance of pBRD4 in TNBC. (**A**) Immunohistochemical images showing pBRD4 positive and negative staining. The line shows 25 µm. Original magnification ×400, (**B**) Kaplan–Meieranalysesof overall survival(OS) and event-free survival(EFS) in a cohort of 132 TNBC patients.

Table 2. Univariate and multivariate Cox analyses in the cohort of 132 TNBC patients.

Parameters		Univariate OS [1] Analysis				Multivariate OS Cox Analysis			
		HR [3]	95% CI [2]		p	HR	95% CI		p
			Lower	Upper			Lower	Upper	
T [4]					0.063				-
	0–1	1.000							
	2–3	2.280	0.957 to 5.433			-	-		
N [5]					0.014				0.100
	-	1.000				1.000			
	+	2.286	1.180 to 4.429			1.983	0.877 to 4.484		
Grade					0.470				-
	L/M [6]	1.000							
	High	1.366	0.586 to 3.182			-	-		
Stage					0.049				0.195
	I–II	1.000				1.000			
	III	2.935	1.006 to 8.564			2.174	0.672 to 7.033		
Ki-67					0.864				
	Low	1.000							
	High	1.091	0.402 to 2.962						
pBRD4					<0.001				<0.001
	Low	1.000				1.000			
	High	5.016	2.155 to 11.676			5.342	2.286 to 12.482		

OS [1]: overall survival; CI [2]: confidence interval; HR [3]: Hazard ratio; T [4] = tumor size; N [5] = lymph node metastases; L/M [6]: low/moderate.

To further evaluate the prognostic value of pBRD4 in TNBC, we stratified our patient cohort by stage. Of note, we observed that relevance of high pBRD4 expression levels as a biomarker predictor of poor outcome was retained in all cases for both OS and EFS, but the significance was particularly marked in the subgroup of TNBC patients with stage III ($p < 0.001$ for OS, and $p = 0.001$ for EFS), compared to those with stages I-II ($p = 0.005$ for OS, and $p = 0.017$ for EFS) (Supplementary Materials Figure S1).

3.3. BRD4 Phosphorylation Is Associated with the Activation Status of the PP2A Pathway

We next studied the molecular mechanisms that could be involved in BRD4 hyperphosphorylation. Due to BRD4 having been previously proposed as a direct target of the tumor suppressor protein phosphatase 2A (PP2A) in TNBC, the activation status of this phosphatase was evaluated in our patient series. The phosphorylation of the PP2A catalytic subunit in its tyrosine 307, as well as the overexpression of endogenous inhibitors such as SET, have been reported as major contributing alterations to inhibit PP2A in human cancer. Thus, we analyzed both pPPP2CA and SET levels in 128 TNBC cases from our cohort with enough material available. High pPPP2CA expression was found in 31 out of 128 cases (24.2%), whereas 17 out of 128 cases (13.3%) showed SET overexpression. Interestingly, we found that high pBRD4 expression was strongly associated with both PP2A hyperphosphorylation ($p < 0.001$) and SET overexpression ($p < 0.001$) (Table 3), which highlights that PP2A inhibition could be a key molecular mechanism to maintain BRD4 phosphorylation in TNBC.

Since pPPP2CA and SET have been described to be associated alterations, we analyzed how many patients had a concomitant PP2A hyperphosphorylation and SET overexpression. As expected, we observed a significant correlation between both alterations ($p < 0.001$), which were found in 12 cases from our series (Table S2). Moreover, we also analyzed the prognostic value of pPPP2CA in our patient cohort. As expected, those patients with high pPPP2CA expression levels showed a significantly worse OS ($p < 0.001$) and EFS ($p < 0.001$) (Figure S2).

Table 3. Association between pBRD4 expression and PP2A activation status in TNBC patients.

pBRD4	No. Cases	No. Low pBRD4(%)		No. High pBRD4(%)		p
pPPP2CA	128	87		41		<0.001
Low	97	85	(97.7)	12	(29.3)	
High	31	2	(2.3)	29	(70.7)	
SET	128	87		41		<0.001
Low	111	87	(100)	24	(58.5)	
High	17	0	(0)	17	(41.5)	

4. Discussion

The TNBC subtype has been previously reported to be particularly sensitive to the treatment with bromodomain inhibitors. In addition, BRD4 hyperphosphorylation has been defined as a molecular alteration that promotes resistance to BRD4 inhibitors, and the tumor suppressor PP2A as the major regulator of BRD4 dephosphorylation. However, the potential clinical impact of this pBRD4 together with the validation of its linking with the PP2A activation status remain to be fully clarified in TNBC patients. It has been recently reported that BRD4 expression is significantly higher in breast cancer tissues than in normal controls, and defines poor prognosis in breast cancer patients [36]. These results would further strengthen our findings in the present study, especially considering that BRD4 phosphorylation has been described as an alteration involved in BRD4 protein stabilization [21]. Moreover, we observed that the prognostic impact of pBRD4 was particularly evident in stage III TNBC patients (Figure S1). This observation, together with the fact that this alteration is associated with recurrence (Table 1), would suggest that BRD4 hyperphosphorylation could be an event with functional relevance in TNBC progression. Thus, its evaluation in a TNBC cohort with metastatic disease would be of high interest in forthcoming studies.

The fact that decreased PP2A activity has been described to induce in vitro BRD4 hyperphosphorylation and resistance to BRD4 inhibition [21] prompted us to analyze the PP2A activation status in our patient cohort. PP2A is a key tumor suppressor commonly deregulated in human cancer [37]. PP2A hyperphosphorylation, as well as upregulation of the endogenous PP2A inhibitors such as SET, has been reported as main molecular mechanisms of PP2A inhibition in many tumors including breast cancer. These alterations have progressively emerged as promising therapeutic targets in this disease [38–44]. Although it has been recently reported that PP2A inhibition is a frequent alteration in breast cancer related with poor outcome and therapy resistance, such studies have been carried out in cohorts including cases with different molecular subtypes [40,45,46]. Therefore, the evaluation of the precise PP2A status in a cohort of TNBC patients as well as its clinical impact in this breast cancer subtype remains still to be performed. Previous works have shown that the PP2A inhibitor CIP2A confers poor outcome in TNBC cells, which has been recently confirmed in the work by Tawab Osman and co-workers [47–49]. These findings would suggest that PP2A inhibition could be of relevance in this breast cancer subtype. In fact, we found in this work that high pPPP2CA were predictor of poor outcome in our TNBC patient cohort (Figure S2). We observed PP2A hyperphosphorylation in 24.2% of cases (31/128) and SET overexpression in 13.3% of cases (17/128). Both alterations were present in 12 patients from our cohort, indicating that 5 patients had SET overexpression without high pPPP2CA expression, and 19 cases only showed high pPPP2CA levels. Thus, 82.9% of cases (34/41) with BRD4 hyperphosphorylated had at least one of the PP2A inhibitory markers altered. Therefore, our results suggest that both PP2A hyperphosphorylation and SET overexpression could be molecular contributing alterations to enhance BRD4 phosphorylation levels in TNBC, but it remains to be experimentally confirmed. Only 2 out of 31 cases with high pPPP2CA had low pBRD4 expression. However, the observation that 7 pBRD4 overexpressing patients without any PP2A inhibitory alteration detected would also indicate the potential existence of alternative PP2A inhibitory alterations or molecular mechanisms distinct that PP2A inhibition that deregulate pBRD4 in this disease.

Altogether, these results are in concordance with the conclusions reported by Shu and co-workers [21] identifying PP2A as the phosphatase responsible of dephosphorylating BRD4. However, they did not observe prognostic value for pBRD4 and discrepancies in clinical impact may be due to sample size and the fact that those authors stratified their cohort by pBRD4 expression using a median split of pBRD4 intensity.

Furthermore, these findings are of therapeutic relevance, since the use of PP2A activators could serve to overcome a foreseeable development of resistance to BRD4 inhibitors in TNBC patients with high pBRD4 levels. In fact, Shu and co-workers showed that the combination of the PP2A activator perphenazine with JQ1 served to overcome resistance to BRD4 inhibitors in TNBC cells [21]. In this line of thinking, FTY720 is an FDA-approved immunosuppressant used to treat multiple sclerosis, which has shown potent antitumor effects in many tumor types [50]. Moreover, FTY720 has been described as a PP2A activating drug through targeting pPPP2CA and SET, which are the PP2A inhibitory alterations reported in this work. Another relevant issue is the fact that BRD4 is expressed in two major isoforms, short and long, that have been reported to play opposite functions as regulators of gene transcription and tumor progression [51]. The antibody used in our work recognizes phosphorylation on S484/488, which is a region present in both BRD4 isoforms. Therefore, we analyzed here by IHC the total levels of pBRD4 expression, corresponding to the contribution of the long and short BRD4 isoforms. However, it would be of high interest to investigate the potential functional and clinical implications derived from the phosphorylation of each BRD4 isoform separately. Altogether, our results show that high pBRD4 levels define a subgroup of TNBC cases with very poor outcomes. Moreover, our findings are consistent with PP2A inhibition as a key molecular mechanism to induce BRD4 hyperphosphorylation in TNBC patients, which could benefit from a future inclusion of PP2A activators and BRD4 inhibitors in clinical protocols. Moreover, it would be of high interest to study the potential benefit derived from the clinical use of PP2A activators to anticipate and overcome the development of resistance to BRD4 inhibition in TNBC.

5. Conclusions

In conclusion, BRD4 hyperphosphorylation is a frequent alteration that associates with patient recurrence and independently predicts shorter OS and EFS in TNBC patients. Moreover, we observe a molecular background based on PP2A inhibition as the potential molecular mechanism that contributes to enhanced pBRD4 levels. Altogether, our findings highlight the clinical impact of pBRD4, as well as the PP2A/pBRD4 signaling axis as a novel therapeutic target in TNBC, which needs to be fully confirmed in forthcoming studies.

Supplementary Materials: The following are available online at https://www.mdpi.com/2072-6694/13/6/1246/s1, Figure S1: Clinical impact of pBRD4 in the cohort of 132 TNBC patients stratified by stage in (A) OS and (B) EFS, Figure S2: Clinical impact of pPPP2CA in the cohort of 132 TNBC patients in (A) OS and (B) EFS, Table S1: Clinical and molecular characteristics in a series of 132 TNBC patients, Table S2: Association between SET and pPPP2CA expression levels in TNBC.

Author Contributions: Conceptualization, I.C., J.G.-F. and F.R.; methodology, M.S.-Á., I.C., A.S., S.Z. and M.L.; software, M.S.-Á., I.C. and C.C.; formal analysis, M.S.-Á., I.C. and M.L.; investigation, M.S.-Á., I.C., A.S., M.L.; C.-M.C., writing—original draft preparation, M.S.-Á., I.C. and C.C.; writing—review and editing, J.M.-G., P.E., J.A. and F.R.; funding acquisition, F.R. and J.G.-F. All authors have read and agreed to the published version of the manuscript.

Funding: This research was funded by PI18/00382 and PI16/01468 grants from "Instituto de Salud Carlos III FEDER". M.S-A. is supported by "Fundación Conchita Rábago de Jiménez Díaz".

Institutional Review Board Statement: The study was conducted according to the guidelines of the Declaration of Helsinki, and approved by the Institutional Review Board of Fundación Jiménez Díaz University Hospital (ref. PIC 13-2016).

Informed Consent Statement: Informed consent was obtained from all subjects involved in the study.

Data Availability Statement: Data sharing is not applicable for this article.

Acknowledgments: We especially thank the Fundación Jiménez Díaz Biobank for their exceptional work in sample collection and organization.

Conflicts of Interest: The authors declare no conflict of interest.

References

1. Siegel, R.L.; Miller, K.D.; Jemal, A. Cancer Statistics, 2019. *CA Cancer J. Clin.* **2019**, *69*, 7–34. [CrossRef]
2. Sorlie, T.; Perou, C.M.; Tibshirani, R.; Aas, T.; Geisler, S.; Johnsen, H.; Hastie, T.; Eisen, M.B.; Van De Rijn, M.; Jeffrey, S.S.; et al. Gene Expression Patterns of Breast Carcinomas Distinguish Tumor Subclasses with Clinical Implications. *Proc. Natl. Acad. Sci. USA* **2001**, *98*, 10869–10874. [CrossRef] [PubMed]
3. Perou, C.M.; Sørlie, T.; Eisen, M.B.; van de Rijn, M.; Jeffrey, S.S.; Rees, C.A.; Pollack, J.R.; Ross, D.T.; Johnsen, H.; Akslen, L.A.; et al. Molecular Portraits of Human Breast Tu-mours. *Nature* **2000**, *406*, 747–752. [CrossRef] [PubMed]
4. Anders, C.; Carey, L.A. Understanding and treating triple-negative breast cancer. *Oncology* **2008**, *22*, 1233–1243. [PubMed]
5. Dent, R.; Trudeau, M.; Pritchard, K.I.; Hanna, W.M.; Kahn, H.K.; Sawka, C.A.; Lickley, L.A.; Rawlinson, E.; Sun, P.; Narod, S.A. Triple-Negative Breast Cancer: Clinical Features and Patterns of Recurrence. *Clin. Cancer Res.* **2007**, *13*, 4429–4434. [CrossRef] [PubMed]
6. Li, X.; Yang, J.; Peng, L.; Sahin, A.A.; Huo, L.; Ward, K.C.; O'Regan, R.; Torres, M.A.; Meisel, J.L. Triple-negative breast cancer has worse overall survival and cause-specific survival than non-triple-negative breast cancer. *Breast Cancer Res. Treat.* **2017**, *161*, 279–287. [CrossRef]
7. Lin, N.U.; Claus, E.; Sohl, J.; Razzak, A.R.; Arnaout, A.; Winer, E.P. Sites of Distant Recurrence and Clinical Outcomes in Patients with Metastatic Triple-Negative Breast Cancer: High Incidence of Central Nervous System Metastases. *Cancer* **2008**, *113*, 2638–2645. [CrossRef] [PubMed]
8. Bareche, Y.; Venet, D.; Ignatiadis, M.; Aftimos, P.; Piccart, M.; Rothe, F.; Sotiriou, C. Unravelling triple-negative breast cancer molecular heterogeneity using an integrative multiomic analysis. *Ann. Oncol.* **2018**, *29*, 895–902. [CrossRef]
9. Lehmann, B.D.; Pietenpol, J.A. Clinical implications of molecular heterogeneity in triple negative breast cancer. *Breast* **2015**, *24*, S36–S40. [CrossRef]
10. Huang, B.; Yang, X.-D.; Zhou, M.-M.; Ozato, K.; Chen, L.-F. Brd4 Coactivates Transcriptional Activation of NF-KB via Specific Binding to Acetylated RelA. *Mol. Cell Biol.* **2009**, *29*, 13. [CrossRef]
11. Zhu, W.; Wu, R.-D.; Lv, Y.-G.; Liu, Y.-M.; Huang, H.; Xu, J.-Q. BRD4 blockage alleviates pathological cardiac hypertrophy through the suppression of fibrosis and inflammation via reducing ROS generation. *Biomed. Pharmacother.* **2020**, *121*, 109368. [CrossRef] [PubMed]
12. Shi, Y.; Liu, J.; Zhao, Y.; Cao, J.; Li, Y.; Guo, F. Bromodomain-Containing Protein 4: A Druggable Target. *Curr. Drug Targets* **2019**, *20*, 1517–1536. [CrossRef]
13. Zuber, J.; Shi, J.; Wang, E.; Rappaport, A.R.; Herrmann, H.; Sison, E.A.; Magoon, D.; Qi, J.; Blatt, K.; Wunderlich, M.; et al. RNAi screen identifies Brd4 as a therapeutic target in acute myeloid leukaemia. *Nat. Cell Biol.* **2011**, *478*, 524–528. [CrossRef]
14. Segura, M.F.; Fontanals-Cirera, B.; Gaziel-Sovran, A.; Guijarro, M.V.; Hanniford, D.; Zhang, G.; Gonzalez-Gomez, P.; Morante, M.; Jubierre, L.; Zhang, W.; et al. BRD4 Sustains Mela-noma Proliferation and Represents a New Target for Epigenetic Therapy. *Cancer Res.* **2013**, *73*, 6264–6276. [CrossRef]
15. Tan, Y.; Wang, L.; Du, Y.; Liu, X.; Chen, Z.; Weng, X.; Guo, J.; Chen, H.; Wang, M.; Wang, X. Inhibition of BRD4 suppresses tumor growth in prostate cancer via the enhancement of FOXO1 expression. *Int. J. Oncol.* **2018**, *53*, 2503–2517. [CrossRef]
16. Zou, Z.; Huang, B.; Wu, X.; Zhang, H.; Qi, J.; Bradner, J.; Nair, S.; Chen, L.-F. Brd4 Maintains Constitutively Active NF-KB in Cancer Cells by Binding to Acetylated RelA. *Oncogene* **2014**, *33*, 2395–2404. [CrossRef] [PubMed]
17. Andrieu, G.; Tran, A.H.; Strissel, K.J.; Denis, G.V. BRD4 Regulates Breast Cancer Dissemination through Jagged1/Notch1 Signaling. *Cancer Res.* **2016**, *76*, 6555–6567. [CrossRef] [PubMed]
18. Nagarajan, S.; Hossan, T.; Alawi, M.; Najafova, Z.; Indenbirken, D.; Bedi, U.; Taipaleenmäki, H.; Ben-Batalla, I.; Scheller, M.; Loges, S.; et al. Bromodomain Protein BRD4 Is Required for Estrogen Receptor-Dependent Enhancer Activation and Gene Transcription. *Cell Rep.* **2014**, *8*, 460–469. [CrossRef]
19. Wu, S.-Y.; Lee, A.-Y.; Lai, H.-T.; Zhang, H.; Chiang, C.-M. Phospho Switch Triggers Brd4 Chromatin Binding and Activator Recruitment for Gene-Specific Targeting. *Mol. Cell* **2013**, *49*, 843–857. [CrossRef] [PubMed]
20. Wang, R.; Cao, X.-J.; Kulej, K.; Liu, W.; Ma, T.; Macdonald, M.; Chiang, C.-M.; Garcia, B.A.; You, J. Uncovering BRD4 hyperphosphorylation associated with cellular transformation in NUT midline carcinoma. *Proc. Natl. Acad. Sci. USA* **2017**, *114*, E5352–E5361. [CrossRef] [PubMed]
21. Shu, S.; Lin, C.Y.; He, H.H.; Witwicki, R.M.; Tabassum, D.P.; Roberts, J.M.; Janiszewska, M.; Huh, S.J.; Liang, Y.; Ryan, J.; et al. Response and Resistance to BET Bromo-domain Inhibitors in Triple-Negative Breast Cancer. *Nature* **2016**, *529*, 413–417. [CrossRef] [PubMed]
22. Zhang, C.; Yuan, W.; Wu, Y.; Wan, X.; Gong, Y. Co-delivery of EGFR and BRD4 siRNA by cell-penetrating peptides-modified redox-responsive complex in triple negative breast cancer cells. *Life Sci.* **2021**, *266*, 118886. [CrossRef] [PubMed]
23. Chang, X.; Sun, D.; Shi, D.; Wang, G.; Chen, Y.; Zhang, K.; Tan, H.; Liu, J.; Liu, B.; Ouyang, L. Design, synthesis, and biological evaluation of quinazolin-4(3H)-one derivatives co-targeting poly(ADP-ribose) polymerase-1 and bromodomain containing protein 4 for breast cancer therapy. *Acta Pharm. Sin. B* **2021**, *11*, 156–180. [CrossRef]

24. Jing, X.; Shao, S.; Zhang, Y.; Luo, A.; Zhao, L.; Zhang, L.; Gu, S.; Zhao, X. BRD4 inhibition suppresses PD-L1 expression in triple-negative breast cancer. *Exp. Cell Res.* **2020**, *392*, 112034. [CrossRef]
25. Tian, Y.; Wang, X.; Zhao, S.; Liao, X.; Younis, M.R.; Wang, S.; Zhang, C.; Lu, G. JQ1-Loaded Polydopamine Nanoplatform Inhibits c-MYC/Programmed Cell Death Ligand 1 to Enhance Photothermal Therapy for Triple-Negative Breast Cancer. *ACS Appl. Mater. Interfaces* **2019**, *11*, 46626–46636. [CrossRef]
26. Zhang, Y.; Xu, B.; Shi, J.; Li, J.; Lu, X.; Xu, L.; Yang, H.; Hamad, N.; Wang, C.; Napier, D.; et al. BRD4 modulates vulnerability of triple-negative breast cancer to targeting of integrin-dependent signaling pathways. *Cell. Oncol.* **2020**, *43*, 1049–1066. [CrossRef]
27. Elston, C.; Ellis, I. Pathological prognostic factors in breast cancer. I. The value of histological grade in breast cancer: Experience from a large study with long-term follow-up. *Histopathology* **1991**, *19*, 403–410. [CrossRef] [PubMed]
28. Wolff, A.C.; Hammond, M.E.H.; Schwartz, J.N.; Hagerty, K.L.; Allred, D.C.; Cote, R.J.; Dowsett, M.; Fitzgibbons, P.L.; Hanna, W.M.; Langer, A.; et al. American Society of Clinical Oncol-ogy/College Of American Pathologists guideline recommendations for immunohistochemical testing of estrogen and proges-terone receptors in breast cancer. *J. Clin. Oncol.* **2010**, *28*, 2784–2795.
29. Wolff, A.C.; Hammond, M.E.H.; Hicks, D.G.; Dowsett, M.; McShane, L.M.; Allison, K.H.; Allred, D.C.; Bartlett, J.M.; Bilous, M.; Fitzgibbons, P.; et al. Recommendations for Human Epidermal Growth Factor Receptor 2 Testing in Breast Cancer: American Society of Clinical Oncology/College of American Pathologists Clinical Practice Guideline Update. *J. Clin. Oncol.* **2013**, *31*, 3997–4013. [CrossRef]
30. Rojo, F.; González-Navarrete, I.; Bragado, R.; Dalmases, A.; Menéndez, S.; Cortes-Sempere, M. Mitogen-activated pro-tein kinase phosphatase-1 in human breast cancer independently predicts prognosis and is repressed by doxorubicin. *Clin. Cancer Res.* **2009**, *15*, 3530–3539. [CrossRef]
31. Dowsett, M.; Nielsen, T.O.; A'Hern, R.; Bartlett, J.; Coombes, R.C.; Cuzick, J.; Ellis, M.; Henry, N.L.; Hugh, J.C.; Lively, T.; et al. Assessment of Ki67 in breast cancer: Rec-ommendations from the International Ki67 in Breast Cancer working group. *J. Natl. Cancer Inst.* **2011**, *103*, 1656–1664. [CrossRef] [PubMed]
32. Goldhirsch, A.; Winer, E.P.; Coates, A.S.; Gelber, R.D.; Piccart-Gebhart, M.; Thürlimann, B.; Senn, H.-J.; Albain, K.S.; André, F.; Bergh, J.; et al. Personalizing the treatment of women with early breast cancer: Highlights of the St Gallen International Expert Consensus on the Primary Therapy of Early Breast Cancer 2013. *Ann. Oncol.* **2013**, *24*, 2206–2223. [CrossRef]
33. Obuchowski, N.A. ROC Analysis. *Am. J. Roentgenol.* **2005**, *184*, 364–372. [CrossRef]
34. Generali, D.; Buffa, F.M.; Berruti, A.; Brizzi, M.P.; Campo, L.; Bonardi, S.; Bersiga, A.; Allevi, G.; Milani, M.; Aguggini, S.; et al. Phosphorylated ERα, HIF-1α, and MAPK Signaling As Predictors of Primary Endocrine Treatment Response and Resistance in Patients With Breast Cancer. *J. Clin. Oncol.* **2009**, *27*, 227–234. [CrossRef] [PubMed]
35. McShane, L.M.; Altman, D.G.; Sauerbrei, W.; Taube, S.E.; Gion, M.; Clark, G.M. Reporting Recommendations for Tumor Marker Prognostic Studies. *J. Clin. Oncol.* **2005**, *23*, 9067–9072. [CrossRef]
36. Zhong, L.; Yang, Z.; Lei, D.; Li, L.; Song, S.; Cao, D.; Liu, Y. Bromodomain 4 is a potent prognostic marker associated with immune cell infiltration in breast cancer. *Basic Clin. Pharmacol. Toxicol.* **2021**, *128*, 169–182. [CrossRef] [PubMed]
37. Westermarck, J.; Hahn, W.C. Multiple pathways regulated by the tumor suppressor PP2A in transformation. *Trends Mol. Med.* **2008**, *14*, 152–160. [CrossRef] [PubMed]
38. Switzer, C.H.; Cheng, R.Y.; Vitek, T.M.; Christensen, D.J.; Wink, D.A.; Vitek, M.P. Targeting SET/I2PP2A oncoprotein functions as a multi-pathway strategy for cancer therapy. *Oncogene* **2011**, *30*, 2504–2513. [CrossRef] [PubMed]
39. Switzer, C.H.; Glynn, S.A.; Ridnour, L.A.; Cheng, R.Y.-S.; Vitek, M.P.; Ambs, S.; Wink, D.A. Nitric oxide and protein phosphatase 2A provide novel therapeutic opportunities in ER-negative breast cancer. *Trends Pharmacol. Sci.* **2011**, *32*, 644–651. [CrossRef] [PubMed]
40. Rincón, R.; Cristóbal, I.; Zazo, S.; Arpí, O.; Menéndez, S.; Manso, R.; Lluch, A.; Eroles, P.; Rovira, A.; Albanell, J.; et al. PP2A inhibition determines poor outcome and doxorubicin resistance in early breast cancer and its activation shows promising therapeutic effects. *Oncotarget* **2015**, *6*, 4299–4314. [CrossRef]
41. Zhao, H.; Li, D.; Zhang, B.; Qi, Y.; Diao, Y.; Zhen, Y.; Shu, X. PP2A as the Main Node of Therapeutic Strategies and Resistance Reversal in Triple-Negative Breast Cancer. *Molecules* **2017**, *22*, 2277. [CrossRef]
42. Liu, C.-Y.; Huang, T.-T.; Chen, Y.-T.; Chen, J.-L.; Chu, P.-Y.; Huang, C.-T.; Wang, W.-L.; Lau, K.-Y.; Dai, M.-S.; Shiau, C.-W.; et al. Targeting SET to restore PP2A activity disrupts an oncogenic CIP2A-feedforward loop and impairs triple negative breast cancer progression. *EBioMedicine* **2019**, *40*, 263–275. [CrossRef] [PubMed]
43. Kim, A.-Y.; Na Yoon, Y.; Leem, J.; Lee, J.-Y.; Jung, K.-Y.; Kang, M.; Ahn, J.; Hwang, S.-G.; Oh, J.S.; Kim, J.-S. MKI-1, a Novel Small-Molecule Inhibitor of MASTL, Exerts Antitumor and Radiosensitizer Activities Through PP2A Activation in Breast Cancer. *Front. Oncol.* **2020**, *10*, 571601. [CrossRef]
44. Farrington, C.C.; Yuan, E.; Mazhar, S.; Izadmehr, S.; Hurst, L.; Allen-Petersen, B.L.; Janghorban, M.; Chung, E.; Wolczanski, G.; Galsky, M.; et al. Protein phosphatase 2A activation as a therapeutic strategy for managing MYC-driven cancers. *J. Biol. Chem.* **2020**, *29*, 757–770. [CrossRef]
45. Chen, P.-M.; Chu, P.-Y.; Tung, S.-L.; Liu, C.-Y.; Tsai, Y.-F.; Lin, Y.-S.; Wang, W.-L.; Wang, Y.-L.; Lien, P.-J.; Chao, T.-C.; et al. Overexpression of phosphoprotein phosphatase 2A predicts worse prognosis in patients with breast cancer: A 15-year follow-up. *Hum. Pathol.* **2017**, *66*, 93–100. [CrossRef] [PubMed]

46. Huang, Y.-H.; Chu, P.-Y.; Chen, J.-L.; Huang, C.-T.; Lee, C.-H.; Lau, K.-Y.; Wang, W.-L.; Wang, Y.-L.; Lien, P.-J.; Tseng, L.-M.; et al. SET Overexpression is Associated with Worse Recurrence-Free Survival in Patients with Primary Breast Cancer Receiving Adjuvant Tamoxifen Treatment. *J. Clin. Med.* **2018**, *7*, 245. [CrossRef]
47. Liu, H.; Qiu, H.; Song, Y.; Liu, Y.; Wang, H.; Lu, M.; Deng, M.; Gu, Y.; Yin, J.; Luo, K.; et al. Cip2a promotes cell cycle progression in triple-negative breast cancer cells by regulating the expression and nuclear export of p27Kip1. *Oncogene* **2016**, *36*, 1952–1964. [CrossRef]
48. Cristóbal, I.; Zazo, S.; Torrejón, B.; Pedregal, M.; Madoz-Gúrpide, J.; Lluch, A.; Eroles, P.; Rovira, A.; Albanell, J.; Garcia-Foncillas, J.; et al. CIP2A confirms its prognostic value in triple-negative breast cancer. *Oncogene* **2017**, *36*, 3357–3358. [CrossRef]
49. Osman, N.T.; Khalaf, M.; Ibraheem, S. Assessment of CIP2A and ROCK-I expression and their prognostic value in breast cancer. *Pol. J. Pathol.* **2020**, *71*, 87–98. [CrossRef]
50. Cristóbal, I.; Madoz-Gúrpide, J.; Manso, R.; González-Alonso, P.; Rojo, F.; García-Foncillas, J. Potential anti-tumor effects of FTY720 associated with PP2A activation: A brief review. *Curr. Med. Res. Opin.* **2016**, *32*, 1137–1141. [CrossRef] [PubMed]
51. Wu, S.-Y.; Lee, C.-F.; Lai, H.-T.; Yu, C.-T.; Lee, J.-E.; Zuo, H.; Tsai, S.Y.; Tsai, M.-J.; Ge, K.; Wan, Y.; et al. Opposing Functions of BRD4 Isoforms in Breast Cancer. *Mol. Cell* **2020**, *78*, 1114–1132.e10. [CrossRef] [PubMed]

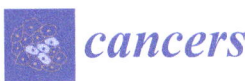

Article

The Novel Oral mTORC1/2 Inhibitor TAK-228 Reverses Trastuzumab Resistance in HER2-Positive Breast Cancer Models

Marta Sanz-Álvarez [1,†], Ester Martín-Aparicio [1,†], Melani Luque [1], Sandra Zazo [1], Javier Martínez-Useros [2], Pilar Eroles [3,4], Ana Rovira [5,6], Joan Albanell [5,6,7], Juan Madoz-Gúrpide [1,*] and Federico Rojo [1,*]

[1] Department of Pathology, Fundación Jiménez Díaz University Hospital Health Research Institute (IIS—FJD, UAM)—CIBERONC, 28040 Madrid, Spain; marta.sanza@quironsalud.es (M.S.-Á.); ester.martin@fjd.es (E.M.-A.); melani.luque@quironsalud.es (M.L.); szazo@fjd.es (S.Z.)
[2] Translational Oncology Division, OncoHealth Institute, Health Research Institute-Fundación Jiménez Díaz (IIS-FJD, UAM), 28040 Madrid, Spain; javier.museros@quironsalud.es
[3] Institute of Health Research INCLIVA-CIBERONC, 46010 Valencia, Spain; Pilar.Eroles@uv.es
[4] Department of Physiology, University of Valencia, 46010 Valencia, Spain
[5] Cancer Research Program, IMIM (Hospital del Mar Research Institute), 08003 Barcelona, Spain; arovira@imim.es (A.R.); 96087@parcdesalutmar.cat (J.A.)
[6] Medical Oncology Department, Hospital del Mar-CIBERONC, 08003 Barcelona, Spain
[7] Department of Experimental and Health Sciences, Faculty of Medicine, Universitat Pompeu Fabra, 08002 Barcelona, Spain
* Correspondence: JMadoz@fjd.es (J.M.-G.); FRojo@fjd.es (F.R.); Tel.: +34-915-504-800 (J.M.-G.); +34-915-504-800 (F.R.)
† These authors contributed equally to this work.

Citation: Sanz-Álvarez, M.; Martín-Aparicio, E.; Luque, M.; Zazo, S.; Martínez-Useros, J.; Eroles, P.; Rovira, A.; Albanell, J.; Madoz-Gúrpide, J.; Rojo, F. The Novel Oral mTORC1/2 Inhibitor TAK-228 Reverses Trastuzumab Resistance in HER2-Positive Breast Cancer Models. Cancers 2021, 13, 2778. https://doi.org/10.3390/cancers13112778

Academic Editor: Giuseppe Curigliano

Received: 26 April 2021
Accepted: 29 May 2021
Published: 3 June 2021

Publisher's Note: MDPI stays neutral with regard to jurisdictional claims in published maps and institutional affiliations.

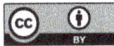

Copyright: © 2021 by the authors. Licensee MDPI, Basel, Switzerland. This article is an open access article distributed under the terms and conditions of the Creative Commons Attribution (CC BY) license (https://creativecommons.org/licenses/by/4.0/).

Simple Summary: Hyperactivation of the PI3K/AKT/mTOR cell signalling pathway is an important and well-described mechanism of trastuzumab resistance in HER2-positive breast cancer. In cell-line models of acquired trastuzumab resistance generated in our laboratory, we demonstrate this type of activation, which is independent of HER2-mediated regulation. We investigate whether the use of specific mTOR inhibitors, a PI3K/AKT/mTOR pathway effector, could lead to decreased activity of the pathway, influencing trastuzumab resistance. We demonstrate that TAK-228, a mTORC1 and mTORC2 inhibitor, can reverse resistance and increasing response to trastuzumab in models of primary and acquired resistance.

Abstract: The use of anti-HER2 therapies has significantly improved clinical outcome in patients with HER2-positive breast cancer, yet a substantial proportion of patients acquire resistance after a period of treatment. The PI3K/AKT/mTOR pathway is a good target for drug development, due to its involvement in HER2-mediated signalling and in the emergence of resistance to anti-HER2 therapies, such as trastuzumab. This study evaluates the activity of three different PI3K/AKT/mTOR inhibitors, i.e., BEZ235, everolimus and TAK-228 in vitro, in a panel of HER2-positive breast cancer cell lines with primary and acquired resistance to trastuzumab. We assess the antiproliferative effect and PI3K/AKT/mTOR inhibitory capability of BEZ235, everolimus and TAK-228 alone, and in combination with trastuzumab. Dual blockade with trastuzumab and TAK-228 was superior in reversing the acquired resistance in all the cell lines. Subsequently, we analyse the effects of TAK-228 in combination with trastuzumab on the cell cycle and found a significant increase in G0/G1 arrest in most cell lines. Likewise, the combination of both drugs induced a significant increase in apoptosis. Collectively, these experiments support the combination of trastuzumab with PI3K/AKT/mTOR inhibitors as a potential strategy for inhibiting the proliferation of HER2-positive breast cancer cell lines that show resistance to trastuzumab.

Keywords: breast cancer; resistance; anti-receptor therapy; trastuzumab; PI3K; mTOR; TAK-228

1. Introduction

Despite ongoing advances in understanding diagnosis and treatment, breast cancer continues to place an enormous burden on healthcare systems worldwide and poses a risk to the lives of many patients. Breast cancer is the second leading cause of cancer deaths among women worldwide, representing 30% of all new cancer diagnoses: More than 2.25 million new cases and around 700,000 deaths were estimated in 2020 [1]. Breast cancer is a heterogeneous disease comprising four major subtypes, each with distinct pathological features and clinical implications [2]. Among those subgroups, HER2-positive breast cancer accounts for 25% of all cases and is associated with high relapse rates and poor prognosis [3,4]. This subtype is characterised by amplifying the *ERBB2/neu* oncogene and/or overexpression of its associated HER2 tyrosine kinase receptor [5]. Despite the absence of a ligand for this transmembrane receptor, HER2 forms homodimers or heterodimers with other HER family members, activating different downstream signalling pathways, including MAPK and PI3K/AKT/mTOR, which ultimately regulate processes, such as cell survival, proliferation, motility and metabolism [6,7]. In 1998, the advent of trastuzumab, the first targeted anti-HER2 therapy and humanised monoclonal antibody against HER2, brought about considerable improvement in the prognosis of metastatic and early-stage HER2-positive breast cancer patients [8,9]. In spite of the efficacy demonstrated by trastuzumab, both alone and in combination with chemotherapy as first-line treatment, primary or acquired resistance emerges within a few months after the start of treatment, and resistance remains one of the main problems in managing these patients [8,10]. Several mechanisms of resistance to trastuzumab have been described in recent decades, such as the expression of splicing variants like p95HER2 [11], heterodimerisation with other RTKs [12–14], Src activation [15] and aberrant activation of the PI3K signalling pathway, most commonly through mutations in PIK3CA and loss of PTEN [16,17]. The intertwining of HER2-mediated signalling and the PI3K pathway takes the form, at the molecular level, that signalling by the HER family is primarily mediated through the PI3K and MAPK cascades [18,19]. As a result, the PI3K/AKT/mTOR signalling pathway has been implicated in the anti-HER2 response [17,20,21], and targeting the PI3K/AKT/mTOR pathway has proven to be a valuable strategy to overcome resistance to HER2-directed therapy [22].

Due to the involvement of the PI3K pathway in both HER2-mediated signalling and in the emergence of resistance to trastuzumab, this network becomes a good target for drug development. Because inhibition of the PI3K/AKT/mTOR axis results in enhanced HER2 signalling in HER2-overexpressing breast cancer, especially increased expression of HER2 and HER3 [23], targeting both pathways could prevent the development of resistance. However, the clonal evolution of cancer itself causes genetic and molecular diversity in patients' tumours that manifests as long-recognised functional and phenotypic heterogeneity. It is, therefore, unclear whether, in a HER2-positive breast cancer subtype scheme, such a therapeutic combination will be effective in different scenarios characterised by small molecular variations, this despite previously published reports in the scientific literature. As reported elsewhere [24], our laboratory generated and characterised several cellular models of trastuzumab-resistant HER2-positive breast cancer lines, covering, albeit to a limited extent, a range of genetic heterogeneity. Moreover, several drugs that are effective against different nodes of the PI3K/AKT/mTOR signalling pathway are available, namely, BEZ235, everolimus, and TAK-228. Different preclinical studies have demonstrated the efficacy of combining trastuzumab with different PI3K/AKT/mTOR inhibitors. For instance, BEZ235, a dual pan-class I PI3K and mTOR kinase inhibitor, has shown antitumor activity in vitro and in vivo in breast cancer models that harbour PI3KCA mutations [25] or are resistant to anti-HER2 therapies [26]. In murine models of HER2-positive mammary tumours, combined therapy with trastuzumab and everolimus, an allosteric mTORC1 inhibitor, obtained better results than either agent alone [27]. Furthermore, in a resistance model generated by the loss of PTEN, trastuzumab combined with everolimus restored sensitivity to trastuzumab and showed greater efficacy than either agent independently [28]. TAK-228 is an ATP-competitive inhibitor that targets both mTORC1 and mTORC2. TAK-

228 has shown efficacy in different preclinical models of breast cancer [29,30]. The aim of our study was to evaluate the efficacy of three different mTOR inhibitors in in vitro models of trastuzumab-resistant breast cancer cells to assess their potential use in both primary resistance and the development of acquired resistance. We show that trastuzumab, in combination with mTOR inhibitors, exerts an antiproliferative effect by inducing alterations in the PI3K/AKT/mTOR and ERK pathways, as well as through the induction of apoptosis and cell cycle arrest in different models of trastuzumab resistance. Our data suggest a potential benefit of using mTOR inhibitors in combination with trastuzumab in acquired resistance.

2. Materials and Methods

2.1. Cell Lines

The effects of trastuzumab on cell growth were studied in a panel of eleven HER2-amplified breast cancer cell lines, including four trastuzumab-conditioned cell lines selected for long-term outgrowth in trastuzumab-containing medium. BT-474 (HTB-20) ductal carcinoma, SK-BR-3 (HTB-30) and AU-565 (CRL-2351) adenocarcinoma, as well as HCC1419 (CRL-2326) and HCC1954 (CRL-2338) ductal carcinoma cell lines, were obtained from the American Type Culture Collection. EFM-192A (ACC-258) and JIMT-1 (ACC-589) ductal carcinoma cells were obtained from the German Tissue Repository DSMZ. Trastuzumab-resistant BT-474.rT3, SK-BR-3.rT1, AU-565.rT2 and EFM-192A.rT1 cell lines were generated as previously described [24]. BT-474, SK-BR-3 and JIMT-1 cells were maintained in DMEM-F12 supplemented with 10% heat-inactivated foetal bovine serum (FBS), 2 mmol/L glutamine, and 1% penicillin G-streptomycin. AU-565, HCC1419 and HCC1954 cells were cultured in RPMI 1640 supplemented with 10% heat-inactivated FBS, 2 mmol/L glutamine, and 1% PSF. EFM-192A cells were grown in RPMI 1640 medium supplemented with 20% heat-inactivated FBS, 2 mmol/L glutamine, and 1% PSF. Cells were maintained at 37 °C with 5% CO_2. All cell lines were checked for authentication every 6 months, either by using the Cell Line Authentication service at LGC Standards (UK) (tracking no: 710259498; 710274855; 710281607; 710272355), or by running a home-made mutational profiling assay.

2.2. Reagents

The recombinant humanised monoclonal HER2 antibody trastuzumab (a concentration of 15 μg/mL was selected as indicated elsewhere [24]) (Herceptin, Genentech, San Francisco, CA, United States) was supplied by the pharmacy of our hospital; BEZ235 (S1009), everolimus (S1120) and TAK-228 (S2811) were obtained from Selleckchem (Selleckchem Spain, Madrid, Spain).

2.3. Determination of the Resistance Rate

Establishment of drug resistance was confirmed by cell proliferation assay, as determined in P100 plates containing 5×10^5 cells for each condition (sensitive and resistant), grown both in the absence and in the presence of trastuzumab for 7 days. The results were processed using the algorithm described by O'Brien, which correlates the rate of growth between the treated and nontreated cells, reflecting the doubling time of the cells [31]. Once resistance was confirmed, cells were maintained in the absence of treatment for 30 days. After this pause, resistance was reconfirmed using the same protocol. Resistant cell lines populations were maintained with 15 μg/mL of trastuzumab in the medium for months. Periodically, vials of both the sensitive (parental) and resistant cell populations (pools and clones) were stored in liquid nitrogen to keep a stock of young cells.

2.4. Cell Proliferation Assays

Cells were seeded in triplicate in P100 plates at a density of 5×10^5 cells per plate and allowed to adhere and enter the growth phase before being treated with or without 15 μg/mL trastuzumab for 7 days in the appropriate culture medium. Cells were then harvested by trypsinisation and counted with trypan blue using the TC20 Automated Cell

Counter (BioRad, Hercules, CA, USA). The appropriate culture media and trastuzumab were replaced every 3 days. All experiments were repeated three times with readings at least in triplicate for each concentration.

2.5. Determination of IC50

To determine the IC50 of the mTOR inhibitors, a panel of HER2-positive breast cancer cell lines was treated with escalating concentrations of BEZ235, everolimus and TAK-228. Proliferation was measured by counting after 7 days of treatment. Viable cells were counted by trypan blue exclusion. IC50 (half the maximal inhibitory concentration) was calculated using SigmaPlot software. Values are mean IC50 from three independent experiments.

2.6. Protein Extraction and Quantification

Cells were washed with 3 mL PBS at RT. Next, cells were scraped in the presence of 150 µL lysis buffer (RIPA, peptidase inhibitor, phosphatase inhibitor) at 4 °C and transferred to a 1.5-mL tube. Cells were incubated in lysis buffer for 20 min at 4 °C and sonicated afterwards. Then the cell lysate was spun at $13,000 \times g$ for 10 min at 4 °C, and the supernatant was retained and stored. Protein extracts were quantified using the Pierce BCA protein assay kit (Thermo Fisher Scientific, Whaltman, MA, USA), following the manufacturer's instructions.

2.7. Western Blotting (WB)

Protein aliquots were prepared at 1 µg/µL in 4× Laemmli loading buffer and boiled at 95 °C for 6 min. Twenty µL of protein extract was loaded in a 10% polyacrylamide gel (SDS-PAGE). Next, proteins were transferred to a nitrocellulose membrane for 1 h at 100 V and 4 °C. The membrane was blocked (5% milk in TBST 1×) for 1 h, washed 3 times for 10 min and then incubated with the primary antibody at RT overnight under agitation. The concentrations used were as follows: HER3 (1:500; Thermo Scientific), p-HER3 Tyr1197 (1:1000), HER2 (1:500), p-HER2 Tyr1221/1222 (1:1000), AKT (1:1000), p-AKT Thr308 (1:300), p-AKT Ser473 (1:500), p44/42 MAPK (ERK1/2) (1:1000), p-p44/42 MAPK (ERK1/2) Thr202/Tyr204 (1:1000), 4E-BP1 (1:500); p-4E-BP1 Thr37/46 (1:500); p-4E-BP1 Thr70 (1:500); S6 ribosomal protein (S6) (1:500); p-S6 ribosomal protein (p-S6) Ser235/236 (1:1000) (Cell Signaling, Danvers, MA, USA) and GAPDH (1:5000; Sigma-Aldrich, St. Louis, MO, USA). All primary antibodies were rabbit, except the anti-HER3, which was mouse; all were monoclonal. Then the membranes were washed 3×10 min in TBST and incubated with a secondary antibody (diluted in 2.5% BSA in TBS 1×) at RT for 1 h. ECL-anti-mouse and ECL-anti-rabbit secondary antibodies attached to peroxidase (HRP; GE Healthcare, Chicago, IL, USA) were used at a concentration of 1:5000. The membranes were washed 3×10 min again, and immeserd in the detection reagent (ECL or ECL Prime, if applicable; Amersham, GE Healthcare) for 1 min, prior to developing on a photographic film. Densitometry and quantification of proteins were carried out using ImageJ software.

2.8. Flow Cytometric Determination of Cell Cycle Arrest and Apoptosis

Before carrying out cell cycle detection and apoptosis, cell lines were synchronised by serum starvation for 24 h. Cell cycle and apoptosis were analysed after treatment with either vehicle (i.e., trastuzumab 15 µg/mL, TAK-228 0.5 µM or both) for 24 and 72 h, respectively. For cell cycle arrest analysis, cells were collected after treatment, washed with PBS and fixed with 70% cold ethanol at −20 °C for at least 2 h. Cells were incubated with 0.5 mg/mL RNase (Sigma-Aldrich) at 37 °C for 30 min, and finally stained with propidium iodide (BD Biosciences, Franklin Lakes, NJ, USA) for 10 min. Apoptosis was assessed with the Annexin-V-FITC Apoptosis Detection Kit (BD Biosciences) according to the manufacturer's instructions. Flow cytometry was performed on a FACS Canto II (BD Biosciences), and data were analysed with FACS Diva software (BD Biosciences).

2.9. Statistical Analysis

All data are expressed as means ± standard deviations for at least three replicates (unless otherwise indicated). Statistical significance was analysed by a two-tailed Student's *t*-test (*: $p < 0.05$, **: $p < 0.01$, ***: $p < 0.001$). This work was performed in accordance with the Reporting Recommendations for Tumour Marker Prognostic Studies (REMARK) guidelines [32].

3. Results

3.1. Development and Characterisation of a Panel of Breast Cancer Cell-Line Models of Acquired Trastuzumab Resistance

To test the efficacy of a combination of HER2 blockade with mTOR inhibition as a potential therapeutic strategy to overcome resistance to trastuzumab in HER2-positive breast cancer cell line (BCCL) models, we first developed four different cellular models with acquired resistance to trastuzumab [24]. Briefly, we used prolonged exposure to moderate doses of the drug to generate novel BCCLs with acquired resistance to trastuzumab, authenticated them based on their molecular profile and their resistance rate was determined. We selected clones for each of the BCCLs and screened them for trastuzumab sensitivity after seven days of treatment (Figure 1). We observed that in all cases, resistant cells showed a higher growth rate in the presence of the drug than the parental sensitive cells. The biochemical analysis of the status of kinase receptors and effectors from different cellular pathways actionable by HER2 signalling revealed differences in phosphorylation levels for several targets between sensitive and resistant lines (Figure S1), as we reported previously [24]. After treatment with trastuzumab, changes occurred in the phosphorylation levels of HER2, AKT (Thr308 and Ser473), ERK1/2, and S6, with more relevant changes between sensitive and resistant populations in the BT474 and AU565 cell lines. This finding was consistent with patterns of molecular alterations commonly described in breast cancer [25]. De novo trastuzumab-resistant cell lines HCC1419, HCC1954 and JIMT-1 were also examined for biochemical changes in the HER2 and PI3K/AKT/mTOR pathways (Figure S2). The most notable signal was the abundant expression of 4E-BP1 in both cell lines, which does not appear to translate into strong activation in either case. Phosphorylation levels of S6 were not elevated either. On the other hand, we observed a slight decrease in AKT phosphorylation levels in the JIMT-1 cell line compared to HCC1954. Overall, the two lines do not show phosphorylation activation signals for either of the two pathways studied.

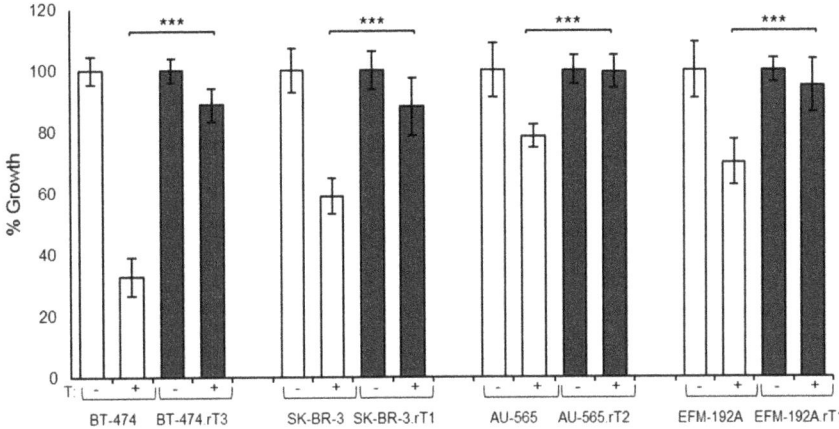

Figure 1. Characterisation of a panel of cell-line models of acquired trastuzumab resistance. Effect of trastuzumab treatment on sensitive and resistant cells. Proliferation was measured after seven days of treatment by trypan blue exclusion. T: Trastuzumab 15 µg/mL. Data are expressed as mean ± SD from ≥ three independent experiments. *** denotes $p \leq 0.001$.

3.2. Effect of Anti-HER2 and MTORC1/2 Treatments on HER2-Positive Breast Cancer Cell Lines (Determination of IC50)

To determine the effects of BEZ235, everolimus and TAK-228 on the inhibition of the PI3K/AKT/mTOR proliferation axis in HER2-positive cells, the panel of eleven cell lines with varying sensitivity to trastuzumab was treated with increasing inhibitor concentrations. After seven days of treatment, cellular proliferation was measured to determine the IC50 for each drug and cell line (Figure S3). In general, a similar sensitivity was observed in all cell lines for every drug, so when treated with any of the three mTOR inhibitors, the proliferation of the eleven cell lines was significantly inhibited at low nanomolar ranges. The determination of sensitivity to BEZ235 showed that all cell lines behaved very similarly when exposed to the treatment, and only the SK-BR-3.rT1 line was more sensitive to this drug than its parental line. The everolimus sensitivity study showed that all the lines were sensitive to treatment at high concentrations. In addition, JIMT-1 was very sensitive to this drug, decreasing its cell proliferation by more than 50% at 1 nM everolimus, and AU-565.rT2 was also found to be more sensitive to treatment than its sensitive parental line. Finally, treatment with TAK-228 showed highly similar sensitivity to treatment in all lines, both trastuzumab-sensitive and trastuzumab-resistant. Based on these results, the IC50 was calculated for each of the lines and for each drug (Table 1). Notably, the IC50 value of everolimus was more heterogeneous between cell lines than the IC50 values of the other two drugs. In addition, the IC50 values of BEZ235 and TAK-228 between the resistant lines and their parents were very similar, though this was not the case for everolimus in AU-565.rT2 and EFM-192A.rT1, which had a significantly lower IC50 value than their respective parental cell lines. The exceptions were the effect of everolimus in HCC1419 and particularly in JIMT-1, which showed at least a 10× increased sensitivity with respect to the other cells. This is probably because different mutations in nodes of the PI3K/AKT/mTOR pathway make some cell lines more sensitive to everolimus than others, which turn out to be more resistant [33].

Table 1. Inhibitory concentrations of mTOR inhibitors as a measure of proliferation inhibition in a panel of breast cancer cell lines.

Cell Line	Proliferation IC50 (nM)			Sensitivity to Trastuzumab
	BEZ235	Everolimus	TAK-228	
BT-474	3.4	3.7	9.4	S
BT-474.rT3	2.4	3.8	6.1	R
SK-BR-3	6.3	3.2	5.3	S
SK-BR-3.rT1	6.4	5.5	8.9	R
AU-565	18.0	7.5	13.1	S
AU-565.rT2	12.8	1.8	9.3	R
EFM-192A	3.6	5.9	5.9	S
EFM-192A.rT1	2.2	1.8	7.6	R
HCC1419	33.2	0.7	6.7	S/R
HCC1954	27.3	23.2	12.8	R
JIMT-1	17.9	0.1	21.0	R

Note: A panel of HER2-positive breast cancer cell lines was treated with escalating concentrations of BEZ235, everolimus and TAK-228. Proliferation was measured by counting cells after seven days of treatment. Viable cells were counted by trypan blue exclusion. IC50 (half-maximal effective concentration) was calculated using the SigmaPlot software. Values are mean IC50 from three independent experiments. BT-474: BT-474 trastuzumab-sensitive cells. BT-474.rT3: BT-474 trastuzumab-resistant cells. SKBR3: SKBR3 trastuzumab-sensitive cells. SK-BR-3.rT1: SK-BR-3 trastuzumab-resistant cells. AU-565: AU-565 trastuzumab-sensitive cells. AU-565.rT2: AU-565 trastuzumab-resistant cells. EFM-192A: EFM-192A trastuzumab-sensitive cells. EFM-192A.rT1: EFM192A trastuzumab-resistant cells.

In view of these results, we considered that combining anti-HER2 therapy with each of these mTOR inhibitors might show a greater antiproliferative effect. For therapeutic studies, the concentration and time of treatments were based on previous reports, and administered as follows: Trastuzumab (15 µg/mL) [15]; BEZ235 (1 nM, 5 nM and 20 nM) [34], everolimus (0.5 nM and 1 nM) [35] and TAK-228 (1 nM and 5 nM) [30].

3.3. Combined Treatment of Trastuzumab and MTORC1/C2 Inhibitor TAK-228 in HER2-Positive Breast Cancer Cell Lines with Acquired Resistance to Trastuzumab

In order to assess the potential synergistic effects of trastuzumab in combination with mTOR inhibitors, we performed viability assays in the four sensitive cell lines, as well as their correspondent resistant models. Overall, the combination of trastuzumab with BEZ235 or everolimus influenced the therapeutic response to a lesser degree than the combination treatment of trastuzumab with TAK-228 because, although it causes a reduction of mTOR activation in the cell lines, cell viability was not affected. In contrast, the combination of trastuzumab with TAK-228 significantly increased the therapeutic response in all cases, suggesting that the decreased mTOR activation status by TAK-228 affects sensitivity to trastuzumab.

The treatment effect of the TAK-228 inhibitor was evaluated using two treatment concentrations (1 nM and 5 nM), as monotherapy and in combination with trastuzumab (Figure 2). A single treatment with TAK-228 showed no effect on cell proliferation in any of the cell lines for either of the two concentrations used. Combination treatment with trastuzumab and TAK-228 5 nM resulted in the reversal of acquired resistance in all lines. BT-474.rT3 cells showed a highly significant decrease in proliferation in the trastuzumab and TAK-228 condition (52%) compared to trastuzumab (84%, p-value < 0.01) and TAK-228 (67%, p-value < 0.01). In addition, a significant decrease in proliferation was also observed in trastuzumab with TAK-228 1 nM combination therapy (77% vs. 84% for trastuzumab and vs. 102% for TAK-228 1 nM, p-value < 0.05). In the SK-BR-3.rT1 line, the combination of trastuzumab and TAK-228 5 nM decreased growth very significantly (44%) compared to treatment with trastuzumab (96%) and TAK-228 (77%, p-value < 0.001). The same effect was observed in the AU-565.rT2 line, with reduced proliferation in combination therapy (64% vs. 100% for trastuzumab, and 84% for TAK-228, p-value < 0.001). Finally, in EFM-192A.rT1, a significant decrease in proliferation was identified trastuzumab plus TAK-228 5 nM combined therapy compared to individual treatments (65%, p-value < 0.01).

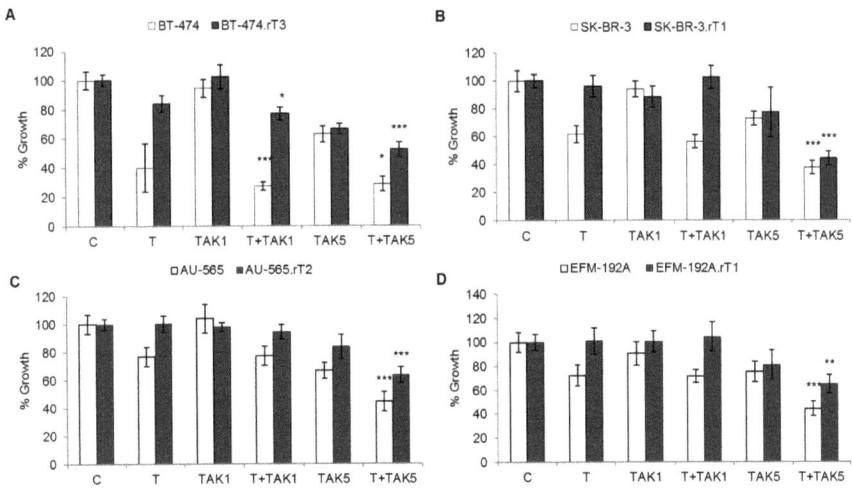

Figure 2. Decrease in mTOR activation status by TAK-228 affects trastuzumab sensitivity. Sensitive and trastuzumab-resistant cells were treated for seven days with DMSO, 15 µg/mL trastuzumab (T), 1 or 5 nM TAK-228 (TAK), or a combination of 15 µg/mL trastuzumab plus 1 or 5 nM TAK-228. Viable cells were then counted by trypan blue exclusion. Viability is presented as a percentage of the DMSO-treated control vector group. Error bars represent standard deviation between replicates ($n \geq 3$). * denotes $p \leq 0.05$, ** denotes $p \leq 0.01$ and *** denotes $p \leq 0.001$. (A) BT-474 sensitive (BT474) and trastuzumab-resistant (BT-474.rT3) cells. (B) SK-BR-3 sensitive (SK-BR-3) and trastuzumab-resistant (SK-BR-3.rT1) cells. (C) AU-565 sensitive (AU565) and trastuzumab-resistant (AU-565.rT2) cells. (D) EFM-192A sensitive (EFM-192A) and trastuzumab-resistant (EFM-192A.rT1) cells.

To test the effect of BEZ235 in combination with trastuzumab on cell proliferation, three concentrations of the drug (1 nM, 5 nM and 20 nM) were selected, all below the IC50 value for all lines. The effect on cell proliferation was assessed in the four trastuzumab-sensitive and trastuzumab-acquired resistance lines (Figure 3). Using a BEZ235 concentration of 20 nM, a significant decrease in proliferation was observed in BT-474.rT3 (19%, p-value < 0.001) and EFM-192A.rT1 (30%, p-value < 0.001) compared to control and trastuzumab treatment conditions. Furthermore, in BT-474.rT3, the combined treatment of BEZ235 plus trastuzumab significantly reversed trastuzumab resistance compared to the trastuzumab treatment condition (45%, p-value < 0.001). In sensitive cell lines, trastuzumab combined with BEZ235 20 nM potentiated the effect of trastuzumab individually, with no significant effect.

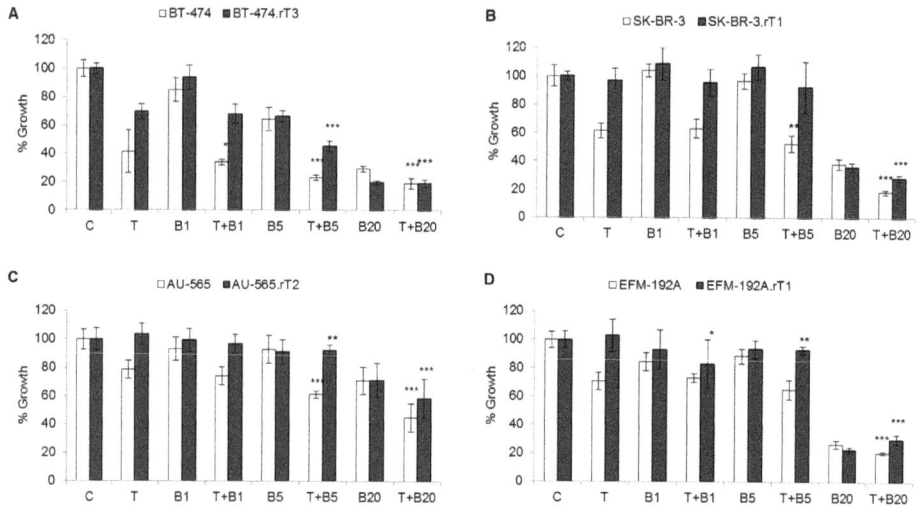

Figure 3. Effect of blocking mTOR activation by BEZ235 on trastuzumab sensitivity in trastuzumab-sensitive and trastuzumab-acquired resistance cell lines. Sensitive and trastuzumab-resistant cells were treated for seven days with DMSO, 15 μg/mL trastuzumab (T), 1, 5 or 20 nM BEZ235 (B), or a combination of 15 μg/mL trastuzumab plus 1, 5 or 20 nM BEZ235. Viable cells were then counted by trypan blue exclusion. Viability is presented as a percentage of the DMSO-treated control vector group. Error bars represent standard deviation between replicates ($n \geq 2$). * denotes $p \leq 0.05$, ** denotes $p \leq 0.01$ and *** denotes $p \leq 0.001$. (**A**) BT-474 sensitive (BT-474) and trastuzumab-resistant (BT-474.rT3) cells. (**B**) SK-BR-3 sensitive (SK-BR-3) and trastuzumab-resistant (SK-BR-3.rT1) cells. (**C**) AU-565 sensitive (AU-565) and trastuzumab-resistant (AU-565.rT2) cells. (**D**) EFM-192A sensitive (EFM-192A) and trastuzumab-resistant (EFM-192A.rT1) cells.

Two concentrations of everolimus (0.5 nM and 1 nM) were selected below the IC50 value in all cell lines (Figure 4). Treatment with either concentration of the drug alone had no effect on cell proliferation in any of the sensitive or acquired-resistant lines. Combination therapy of trastuzumab with 0.5 nM everolimus showed only slightly stronger effects than trastuzumab alone on proliferation in most cell lines, both sensitive and resistant. However, in the combined condition consisting of trastuzumab and everolimus 1 nM, a reversal of trastuzumab resistance was observed, very significantly decreasing proliferation in the BT-474.rT3 (20%, p-value = 0.003) and EFM-192A.rT1 (42%, p-value = 0.005) lines, compared to trastuzumab-alone treatment. Furthermore, this treatment combination enhanced the effect of trastuzumab in the four sensitive lines (i.e., BT-474 (13%), SK-BR-3 (26%), AU-565 (35%) and EFM-192 A (31%)), decreasing their proliferation compared to the single-treatment conditions, without being statistically significant (Figure 4).

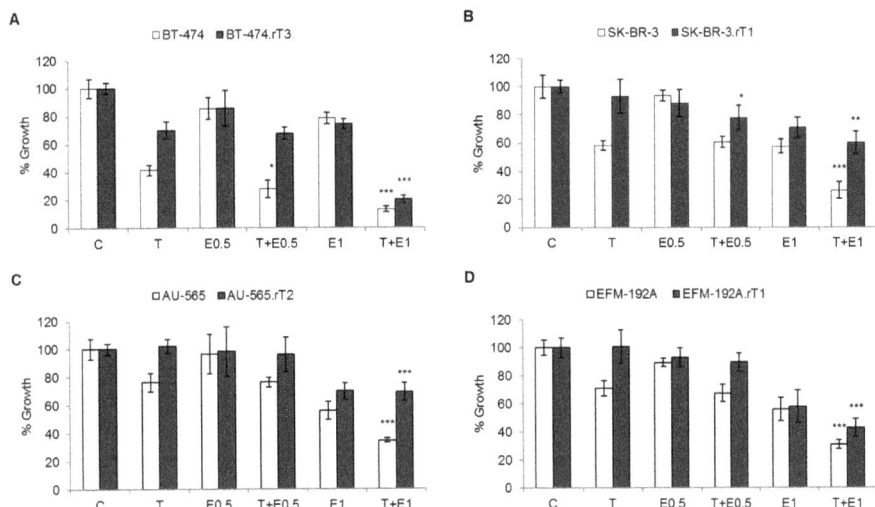

Figure 4. Effect of blocking mTOR activation by everolimus on trastuzumab sensitivity in trastuzumab-sensitive and trastuzumab-acquired resistance cell lines. Sensitive and trastuzumab-resistant cells were treated for seven days with DMSO, 15 µg/mL trastuzumab (T), 0.5 or 1 nM everolimus (E), or a combination of 15 µg/mL trastuzumab plus 0.5 or 1 nM everolimus. Viable cells were then counted by trypan blue exclusion. Viability is presented as a percentage of the DMSO-treated control vector group. Error bars represent standard deviation between replicates ($n \geq 2$). * denotes $p \leq 0.05$, ** denotes $p \leq 0.01$ and *** denotes $p \leq 0.001$. (**A**) BT-474 sensitive (BT474) and trastuzumab-resistant (BT-474.rT3) cells. (**B**) SK-BR-3 sensitive (SK-BR3) and trastuzumab-resistant (SK-BR-3.rT1) cells. (**C**) AU-565 sensitive (AU-565) and trastuzumab-resistant (AU-565.rT2) cells. (**D**) EFM-192A sensitive (EFM192A) and trastuzumab-resistant (EFM-192A.rT1) cells.

3.4. Potentiation Effect between Trastuzumab and mTORC1/2 Inhibitor TAK-228 in Breast Cancer Cell Lines with Primary Trastuzumab Resistance

The effects of drug combinations on BCCLs with primary resistance to trastuzumab were markedly dependent on each particular cell line (but less so on the nature of the inhibitor, Figure S4). In HCC1419, the combination of trastuzumab with any of the inhibitors had a greater effect than treatment with the inhibitor alone but was generally not effective with respect to treatment with trastuzumab, possibly because at baseline these cells are somewhat sensitive to trastuzumab. In the case of HCC1954, a significant effect was observed in the combination of trastuzumab with any inhibitor, both with respect to trastuzumab and the inhibitor alone. However, JIMT-1 cells showed minimal response to the different treatments, except for a small decrease in cell proliferation, due to the effect of the combination of trastuzumab with TAK-228.

Treatment with BEZ235 at any of the three concentrations tested in combination with trastuzumab resulted in a significant decrease in proliferation in the HCC1954 line. A 65% decrease in proliferation was observed in the BEZ235 1 nM plus trastuzumab condition compared to the single-treatment conditions (p-value < 0.001). In the BEZ235 5 nM plus trastuzumab combination, 16% proliferation was identified compared to BEZ235 5 nM treatment (29%) and trastuzumab treatment (87%), with a significant reduction in proliferation (p-value < 0.01). Finally, 8% proliferation was observed in the BEZ235 20 nM plus trastuzumab combination, compared to the single treatments (p-value < 0.01). JIMT1 cell proliferation was not affected by any of the treatment conditions.

For everolimus, two concentrations (0.5 nM and 1 nM) were selected below the IC50 value in the cell lines, except in JIMT-1. Its effect on cell proliferation was evaluated in the untreated condition, treatment with trastuzumab 15 µg/mL, everolimus 0.5 nM or 1 nM and the combination of both treatments at the two selected everolimus concentrations (Figure S4). Treatment with everolimus at 0.5 nM demonstrated a significant effect on cell proliferation in the HCC1954 line, in combined treatment with trastuzumab (59%, compared to 84%, *p*-value < 0.01), reversing trastuzumab resistance. In addition, treatment with everolimus 1 nM significantly reduced the proliferation of this line (12%, *p*-value < 0.001). In the JIMT-1 cell line, treatment with everolimus 0.5 nM, both alone and in combination with trastuzumab, showed no effect on cell proliferation, while treatment with everolimus 1 nM resulted in a significant reduction in cell proliferation (44%, *p*-value < 0.01).

The treatment effect of the TAK-228 inhibitor was evaluated using two treatment concentrations, 1 nM and 5 nM, in monotherapy and in combination with trastuzumab. This resistance reversal effect was also observed in the primary resistant line HCC1954. Combination therapy with trastuzumab and 5 nM TAK-228 significantly reduced cell proliferation compared to trastuzumab (57% vs. 85%, *p*-value < 0.001) and TAK-228 (57% vs. 81%, *p*-value < 0.001). Cell proliferation of the JIMT-1 line was not modified by any of the treatment conditions tested.

3.5. Downregulation of PI3K/AKT/mTOR and MAPK Signalling by the Combination of Trastuzumab with TAK-228 in HER2-Positive Breast Cancer Cell Lines

Since treatment with the inhibitor TAK-228 was shown to reverse trastuzumab resistance in the four cell lines with acquired resistance in combination with trastuzumab, the effect of the combination of both treatments on inhibition of the PI3K/AKT/mTOR pathway was evaluated. The molecular effect of the treatment was assessed by analysing the phosphorylation of the effector proteins of the two mTOR complexes: p-S6 (Ser235/236), p-4E-BP1 (Thr37/46) and p-4E-BP1 (Thr70) of the mTORC1 complex; and p-AKT (Ser473) of the mTORC2 complex, as well as their total forms; in addition, the analysis of the phosphorylated form of ERK was included. Protein expression profiling was performed after 24 h of treatment with trastuzumab 15 µg/mL, or treatment with TAK-228 5 nM, with TAK-228 50 nM, or the combination of trastuzumab plus TAK-228 at the two concentrations above, as well as the control condition.

Combination treatment of trastuzumab with TAK-228 (at either of the two concentrations tested) resulted in a decrease in AKT phosphorylation levels (Ser473) in the BT-474 line, but not in the BT-474.rT3 line (Figure 5A). In both lines, combined treatment with TAK-228 5 nM plus trastuzumab resulted in a significant reduction in p-S6 (Ser235/236) compared to the monotherapy condition, although this reduction was not observed in the two phosphorylated forms of 4E-BP1. In the 50 nM TAK-228 treatment condition, combination with trastuzumab induced disappearance of p-S6 (Ser235/236) and a significant reduction of p-4E-BP1 (Thr37/46 and Thr70) levels in both sensitive and resistant cells. In addition, only in the sensitive line did we observe that TAK-228 combined with trastuzumab resulted in a decrease in the phosphorylated form p-ERK1/2 (Thr202/Tyr204) compared to the levels detected in the single-treatment conditions. Furthermore, the combination of trastuzumab plus TAK-228 5 nM in the sensitive cell line induced a decrease in HER2 phosphorylation levels, while in the BT-474.rT3 line, it was necessary to increase the concentration of the inhibitor to 50 nM (in combination with trastuzumab) to observe the same effect in reduced p-HER2 levels. In both lines, TAK-228 5 nM increased p-HER3, as previously described, and combined treatment with both concentrations of TAK-228 reduced phosphorylation only in the resistant line.

In SK-BR-3 and SK-BR-3.rT1 lines, combined treatment consisting of TAK-228 50 nM and trastuzumab reduced p-AKT levels (Ser473) compared to baseline and trastuzumab treatment, with no change in total form expression (Figure 5B). In both lines, treatment with TAK-228 plus trastuzumab was also found to decrease S6 (Ser235/236) phosphorylation compared to levels detected in the treatment conditions alone. In addition, the 50 nM TAK-228 treatment condition and the trastuzumab combination condition resulted in a highly significant decrease in S6 (Ser235/236) activation, as did the phosphorylated forms of 4E-BP1 (Thr37/46 and Thr70). It is also noteworthy that the total forms of S6 and 4E-BP1 were affected by treatment with TAK-228 50 nM and the combination with trastuzumab. Treatment of both sensitive and resistant cells with TAK-228 alone or in combination with trastuzumab induced an increment in HER2 and HER3 phosphorylation.

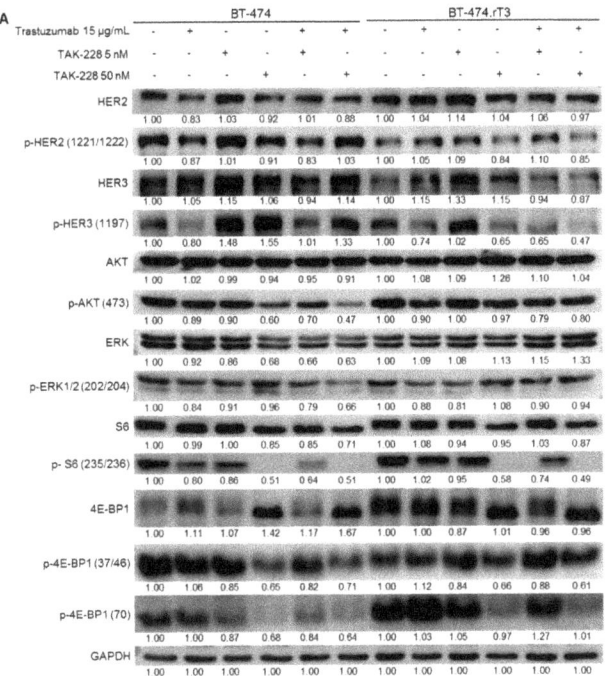
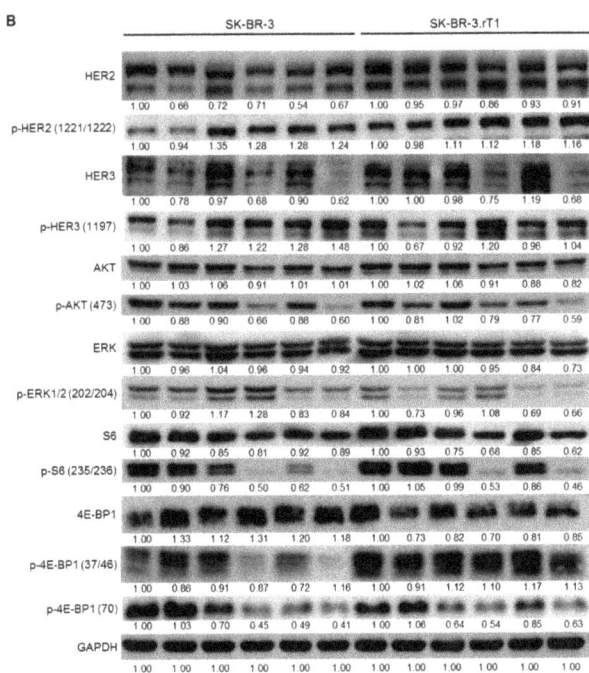

Figure 5. Cont.

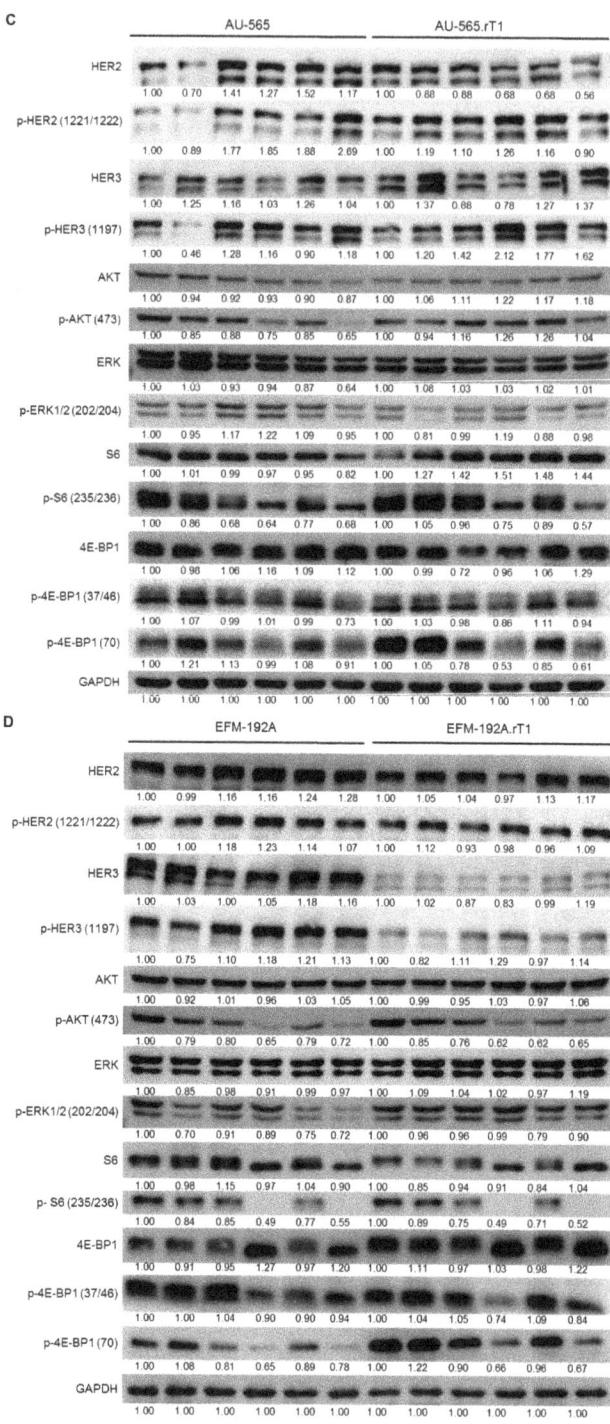

Figure 5. (**A**) Inhibition of p-S6 (Ser235/236) in trastuzumab-sensitive and -resistant BT-474 cells treated with a combination of trastuzumab and TAK-228. Sensitive and trastuzumab-resistant cells

were treated for 24 h with DMSO, 15 µg/mL trastuzumab (T), 5 and 50 nM TAK-228 (TAK), or a combination of 15 µg/mL trastuzumab plus 5 or 50 nM TAK-228. Whole-cell protein extracts were analysed with the indicated antibodies. Images are representative of three independent experiments. (**B**) Inhibition of p-S6 (Ser235/236) in trastuzumab-sensitive and -resistant SK-BR-3 cells treated with a combination of trastuzumab and TAK-228. Sensitive and trastuzumab-resistant cells were treated for 24 h with DMSO, 15 µg/mL trastuzumab (T), 5 and 50 nM TAK-228 (TAK), or a combination of 15 µg/mL trastuzumab plus 5 or 50 nM TAK-228. Whole-cell protein extracts were analysed with the indicated antibodies. Images are representative of three independent experiments. (**C**) Inhibition of p-S6 (Ser235/236) in trastuzumab-sensitive and -resistant AU-565 cells treated with a combination of trastuzumab and TAK-228. Sensitive and trastuzumab-resistant cells were treated for 24 h with DMSO, 15 µg/mL trastuzumab (T), 5 and 50 nM TAK-228 (TAK), or a combination of 15 µg/mL trastuzumab plus 5 or 50 nM TAK-228. Whole-cell protein extracts were analysed with the indicated antibodies. Images are representative of three independent experiments. (**D**) Inhibition of p-S6 (Ser235/236) in trastuzumab-sensitive and -resistant EFM-192A cells treated with a combination of trastuzumab and TAK-228. Sensitive and trastuzumab-resistant cells were treated for 24 h with DMSO, 15 µg/mL trastuzumab (T), 5 and 50 nM TAK-228 (TAK), or a combination of 15 µg/mL trastuzumab plus 5 or 50 nM TAK-228. Whole-cell protein extracts were analysed with the indicated antibodies. Images are representative of three independent experiments.

In AU-565 and AU-565.rT2 lines, treatment with TAK-228 in combination with trastuzumab resulted in decreased phosphorylation of AKT (Ser473) and S6 (Ser235/236) (Figure 5C). In addition, single TAK-228 treatment lowered the level of p-S6 (Ser235/236) compared to baseline. As in the sensitive and resistant SK-BR-3 lines, the total form of 4E-BP1 decreased in the presence of TAK-228 treatment at either of the two concentrations tested and in combination with trastuzumab, as did the phosphorylated form of 4E-BP1 (Thr37/46). In these lines, the phosphorylation levels of 4E-BP1 (Thr70) are almost undetectable, and no differences between treatment conditions were in evidence. We observed an increase in p-HER2 levels in AU-565 cells when treated with TAK-228 at 5 or 50 nM in combination with trastuzumab. However, TAK-228 50 nM plus trastuzumab in the resistant cell line induced a reduction in phosphorylation levels. Regarding the levels of HER3 phosphorylation, we did not observe a decrease with the different combinatorial treatments in either cell line.

Similarly, in the EFM-192A and EFM-192A.rT1 lines, treatment with TAK-228 at 5 nM and 50 nM and combination with trastuzumab resulted in inhibition of the PI3K/AKT/mTOR pathway (Figure 5D). In both lines, p-AKT (Ser473) levels were found to decrease in the presence of trastuzumab with TAK-228 (at both concentrations) compared to single treatments. In the EFM-192A line, a decrease in p-AKT (Ser473) levels was also observed in the presence of TAK-228 50 nM. In both lines, the combined treatment with TAK-228 50 nM caused a disappearance of p-S6, as well as a decrease in total protein levels. Finally, the EFM19-2A.rT1 line under baseline conditions showed significant activation of p-4E-BP1 (Thr70) compared to its parental line, with very similar levels of total 4E-BP1. Combination treatment with trastuzumab plus TAK-228 50 nM resulted in inhibition of this p-4E-BP1 (Thr70) activation to levels below those of trastuzumab or TAK-228 monotherapy. In addition, as observed in the other cell lines, the levels of the total 4E-BP1 form decreased in the presence of TAK-228 compared to baseline. In the EFM-192A line, as in BT474, combined treatment of trastuzumab with TAK-228 at both concentrations resulted in decreased levels of ERK1/2 (Thr202/Tyr204) phosphorylation compared to levels observed in the single-treatment conditions. In the EFM-192A and EFM-192A.rT1 cells, single or combined treatments did not induce significant changes in HER2 phosphorylation levels. Additionally, we observed an increase in HER3 phosphorylation with the single TAK-228 treatment, though the addition of trastuzumab did not produce a decrease in those levels.

The molecular effect of TAK-228 on the two lines with primary resistance to trastuzumab (i.e., HCC1954 and JIMT-1) was also studied under the treatment conditions mentioned above. In the presence of combined treatment at both concentrations, the HCC1954 line showed a slight decrease in AKT phosphorylation (Ser473) (Figure S5). It was also observed that p-S6 (Ser235/236) was significantly decreased by treatment with TAK-228 at both concentrations, independent of trastuzumab. The same was true for the full form of 4E-BP1 and its phosphorylated form, p-4EBP1 (Thr37/46). In this line, phosphorylation levels of p-4EBP1 (Thr70) were almost undetectable, so no differences between treatments could be assessed. In the JIMT-1 line, only treatment with TAK-228 at either concentration resulted in a trastuzumab-independent decrease in p-S6 (Ser235/236). No changes were observed in 4E-BP1 or its phosphorylated forms, nor in AKT and its phosphorylated form. The original WB images can be found as Supplementary Material (Figure S6).

In summary, the combined treatment decreased the phosphorylation levels of HER2/HER3, diminished PI3K/AKT/mTOR signalling and limited ERK phosphorylation, as a direct consequence of the TAK-228 mechanism of action.

3.6. Cell-Cycle and Apoptosis Analysis in Trastuzumab-Resistant Breast Cancer Cell Lines Treated with Trastuzumab and TAK-228

The results of resistance reversal obtained in cell proliferation assays with the combination of trastuzumab plus TAK-228 led us to investigate whether the treatment would also have an impact on cell cycle control, as well as on apoptosis induction. We firstly checked cell viability at shorter times, after treatment with trastuzumab in combination with different concentrations of TAK-228, to discard a deleterious effect. Cell cycle arrest was analysed after treatment with trastuzumab, TAK-228 and the combination of both for 24 h, in the cell lines SK-BR-3, AU-565 and EFM-192A, as well as in their corresponding resistant lines, SK-BR-3.rT1, AU-565.rT2 and EFM-192A.rT1 (Figure 6A). We observed a significant increase in the G0/G1 phase signal in SK-BR-3 and SK-BR-3.rT1 cells treated with the mTOR inhibitor alone ($p = 0.004$, $p = 0.009$, respectively), and the combination with trastuzumab improved the cell cycle delay ($p = 0.004$, $p = 0.006$, respectively). AU-565 and EFM-192A lines showed an increase in G0/G1 arrest with trastuzumab ($p = 0.04$, $p = 0.007$, respectively) and TAK-228 ($p = 0.006$, $p = 0.005$, respectively) treatment alone, but the effect was enhanced with the combined treatment ($p = 0.004$, $p = 0.001$, respectively). However, in the corresponding resistant lines AU-565.rT2 and EFM-192A.rT1, only TAK-228 ($p = 0.001$, $p = 0.03$, respectively) and both treatments ($p = 0.0005$, $p = 0.01$, respectively) were able to significantly induce cell cycle arrest. No significant changes were detected in the cell lines BT-474 and BT-474.rT3.

Apoptosis was determined by positive staining with annexin V by flow cytometry, including both early and late apoptosis. We analysed the apoptotic effect of each treatment as a single agent and in combination in the BT-474, BT-474.rT3, SK-BR-3 and SK-BR-3.rT1 cell lines (Figure 6B). In BT474 and BT-474.rT3 we observed a significant increase in cell death with TAK-228 alone ($p = 0.02$, $p = 0.0001$, respectively), but the combination of both drugs ($p = 0.012$, $p = 0.0001$) showed a greater rise in cell death. Furthermore, treatment of BT-474.rT3 cells with trastuzumab alone induced a significant increase in the percentage of apoptotic cells ($p = 0.03$). In SK-BR-3 and SK-BR-3.rT1 cell lines trastuzumab did not significantly affect the percentage of apoptotic cells, though the treatment with TAK-228 ($p = 0.013$, $p = 0.021$) or the combination of the two led to a significant increase in cell death.

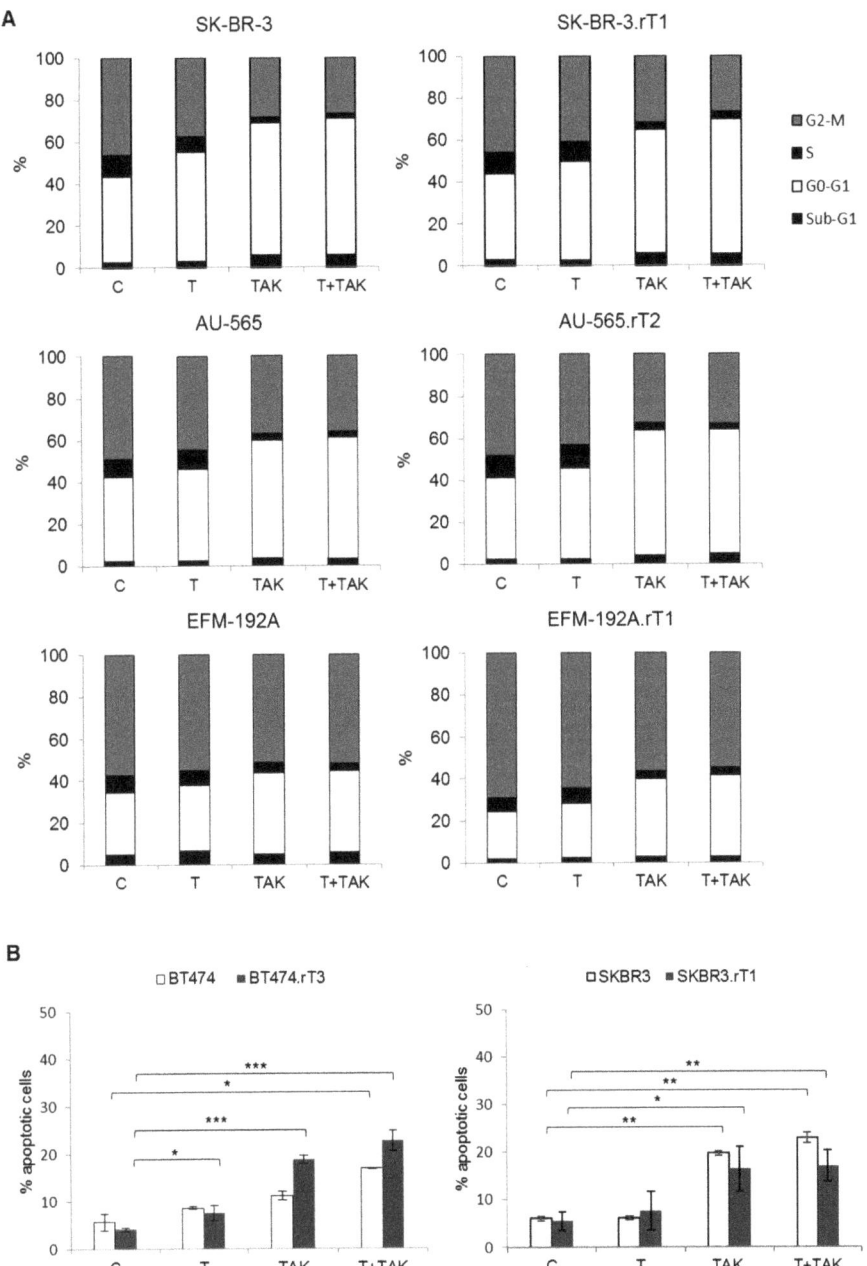

Figure 6. (A) Cell cycle arrest induced by trastuzumab and TAK-228 in trastuzumab-sensitive and -resistant cell lines. Cell lines were treated with 15 µg/mL trastuzumab (T), 0.5 µM TAK-228 (TAK) or a combination (T+TAK). Cell cycle arrest was analysed by flow cytometry after 24 h. (B) Apoptosis induced by trastuzumab and TAK-228 in trastuzumab sensitive and resistant cell lines. Cell lines were treated with 15 µg/mL trastuzumab (T), 0.5 µM TAK-228 (TAK) or the combination (T+TAK). Apoptosis was measured after 72 h by Annexin V positive staining by flow cytometry. Data are expressed as mean ± SD from three independent experiments. * denotes $p \leq 0.05$, ** denotes $p \leq 0.01$ and *** denotes $p \leq 0.001$.

4. Discussion

The development of anti-HER2 targeted therapies to treat patients with HER2-positive breast cancer has proved to be effective in survival in both early and advanced settings. For this reason, trastuzumab has been the standard treatment for HER2-positive breast cancer for more than two decades. Despite this advance, almost all patients eventually experience disease progression on trastuzumab-based therapy, due to de novo or acquired resistance. Aside from alterations in the receptor itself, one mechanism that trastuzumab interferes with HER2 signalling is inhibition of the PI3K/AKT/mTOR signalling pathway [36]. As a logical consequence, among the many causes that have been associated with resistance to anti-HER2 therapies in breast cancer, dysregulations in the signalling of the PI3K/AKT/mTOR pathway seem to play an important role [17,21], as we confirmed in our cellular models of acquired resistance (Figure 1 and Figure S1). As we can see in Figure S1 and as previously reported by our group [24], the acquisition of resistance to trastuzumab in these four HER2-positive breast cancer cell lines was associated with an increase in the amounts of p-ERK, p-AKT and p-S6, suggesting a higher level of activation of their PI3K and MAPK pathways and a plausible association with mechanisms of resistance generation in these cell line models. This finding is consistent with previous reports of a correlation between increased activation of the PI3K/AKT pathway and resistance to trastuzumab [31]. Mechanistically, PI3K activation, followed by AKT activation, triggers the release of mTOR from the mTORC1 complex, which in turn activates the S61 and 4E-BP1 proteins. In addition, the complex itself has a negative feedback mechanism, which inactivates AKT [37]. The mTOR protein also localises to the mTORC2 complex, exhibiting direct AKT-activation capability at the Ser473 residue, leading to AKT and BAD activation [38]. Unlike the mTORC1 complex, the activation of this complex appears to be AKT-independent and controlled by RAS/MAPKs [37,38]. At the same time, it has been previously described that PI3K/AKT/mTOR pathway inhibition may result in the activation of compensatory pathways that could reduce the antiproliferative activity of these inhibitors [23,39–41]. From a clinical point of view, due to the involvement of this pathway in both HER2-mediated signalling and in the emergence of resistance to HER2-targeted therapies, such as trastuzumab, it would therefore be very interesting to consider inhibiting or modulating this pathway. Because inhibition of the PI3K/AKT/mTOR axis results in enhanced HER2 signalling in HER2-overexpressing breast cancer, especially in increased expression of HER2 and HER3 [23], targeting both pathways could prevent the development of resistance.

However, given the importance of this network in the cellular processes of proliferation, differentiation and apoptosis, its inhibition can be expected to be compensated by hyperactivation of alternative molecular pathways, which would offer the tumour cells escape routes to continue oncogenesis and would eventually lead to the therapy failure. Therefore, it seems logical to test different inhibitors of the pathway, from PI3K to AKT to mTOR (both the mTORC1 and mTORC2 complexes) together with trastuzumab, to see which combination is most effective in controlling tumorigenesis and preventing the development of resistance. We decided to test three different inhibitors covering a broad spectrum of effectors in the pathway, from PI3K to the two mTOR complexes, to ensure the effective blockade of the pathway. One strategy has focused on inhibiting the HER2 signalling pathway more effectively with dual blockade approach. The combined use of trastuzumab and mTOR inhibitors has been shown to be more effective to treat HER2-positive breast cancer than single agents [27]. In addition, receptor tyrosine kinase-dependent ERK1 and ERK2 activation following PI3K/AKT/mTOR inhibition have also been described in preclinical models of HER2-positive breast tumours [23,42]. In these cases, the combination of PI3K/AKT/mTOR inhibitors with an anti-HER2 drug or a MEK inhibitor was more effective than single treatments.

The availability of four cellular models of acquired resistance to trastuzumab over an extended period of time (as well as models of primary resistance), in which we had observed hyperactivation of PI3K/AKT/mTOR pathway markers, led us to explore whether combined suppression of HER2 and PI3K/AKT/mTOR signalling was necessary to achieve optimal therapeutic efficacy, given that there are few such studies in the literature. BEZ235 is an inhibitor of the PI3K/AKT/mTOR pathway with a dual inhibitory capacity of PI3K and mTOR due to the high similarity of the tyrosine kinase domains of both proteins. The combination of trastuzumab plus BEZ235 targets those cells with alterations in the PI3K/AKT/mTOR signalling pathway, due to loss of PTEN or activating mutations in PI3K, while maintaining therapeutic pressure on other cells in the same heterogeneous population that are still sensitive to HER2-targeted drugs [43]. Our results confirm that the addition of BEZ235 overcame resistance to the trastuzumab-only regimen in the sensitive cell lines, some acquired-resistant cells, and in some cells with primary resistance (Figure 3), probably due to its inactivation effect on AKT, S6 and 4E-BP1 phosphorylation [25]. Similarly, several in vivo and in vitro models have shown the efficacy of this combination in restoring sensitivity to HER2-targeted therapy [44,45]. Our results demonstrate that the combination with trastuzumab and BEZ235 significantly results in the reversal of trastuzumab resistance in the primary resistant line HCC1954 (Figure S4). This cell line has an activating H1047R mutation in PI3K, which likely makes it significantly susceptible to BEZ235 treatment [46], and consequently, the combination of BEZ235 with trastuzumab can reverse trastuzumab resistance. However, this did not occur in the JIMT-1 line. This line not only showed loss of PTEN, but also overexpression of mucin 4, which has been described as a mechanism of trastuzumab resistance in breast cancer [47]. The limited effect of trastuzumab plus BEZ235 combination therapy in reversing trastuzumab resistance in the acquired resistance cell lines may be because this dual inhibitor only blocks the action of the mTORC1 complex and not the mTORC2 complex. This results in activation of AKT (Ser473) by the mTORC2 complex and overactivation of the pathway, which may not be affected by PI3K inhibition [39]. In addition, dual PI3K/mTOR inhibition by this drug has been reported to produce compensatory ERK activation, due to activation of receptor tyrosine kinases, such as IGF-1R [23,41]. Despite encouraging results in in vitro and preclinical animal models, few clinical trials with BEZ235 in combination with trastuzumab have been conducted, mainly due to the toxicity of the inhibitor, which causes frequent adverse effects in patients, and high variability in responses to the high doses at which treatment is required.

Everolimus is a rapamycin derivative with mTORC1 complex inhibitory capacity, approved by the FDA to treat postmenopausal patients with ER-positive and HER2-negative metastatic breast cancer. Early phase I trials demonstrated that this drug, in combination with trastuzumab, resulted in decreased cell proliferation in trastuzumab-sensitive cell lines [48]. These results were not confirmed in patient cohorts, such as the phase III BOLERO-1 trial [49], but were confirmed in other trials, such as BOLERO-3 [50]. Given that the patient safety profile of everolimus is superior to that of BEZ235, our results at the cellular level are of interest, although its antiproliferative effects were not as pronounced (Figure 4). This difference between everolimus and BEZ235 in terms of cell growth reflects the different mechanisms of action of the drugs in cell lines with different mutational profiles, as reported previously [25]. Over a decade ago, it was proven that the combination of trastuzumab with everolimus can rescue cancer cells from trastuzumab resistance caused by alterations in the PI3K/AKT/mTOR signalling pathway, with greater efficacy than either agent alone [28]. This is achieved by blocking 4E-BP1 and S6 activation, as well as suppressing AKT activation (which everolimus itself phosphorylates and activates in a feedback loop). Our results showed that the combined treatment of trastuzumab and everolimus in trastuzumab-sensitive lines potentiates, although not significantly, the inhibitory effect of trastuzumab on cell proliferation. However, the combination showed no effect in lines with acquired trastuzumab resistance. Notably, our results demonstrate that in the primary resistant line HCC1954, both combination therapy and individual treatment with everolimus had an impact on cell viability, statistically significantly reversing primary trastuzumab resistance (Figure S4). This may be because the HCC1954 line has the PI3K activating mutation H1047R [31]. But this reversal did not occur in the JIMT-1 line, which has loss of PTEN. In other preclinical models of trastuzumab resistance, trastuzumab and everolimus (or rapamycin) combined therapy obtained better results than either agent alone [27]. Today, combining everolimus with anti-HER2 drugs to decrease tumour activity in HER-2-overexpressing patients with resistance to trastuzumab-based therapy for metastatic breast cancer has proven to be a useful clinical strategy, which has been confirmed in numerous clinical trials [48,51,52]. The limited effect of everolimus observed in our results could be because this dual inhibitor, like BEZ235, is only capable of inhibiting the mTORC1 complex. In addition, inhibition of mTORC1 causes a reactivation loop in the PI3K/AKT/mTOR signalling cascade, due to inhibition of S6, which negatively regulates PI3K activation [53].

Our most conclusive results in cellular models, however, were obtained with the combination of trastuzumab plus TAK-228. TAK-228 is a competitive inhibitor of the ATP domain of mTOR that can simultaneously block the activity of the mTORC1 and mTORC2 complexes. In the three primary trastuzumab-resistant lines and the four lines with acquired resistance, dual blockade of the HER2 and PI3K pathways significantly increased the therapeutic response. In sensitive lines, the association of TAK-228 with trastuzumab significantly decreased cell proliferation and demonstrated, at the molecular level, an ability to block both mTOR complexes, decreasing phosphorylation of all the effectors analysed. Therefore, TAK-228 potentiates the inhibitory effect of trastuzumab on the PI3K/AKT/mTOR pathway (Figure 2). Our results demonstrate that treatment with trastuzumab in combination with TAK-228 results in a statistically significant decrease in cell proliferation in all lines with acquired resistance, and reverses resistance to trastuzumab. Furthermore, at the molecular level, trastuzumab plus TAK-228 combination treatment proves superior to individual treatments, decreasing the activation of PI3K/AKT/mTOR pathway effectors that trastuzumab alone was unable to inhibit. In the primary trastuzumab-resistant cell line, HCC1954, treatment with trastuzumab plus TAK-228 also significantly reversed trastuzumab resistance (Figure S4). The effect at the molecular level shows that TAK-228 can block mTORC1, decreasing phosphorylation of S6 and 4E-BP1, but not the mTORC2 complex, because it does not decrease AKT (Ser473) activation. This effect is different from that reported in the literature for TAK-228 treatment in combination with lapatinib, which causes complete inhibition of S6, 4E-BP1 and AKT (Ser473) phosphorylation in the HCC1954 line [30]. The JIMT-1 line, however, is not affected by any TAK-228 plus trastuzumab treatment condition, which supports the data presented above indicating that this line, in addition to the loss of PTEN, could present mutations in MUC4 that stabilise the HER2/HER3 heterodimer, thus making inhibition with this type of drug useless for reversing resistance [47]. Furthermore, no molecular modification of its phosphorylation pattern was observed with treatment, suggesting that this cell line exhibits a PI3K/AKT/mTOR-independent mechanism of resistance to trastuzumab that results in activation of the pathway even in the presence of specific inhibitors. TAK-228 has shown efficacy in preclinical models of resistant breast cancer when combined with different anti-HER2 therapies [29,30]. In a preclinical model with HER2-positive breast cancer patient-derived xenografts, TAK-228 sensitised tumours to trastuzumab, so that the combination of both drugs strongly suppressed tumour growth [54]. Given that this and other preclinical trials have shown that combination treatment of the dual mTOR inhibitor TAK-228 with trastuzumab is more potent in treating HER2-positive breast cancers than either agent alone, it is hoped that in the coming years, we will see clinical trials that comprehensively translate the biology of these cancers and subsequently explore targeted therapy strategies. Clinical trials combining TAK-228 with other drugs (such as letrozole, alisertib or paclitaxel) are still under way in solid tumours, including breast cancer.

Sensitivity to trastuzumab is related to activating alterations of the PI3K/AKT/mTOR pathway (either by PIK3CA mutations [55], low/loss of expression of PTEN [56] or both). As described above, biochemical analysis of HER2 and PI3K/AKT/mTOR pathway targets confirmed that trastuzumab treatment partially suppressed pathway signalling in sensitive lines, which lack activating alterations in the PI3K/AKT/mTOR pathway (Figure S1).

HCC1954 and JIMT-1 cell lines were found to harbour activating alterations of the PI3K pathway, whereas the sensitive cell lines were not (BT-474 presents a nonactivating K111N PIK3CA mutation [55]). In the case of primary resistant lines, which do have activating alterations in the pathway, less phosphorylation is reported to be affected. Treatment with TAK-228 (alone or in combination with trastuzumab) resulted in even greater inhibition of these signals in most cell lines. However, in HER2-positive cell lines with primary resistance to trastuzumab and PI3K mutations, treatment with TAK-228 was shown not to affect cell proliferation, in contrast to treatment with BEZ235. These data suggest that in the presence of PI3K activating point mutations, treatment with BEZ235 in combination with trastuzumab may be superior to combination treatment with TAK-228 plus anti-HER2 therapy [25,44,46]. The mutational status of PI3K and expression of PTEN of the cell lines have been previously described (Cosmic Database) [31].

Here, we demonstrate that dual blockade of HER2 and PI3K/AKT/mTOR signalling is effective in improving the therapeutic response in HER2-positive breast cell lines with long-term induced resistance to trastuzumab. The combination of trastuzumab with TAK-228 significantly increased the therapeutic response in all the cases (Figure 2A), suggesting that a decrease in mTOR activation status by TAK-228, as determined by the reduction in phosphorylation levels of S6 and 4E-BP1 (Figure 5), affects trastuzumab sensitivity. One limitation to our study is that we have considered resistance in single trastuzumab treatment models, when the current therapeutic protocol establishes first-line treatment with trastuzumab in combination with pertuzumab (a second monoclonal antibody) for HER2-positive breast cancer. To address this limitation, we have generated four de novo models of HER2-positive cell lines with acquired resistance to trastuzumab plus pertuzumab combination therapy. It will be interesting to see whether some of these models also exhibit the PI3K/AKT/mTOR pathway hyperactivation characteristic of the models presented here, and if so, whether ablation of this signal by dual treatment with inhibitors, such as TAK-228 (or others) are effective in treating this refractory cancer.

5. Conclusions

In summary, our results obtained in models of sensitive breast cancer cell lines, lines with acquired resistance, and lines with primary resistance to trastuzumab, exposed to combination therapy with specific inhibitors of the PI3K/AKT/mTOR signalling pathway plus trastuzumab, suggest that this combination therapy favours the reversal of trastuzumab resistance. Inhibition of the PI3K/AKT/mTOR pathway using the mTORC1 and mTORC2 inhibitor, TAK-228, can reverse acquired resistance to trastuzumab in all models generated and in some primary resistant lines. When combined with trastuzumab, treatment with the inhibitor TAK-228 has been shown to be superior to the other two inhibitors tested, BEZ235 and everolimus, in reversing acquired trastuzumab resistance. However, in the presence of PI3K activating mutations, single and combined treatment with BEZ235 has been shown to be superior to treatment with TAK-228 and everolimus.

Supplementary Materials: The following are available online at https://www.mdpi.com/article/10.3390/cancers13112778/s1: Figure S1. Immunoblotting analysis of trastuzumab-sensitive and -resistant cells. Cell lines were treated with 15 µg/mL trastuzumab for 24 h. Whole-cell protein extracts were analysed with the indicated antibodies. Images are representative of three independent experiments. C, control culture medium; T, trastuzumab 15 µg/mL. Figure S2. Characterisation of a panel of cell line models of de novo trastuzumab resistance. (A) Effect of trastuzumab treatment on primary resistant cells. Proliferation was measured after seven days of treatment by trypan blue exclusion. Data are expressed as mean +/− SD from ≥ three independent experiments. * denotes $p \leq 0.05$, ** denotes $p \leq 0.01$ and *** denotes $p \leq 0.001$. (B) Immunoblotting analysis of primary resistant cell lines. Whole-cell protein extracts were analysed with the indicated antibodies. Images are representative of three independent experiments. Figure S3. Effect of increasing concentration of PI3K/AKT/mTOR inhibitors over seven days of treatment on cell lines BT-474, BT-474.rT3, SK-BR-3, SK-BR-3.rT1, AU-565, AU-565.rT2, EFM-192A, EFM-192A.rT1, HCC1954 and JIMT-1. Figure S4. Effects of decrease in mTOR activation on trastuzumab sensitivity in primary resistant cell lines.

Trastuzumab resistant cells were treated for seven days with DMSO, 15 μg/mL trastuzumab (T), 1 or 5 nM BEZ235 (B), 0.5 or 1 nM everolimus (E), 1 or 5 nM TAK-228 (I), or a combination of 15 μg/mL trastuzumab plus each mTOR inhibitor. Viable cells were then counted by trypan blue exclusion. Viability is presented as a percentage of the DMSO-treated control vector group. Error bars represent standard deviation between replicates ($n \geq 3$). * denotes $p \leq 0.05$, ** denotes $p \leq 0.01$ and *** denotes $p \leq 0.001$. (A) HCC1419 trastuzumab-sensitive/resistant cells. (B) HCC1954 trastuzumab-resistant cells. (C) JIMT-1 trastuzumab-resistant cells. Figure S5. Biochemical analyses of primary trastuzumab-resistant cells treated with trastuzumab and TAK-228. HCC1954 and JIMT-1 cells were treated for 24 h with DMSO, 15 μg/mL trastuzumab (T), 5 and 50 nM TAK-228 (I), or a combination of 15 μg/mL trastuzumab plus 5 or 50 nM TAK-228. Whole-cell protein extracts were analysed with the indicated antibodies. Images are representative of three independent experiments. Figure S6: Uncropped Western blot images.

Author Contributions: Conception and design: J.M.-G., F.R. Development of methodology: M.S.-Á., E.M.-A., S.Z., J.M.-G., F.R. Acquisition of data: M.S.-Á., E.M.-A., M.L., S.Z., J.M.-U. Analysis and interpretation of data: M.S.-Á., E.M.-A., M.L., S.Z., J.M.-U., J.M.-G., F.R. Writing, review, and/or revision of the manuscript: M.S.-Á., P.E., A.R., J.A., J.M.-G., F.R. Administrative, technical, or material support: M.S.-Á., E.M.-A., M.L., S.Z. Study supervision: J.M.-G., F.R. All authors have read and agreed to the published version of the manuscript.

Funding: The present work was supported by grants from the Spanish Ministry of Economy and Competitiveness (MINECO) with European Regional Development Fund (ERDF) funding through the Institute of Health Carlos III (AES Program, grants PI18/00382, PI18/00006 and PI18/01219; CIBERONC, Biomedical Research Networking Centre for Cancer). M.S.-Á. was supported by a Jiménez Díaz predoctoral research grant funded by the Fundación Conchita Rábago de Jiménez Díaz.

Institutional Review Board Statement: Not applicable.

Informed Consent Statement: Not applicable.

Data Availability Statement: Data sharing is not applicable to this article.

Acknowledgments: We thank Oliver Shaw for language editing.

Conflicts of Interest: The authors declare no competing financial interests.

References

1. Sung, H.; Ferlay, J.; Siegel, R.L.; Laversanne, M.; Soerjomataram, I.; Jemal, A.; Bray, F. Global cancer statistics 2020: Globocan estimates of incidence and mortality worldwide for 36 cancers in 185 countries. *CA Cancer J. Clin.* **2021**, *71*, 209–249. [CrossRef] [PubMed]
2. Perou, C.M.; Sorlie, T.; Eisen, M.B.; van de Rijn, M.; Jeffrey, S.S.; Rees, C.A.; Pollack, J.R.; Ross, D.T.; Johnsen, H.; Akslen, L.A.; et al. Molecular portraits of human breast tumours. *Nature* **2000**, *406*, 747–752. [CrossRef]
3. Slamon, D.J.; Clark, G.M.; Wong, S.G.; Levin, W.J.; Ullrich, A.; McGuire, W.L. Human breast cancer: Correlation of relapse and survival with amplification of the HER-2/neu oncogene. *Science* **1987**, *235*, 177–182. [CrossRef]
4. Nguyen, P.L.; Taghian, A.G.; Katz, M.S.; Niemierko, A.; Abi Raad, R.F.; Boon, W.L.; Bellon, J.R.; Wong, J.S.; Smith, B.L.; Harris, J.R. Breast cancer subtype approximated by estrogen receptor, progesterone receptor, and HER-2 is associated with local and distant recurrence after breast-conserving therapy. *J. Clin. Oncol.* **2008**, *26*, 2373–2378. [CrossRef]
5. Slamon, D.J.; Godolphin, W.; Jones, L.A.; Holt, J.A.; Wong, S.G.; Keith, D.E.; Levin, W.J.; Stuart, S.G.; Udove, J.; Ullrich, A.; et al. Studies of the HER-2/neu proto-oncogene in human breast and ovarian cancer. *Science* **1989**, *244*, 707–712. [CrossRef]
6. Moasser, M.M. The oncogene HER2: Its signaling and transforming functions and its role in human cancer pathogenesis. *Oncogene* **2007**, *26*, 6469–6487. [CrossRef] [PubMed]
7. Klapper, L.N.; Glathe, S.; Vaisman, N.; Hynes, N.E.; Andrews, G.C.; Sela, M.; Yarden, Y. The ErbB-2/HER2 oncoprotein of human carcinomas may function solely as a shared coreceptor for multiple stroma-derived growth factors. *Proc. Natl. Acad. Sci. USA* **1999**, *96*, 4995–5000. [CrossRef] [PubMed]
8. Slamon, D.J.; Leyland-Jones, B.; Shak, S.; Fuchs, H.; Paton, V.; Bajamonde, A.; Fleming, T.; Eiermann, W.; Wolter, J.; Pegram, M.; et al. Use of chemotherapy plus a monoclonal antibody against HER2 for metastatic breast cancer that overexpresses HER2. *N. Engl. J. Med.* **2001**, *344*, 783–792. [CrossRef]
9. Romond, E.H.; Perez, E.A.; Bryant, J.; Suman, V.J.; Geyer, C.E., Jr.; Davidson, N.E.; Tan-Chiu, E.; Martino, S.; Paik, S.; Kaufman, P.A.; et al. Trastuzumab plus adjuvant chemotherapy for operable HER2-positive breast cancer. *N. Engl. J. Med.* **2005**, *353*, 1673–1684. [CrossRef] [PubMed]

10. Seidman, A.D.; Fornier, M.N.; Esteva, F.J.; Tan, L.; Kaptain, S.; Bach, A.; Panageas, K.S.; Arroyo, C.; Valero, V.; Currie, V.; et al. Weekly trastuzumab and paclitaxel therapy for metastatic breast cancer with analysis of efficacy by HER2 immunophenotype and gene amplification. *J. Clin. Oncol.* **2001**, *19*, 2587–2595. [CrossRef]
11. Scaltriti, M.; Rojo, F.; Ocaña, A.; Anido, J.; Guzman, M.; Cortes, J.; Di Cosimo, S.; Matias-Guiu, X.; Ramon y Cajal, S.; Arribas, J.; et al. Expression of p95HER2, a truncated form of the HER2 receptor, and response to anti-HER2 therapies in breast cancer. *J. Natl. Cancer Inst.* **2007**, *99*, 628–638. [CrossRef]
12. Lu, Y.H.; Zi, X.L.; Zhao, Y.H.; Mascarenhas, D.; Pollak, M. Insulin-like growth factor-i receptor signaling and resistance to trastuzumab (herceptin). *J. Natl. Cancer Inst.* **2001**, *93*, 1852–1857. [CrossRef]
13. Sergina, N.V.; Rausch, M.; Wang, D.; Blair, J.; Hann, B.; Shokat, K.M.; Moasser, M.M. Escape from her-family tyrosine kinase inhibitor therapy by the kinase-inactive HER3. *Nature* **2007**, *445*, 437–441. [CrossRef]
14. Shattuck, D.L.; Miller, J.K.; Carraway, K.L., 3rd; Sweeney, C. Met receptor contributes to trastuzumab resistance of HER2-overexpressing breast cancer cells. *Cancer Res.* **2008**, *68*, 1471–1477. [CrossRef]
15. Zhang, S.; Huang, W.C.; Li, P.; Guo, H.; Poh, S.B.; Brady, S.W.; Xiong, Y.; Tseng, L.M.; Li, S.H.; Ding, Z.; et al. Combating trastuzumab resistance by targeting src, a common node downstream of multiple resistance pathways. *Nat. Med.* **2011**, *17*, 461–469. [CrossRef] [PubMed]
16. Berns, K.; Hijmans, E.M.; Mullenders, J.; Brummelkamp, T.R.; Velds, A.; Heimerikx, M.; Kerkhoven, R.M.; Madiredjo, M.; Nijkamp, W.; Weigelt, B.; et al. A large-scale rnai screen in human cells identifies new components of the p53 pathway. *Nature* **2004**, *428*, 431–437. [CrossRef] [PubMed]
17. Nagata, Y.; Lan, K.H.; Zhou, X.; Tan, M.; Esteva, F.J.; Sahin, A.A.; Klos, K.S.; Li, P.; Monia, B.P.; Nguyen, N.T.; et al. Pten activation contributes to tumor inhibition by trastuzumab, and loss of pten predicts trastuzumab resistance in patients. *Cancer Cell* **2004**, *6*, 117–127. [CrossRef]
18. Sliwkowski, M.X.; Lofgren, J.A.; Lewis, G.D.; Hotaling, T.E.; Fendly, B.M.; Fox, J.A. Nonclinical studies addressing the mechanism of action of trastuzumab (herceptin). *Semin. Oncol.* **1999**, *26*, 60–70. [PubMed]
19. Baselga, J.; Albanell, J.; Molina, M.A.; Arribas, J. Mechanism of action of trastuzumab and scientific update. *Semin. Oncol.* **2001**, *28*, 4–11. [CrossRef]
20. Kataoka, Y.; Mukohara, T.; Shimada, H.; Saijo, N.; Hirai, M.; Minami, H. Association between gain-of-function mutations in PIK3CA and resistance to HER2-targeted agents in HER2-amplified breast cancer cell lines. *Ann. Oncol. Off. J. Eur. Soc. Med. Oncol. ESMO* **2010**, *21*, 255–262. [CrossRef]
21. Berns, K.; Horlings, H.M.; Hennessy, B.T.; Madiredjo, M.; Hijmans, E.M.; Beelen, K.; Linn, S.C.; Gonzalez-Angulo, A.M.; Stemke-Hale, K.; Hauptmann, M.; et al. A functional genetic approach identifies the PI3K pathway as a major determinant of trastuzumab resistance in breast cancer. *Cancer Cell* **2007**, *12*, 395–402. [CrossRef] [PubMed]
22. Junttila, T.T.; Akita, R.W.; Parsons, K.; Fields, C.; Phillips, G.D.L.; Friedman, L.S.; Sampath, D.; Sliwkowski, M.X. Ligand-independent HER2/HER3/PI3K complex is disrupted by trastuzumab and is effectively inhibited by the PI3K inhibitor GDC-0941. *Cancer Cell* **2009**, *15*, 429–440. [CrossRef] [PubMed]
23. Serra, V.; Scaltriti, M.; Prudkin, L.; Eichhorn, P.J.; Ibrahim, Y.H.; Chandarlapaty, S.; Markman, B.; Rodriguez, O.; Guzman, M.; Rodriguez, S.; et al. PI3K inhibition results in enhanced HER signaling and acquired ERK dependency in HER2-overexpressing breast cancer. *Oncogene* **2011**, *30*, 2547–2557. [CrossRef]
24. Zazo, S.; Gonzalez-Alonso, P.; Martin-Aparicio, E.; Chamizo, C.; Cristobal, I.; Arpi, O.; Rovira, A.; Albanell, J.; Eroles, P.; Lluch, A.; et al. Generation, characterization, and maintenance of trastuzumab-resistant HER2+ breast cancer cell lines. *Am. J. Cancer Res.* **2016**, *6*, 2661–2678.
25. Serra, V.; Markman, B.; Scaltriti, M.; Eichhorn, P.J.; Valero, V.; Guzman, M.; Botero, M.L.; Llonch, E.; Atzori, F.; Di Cosimo, S.; et al. NVP-BEZ235, a dual PI3K/mtor inhibitor, prevents PI3K signaling and inhibits the growth of cancer cells with activating PI3K mutations. *Cancer Res.* **2008**, *68*, 8022–8030. [CrossRef]
26. Dey, N.; Sun, Y.; Carlson, J.H.; Wu, H.; Lin, X.; Leyland-Jones, B.; De, P. Anti-tumor efficacy of BEZ235 is complemented by its anti-angiogenic effects via downregulation of PI3K-mtor-hif1alpha signaling in HER2-defined breast cancers. *Am. J. Cancer Res.* **2016**, *6*, 714–746.
27. Miller, T.W.; Forbes, J.T.; Shah, C.; Wyatt, S.K.; Manning, H.C.; Olivares, M.G.; Sanchez, V.; Dugger, T.C.; de Matos Granja, N.; Narasanna, A.; et al. Inhibition of mammalian target of rapamycin is required for optimal antitumor effect of HER2 inhibitors against HER2-overexpressing cancer cells. *Clin. Cancer Res.* **2009**, *15*, 7266–7276. [CrossRef]
28. Lu, C.H.; Wyszomierski, S.L.; Tseng, L.M.; Sun, M.H.; Lan, K.H.; Neal, C.L.; Mills, G.B.; Hortobagyi, G.N.; Esteva, F.J.; Yu, D. Preclinical testing of clinically applicable strategies for overcoming trastuzumab resistance caused by pten deficiency. *Clin. Cancer Res.* **2007**, *13*, 5883–5888. [CrossRef]
29. Gökmen-Polar, Y.; Liu, Y.; Toroni, R.A.; Sanders, K.L.; Mehta, R.; Badve, S.; Rommel, C.; Sledge, G.W., Jr. Investigational drug MLN0128, a novel TORC1/2 inhibitor, demonstrates potent oral antitumor activity in human breast cancer xenograft models. *Breast Cancer Res. Treat.* **2012**, *136*, 673–682. [CrossRef]
30. Garcia-Garcia, C.; Ibrahim, Y.H.; Serra, V.; Calvo, M.T.; Guzman, M.; Grueso, J.; Aura, C.; Perez, J.; Jessen, K.; Liu, Y.; et al. Dual MTORC1/2 and HER2 blockade results in antitumor activity in preclinical models of breast cancer resistant to anti-HER2 therapy. *Clin. Cancer Res.* **2012**, *18*, 2603–2612. [CrossRef]

31. O'Brien, N.A.; Browne, B.C.; Chow, L.; Wang, Y.; Ginther, C.; Arboleda, J.; Duffy, M.J.; Crown, J.; O'Donovan, N.; Slamon, D.J. Activated phosphoinositide 3-kinase/AKT signaling confers resistance to trastuzumab but not lapatinib. *Mol. Cancer Ther.* **2010**, *9*, 1489–1502. [CrossRef]
32. McShane, L.M.; Altman, D.G.; Sauerbrei, W.; Taube, S.E.; Gion, M.; Clark, G.M. Statistics Subcommittee of the NCI-EORTC Working Group on Cancer Diagnostics; Reporting recommendations for tumor marker prognostic studies. *J. Clin. Oncol.* **2005**, *23*, 9067–9072. [CrossRef] [PubMed]
33. Hurvitz, S.; Kalous, O.; Conklin, D.; Desai, A.; Dering, J.; Anderson, L.; O'Brien, N.; Kolarova, T.; Finn, R.; Linnartz, R.; et al. In vitro activity of the mtor inhibitor everolimus, in a large panel of breast cancer cell lines and analysis for predictors of response. *Breast Cancer Res. Treat.* **2015**, *149*, 669–680. [CrossRef] [PubMed]
34. Brachmann, S.M.; Hofmann, I.; Schnell, C.; Fritsch, C.; Wee, S.; Lane, H.; Wang, S.; Garcia-Echeverria, C.; Maira, S.-M. Specific apoptosis induction by the dual PI3K/mTor inhibitor NVP-BEZ235 in HER2 amplified and PIK3CA mutant breast cancer cells. *Proc. Natl. Acad. Sci. USA* **2009**, *106*, 22299–22304. [CrossRef]
35. Yunokawa, M.; Koizumi, F.; Kitamura, Y.; Katanasaka, Y.; Okamoto, N.; Kodaira, M.; Yonemori, K.; Shimizu, C.; Ando, M.; Masutomi, K.; et al. Efficacy of everolimus, a novel mtor inhibitor, against basal-like triple-negative breast cancer cells. *Cancer Sci.* **2012**, *103*, 1665–1671. [CrossRef]
36. Yakes, F.M.; Chinratanalab, W.; Ritter, C.A.; King, W.; Seelig, S.; Arteaga, C.L. Herceptin-induced inhibition of phosphatidylinositol-3 kinase and akt is required for antibody-mediated effects on p27, cyclin d1, and antitumor action. *Cancer Res.* **2002**, *62*, 4132–4141.
37. Guertin, D.A.; Sabatini, D.M. Defining the role of mTor in cancer. *Cancer Cell* **2007**, *12*, 9–22. [CrossRef] [PubMed]
38. Hernandez-Aya, L.F.; Gonzalez-Angulo, A.M. Targeting the phosphatidylinositol 3-kinase signaling pathway in breast cancer. *Oncologist* **2011**, *16*, 404–414. [CrossRef]
39. O'Reilly, K.E.; Rojo, F.; She, Q.B.; Solit, D.; Mills, G.B.; Smith, D.; Lane, H.; Hofmann, F.; Hicklin, D.J.; Ludwig, D.L.; et al. mTor inhibition induces upstream receptor tyrosine kinase signaling and activates akt. *Cancer Res.* **2006**, *66*, 1500–1508. [CrossRef]
40. Chandarlapaty, S.; Sawai, A.; Scaltriti, M.; Rodrik-Outmezguine, V.; Grbovic-Huezo, O.; Serra, V.; Majumder, P.K.; Baselga, J.; Rosen, N. AKT inhibition relieves feedback suppression of receptor tyrosine kinase expression and activity. *Cancer Cell* **2011**, *19*, 58–71. [CrossRef]
41. Carracedo, A.; Ma, L.; Teruya-Feldstein, J.; Rojo, F.; Salmena, L.; Alimonti, A.; Egia, A.; Sasaki, A.T.; Thomas, G.; Kozma, S.C.; et al. Inhibition of mTORC1 leads to MAPK pathway activation through a PI3K-dependent feedback loop in human cancer. *J. Clin. Investig.* **2008**, *118*, 3065–3074. [CrossRef]
42. Rodrik-Outmezguine, V.S.; Chandarlapaty, S.; Pagano, N.C.; Poulikakos, P.I.; Scaltriti, M.; Moskatel, E.; Baselga, J.; Guichard, S.; Rosen, N. mTor kinase inhibition causes feedback-dependent biphasic regulation of AKT signaling. *Cancer Discov.* **2011**, *1*, 248–259. [CrossRef] [PubMed]
43. O'Brien, N.A.; McDonald, K.; Tong, L.; von Euw, E.; Kalous, O.; Conklin, D.; Hurvitz, S.A.; di Tomaso, E.; Schnell, C.; Linnartz, R.; et al. Targeting PI3K/mTor overcomes resistance to HER2-targeted therapy independent of feedback activation of AKT. *Clin. Cancer Res.* **2014**, *20*, 3507–3520. [CrossRef]
44. Eichhorn, P.J.A.; Gili, M.; Scaltriti, M.; Serra, V.; Guzman, M.; Nijkamp, W.; Beijersbergen, R.L.; Valero, V.; Seoane, J.; Bernards, R.; et al. Phosphatidylinositol 3-kinase hyperactivation results in lapatinib resistance that is reversed by the mTor/phosphatidylinositol 3-kinase inhibitor NVP-BEZ235. *Cancer Res.* **2008**, *68*, 9221–9230. [CrossRef] [PubMed]
45. Brünner-Kubath, C.; Shabbir, W.; Saferding, V.; Wagner, R.; Singer, C.F.; Valent, P.; Berger, W.; Marian, B.; Zielinski, C.C.; Grusch, M.; et al. The PI3 kinase/mTOR blocker NVP-BEZ235 overrides resistance against irreversible ErbB inhibitors in breast cancer cells. *Breast Cancer Res. Treat.* **2011**, *129*, 387–400. [CrossRef] [PubMed]
46. Chakrabarty, A.; Rexer, B.N.; Wang, S.E.; Cook, R.S.; Engelman, J.A.; Arteaga, C.L. H1047r phosphatidylinositol 3-kinase mutant enhances HER2-mediated transformation by heregulin production and activation of HER3. *Oncogene* **2010**, *29*, 5193–5203. [CrossRef] [PubMed]
47. Nagy, P.; Friedlander, E.; Tanner, M.; Kapanen, A.I.; Carraway, K.L.; Isola, J.; Jovin, T.M. Decreased accessibility and lack of activation of ErbB2 in jimt-1, a herceptin-resistant, MUC4-expressing breast cancer cell line. *Cancer Res.* **2005**, *65*, 473–482.
48. Andre, F.; Campone, M.; O'Regan, R.; Manlius, C.; Massacesi, C.; Sahmoud, T.; Mukhopadhyay, P.; Soria, J.C.; Naughton, M.; Hurvitz, S.A. Phase i study of everolimus plus weekly paclitaxel and trastuzumab in patients with metastatic breast cancer pretreated with trastuzumab. *J. Clin. Oncol.* **2010**, *28*, 5110–5115. [CrossRef]
49. Hurvitz, S.A.; Andre, F.; Jiang, Z.; Shao, Z.; Mano, M.S.; Neciosup, S.P.; Tseng, L.M.; Zhang, Q.; Shen, K.; Liu, D.; et al. Combination of everolimus with trastuzumab plus paclitaxel as first-line treatment for patients with HER2-positive advanced breast cancer (BOLERO-1): A phase 3, randomised, double-blind, multicentre trial. *Lancet Oncol.* **2015**, *16*, 816–829. [CrossRef]
50. Andre, F.; O'Regan, R.; Ozguroglu, M.; Toi, M.; Xu, B.; Jerusalem, G.; Masuda, N.; Wilks, S.; Arena, F.; Isaacs, C.; et al. Everolimus for women with trastuzumab-resistant, HER2-positive, advanced breast cancer (BOLERO-3): A randomised, double-blind, placebo-controlled phase 3 trial. *Lancet Oncol.* **2014**, *15*, 580–591. [CrossRef]
51. Baselga, J.; Campone, M.; Piccart, M.; Burris, H.A., 3rd; Rugo, H.S.; Sahmoud, T.; Noguchi, S.; Gnant, M.; Pritchard, K.I.; Lebrun, F.; et al. Everolimus in postmenopausal hormone-receptor-positive advanced breast cancer. *N. Engl. J. Med.* **2012**, *366*, 520–529. [CrossRef]

52. André, F.; Hurvitz, S.; Fasolo, A.; Tseng, L.M.; Jerusalem, G.; Wilks, S.; O'Regan, R.; Isaacs, C.; Toi, M.; Burris, H.; et al. Molecular alterations and everolimus efficacy in human epidermal growth factor receptor 2-overexpressing metastatic breast cancers: Combined exploratory biomarker analysis from BOLERO-1 and BOLERO-3. *J. Clin. Oncol.* **2016**, *34*, 2115–2124. [CrossRef] [PubMed]
53. Wilson-Edell, K.A.; Yevtushenko, M.A.; Rothschild, D.E.; Rogers, A.N.; Benz, C.C. mTORC1/C2 and pan-HDAC inhibitors synergistically impair breast cancer growth by convergent AKT and polysome inhibiting mechanisms. *Breast Cancer Res. Treat.* **2014**, *144*, 287–298. [CrossRef] [PubMed]
54. Hsu, P.Y.; Wu, V.S.; Kanaya, N.; Petrossian, K.; Hsu, H.K.; Nguyen, D.; Schmolze, D.; Kai, M.; Liu, C.Y.; Lu, H.; et al. Dual mTOR kinase inhibitor MLN0128 sensitizes HR$^+$/HER2$^+$ breast cancer patient-derived xenografts to trastuzumab or fulvestrant. *Clin. Cancer Res.* **2018**, *24*, 395–406. [CrossRef] [PubMed]
55. Zhang, H.; Liu, G.; Dziubinski, M.; Yang, Z.; Ethier, S.P.; Wu, G. Comprehensive analysis of oncogenic effects of PIK3CA mutations in human mammary epithelial cells. *Breast Cancer Res. Treat.* **2008**, *112*, 217–227. [CrossRef]
56. Hu, X.; Stern, H.M.; Ge, L.; O'Brien, C.; Haydu, L.; Honchell, C.D.; Haverty, P.M.; Peters, B.A.; Wu, T.D.; Amler, L.C.; et al. Genetic alterations and oncogenic pathways associated with breast cancer subtypes. *Mol. Cancer Res.* **2009**, *7*, 511–522. [CrossRef]

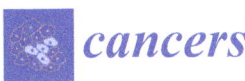

Article

Downregulation of Snail by DUSP1 Impairs Cell Migration and Invasion through the Inactivation of JNK and ERK and Is Useful as a Predictive Factor in the Prognosis of Prostate Cancer

Desirée Martínez-Martínez [1], María-Val Toledo Lobo [2,3], Pablo Baquero [4], Santiago Ropero [4], Javier C. Angulo [5], Antonio Chiloeches [4] and Marina Lasa [1,*]

1. Departamento de Bioquímica-Instituto de Investigaciones Biomédicas "Alberto Sols", Universidad Autónoma de Madrid-Consejo Superior de Investigaciones Científicas, E-28029 Madrid, Spain; desiree.martinez@edu.uah.es
2. Departamento de Biomedicina y Biotecnología, Universidad de Alcalá, E-28805 Madrid, Spain; mval.toledo@uah.es
3. IRYCIS, Instituto de Investigaciones Sanitarias Ramón y Cajal, E-28034 Madrid, Spain
4. Departamento de Biología de Sistemas, Unidad de Bioquímica y Biología Molecular, Facultad de Medicina, Universidad de Alcalá, E-28805 Madrid, Spain; pablo.baquero@uah.es (P.B.); santiago.ropero@uah.es (S.R.); antonio.chiloeches@uah.es (A.C.)
5. Servicio de Urología, Hospital Universitario de Getafe, E-28905 Madrid, Spain; javier.angulo@salud.madrid.org
* Correspondence: mlasa@iib.uam.es

Simple Summary: The role of dual specificity phosphatase 1 (DUSP1) in metastasis-associated processes in prostate cancer and its impact on patient outcome remains to be elucidated. Our results reveal that this phosphatase reduces Snail expression and impairs cell migration and invasion in prostate cancer cells through a mechanism involving the inhibition of DUSP1 molecular targets, c-Jun N-terminal kinase (JNK) and extracellular-signal-regulated kinase (ERK). In clinical samples, we evidence an inverse correlation between DUSP1 expression and Snail levels, which are further associated with JNK and ERK activation. Importantly, patients with the pattern DUSP1$_{high}$/activated JNK$_{low}$/activated ERK$_{low}$/Snail$_{low}$ exhibit a longer time to progression and a better outcome than those with the opposite pattern. All these findings highlight new opportunities to improve current therapeutic strategies for the diagnosis and treatment of prostate cancer.

Abstract: Dual specificity phosphatase 1 (DUSP1) is crucial in prostate cancer (PC), since its expression is downregulated in advanced carcinomas. Here, we investigated DUSP1 effects on the expression of mesenchymal marker Snail, cell migration and invasion, analyzing the underlying mechanisms mediated by mitogen-activated protein kinases (MAPKs) inhibition. To this purpose, we used different PC cells overexpressing or lacking DUSP1 or incubated with MAPKs inhibitors. Moreover, we addressed the correlation of DUSP1 expression with Snail and activated MAPKs levels in samples from patients diagnosed with benign hyperplasia or prostate carcinoma, studying its implication in tumor prognosis and survival. We found that DUSP1 downregulates Snail expression and impairs migration and invasion in PC cells. Similar results were obtained following the inhibition of c-Jun N-terminal kinase (JNK) and extracellular-signal-regulated kinase (ERK). In clinical samples, we evidenced an inverse correlation between DUSP1 expression and Snail levels, which are further associated with JNK and ERK activation. Consequently, the pattern DUSP1$_{high}$/activated JNK$_{low}$/activated ERK$_{low}$/Snail$_{low}$ is associated with an overall extended survival of PC patients. In summary, the ratio between DUSP1 and Snail expression, with additional JNK and ERK activity measurement, may serve as a potential biomarker to predict the clinical outcome of PC patients. Furthermore, DUSP1 induction or inhibition of JNK and ERK pathways could be useful to treat PC.

Keywords: DUSP1; MAPK; Snail; prostate cancer; migration and invasion; patient survival; biomarkers

Citation: Martínez-Martínez, D.; Toledo Lobo, M.-V.; Baquero, P.; Ropero, S.; Angulo, J.C.; Chiloeches, A.; Lasa, M. Downregulation of Snail by DUSP1 Impairs Cell Migration and Invasion through the Inactivation of JNK and ERK and Is Useful as a Predictive Factor in the Prognosis of Prostate Cancer. *Cancers* **2021**, *13*, 1158. https://doi.org/10.3390/cancers13051158

Academic Editors: Ion Cristóbal and Marta Rodríguez

Received: 1 February 2021
Accepted: 3 March 2021
Published: 8 March 2021

Publisher's Note: MDPI stays neutral with regard to jurisdictional claims in published maps and institutional affiliations.

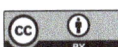

Copyright: © 2021 by the authors. Licensee MDPI, Basel, Switzerland. This article is an open access article distributed under the terms and conditions of the Creative Commons Attribution (CC BY) license (https://creativecommons.org/licenses/by/4.0/).

1. Introduction

Prostate cancer is one of the most frequently diagnosed cancers in men worldwide and is the second leading cause of cancer-related deaths among males [1]. The majority of the deaths associated with this type of tumors are related to metastasis, in which the so-called epithelial–mesenchymal transition (EMT) is one of the most important events involved [2]. EMT is a cell plasticity program that plays very important roles during embryonic development and can be reactivated in adult physiological situations to maintain epithelial homeostasis in order to guarantee tissue integrity and organ function [3,4]. Moreover, EMT also has important roles in pathological processes such as cancer metastasis. This process is defined by a loss of epithelial cell-specific characteristics, such as polarity and cohesiveness, and by an acquisition of a mesenchymal-like morphology with increased motility [5]. The abnormal activation of EMT in cancer disrupts the intercellular junctions, causing the dissociation of surrounding cells and the acquisition of migratory phenotype. Thus, EMT is often associated with the invasion and metastatic ability of tumor cells. In agreement with this, a large amount of evidence have shown that metastatic cells display a decreased expression of epithelial markers and an increased expression of mesenchymal markers both in vitro and in vivo [4]. One of the hallmarks of the EMT is the overexpression of Snail, which is a transcription factor that downregulates the expression of epithelial genes and upregulates the expression of mesenchymal genes, ultimately leading to increased migration and invasion [6]. Thus, Snail overexpression has been found in the invasive fronts of several human tumors derived from epithelial cells, including hepatocellular, breast, or thyroid carcinomas, among others [7–11]. Accordingly, Snail is widely associated with invasiveness, metastasis, tumor recurrence, and poor prognosis [7–9]. In particular, metastatic prostate cancer cells display typical features of EMT, and Snail plays an important role in the regulation of cell polarity, the expression of epithelial and mesenchymal markers, as well as migration and invasion [2,12]. Consistently, Snail expression increases with prostate cancer progression from benign to bone metastatic tumors [13–15]. From a molecular point of view, several studies in different tumor contexts have demonstrated that the expression and activity of Snail can be regulated by multiple molecular mechanisms, including transcriptional regulation and post-translational modifications. In this sense, one of the most important mechanisms that affects Snail stability involves its export from the nucleus and its subsequent degradation by the proteasome in the cytosol [16]. Furthermore, it has been demonstrated that mitogen-activated protein kinase (MAPK) activation results in an increase of Snail protein levels, which in turn regulate the expression of EMT-associated genes [16].

Dual specificity phosphatase 1 (DUSP1) acts as a tumor suppressor by negatively regulating MAPK activity in different tumors, including prostate cancer. Thus, we and others have previously demonstrated that the expression of this phosphatase decreases with prostate tumor progression. Whereas DUSP1 levels are high in benign prostatic hyperplasia (BPH) and hormone-sensitive prostatic adenocarcinoma (HS-PC), the expression of this phosphatase is almost absent in hormone-refractory prostatic adenocarcinoma (HR-PC) [17,18]. Consistently, DUSP1 overexpression in androgen-independent prostate cancer cells promotes apoptosis through inhibition of the p38 mitogen-activated protein kinase (p38MAPK)/nuclear factor-kappaB (NF-kB) signaling pathway [17]. Moreover, DUSP1 is also involved in the pro-apoptotic effects of the chemopreventive molecule resveratrol in prostate cancer cells [19]. In addition, it has been reported that DUSP1 inhibits cell migration, invasion, and metastasis in other cancer types [20–24]. However, despite all these studies showing DUSP1 as an apoptosis inducer in prostate cancer, the role of this phosphatase in cell migration and invasion in these kind of tumors remains largely unknown. Therefore, in this work, we aimed to investigate whether DUSP1 is involved in the motility of prostate cancer cells and whether this protein regulates the signaling pathways that control these processes. In brief, our results demonstrate that DUSP1 decreases Snail expression as well as cell migration and invasion in prostate tumor cells. Moreover, our data also support that DUSP1 regulates both processes, together with Snail expression, through the inactivation of c-Jun N-terminal kinase (JNK) and extracellular-signal-regulated kinase (ERK). Importantly, we also elucidate a new molecular pattern, which might be useful as a prognosis biomarker for prostate cancer monitoring. This molecular signature is characterized by an inverse correlation between DUSP1 and Snail levels with an additional activation of JNK and ERK pathways. Finally, our results show that expression of DUSP1 and Snail, as well as levels of active ERK and JNK correlate with time of progression and with exitus rate. In line with this, those patients with high DUSP1 expression, low JNK and ERK activities, and low Snail expression exhibit a longer time until they reach metastatic disease, a better outcome, and a lower exitus rate than those with the opposite expression pattern (DUSP1$_{low}$/activated JNK$_{high}$/activated ERK$_{high}$/Snail$_{high}$). Importantly, we consider that our findings suggest new opportunities to improve current strategies for the diagnosis and treatment of prostate cancer.

2. Materials and Methods

2.1. Cell Lines, Inhibitors, Plasmids, Cell Transfection and Luciferase Assay

DU145 and PC3 androgen-independent prostate cancer cells were purchased from the American Tissue Culture Collection (Manassas, UA, USA) and were cultured as recommended. The inhibitors were U0126 (Promega Biotech Ibérica, Madrid, Spain), SB203580, SP600125, and MG132 (Calbiochem, Merck Chemicals, Barcelona, Spain). The pCMV-DUSP1 and the Snail-Luc reporter plasmids were previously described [25,26]. For overexpression and siRNA experiments, cells were transiently transfected as previously described [19]. Luciferase assays were performed as in [27], being the luciferase levels normalized to those of renilla, and expressed as the induction over the controls.

2.2. Western Blot Analyses and Immunofluorescence Staining

Western blot analyses were performed as described in [27]. The antibodies were anti-DUSP1, anti-p38MAPK, anti-JNK1, and anti-ERK2 (Santa Cruz Biotechnology, Heidelberg, Germany); anti-phospho-p38MAPK (pp38MAPK), anti-phospho-ERK (pERK), and anti-Snail (Cell Signalling Technology, Izasa S.A., Barcelona, Spain); anti-phospho-pJNK (pJNK) (Promega Biotech Ibérica, Madrid, Spain); anti-Tubulin (Sigma Aldrich, Madrid, Spain); peroxidase-conjugated secondary antibodies (GE Healthcare Europe GMBH, Barcelona, Spain). Tubulin was utilized as a loading control for Western blotting analysis. Relative protein levels compared to tubulin were analyzed by Image J software and plotted.

Immunofluorescence staining was performed as previously described [28]. Briefly, cells cultured on coverslips were fixed, permeabilized, blocked and, after several washes, stained for Snail with the specific antibody, followed by the anti-rabbit Alexa Fluor® 488 secondary antibody (BD Biosciences, Franklin Lakes, NJ, USA). Samples were mounted using ProLong® Gold Antifade Mountant with DAPI (Invitrogen, Life Technologies, Carlsbad, CA, USA), and fluorescence visualization was performed by ICTS "NANBIOSIS", more specifically by the Confocal Microscopy Service (Ciber in Bioengineering, Biomaterials & Nanomedicine (CIBER-BNN)) at the Alcalá University.

2.3. Cell Migration and Invasion Assays

Cell migration was examined by wound-healing assays. After transfection/treatment of cells, scratches were made using sterile 200 µL-pipette tips, and bright-field microphotographs were taken at different times. The percentages of cell migration were quantitated, by the ImageJ software, measuring the width of the cell-free zone immediately after making the scratch, and at different times after scratching. Migration velocities represented the average velocities at which the cells moved into the gap.

Cell invasion was examined in Matrigel-coated transwells (BD Biosciences, Franklin Lakes, NJ, USA) as previously described [29]. The number of cells loaded onto the surface of each Matrigel-coated transwell was 100,000 in DUSP1 overexpression and MAPK inhibitors experiments, and 50,000 in DUSP1 silencing experiments. Invaded cells were stained with crystal violet, and three different cell fields of each well were photographed under a phase contrast microscope (Nikon TS100). Changes in cell invasion were expressed as percentages of the corresponded controls.

2.4. Experimental Subjects and Immunohistochemistry of Prostate Tissues

Paraffin-embedded samples from patients diagnosed with BPH ($n = 9$) or PC ($n = 35$) were used (Table 1). Five-micron thick sections from samples were incubated overnight at room temperature with each primary antibody (anti-DUSP1 and anti-Snail1, clone G7 (Santa Cruz Biotechnology, Heidelberg, Germany); anti-pJNK (Promega, Promega Biotech Ibérica, Madrid, Spain); anti-pERK (Cell Signalling Technology, Izasa S.A., Barcelona, Spain)). Afterwards, samples were washed and sequentially incubated with the biotin free, peroxidase-detection system (polymer-based detection kit, MasVision™, Master Diagnostica, Spain). Nuclei were stained with Caracci's hematoxylin. Samples were dehydrated and mounted with DePex. The intensity of the immunostaining was evaluated by two independent observers who were blinded to patient clinical information through a system of subjective gradation. Immunostaining scores were ranged into four categories based on the staining pattern of the majority of tumor cells in the whole section, which were grouped into two main categories for statistical purposes (0–1: negative/low staining; 2–3: moderate/high staining).

Table 1. Clinical data of prostate cancer patients ($n = 35$).

CLINICAL DATA	n
Age (median = 65)	
<65	15
≥65	20
Gleason grade	
≤7	13
>7	22
Invasivity (T)	
T1	5
T2	11
T3	15
T4	4
Metastatic disease at diagnostic (M)	
M0	31
M1	4
Response to androgen blockade	
Hormone-responsive (HS)	20
Hormone-refractory (HR)	15
OUTCOME	n
Alive	22
Exitus	13
PROGRESSION	months
Median survival	16
Time to biochemical progression	15
Time to clinical progression	50

2.5. Statistical Analyses

In the experiments with cell lines, all data were expressed as means ± SEM. Student's *t* test was performed using the SSC-Stat software (V2.18, University of Reading, UK). In the immunohistochemistry assays, GraphPad Prisma 3.0 software was used for statistical purposes. Immunostaining score and clinical data were analyzed using one-way ANOVA and either the Bonferroni's or Dunnet´s multiple comparison tests. The correlation among markers was analyzed using the Pearson´s test (95% confidence interval). Log-rank test and survival curves were used to determine the relationship among markers and time to clinical progression. The statistical significance of difference between groups was expressed by asterisks (* $0.01 < p < 0.05$; ** $0.001 < p < 0.01$; *** $p < 0.001$).

3. Results

3.1. DUSP1 Downregulates Snail Expression and Impairs Cell Migration and Invasion in Prostate Cancer Cells

To study the role of DUSP1 in the migration and invasion of prostate cancer cells, we first analyzed the effect of DUSP1 knockdown on Snail expression in DU145 cells. DUSP1 silencing efficiency was tested by measuring its protein levels, observing a significant decrease in DUSP1-deficient cells (Figure 1a). The results showed an increase in Snail levels both at a transcriptional (Figure 1b) and at a protein level (Figure 1c). Consistently, DUSP1-deficient cells significantly displayed an enhanced capacity of both cell migration (Figure 1d–f) and invasion (Figure 1g,h). Conversely, cells overexpressing DUSP1 showed a significant increase in protein levels (Figure 1i), significantly reduced Snail expression levels (Figure 1j,k), were less migratory (Figure 1l–n), and displayed limited cell invasion (Figure 1o,p). Similar results were obtained from experiments performed in PC3 cells, thus ruling out the cell-type specific effects of this phosphatase (Figure S1 in Supplementary Materials). All these results indicate that DUSP1 downregulates Snail expression, which in turn results in a further decrease in migration and invasion of prostate cancer cells.

3.2. The Inhibition of JNK and ERK Downregulates Snail Expression, Cell Migration and Invasion

Given that DUSP1 is able to dephosphorylate and inhibit different MAPK signaling pathways, we next investigated which of them were involved in the effects of this phosphatase on Snail expression, cell migration, and invasion in DU145 cells. Our results confirmed that p38MAPK, JNK, and ERK were targets of this phosphatase, since the abrogation of its expression activated these three MAPKs (Figure 2a). In addition, the inhibitory effect of DUSP1 on MAPK's activities was confirmed by monitoring the levels of their phosphorylated forms in cells overexpressing this phosphatase (data not shown).

Further analysis of Snail expression after inactivation of these MAPKs was performed upon treatment of cells with specific inhibitors. The efficiency of selective inhibition of MAPK activity by SB203580 (p38MAPK inhibitor), SP600125 (JNK inhibitor), or U0126 (MEK inhibitor) was confirmed by measuring MAPK phosphorylation levels in cells incubated with these compounds (Figure S2 in Supplementary Materials). Moreover, the inhibition of these MAPKs differently affected cell proliferation and survival [17] (unpublished results). Regarding Snail expression, the inhibition of p38MAPK with SB203580 did not affect Snail expression (Figure 2b,c). In contrast, treatment with either SP600125 or U0126 achieved a significant reduction in Snail levels (Figure 2b), although only ERK inhibition exerted its effects at a transcriptional level (Figure 2c). Moreover, the effect of JNK and ERK inhibition on Snail proteasomal degradation was assessed, and the analysis of these data revealed that the reduction in Snail levels achieved by SP600125 or U0126 was reversed by the inhibitor MG132 (Figure 2d), suggesting that Snail regulation by JNK or ERK pathways is proteasome dependent.

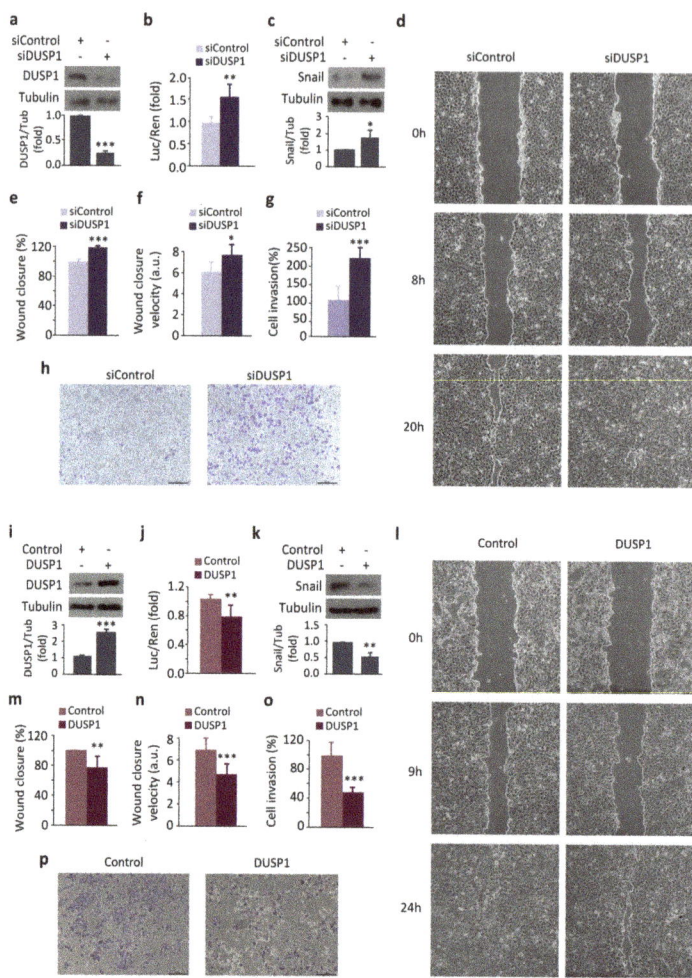

Figure 1. DUSP1 downregulates Snail expression and impairs cell migration and invasion in DU145 cells. (**a**) Cells were transfected for 48 h with the control siRNA (siControl) or the DUSP1 siRNA (siDUSP1) and expression levels of DUSP1 and Tubulin were determined by western blotting. (**b**) Cells were transfected for 48 h with the siControl or the siDUSP1 together with the Snail-Luc plasmid and luciferase activity was measured in cell extracts. (**c**) Cells were transfected as in *a* and expression levels of Snail and Tubulin were determined by western blotting. (**d–f**) Wound healing assay and measurement of wound closure area and velocity in cells transfected as in *a*. (**g,h**) Invasion capacity using transwell assays in cells transfected as in *a*. (**i**) Cells were transfected with a control vector (Control) or a vector encoding DUSP1 (DUSP1) and expression levels of DUSP1 and Tubulin were determined by western blotting. (**j**) Cells were transfected for 48 h with the Control or the DUSP1 vectors together with the Snail-Luc plasmid and luciferase activity was measured in cell extracts. (**k**) Cells were transfected with the Control or the DUSP1 vectors and expression levels of Snail and Tubulin were determined by western blotting. (**l–n**) Wound healing assay and measurement of wound closure area and velocity in cells transfected as in *i*. (**o,p**) Invasion capacity using transwell assays in cells transfected as in *i*. For all the results, data are shown as the mean ± SEM of at least three independent experiments. For migration and invasion assays, pictures are from one representative experiment of three with similar results. Student's *t* test: * $0.01 < p < 0.05$; ** $0.001 < p < 0.01$; *** $p < 0.001$.

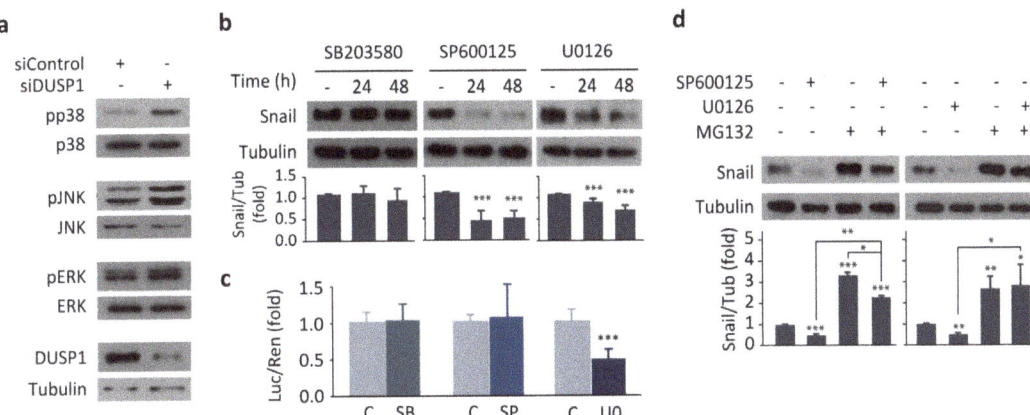

Figure 2. The inhibition of JNK and ERK downregulates Snail expression in DU145 cells. (**a**) Cells were transfected for 48 h with the siControl or the siDUSP1 and expression levels of DUSP1, phosphorylated MAPKs (pp38, pJNK, pERK), total MAPKs and Tubulin were determined by western blotting. (**b**) Cells were incubated at different times in the absence or presence of 1 µM SB203580 (SB), 10 µM SP600125 (SP) or 20 µM U0126 (U0), and expression levels of Snail and Tubulin were determined by western blotting. (**c**) Cells were transfected with the Snail-Luc plasmid, incubated for 48 h as in *b* and luciferase activity was assayed in cell extracts. (**d**) Cells were incubated for 48 h with 10 µM SP600125 or 20 µM U0126, treated in the absence or presence of 10 µM MG132 for the last 4 h and expression levels of Snail and Tubulin were determined by western blotting. For all the results, data are shown as the mean ± SEM of at least three independent experiments. Student's t test: * $0.01 < p < 0.05$; ** $0.001 < p < 0.01$; *** $p < 0.001$.

Additionally, both JNK and ERK inhibition reduced cell migration (Figure 3a–f) and invasion (Figure 3g–j), mimicking the results obtained following DUSP1 overexpression (Figure 1j–n). In contrast, p38MAPK inhibition did not affect cell migration (Figure S3 in Supplementary Materials), suggesting that this kinase is supporting other processes in prostate cancer progression. All these results, together with those showed in Figure 1, demonstrate that both pharmacological inhibition of JNK or ERK and DUSP1 overexpression exert similar effects on Snail expression, cell migration, and invasion, suggesting that this phosphatase regulates these processes by specifically targeting these two pathways.

3.3. Snail Subcellular Location Is Regulated by the Phosphatase DUSP1 and JNK and ERK Signaling Pathways

One of the most common molecular mechanisms by which Snail expression is downregulated involves its nuclear export to the cytoplasm and its subsequent proteasomal degradation. Since we demonstrated that JNK and ERK inhibition decreased Snail expression by affecting its proteasomal degradation (Figure 2d), we next analyzed Snail location upon treatment with the specific MAPKs inhibitors. As expected, our results showed that SP600125 and U0126 induced a more diffuse location of Snail with an increase in the cytosolic compartment (Figure 4).

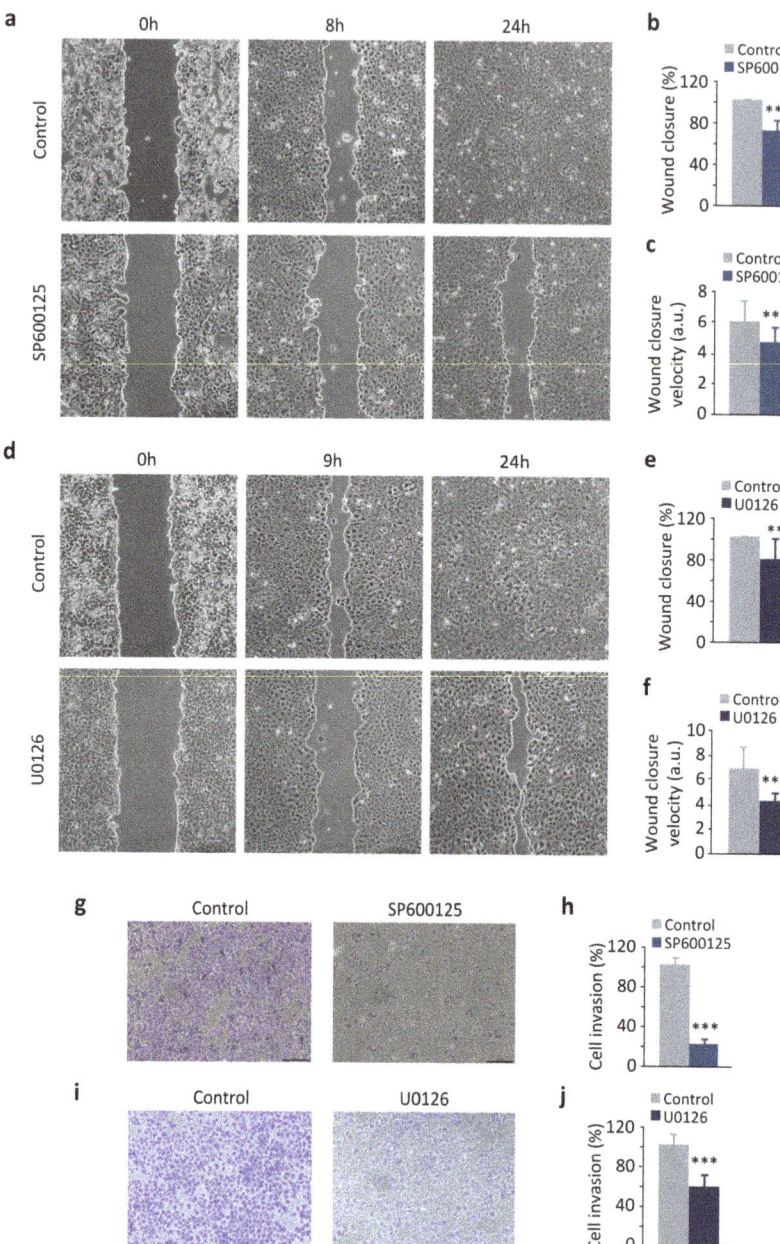

Figure 3. The inhibition of JNK and ERK decreases migration and invasion in DU145 cells. (**a–f**) Wound healing assay and measurement of wound closure area and velocity in cells incubated for 48 h with 10 µM SP600125 (**a–c**) or 20 µM U0126 (**d–f**). (**g–j**) Invasion capacity using transwell assays in cells incubated as above. For all the results, data are shown as the mean ± SEM of at least three independent experiments. Pictures are from one representative experiment of three with similar results. Student's t test: ** $0.001 < p < 0.01$; *** $p < 0.001$.

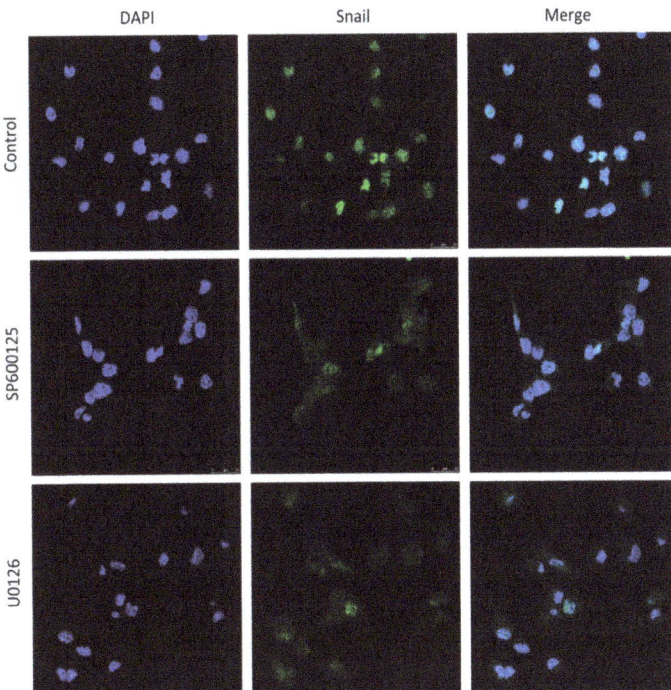

Figure 4. Snail subcellular location is regulated by the JNK and ERK signaling pathways. DU145 cells were incubated for 48 h with 10 µM SP600125 or 20 µM U0126 and Snail subcellular location was determined by immunofluorescence as described in Material and methods. DAPI was used to identify the nuclei. Pictures are from one representative experiment of three with similar results.

Consistently, DUSP1 overexpression also induced a predominantly cytosolic location of Snail, while DUSP1 knockdown maintained this transcription factor in the nucleus (Figure 5). These results reveal that both DUSP1 overexpression and JNK or ERK inhibition induce the export of Snail from the nucleus to the cytoplasm; hence, these data strengthen our hypothesis that this phosphatase exerts its effects on Snail subcellular location through the downregulation of these MAPKs.

3.4. JNK and ERK Cooperatively Regulate Snail Expression, Cell Migration and Invasion

Given that DUSP1 impaired the activity of JNK and ERK (Figure 2a), and that the individual inhibition of these MAPKs downregulated Snail expression (Figure 2b), as well as cell migration and invasion (Figure 3), we further studied whether these MAPKs cooperated in the regulation of these events in our prostate cancer cells. Interestingly, the combination of SP600125 and U0126 significantly achieved a higher reduction in Snail expression than the single treatments in DU145 cells (Figure 6a).

Notably, cells treated with SP600125 plus U0126 were even less migratory (Figure 6b–d) and displayed less invasion capacity (Figure 6e,f) compared to cells treated with the single agents. To further strengthen these results, we extended our study, performing similar experiments in PC3 cells. As expected, our results showed that JNK and ERK cooperatively regulated Snail expression and cell migration also in these cells (Figure S4 in Supplementary Materials). All these results indicate that the dual inhibition of JNK and ERK pathways in prostate cancer cells is more effective in decreasing Snail expression, cell migration, and invasion than blocking each pathway independently. Altogether, these results suggest once again that DUSP1 regulates these events through a dual inhibition of both JNK and ERK pathways.

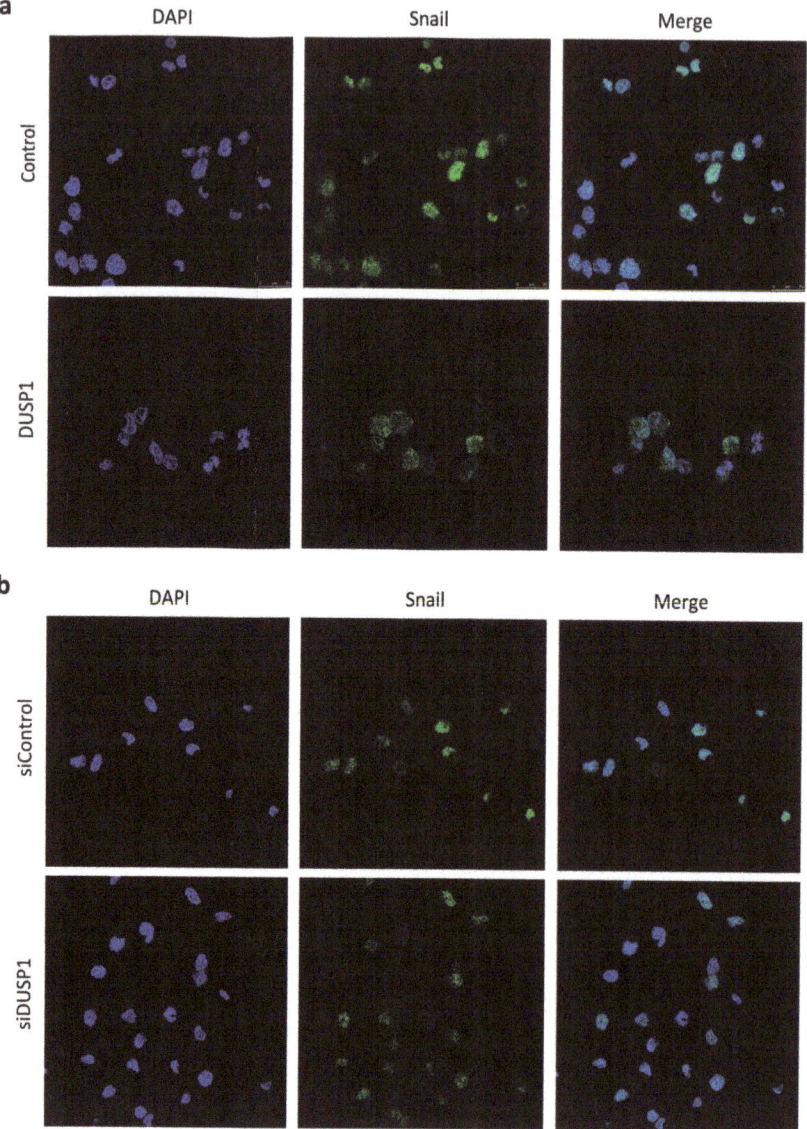

Figure 5. Snail subcellular location is regulated by the phosphatase DUSP1. (**a**) DU145 cells were transfected for 48 h with the Control or the DUSP1 vectors. (**b**) Cells were transfected for 48 h with the siControl or the siDUSP1. In both set of experiments, Snail subcellular location was determined by immunofluorescence as described in Material and methods. DAPI was used to identify the nuclei. Pictures are from one representative experiment of three with similar results.

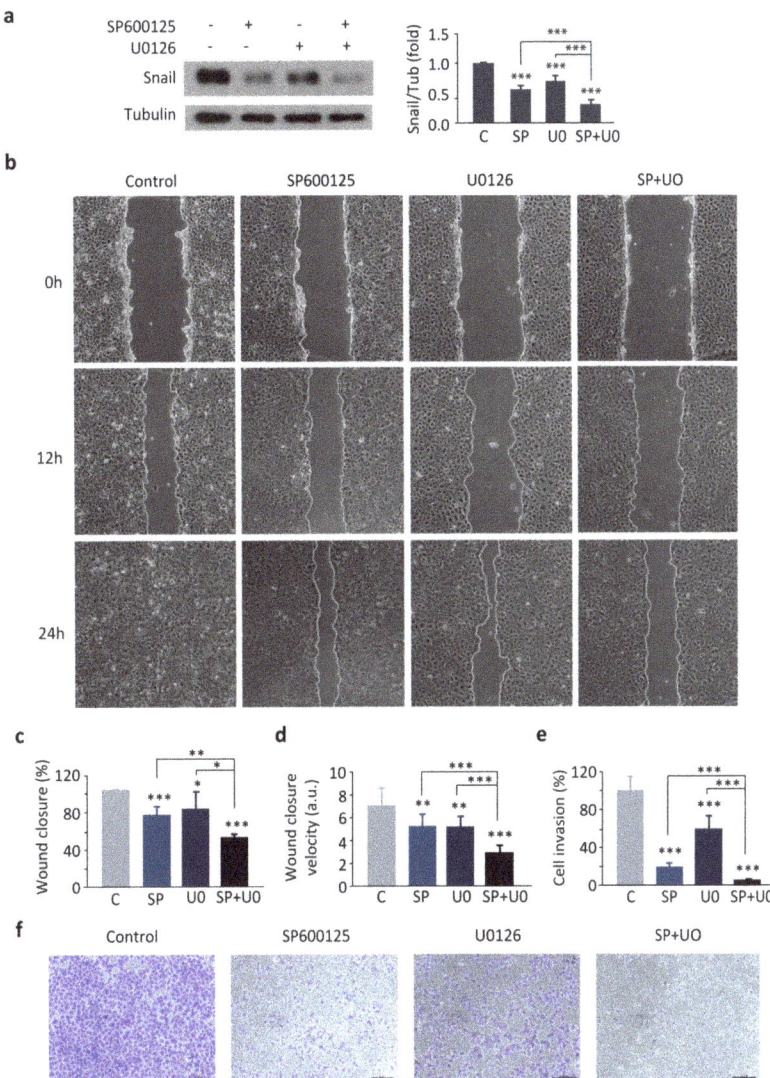

Figure 6. JNK and ERK cooperatively regulate Snail expression, cell migration and invasion in DU145 cells. Cells were incubated in the absence (C) or presence of 10 μM SP600125 (SP, 24 h) and 20 μM U0126 (U0, 48 h). (**a**) Expression levels of Snail and Tubulin were determined by western blotting. (**b–d**) Wound healing assay and measurement of wound closure area and velocity. (**e,f**) Invasion capacity using transwell assays. For all the results, data are shown as the mean ± SEM of at least three independent experiments. For migration and invasion assays, pictures are from one representative experiment of three with similar results. Student's t test: * $0.01 < p < 0.05$; ** $0.001 < p < 0.01$; *** $p < 0.001$.

3.5. DUSP1 Expression Inversely Correlates with Snail Levels and Activated JNK and ERK in Human Prostate Samples

To investigate whether our results obtained from the experiments performed with the cell lines were clinically relevant, we next analyzed the expression levels of DUSP1 and Snail in a series of samples from patients with BPH, HS-PC, and HR-PC (Table 1). Prostatic glands from BPH samples showed a high expression of DUSP1 (Figure 7a-I) and a weak expression of Snail (Figure 7a-X). In prostate cancer samples, DUSP1 expression was high in HS-PC (Figure 7a-II), whereas low or no signal for Snail was detected (Figure 7a-XI). Conversely, HR-PC samples showed a weak or even undetectable DUSP1 expression (Figure 7a-III) but a moderate to strong signal for Snail (Figure 7a-XII). Consequently, the immunohistochemical analyses demonstrated an inverse correlation between DUSP1 and Snail, with a DUSP1$_{high}$/Snail$_{low}$ pattern in both BPH and HS-PC samples, and a DUSP1$_{low}$/Snail$_{high}$ pattern in HR-PC samples. Importantly, results from the Pearson´s Test confirmed the inverse correlation between DUSP1 and Snail expression (Figure 7b).

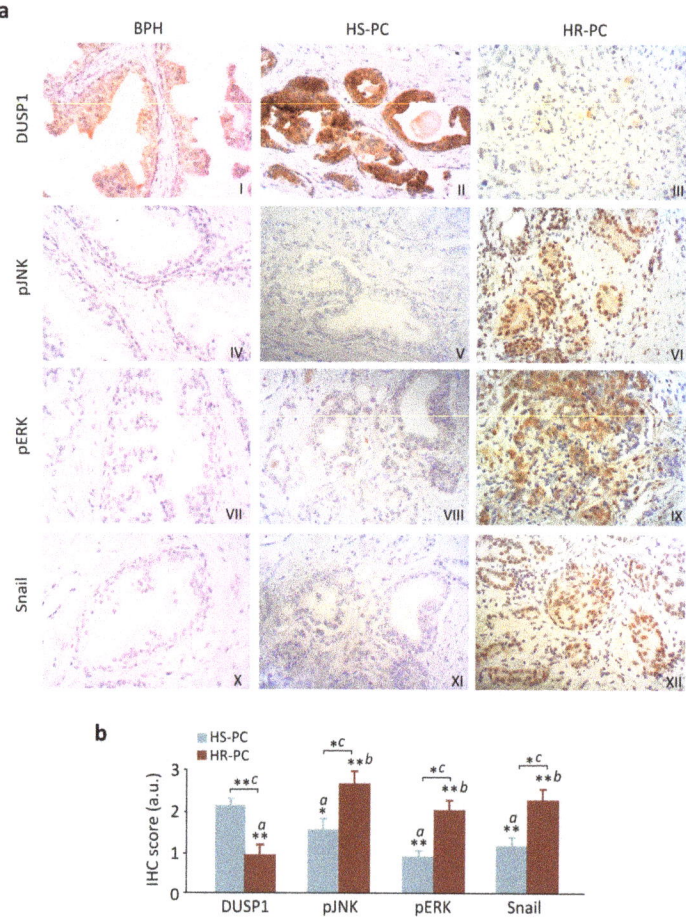

Figure 7. DUSP1 expression inversely correlates with Snail levels and activated JNK and ERK in human prostate samples. (**a**) Immunohistochemical analysis of expression levels of DUSP1 (I–III), phosphorylated JNK (pJNK, IV–VI), phosphorylated ERK (pERK, VII–IX) and Snail (X–XII) from human prostate cancer samples. Micrographs were taken at 200× magnification and show serial sections from the same gland stained with each one of the four used antibodies. (**b**) Immunohistochemical score for DUSP1, pJNK, pERK and Snail in samples from HS-PC and HR-PC. The statistical analysis was performed with One-way ANOVA and Dunnet´s multiple comparison test, and asterisks show the statistical significance of differences between the groups (*a*: comparison with DUSP1 from HS-PC samples; *b*: comparison with DUSP1 from HR-PC samples; *c*: HS-PC vs HR-PC for each marker), * $0.01 < p < 0.05$; ** $0.001 < p < 0.01$.

Since our data in prostate cancer cells revealed that DUSP1 inhibits JNK and ERK (Figure 2a) and these MAPKs negatively regulated Snail expression (Figure 2b–d), we also analyzed the levels of activated JNK and ERK (pJNK and pERK) in patient samples. Accordingly, our results indicated that the levels of active JNK and ERK were low in BPH samples (Figure 7a-IV,VII). Moreover, an inverse correlation was also detected for PC samples, with a $DUSP1_{high}/pJNK_{low}/pERK_{low}$ pattern in samples from HS-PC patients (Figure 7a-II,V,VIII) and a $DUSP1_{low}/pJNK_{high}/pERK_{high}$ pattern in HR-PC samples (Figure 7a-III,VI,IX). As in previous results, the Pearson´s Test confirmed these inverse correlations (Figure 7b).

In all cases, subcellular localization for DUSP1 and pERK was mainly cytosolic, while Snail was located in the cell nucleus. Regarding pJNK subcellular expression, it was predominantly nuclear, although a mild-to-moderate signal for this marker was also observed in cytosol (Figure S5 in Supplementary Materials). Moreover, a compilation of different IHC images for each marker can be observed in Figure S6 in Supplementary Materials.

3.6. The Relationship of DUSP1 and Snail Levels and JNK and ERK Activities Are Associated with Disease Progression and Clinical Outcome in Patients with Prostate Cancer

Since we observed a differential expression of DUSP1, Snail, and the active forms of JNK and ERK in samples from prostate cancer patients at different stages, we next studied the interrelation between the levels of these proteins and some of the most important clinical parameters. Firstly, we analyzed the correlation of expression patterns of DUSP1, Snail, and activated JNK and ERK with either Gleason score (Figure 8a) or American Joint Committee on Cancer (AJCC) group staging at diagnosis [30] (Figure 8b), and no correlation was observed in any of these cases. In contrast, we did observe a significant correlation when we compared the levels of DUSP1, Snail, and activated JNK and ERK with both the disease progression and the clinical outcome (Figure 8c–e). Thus, shorter intervals to clinical progression were related with lower DUSP1 expression and higher levels of activated JNK (*log-rank*, $p = 0.0237$) and ERK (*log-rank*, $p = 0.0005$) (Figure 8c), although we did not observe correlation of time to clinical progression with lower DUSP1 expression and higher levels of Snail (Figure 8c). Despite this, the combined pattern $DUSP1_{low}/pJNK_{high}/pERK_{high}/Snail_{high}$ was strongly related with overall time to clinical progression (*log-rank*, $p = 0.0002$) (Figure 8d). More importantly, our data also evidenced a significant relationship between the expression pattern of these proteins and exitus (Figure 8e). Indeed, the median overall survival of patients with the combined pattern $DUSP1_{low}/pJNK_{high}/pERK_{high}/Snail_{high}$ was 29 months, compared to 79 months in patients with $DUSP1_{high}/pJNK_{low}/pERK_{low}/Snail_{low}$.

Collectively, all the results in human prostate samples reveal the existence of an inverse correlation between DUSP1 expression and the levels of Snail and activated JNK and ERK (negative correlation at Pearson´s test, $p < 0.001$), supporting our experiments in prostate cancer cells which demonstrate that DUSP1 downregulates Snail expression. In addition, our results indicate that low levels of DUSP1 and high levels of pJNK ($p < 0.02$) and pERK ($p < 0.0005$), but not Snail ($p > 0.05$), are related to shorter intervals to clinical progression. Finally, and more interestingly, we evidence that the levels of all proteins tested are related to clinical outcome, suggesting that the ratio between the expression of DUSP1, Snail, and activated JNK and ERK is an important marker for diagnostic purposes in prostate cancer.

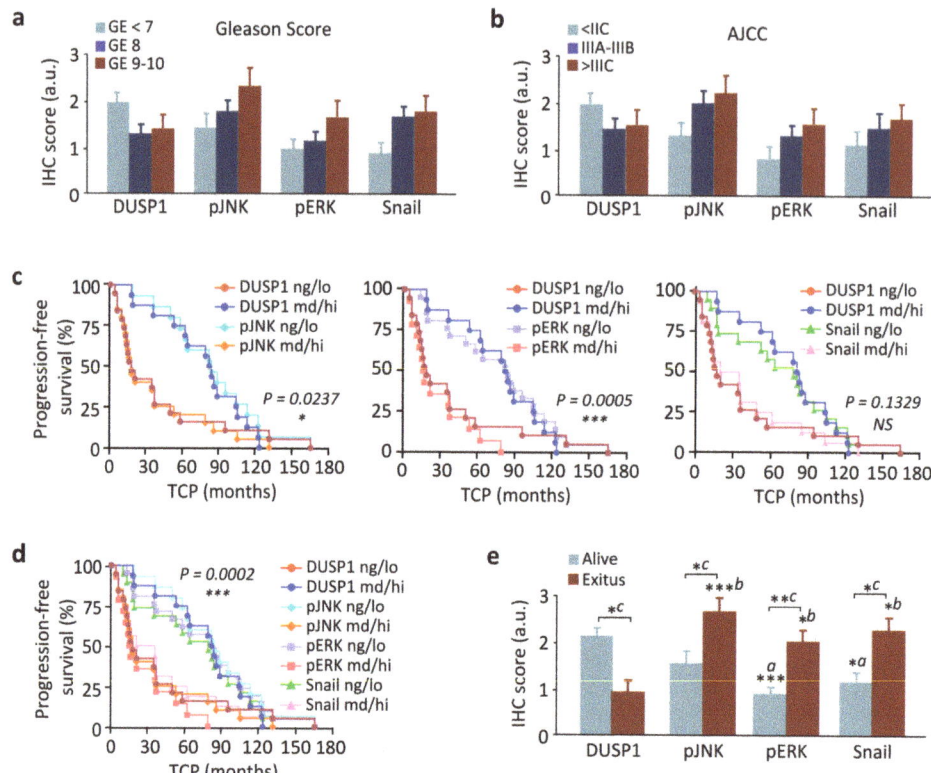

Figure 8. The relationship of DUSP1 and Snail levels and JNK and ERK activities are associated with disease progression and clinical outcome in patients with prostate cancer. (**a**,**b**) Immunohistochemical score for DUSP1, phosphorylated JNK and ERK (pJNK and pERK) and Snail in samples ranged into three categories based on their Gleason Score (**a**) or AJCC group staging at diagnosis (**b**). (**c**) Progression-free survival of patients showing immunohistochemical score for DUSP1/pJNK, DUSP1/pERK or DUSP1/Snail. Samples were ranged into two categories based on the staining pattern of the majority of tumor cells in the whole section (negative/low (ng/lo); moderate/high (md/hi)). (**d**) Progression-free survival of patients showing immunohistochemical score for DUSP1/pJNK/pERK/Snail. Samples were ranged into two categories as described in *c*. (**e**) Immunohistochemical score for DUSP1, pJNK, pERK and Snail in samples from patients either alive or dead. The statistical analysis was performed with One-way ANOVA and Dunnet´s multiple comparison test, and asterisks show the statistical significance of differences between the groups (*a*: comparison with DUSP1 from HS-PC samples; *b*: comparison with DUSP1 from HR-PC samples; *c*: HS-PC vs HR-PC for each marker). *TCP, Time to clinical progression*, * $0.01 < p < 0.05$; ** $0.001 < p < 0.01$; *** $p < 0.001$.

4. Discussion

DUSP1 expression has been previously related to different stages of human prostate carcinomas. In line with this, the expression of this phosphatase is high in BPH and HS-PC, but it is lost in later stages, such as HR-PC [17]. Furthermore, DUSP1 overexpression in androgen-independent prostate cancer cells induces apoptosis through both p38MAPK and NF-kB dependent mechanisms [17]. Here, we show for the first time that this phosphatase plays an additional anti-tumorigenic role in prostate cancer cells, since it decreases the expression levels of the EMT master regulator, Snail, and inhibits cell migration and invasion through the inactivation of JNK and ERK. Interestingly, we also demonstrate a correlation between the expression levels of DUSP1 and Snail and the activity of JNK and

ERK in samples from prostate cancer patients, discovering a novel approach to predict the prognosis and outcome of this disease.

Previous studies have shown that the overexpression of Snail in prostate cancer cells is associated with an increased cell migration and invasion, while its silencing induces a decrease in these processes [31]. In agreement with this, here, we demonstrate that DUSP1 downregulates Snail expression and inhibits migration and invasion in prostate cancer cells. Our data are similar to those observed in different types of tumors, in which DUSP1 suppresses cell migration, cell invasion, metastasis, and/or angiogenesis by inhibiting either ERK [21,23], JNK [22,24], or p38MAPK [20]. Consistently with DUSP1 effects on MAPK activity, the ERK pathway is one of the major oncogenic signals in human cancers because its activation leads to an increase in proliferation, invasion, and metastasis [32]. Particularly in prostate cancer, the ERK pathway is often hyperactivated [33], acts as an inducer of cell migration and invasion [34,35] through a Snail-mediated mechanism [36], and is involved in the effects of different molecules on these processes [37–39]. In addition, the JNK pathway has also been described to be important as a pro-tumorigenic signal through Snail regulation in different tumors [40–42]. Regarding prostate cancer, it has been previously described that JNK activity is related to elevated cell migration and invasion [43] and controls tumor growth in DU145 prostate carcinoma xenografts [44], although the involvement of Snail in these processes is still unknown. Our results are in agreement with all these data, since we demonstrate that the effects of DUSP1 on Snail levels, cell migration, and cell invasion are similar to those observed upon specific inhibition of the ERK and JNK pathways. By contrast, our findings evidence that p38MAPK is not involved in the regulation of these processes by DUSP1. Although several reports have showed that this kinase promotes cancer by enhancing migration in tumor cells [45], we demonstrate that the pro-tumorigenic role of p38MAPK in prostate cancer is more related to its effects on cell apoptosis [17] than to those involved in cell migration and invasion. Overall, all these data suggest that the role that DUSP1 plays as a tumor suppressor in prostate cancer is complex and depends on the specific inactivation of one or the other MAPK, which ultimately controls either cell apoptosis, or cell migration and invasion.

The regulatory mechanisms that control the cellular levels of Snail are very complex and involve changes at the transcriptional level or post-translational modifications, which affect its location in the cell nucleus and/or cytosol, as well as its susceptibility to degradation [16]. Here, we show for the first time that DUSP1 expression regulates the transcription of Snail. Moreover, only the concomitant ERK inhibition affects Snail expression at this level, while JNK controls it exclusively at protein level. Similar data in other cancer cell contexts have shown that the activation of Snail transcription requires an active ERK pathway [46], whereas no data on JNK involvement in this process have been reported. Regarding the regulation of Snail at a protein level, several mechanisms control the migration and invasion of prostate cancer cells by modulating the location and stability of this transcription factor. In this regard, one of the most common regulatory mechanisms is the phosphorylation of Snail by glycogen synthase kinase 3 beta (GSK-3β), which induces its nuclear export to cytosol and marks this protein for degradation in prostate cancer [47–49]. Interestingly, active ERK phosphorylates and inhibits GSK-3β, maintaining Snail in an active non-phosphorylated state and located at the cell nucleus [50]. Thus, the location of Snail in the cytosol promoted by DUSP1-dependent ERK inactivation is a possible mechanism that explains the decrease of Snail levels following DUSP1 overexpression. However, other regulatory mechanisms of Snail expression, independent of GSK-3β, have been previously identified in different tumors. For example, in hepatocarcinoma and breast cancer cells, the JNK pathway upregulates the lysil oxidase-2 (LOXL-2) [51], which oxidizes Snail, preventing its phosphorylation by GSK-3β [52]. In prostate cancer cells, elevated levels of LOXL-2 have been detected [53], supporting the possible involvement of this protein in the effects of the JNK pathway on the prostatic carcinogenesis. Alternatively, our group has previously shown that Snail expression is regulated by ERK and an autocrine loop involving transforming growth factor beta (TGFβ)/Src/focal adhesion kinase (FAK) complex in thyroid cancer cells [28]. Similarly, other authors have demonstrated that FAK activation induces Snail expression and enhances mesothelial cell migration, promoting peritoneal metastasis from ovarian cancer [54]. Moreover, the JNK pathway activates migration by inducing the phosphorylation of paxillin, which is an adaptor protein related to FAK activation in different cancer cells [55,56]. In this regard, DUSP22, a member of the DUSP1 family which reduces JNK activation, negatively regulates cell migration through FAK dephosphorylation and inactivation in lung cancer cells [57]. Given that FAK and paxillin expression is elevated in prostate cancer and both proteins are associated with tumor progression, lymph node metastasis, and/or shortened survival [58,59], it is also plausible that in our cancer model, the paxillin/FAK pathway could contribute to the regulation of Snail expression by ERK and JNK. However, due to the difference between ERK- and JNK-dependent mechanisms, further research is required to investigate the molecular mechanisms underlying Snail regulation by these kinases.

Interestingly, we also demonstrate in this work the existence of an inverse correlation between DUSP1 and Snail expression levels in patients with different stages of prostate cancer. Importantly, in BPH and HS-PC samples, high levels of this phosphatase and low or none Snail expression were detected, while in HR-PC samples, either low or no DUSP1 expression and high Snail levels were observed. In agreement with our results, an increase in Snail expression has been related to disease progression, since there are higher levels of this protein in bone metastasis from prostate cancer compared to BPH samples [13–15]. Furthermore, other studies indicate that 66% of patients with prostatic adenocarcinoma show elevated Snail levels [60]. Here, we add new related information, demonstrating for the first time that Snail expression in patient samples is inversely correlated with DUSP1 levels and directly correlated with activated ERK and JNK pathways. In addition, the increase of active ERK in samples of HR-PC compared to those of HS-PC or BPH observed in our study is coincident with previous works. Accordingly, higher levels of phosphorylated ERK are found in samples obtained from tumors in advanced or metastatic phase, with respect to more localized tumors or BPH samples [61,62]. However, to our knowledge, this is the first study showing that the level of activated JNK is increased in prostate tumors with a more invasive phenotype, as previously seen in breast and urothelial carcinomas [63,64]. All these data obtained from the experiments carried out with patient samples confirm the results derived from our experimental cell line models and suggest that DUSP1 regulates prostate tumor progression by controlling Snail expression through ERK and JNK inactivation.

The presence of Snail has been strongly associated in prostate tumors with a high Gleason score [13,60] but not with other parameters such as the risk of recurrence or the Stage T [13]. In fact, no significant differences have been previously found in Snail expression in non-metastatic, non-recurrent cancer, recurrent cancer, or metastatic cancer at the time of diagnosis, suggesting that increased Snail expression is a relatively early event in the progress of the disease [13]. Most of the samples we analyzed in this study were locally advanced cancers. In fact, just one of our samples was graded as Gleason 6. Intermediate-risk Gleason grade 7 is usually considered as an individual group between grade 6 or lower and grade 8 or higher. Previous studies focused on the differences among the lower and the higher grades, but usually, no significant differences among grade 7 and higher grades were reported. When we correlated the expression of DUSP1, Snail, and activated ERK and JNK to clinical information, we found that their expression patterns did not correlate with either Gleason score or AJCC group staging at diagnosis. However, our results demonstrate that the pattern $DUSP1_{low}/pJNK_{high}/pERK_{high}/Snail_{high}$ is closely related with a worse survival. This observation is in agreement with previous data showing that DUSP1 expression correlates with better prognosis in glioblastoma [22] and with other studies where the association of Snail expression with a worse prognosis in prostate cancer was reported [13]. Therefore, since low DUSP1 expression and high levels of Snail and activated JNK and ERK are positively associated with final outcome (death), we can conclude that besides the overall immunohistochemical profile, high levels of Snail might be considered an independent indicator of bad prognosis that is predictive for worst outcome independently of time to progression. Moreover, since the expression pattern DUSP1$_{high}$/pJNK$_{low}$/pERK$_{low}$/Snail$_{low}$ is associated with an overall extended survival of patients and decreased cell migration and invasion, our results suggest that therapies based on DUSP1 induction combined with ERK and/or JNK inhibition may be promising in the treatment of metastatic prostate cancer.

5. Conclusions

Our study provides new insights about the molecular mechanisms underlying the effects of the phosphatase DUSP1 on metastasis-associated events in prostate cancer (Figure 9). In summary, our experiments show that the overexpression of this phosphatase downregulates Snail levels and decreases cell migration and invasion, whereas DUSP1 silencing shows opposite effects. Moreover, we demonstrate that DUSP1 inactivates JNK and ERK pathways. Interestingly, the inhibition of these two kinases leads to similar effects on Snail expression, cell migration, and invasion to those observed following the overexpression of this phosphatase. In addition, JNK and ERK cooperate to regulate Snail levels, cell migration, and invasion through different mechanisms. Strikingly, we also demonstrate in human prostate tissue samples an inverse correlation between DUSP1 levels and both active JNK and ERK, as well as Snail expression. Thus, we show that the expression pattern DUSP1$_{high}$/pJNK$_{low}$/pERK$_{low}$/Snail$_{low}$ is associated with the overall extended survival of patients. Based on all these data, we conclude that the ratio between the expression levels of DUSP1 and Snail could be an important biomarker for diagnostic purposes in prostate cancer, as they may serve for identifying patients at risk for an unfavorable clinical outcome. In addition, our results strongly suggest that the induction of DUSP1 or the inhibition of ERK and JNK pathways could be useful as a therapeutic approach to treat prostate cancer.

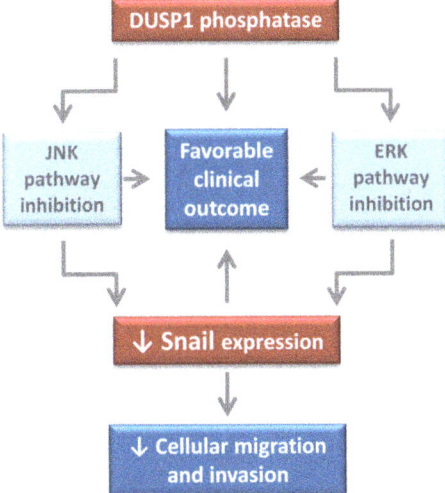

Figure 9. The phosphatase DUSP1 regulates metastasis-associated events in prostate cancer. This study demonstrate that DUSP1 overexpression downregulates Snail levels and decreases cell migration and invasion. Moreover, DUSP1 inactivates ERK and JNK pathways, whose inhibition exert similar effects on Snail expression, cell migration and invasion than overexpression of the phosphatase. In addition, JNK and ERK cooperate to regulate Snail expression, cell migration and invasion through different mechanisms. Finally, in clinical samples, the expression pattern DUSP1$_{high}$/activeJNK$_{low}$/activeERK$_{low}$/Snail$_{low}$ is associated with overall extended survival of patients and may serve as potential biomarker for identifying patients with favorable clinical outcome.

Supplementary Materials: The following are available online at https://www.mdpi.com/2072-6694/13/5/1158/s1, Figure S1: The phosphatase DUSP1 regulates Snail expression and migration in PC3 cells; Figure S2: The MAPKs selective inhibitors reduce MAPK activation; Figure S3: The inhibition of p38MAPK does not affect cell migration; Figure S4: JNK and ERK cooperatively regulate Snail expression and migration in PC3 cells; Figure S5: Immunohistochemical analysis showing details of subcellular localization of DUSP1, pERK, pJNK and Snail levels in samples from BPH, HS-PC and HR-PC selected from Figure 7; Figure S6: Immunohistochemical analysis of expression levels of DUSP1, pERK, pJNK and Snail in samples from three different patients diagnosed with BPH, HS-PC or HR-PC.

Author Contributions: Conceptualization, M.L. and A.C.; methodology, M.L., A.C., P.B., D.M.-M. and M.-V.T.L.; formal analysis, M.L., A.C., D.M.-M., M.-V.T.L. and S.R.; investigation, M.L., D.M.-M. and M.-V.T.L.; resources, M.L., A.C., P.B., M.-V.T.L., S.R., and J.C.A.; writing—original draft preparation, M.L., A.C. and M.-V.T.L.; writing—review and editing, M.L., A.C., P.B., M.-V.T.L., S.R. and J.C.A.; funding acquisition, A.C., P.B. and M.L. All authors have read and agreed to the published version of the manuscript.

Funding: D.M.-M. was recipient of grants from UAM ("Post-Master Program of Dpt. Biochemistry) and from Comunidad de Madrid ("Ayudas para la contratación de investigadores predoctorales y postdoctorales, ref. PEJD-2018-PRE/BMD-8987). P.B. was recipient of a grant from Comunidad de Madrid ("Atracción al Talento Investigador", ref. 2017-T1/BMD-5704).

Institutional Review Board Statement: The study involving human specimens was conducted according to the guidelines of the Declaration of Helsinki, and approved by the Ethics Committee of Hospital Universitario de Getafe (A17-11 of 10/27/2011).

Informed Consent Statement: Informed consent was obtained from all subjects involved in the study.

Data Availability Statement: No new data were created or analyzed in this study. Data sharing is not applicable to this article.

Acknowledgments: We are grateful to J. Renart (Instituto de Investigaciones Biomédicas "Alberto Sols", Madrid, Spain), and Clark (University of Birmingham, UK) for providing Snail-Luc, and pCMVDUSP1 plasmids, respectively. We are grateful to Larriba and Ferrer for their help with cell invasion assays. We thank I. Trabado (Universidad de Alcalá, Spain) for technical help.

Conflicts of Interest: The authors declare no conflict of interest.

References

1. Bray, F.; Ferlay, J.; Soerjomataram, I.; Siegel, R.L.; Torre, L.A.; Jemal, A. Global cancer statistics 2018: GLOBOCAN estimates of incidence and mortality worldwide for 36 cancers in 185 countries. *CA Cancer J. Clin.* **2018**, *68*, 394–424. [CrossRef]
2. Odero-Marah, V.; Hawsawi, O.; Henderson, V.; Sweeney, J. Epithelial-Mesenchymal Transition (EMT) and Prostate Cancer. *Adv. Exp. Med. Biol.* **2018**, *1095*, 101–110. [CrossRef] [PubMed]
3. Pei, D.; Shu, X.; Gassama-Diagne, A.; Thiery, J.P. Mesenchymal-epithelial transition in development and reprogramming. *Nat. Cell Biol.* **2019**, *21*, 44–53. [CrossRef] [PubMed]
4. Nieto, M.A.; Huang, R.Y.; Jackson, R.A.; Thiery, J.P. Emt: 2016. *Cell* **2016**, *166*, 21–45. [CrossRef]
5. Thiery, J.P.; Acloque, H.; Huang, R.Y.; Nieto, M.A. Epithelial-mesenchymal transitions in development and disease. *Cell* **2009**, *139*, 871–890. [CrossRef]
6. Lamouille, S.; Xu, J.; Derynck, R. Molecular mechanisms of epithelial-mesenchymal transition. *Nat. Rev. Mol. Cell Biol.* **2014**, *15*, 178–196. [CrossRef] [PubMed]
7. Sugimachi, K.; Tanaka, S.; Kameyama, T.; Taguchi, K.; Aishima, S.; Shimada, M.; Sugimachi, K.; Tsuneyoshi, M. Transcriptional repressor snail and progression of human hepatocellular carcinoma. *Clin. Cancer Res.* **2003**, *9*, 2657–2664. [PubMed]
8. Perez-Mancera, P.A.; Perez-Caro, M.; Gonzalez-Herrero, I.; Flores, T.; Orfao, A.; de Herreros, A.G.; Gutierrez-Adan, A.; Pintado, B.; Sagrera, A.; Sanchez-Martin, M.; et al. Cancer development induced by graded expression of Snail in mice. *Hum. Mol. Genet.* **2005**, *14*, 3449–3461. [CrossRef]
9. Peinado, H.; Olmeda, D.; Cano, A. Snail, Zeb and bHLH factors in tumour progression: An alliance against the epithelial phenotype? *Nat. Rev. Cancer* **2007**, *7*, 415–428. [CrossRef]
10. Christofori, G. New signals from the invasive front. *Nature* **2006**, *441*, 444–450. [CrossRef]
11. Hardy, R.G.; Vicente-Duenas, C.; Gonzalez-Herrero, I.; Anderson, C.; Flores, T.; Hughes, S.; Tselepis, C.; Ross, J.A.; Sanchez-Garcia, I. Snail family transcription factors are implicated in thyroid carcinogenesis. *Am. J. Pathol.* **2007**, *171*, 1037–1046. [CrossRef] [PubMed]
12. Smith, B.N.; Odero-Marah, V.A. The role of Snail in prostate cancer. *Cell Adhes Migr.* **2012**, *6*, 433–441. [CrossRef]

13. Heeboll, S.; Borre, M.; Ottosen, P.D.; Dyrskjot, L.; Orntoft, T.F.; Torring, N. Snail1 is over-expressed in prostate cancer. *APMIS* **2009**, *117*, 196–204. [CrossRef]
14. Fawzy, A.I.; Gayyed, M.F.; Elsaghir, G.A.; Elbadry, M.S. Expression of Snail transcription factor in prostatic adenocarcinoma in Egypt: Correlation with Maspin protein expression and clinicopathologic variables. *Int. J. Clin. Exp. Pathol.* **2013**, *6*, 1558–1566.
15. Beach, S.; Tang, H.; Park, S.; Dhillon, A.S.; Keller, E.T.; Kolch, W.; Yeung, K.C. Snail is a repressor of RKIP transcription in metastatic prostate cancer cells. *Oncogene* **2008**, *27*, 2243–2248. [CrossRef] [PubMed]
16. Kaufhold, S.; Bonavida, B. Central role of Snail1 in the regulation of EMT and resistance in cancer: A target for therapeutic intervention. *J. Exp. Clin. Cancer Res.* **2014**, *33*, 62. [CrossRef] [PubMed]
17. Gil-Araujo, B.; Toledo Lobo, M.V.; Gutierrez-Salmeron, M.; Gutierrez-Pitalua, J.; Ropero, S.; Angulo, J.C.; Chiloeches, A.; Lasa, M. Dual specificity phosphatase 1 expression inversely correlates with NF-kappaB activity and expression in prostate cancer and promotes apoptosis through a p38 MAPK dependent mechanism. *Mol. Oncol.* **2014**, *8*, 27–38. [CrossRef]
18. Rauhala, H.E.; Porkka, K.P.; Tolonen, T.T.; Martikainen, P.M.; Tammela, T.L.; Visakorpi, T. Dual-specificity phosphatase 1 and serum/glucocorticoid-regulated kinase are downregulated in prostate cancer. *Int. J. Cancer* **2005**, *117*, 738–745. [CrossRef] [PubMed]
19. Martinez-Martinez, D.; Soto, A.; Gil-Araujo, B.; Gallego, B.; Chiloeches, A.; Lasa, M. Resveratrol promotes apoptosis through the induction of dual specificity phosphatase 1 and sensitizes prostate cancer cells to cisplatin. *Food Chem. Toxicol.* **2019**, *124*, 273–279. [CrossRef] [PubMed]
20. Zhang, X.; Hyer, J.M.; Yu, H.; D'Silva, N.J.; Kirkwood, K.L. DUSP1 phosphatase regulates the proinflammatory milieu in head and neck squamous cell carcinoma. *Cancer Res.* **2014**, *74*, 7191–7197. [CrossRef] [PubMed]
21. Shen, J.; Zhou, S.; Shi, L.; Liu, X.; Lin, H.; Yu, H.; Liang, X.; Tang, J.; Yu, T.; Cai, X. DUSP1 inhibits cell proliferation, metastasis and invasion and angiogenesis in gallbladder cancer. *Oncotarget* **2017**, *8*, 12133–12144. [CrossRef]
22. Arrizabalaga, O.; Moreno-Cugnon, L.; Auzmendi-Iriarte, J.; Aldaz, P.; Ibanez de Caceres, I.; Garros-Regulez, L.; Moncho-Amor, V.; Torres-Bayona, S.; Pernia, O.; Pintado-Berninches, L.; et al. High expression of MKP1/DUSP1 counteracts glioma stem cell activity and mediates HDAC inhibitor response. *Oncogenesis* **2017**, *6*, 401. [CrossRef] [PubMed]
23. Kho, D.H.; Uddin, M.H.; Chatterjee, M.; Vogt, A.; Raz, A.; Wu, G.S. GP78 Cooperates with Dual-Specificity Phosphatase 1 to Stimulate Epidermal Growth Factor Receptor-Mediated Extracellular Signal-Regulated Kinase Signaling. *Mol. Cell Biol.* **2019**, *39*. [CrossRef] [PubMed]
24. Pan, S.; Shen, M.; Zhou, M.; Shi, X.; He, R.; Yin, T.; Wang, M.; Guo, X.; Qin, R. Long noncoding RNA LINC01111 suppresses pancreatic cancer aggressiveness by regulating DUSP1 expression via microRNA-3924. *Cell Death Dis.* **2019**, *10*, 883. [CrossRef] [PubMed]
25. Lasa, M.; Gil-Araujo, B.; Palafox, M.; Aranda, A. Thyroid hormone antagonizes tumor necrosis factor-alpha signaling in pituitary cells through the induction of dual specificity phosphatase 1. *Mol. Endocrinol.* **2010**, *24*, 412–422. [CrossRef]
26. Espada, J.; Peinado, H.; Lopez-Serra, L.; Setien, F.; Lopez-Serra, P.; Portela, A.; Renart, J.; Carrasco, E.; Calvo, M.; Juarranz, A.; et al. Regulation of SNAIL1 and E-cadherin function by DNMT1 in a DNA methylation-independent context. *Nucleic Acids Res.* **2011**, *39*, 9194–9205. [CrossRef]
27. Chiloeches, A.; Sanchez-Pacheco, A.; Gil-Araujo, B.; Aranda, A.; Lasa, M. Thyroid hormone-mediated activation of the ERK/dual specificity phosphatase 1 pathway augments the apoptosis of GH4C1 cells by down-regulating nuclear factor-kappaB activity. *Mol. Endocrinol.* **2008**, *22*, 2466–2480. [CrossRef] [PubMed]
28. Baquero, P.; Jimenez-Mora, E.; Santos, A.; Lasa, M.; Chiloeches, A. TGFbeta induces epithelial-mesenchymal transition of thyroid cancer cells by both the BRAF/MEK/ERK and Src/FAK pathways. *Mol. Carcinog.* **2016**, *55*, 1639–1654. [CrossRef]
29. Baquero, P.; Sanchez-Hernandez, I.; Jimenez-Mora, E.; Orgaz, J.L.; Jimenez, B.; Chiloeches, A. (V600E)BRAF promotes invasiveness of thyroid cancer cells by decreasing E-cadherin expression through a Snail-dependent mechanism. *Cancer Lett.* **2013**, *335*, 232–241. [CrossRef] [PubMed]
30. Buyyounouski, M.K.; Choyke, P.L.; McKenney, J.K.; Sartor, O.; Sandler, H.M.; Amin, M.B.; Kattan, M.W.; Lin, D.W. Prostate cancer—Major changes in the American Joint Committee on Cancer eighth edition cancer staging manual. *CA Cancer J. Clin.* **2017**, *67*, 245–253. [CrossRef]
31. Osorio, L.A.; Farfan, N.M.; Castellon, E.A.; Contreras, H.R. SNAIL transcription factor increases the motility and invasive capacity of prostate cancer cells. *Mol. Med. Rep.* **2016**, *13*, 778–786. [CrossRef]
32. Guo, Y.J.; Pan, W.W.; Liu, S.B.; Shen, Z.F.; Xu, Y.; Hu, L.L. ERK/MAPK signalling pathway and tumorigenesis. *Exp. Ther. Med.* **2020**, *19*, 1997–2007. [CrossRef]
33. Yu, C.; Hu, K.; Nguyen, D.; Wang, Z.A. From genomics to functions: Preclinical mouse models for understanding oncogenic pathways in prostate cancer. *Am. J. Cancer Res.* **2019**, *9*, 2079–2102.
34. Kwegyir-Afful, A.K.; Bruno, R.D.; Purushottamachar, P.; Murigi, F.N.; Njar, V.C. Galeterone and VNPT55 disrupt Mnk-eIF4E to inhibit prostate cancer cell migration and invasion. *FEBS J.* **2016**, *283*, 3898–3918. [CrossRef] [PubMed]
35. Chen, P.S.; Shih, Y.W.; Huang, H.C.; Cheng, H.W. Diosgenin, a steroidal saponin, inhibits migration and invasion of human prostate cancer PC-3 cells by reducing matrix metalloproteinases expression. *PLoS ONE* **2011**, *6*, e20164. [CrossRef] [PubMed]
36. Randle, D.D.; Clarke, S.; Henderson, V.; Odero-Marah, V.A. Snail mediates invasion through uPA/uPAR and the MAPK signaling pathway in prostate cancer cells. *Oncol. Lett.* **2013**, *6*, 1767–1773. [CrossRef] [PubMed]

37. Hawsawi, O.; Henderson, V.; Burton, L.J.; Dougan, J.; Nagappan, P.; Odero-Marah, V. High mobility group A2 (HMGA2) promotes EMT via MAPK pathway in prostate cancer. *Biochem. Biophys. Res. Commun.* **2018**, *504*, 196–202. [CrossRef]
38. Ardura, J.A.; Gutierrez-Rojas, I.; Alvarez-Carrion, L.; Rodriguez-Ramos, M.R.; Pozuelo, J.M.; Alonso, V. The secreted matrix protein mindin increases prostate tumor progression and tumor-bone crosstalk via ERK 1/2 regulation. *Carcinogenesis* **2019**, *40*, 828–839. [CrossRef]
39. Zhang, Y.P.; Liu, K.L.; Yang, Z.; Lu, B.S.; Qi, J.C.; Han, Z.W.; Yin, Y.W.; Zhang, M.; Chen, D.M.; Wang, X.W.; et al. The involvement of FBP1 in prostate cancer cell epithelial mesenchymal transition, invasion and metastasis by regulating the MAPK signaling pathway. *Cell Cycle* **2019**, *18*, 2432–2446. [CrossRef]
40. Zhan, X.; Feng, X.; Kong, Y.; Chen, Y.; Tan, W. JNK signaling maintains the mesenchymal properties of multi-drug resistant human epidermoid carcinoma KB cells through snail and twist1. *BMC Cancer* **2013**, *13*, 180. [CrossRef]
41. Choi, Y.; Ko, Y.S.; Park, J.; Choi, Y.; Kim, Y.; Pyo, J.S.; Jang, B.G.; Hwang, D.H.; Kim, W.H.; Lee, B.L. HER2-induced metastasis is mediated by AKT/JNK/EMT signaling pathway in gastric cancer. *World J. Gastroenterol.* **2016**, *22*, 9141–9153. [CrossRef]
42. Kim, J.H.; Shim, J.W.; Eum, D.Y.; Kim, S.D.; Choi, S.H.; Yang, K.; Heo, K.; Park, M.T. Downregulation of UHRF1 increases tumor malignancy by activating the CXCR4/AKT-JNK/IL-6/Snail signaling axis in hepatocellular carcinoma cells. *Sci. Rep.* **2017**, *7*, 2798. [CrossRef] [PubMed]
43. Xu, R.; Hu, J. The role of JNK in prostate cancer progression and therapeutic strategies. *Biomed. Pharmacother.* **2020**, *121*, 109679. [CrossRef]
44. Ennis, B.W.; Fultz, K.E.; Smith, K.A.; Westwick, J.K.; Zhu, D.; Boluro-Ajayi, M.; Bilter, G.K.; Stein, B. Inhibition of tumor growth, angiogenesis, and tumor cell proliferation by a small molecule inhibitor of c-Jun N-terminal kinase. *J. Pharmacol. Exp. Ther.* **2005**, *313*, 325–332. [CrossRef]
45. Martinez-Limon, A.; Joaquin, M.; Caballero, M.; Posas, F.; de Nadal, E. The p38 Pathway: From Biology to Cancer Therapy. *Int. J. Mol. Sci.* **2020**, *21*, 1913. [CrossRef] [PubMed]
46. Barbera, M.J.; Puig, I.; Dominguez, D.; Julien-Grille, S.; Guaita-Esteruelas, S.; Peiro, S.; Baulida, J.; Franci, C.; Dedhar, S.; Larue, L.; et al. Regulation of Snail transcription during epithelial to mesenchymal transition of tumor cells. *Oncogene* **2004**, *23*, 7345–7354. [CrossRef] [PubMed]
47. Wang, H.; Fang, R.; Wang, X.F.; Zhang, F.; Chen, D.Y.; Zhou, B.; Wang, H.S.; Cai, S.H.; Du, J. Stabilization of Snail through AKT/GSK-3beta signaling pathway is required for TNF-alpha-induced epithelial-mesenchymal transition in prostate cancer PC3 cells. *Eur. J. Pharmacol.* **2013**, *714*, 48–55. [CrossRef] [PubMed]
48. Fang, F.; Chen, S.; Ma, J.; Cui, J.; Li, Q.; Meng, G.; Wang, L. Juglone suppresses epithelial-mesenchymal transition in prostate cancer cells via the protein kinase B/glycogen synthase kinase-3beta/Snail signaling pathway. *Oncol. Lett.* **2018**, *16*, 2579–2584. [CrossRef] [PubMed]
49. Liu, Z.C.; Wang, H.S.; Zhang, G.; Liu, H.; Chen, X.H.; Zhang, F.; Chen, D.Y.; Cai, S.H.; Du, J. AKT/GSK-3beta regulates stability and transcription of snail which is crucial for bFGF-induced epithelial-mesenchymal transition of prostate cancer cells. *Biochim. Biophys. Acta* **2014**, *1840*, 3096–3105. [CrossRef]
50. McCubrey, J.A.; Fitzgerald, T.L.; Yang, L.V.; Lertpiriyapong, K.; Steelman, L.S.; Abrams, S.L.; Montalto, G.; Cervello, M.; Neri, L.M.; Cocco, L.; et al. Roles of GSK-3 and microRNAs on epithelial mesenchymal transition and cancer stem cells. *Oncotarget* **2017**, *8*, 14221–14250. [CrossRef]
51. Wu, S.; Zheng, Q.; Xing, X.; Dong, Y.; Wang, Y.; You, Y.; Chen, R.; Hu, C.; Chen, J.; Gao, D.; et al. Matrix stiffness-upregulated LOXL2 promotes fibronectin production, MMP9 and CXCL12 expression and BMDCs recruitment to assist pre-metastatic niche formation. *J. Exp. Clin. Cancer Res.* **2018**, *37*, 99. [CrossRef] [PubMed]
52. de Herreros, A.G.; Peiro, S.; Nassour, M.; Savagner, P. Snail family regulation and epithelial mesenchymal transitions in breast cancer progression. *J. Mammary Gland. Biol. Neoplasia* **2010**, *15*, 135–147. [CrossRef] [PubMed]
53. Xie, P.; Yu, H.; Wang, F.; Yan, F.; He, X. Inhibition of LOXL2 Enhances the Radiosensitivity of Castration-Resistant Prostate Cancer Cells Associated with the Reversal of the EMT Process. *Biomed. Res. Int.* **2019**, *2019*, 4012590. [CrossRef] [PubMed]
54. Li, X.; Tang, M.; Zhu, Q.; Wang, X.; Lin, Y.; Wang, X. The exosomal integrin alpha5beta1/AEP complex derived from epithelial ovarian cancer cells promotes peritoneal metastasis through regulating mesothelial cell proliferation and migration. *Cell Oncol.* **2020**, *43*, 263–277. [CrossRef]
55. Huang, C.; Rajfur, Z.; Borchers, C.; Schaller, M.D.; Jacobson, K. JNK phosphorylates paxillin and regulates cell migration. *Nature* **2003**, *424*, 219–223. [CrossRef]
56. Lopez-Colome, A.M.; Lee-Rivera, I.; Benavides-Hidalgo, R.; Lopez, E. Paxillin: A crossroad in pathological cell migration. *J. Hematol. Oncol.* **2017**, *10*, 50. [CrossRef]
57. Li, J.P.; Fu, Y.N.; Chen, Y.R.; Tan, T.H. JNK pathway-associated phosphatase dephosphorylates focal adhesion kinase and suppresses cell migration. *J. Biol. Chem.* **2010**, *285*, 5472–5478. [CrossRef] [PubMed]
58. Rovin, J.D.; Frierson, H.F., Jr.; Ledinh, W.; Parsons, J.T.; Adams, R.B. Expression of focal adhesion kinase in normal and pathologic human prostate tissues. *Prostate* **2002**, *53*, 124–132. [CrossRef] [PubMed]
59. Zheng, Q.S.; Chen, S.H.; Wu, Y.P.; Chen, H.J.; Chen, H.; Wei, Y.; Li, X.D.; Huang, J.B.; Xue, X.Y.; Xu, N. Increased Paxillin expression in prostate cancer is associated with advanced pathological features, lymph node metastases and biochemical recurrence. *J. Cancer* **2018**, *9*, 959–967. [CrossRef]

60. Wen, Y.C.; Chen, W.Y.; Lee, W.J.; Yang, S.F.; Lee, L.M.; Chien, M.H. Snail as a potential marker for predicting the recurrence of prostate cancer in patients at stage T2 after radical prostatectomy. *Clin. Chim. Acta* **2014**, *431*, 169–173. [CrossRef] [PubMed]
61. Li, S.; Fong, K.W.; Gritsina, G.; Zhang, A.; Zhao, J.C.; Kim, J.; Sharp, A.; Yuan, W.; Aversa, C.; Yang, X.J.; et al. Activation of MAPK Signaling by CXCR7 Leads to Enzalutamide Resistance in Prostate Cancer. *Cancer Res.* **2019**, *79*, 2580–2592. [CrossRef] [PubMed]
62. Nickols, N.G.; Nazarian, R.; Zhao, S.G.; Tan, V.; Uzunangelov, V.; Xia, Z.; Baertsch, R.; Neeman, E.; Gao, A.C.; Thomas, G.V.; et al. MEK-ERK signaling is a therapeutic target in metastatic castration resistant prostate cancer. *Prostate Cancer Prostatic Dis.* **2019**, *22*, 531–538. [CrossRef] [PubMed]
63. Sahu, S.K.; Garding, A.; Tiwari, N.; Thakurela, S.; Toedling, J.; Gebhard, S.; Ortega, F.; Schmarowski, N.; Berninger, B.; Nitsch, R.; et al. JNK-dependent gene regulatory circuitry governs mesenchymal fate. *EMBO J.* **2015**, *34*, 2162–2181. [CrossRef]
64. Shimada, K.; Nakamura, M.; Ishida, E.; Higuchi, T.; Tanaka, M.; Ota, I.; Konishi, N. c-Jun NH2 terminal kinase activation and decreased expression of mitogen-activated protein kinase phosphatase-1 play important roles in invasion and angiogenesis of urothelial carcinomas. *Am. J. Pathol.* **2007**, *171*, 1003–1012. [CrossRef] [PubMed]

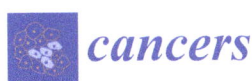

Article

NEK1 Phosphorylation of YAP Promotes Its Stabilization and Transcriptional Output

Md Imtiaz Khalil [1], Ishita Ghosh [1], Vibha Singh [1], Jing Chen [2], Haining Zhu [2] and Arrigo De Benedetti [1,*]

[1] Department of Biochemistry and Molecular Biology, LSU Health Sciences Center, Shreveport, LA 71130, USA; mkhal2@lsuhsc.edu (M.I.K.); ighosh@lsuhsc.edu (I.G.); Vibha.Singh@utdallas.edu (V.S.)

[2] Department of Molecular and Cellular Biochemistry and Proteomics Core, Center for Structural Biology, University of Kentucky, Lexington, KY 40506, USA; jchen4@email.uky.edu (J.C.); haining@uky.edu (H.Z.)

* Correspondence: adeben@lsuhsc.edu; Tel.: +1-31-8675-5668

Received: 3 November 2020; Accepted: 4 December 2020; Published: 7 December 2020

Simple Summary: We earlier described the involvement of the TLK1>NEK1>ATR>Chk1 axis as a key determinant of cell cycle arrest in androgen-dependent prostate cancer (PCa) cells after androgen deprivation. We now report that the TLK1>NEK1 axis is also involved in stabilization of yes-associated protein 1 (YAP1), the transcriptional co-activator in the Hippo pathway, presumably facilitating reprogramming of the cells toward castration-resistant PCa (CRPC). NEK1 interacts with YAP1 physically resulting in its phosphorylation of 6 residues, which enhance its stability and activity. Analyses of cancer Protein Atlas and TCGA expression panels revealed a link between activated NEK1 and YAP1 expression and several YAP transcription targets.

Abstract: Most prostate cancer (PCa) deaths result from progressive failure in standard androgen deprivation therapy (ADT), leading to metastatic castration-resistant PCa (mCRPC); however, the mechanism and key players leading to this are not fully understood. While studying the role of tousled-like kinase 1 (TLK1) and never in mitosis gene A (NIMA)-related kinase 1 (NEK1) in a DNA damage response (DDR)-mediated cell cycle arrest in LNCaP cells treated with bicalutamide, we uncovered that overexpression of wt-NEK1 resulted in a rapid conversion to androgen-independent (AI) growth, analogous to what has been observed when YAP1 is overexpressed. We now report that overexpression of wt-NEK1 results in accumulation of YAP1, suggesting the existence of a TLK1>NEK1>YAP1 axis that leads to adaptation to AI growth. Further, YAP1 is co-immunoprecipitated with NEK1. Importantly, NEK1 was able to phosphorylate YAP1 on six residues in vitro, which we believe are important for stabilization of the protein, possibly by increasing its interaction with transcriptional partners. In fact, knockout (KO) of NEK1 in NT1 PCa cells resulted in a parallel decrease of YAP1 level and reduced expression of typical YAP-regulated target genes. In terms of cancer potential implications, the expression of NEK1 and YAP1 proteins was found to be increased and correlated in several cancers. These include PCa stages according to Gleason score, head and neck squamous cell carcinoma, and glioblastoma, suggesting that this co-regulation is imparted by increased YAP1 stability when NEK1 is overexpressed or activated by TLK1, and not through transcriptional co-expression. We propose that the TLK1>NEK1>YAP1 axis is a key determinant for cancer progression, particularly during the process of androgen-sensitive to -independent conversion during progression to mCRPC.

Keywords: tousled-like kinase (TLK); NIMA-related kinase 1 (NEK1); yes-associated protein 1 (YAP1); thioridazine (THD); MS-determined phosphopeptides

1. Introduction

The founding member of the NIMA (never in mitosis gene A) family of protein kinases was originally identified in *Aspergillus nidulans* as a protein kinase essential for mitosis [1], and expression of a dominant-negative mutant of NIMA results in G2 arrest in vertebrate cells [2]. NIMA-related kinases (NEKs) have adapted to a variety of cellular functions in addition to mitosis [3]. In human cells, 11 NEKs were identified that are involved in several functions. For example, NEK2 is critical for centrosome duplication [3], whereas NEK6, 7, and 9 are regulators of the mitotic spindle and cytokinesis [4]. NEK1, NEK4, NEK8, NEK10, and NEK11 have been linked to the DNA damage response (DDR) and DNA repair pathways as well as ciliogenesis [3]. NEK1 mediates Chk1 activation likely by modulating the ATRIP/ATR interaction and activity [5], although this may be controversial [6]. NEK1 activity and relocalization to nuclei were reported to increase upon a variety of genotoxic stresses [5,7]. A defect in DNA repair in NEK1-deficient cells is suggested by the persistence of Double Strand Breaks (DSBs) after low-dose ionizing radiation (IR). NEK1-deficient cells fail to activate the checkpoint kinases Chk1 and Chk2, and fail to arrest properly at G1/S- or G2/M-phase checkpoints after DNA damage [8]. NEK1-deficient cells suffer major errors in mitotic chromosome segregation and cytokinesis, and become aneuploid [9]. Genomic instability is also manifested in NEK1$^{+/-}$ mice, which later in life develop lymphomas with a higher incidence than wild type littermates [9]. NEK1 is also known to negatively regulate apoptosis by phosphorylating VDAC1, regulating the closure of the anion channel of the mitochondrial membrane, which promotes survival of renal cell carcinoma [10–12]. Loss of function mutation of NEK1 leads to DNA damage accumulation in the motorneurons that may lead to several neurodegenerative diseases such as amyotrophic lateral sclerosis (ALS) [13,14]. NEK1 is associated with primary cilia and centrosomes [15,16], which was reported to be implicated in the development of polycystic kidney disease (PKD) when there is a NEK1 deficiency [17]. However, the precise mechanism leading to PKD due to NEK1 insufficiency is not clear, but a clue came from the discovery that NEK1 interacts with and phosphorylates TAZ, involved in the E3 ligase complex, which regulates the stability of polycystin 2 [18]. TAZ is also a paralog of yes-associated protein (YAP), a transcriptional coactivator that mediates many functions in normal development and in disease pathology, such as cancer progression, including prostate cancer [19–22].

We recently uncovered a new DDR axis involving the protein kinase tousled-like kinase (TLK)1 as an early mediator of the DDR. TLK1 serves as an upstream activator of NEK1>ATR>Chk1 [6,23], which has important implications during the early stages of prostate cancer (PCa) progression to androgen independence (AI) [24,25]. We found that overexpression of wt-NEK1 (but not the T141A kinase-hypoactive mutant that cannot be phosphorylated by TLK1) hastens the progression of LNCaP cells to androgen-independent growth [24]. The protective cell cycle arrest mediated by the TLK1>NEK1 DDR pathway seems insufficient to explain the rapid growth recovery observed in bicalutamide-treated cells when NEK1 is overexpressed, and suggests that NEK1 may have additional functions. We suspected that it may regulate the Hippo pathway, as it was reported that ectopic expression of YAP is sufficient to convert LNCaP cells from androgen-sensitive (AS) to AI in vitro [19]. NEK1 was also found to phosphorylate TAZ specifically at S309 [18], and this was related to increased CTGF expression (one of TAZ/YAP transcriptional targets). TLKs may regulate the Hippo pathway through their activity on NEK1 upstream of YAP/TAZ. YAP/TAZ (60% identical) are the main effectors of the Hippo signaling pathway. This pathway is involved in regulating organ size through controlling multiple cellular functions including cell proliferation and apoptosis [26]. The Hippo pathway responds to a variety of signals, including cell–cell contact, mechano-transduction [21], and apico–basal polarity [20,26]. When the Hippo pathway is activated, kinases MST1/2 and LATS1/2 phosphorylate and inactivate YAP and TAZ. YAP and TAZ are transcriptional co-activators but lack DNA binding activity. Upon phosphorylation by MST and LATS kinases, they are sequestered in the cytoplasm, ubiquitylated by the β-TrCP ubiquitin ligase, and marked for proteasomal degradation (reviewed in [20]). YAP/TAZ are usually inhibited by cell–cell contact in normal tissues [26], while over-activation of YAP/TAZ through aberrant regulation of the Hippo pathway has been noted in many types of tumors. This is associated with the acquisition of malignant traits, including resistance to anticancer therapies; maintenance of cancer stem cells; distant metastasis [26]; and, in prostate, adenocarcinoma progression [27,28]. When the Hippo core kinases are "off", YAP/TAZ translocate into the nucleus, binds to TEAD1–4, and activates the transcription of TEAD downstream target genes, leading to multiple oncogenic activities, including loss of contact inhibition, cell proliferation, epithelial–mesenchymal transition, and resistance to apoptosis. In PCa, YAP has been identified as an Androgen Receptor-binding partner that colocalizes with AR in both androgen-dependent and androgen-independent manners in castration-resistant PCa (CRPC) patients [27]. YAP is also found to be upregulated in AI-LNCaP-C4-2 cells and, when expressed ectopically in LNCaP cells, it activates AR signaling and confers castration resistance. Knockdown of YAP greatly reduces the rates of migration and invasion of LNCaP, and YAP-activated androgen receptor signaling is sufficient to promote LNCaP cells from an AS to an AI state in vitro, while YAP conferred castration resistance in vivo [19]. It was also recently determined that ERG (and the common *TMPRSS2–ERG* fusion) activates the transcriptional program regulated by YAP1, and that prostate-specific activation of either ERG or YAP1 in mice induces similar transcriptional changes and results in age-related prostate tumors [29]. However, it has remained unclear as to what the upstream activators of the Hippo pathway are in PCa, and we show in this report that TLKs have a role in this process via activation and induced stabilization of YAP from elevated phosphorylation by NEK1.

2. Materials and Methods

2.1. Plasmids and Antibodies

Wild type human full length NEK1 mammalian expression plasmid was purchased from Origene (MR216282). NEK1 T141A variant was generated by site-directed mutagenesis, as previously described [23]. Generation of His-tagged N-terminal NEK1 (aa 1–480) bacterial expression plasmid was conducted as previously described. Human full length MK5 bacterial expression plasmid was purchased from Vector Builder. The following antibodies were used in this study: mouse anti-YAP (Santa Cruz Biotechnology, SCBT, Dallas, TX, USA, cat# sc101199), rabbit anti-phospho-YAP (Cell Signaling Technology, CST, Dallas, TX, USA, cat# 13008), mouse anti-NEK1 (SCBT, cat# sc 398813, Dallas, TX, USA), rabbit anti-phospho-NEK1 pT141 (lab-generated), rabbit anti-phospho-tyrosine (CST, cat# 8954S, Dallas, TX, USA), HRP-conjugated anti-β-tubulin (SCBT, Dallas, TX, USA, cat# sc-23949), mouse IgG (SCBT, Dallas, TX, USA, cat# sc-2025), and rabbit anti-actin (Abcam, Cambridge, MA, USA, cat# ab1801).

2.2. Cell Culture

Human embryonic kidney HEK293 and HeLa cells were cultured in Dulbecco Modified Eagle Medium (DMEM) supplemented with 10% Fetal Bovine Serum (FBS) and 1% penicillin/streptomycin. HEK293T cells were cultured in D10 medium containing 10% FBS, 0.25% penicillin/streptomycin, and 1% glutamine in DMEM media. LNCaP cells were cultured in Roswell Park Memorial Institute (RPMI) 1640 supplemented with 10% FBS and 1% penicillin/streptomycin. NT1 cells were a kind gift from Dr. Xiuping Yu (Department of Biochemistry, Louisiana State University Health Sciences Center Shreveport) and cultured according to the published literature [30]. All other cells were purchased from American Type Culture Collection (ATCC). All the cells were maintained in a humidified incubator at 37 °C with 5% CO_2.

2.3. Cell Treatment

LNCaP or HeLa or NT1 cells were plated as 5×10^5 cells per well in a 6-well plate and grown until 70–80% confluency. Cells were treated with either 10 µM of either bicalutamide (Selleckchem, Houston, TX, USA, cat# S1190), thioridazine (THD; Sigma Aldrich, St. Louis, MO, USA, cat# T9025 or J54 [31], or in combination with both bicalutamide and THD for 24 h. After the treatment, cells were harvested for Western blotting (WB) analysis or qPCR analysis.

2.4. Cell Transfection

LNCaP cells were transfected with either wild type mouse full-length NEK1 or NEK1 T141A variant, as previously described [23]. TLK1 shRNA (ATTACTTCATCTGCTTGGTAGAGGTGGCT) was obtained from origene (Rockville, MD, USA, cat# TR320623). HeLa cells were plated as 10^5 cells per well in a 6-well plate 24 h before shRNA transfection. Transfection was conducted using 140 nM and 280 nM of TLK1 shRNA by lipofectamine 3000 (Thermo Scientific, Waltham, MA, USA, cat# L3000-015) reagent for 24 h, following the manufacturer's protocol, and subsequently selected the cells with 1 µg/mL of puromycin for 7 days. Puromycin-selected cells were harvested and knockdown efficiency was determined by WB.

2.5. Co-immunoprecipitation (co-IP)

Cells were lysed by sonication in 1X RIPA lysis buffer (SCBT, Dallas, TX, USA, cat# 24948). A total of 50 µL of equilibrated protein A/G agarose (SCBT, Dallas, TX, USA, cat# sc-2003) was incubated with either mouse anti-NEK1 antibody or mouse IgG antibody at 4 °C for 4 h with rotation. A total of 500 µg of protein lysate was added to the reaction and incubated overnight at 4 °C. Beads were washed thrice and eluted with 25 µL of 2X SDS-Laemmli buffer, and the entire volume was loaded into SDS-PAGE gel for WB analysis.

2.6. Generation of NT1 NEK1 Knockout (KO) Cells Lines

NT1 NEK1 KO clones were generated by lentiviral infection using NEK1 CRISPR gRNA (AAGGAGAGAAGTTGCTGTAT) cloned into pLentiCRISPR V2 vector backbone from Genscript (Piscataway, NJ, USA). Lentivirus containing NEK1 CRISPR gRNA was packaged using HEK293T cells. NT1 cells were infected with lentivirus using polybrene transfection reagent following standard protocol. After 72 h of infection, cells were supplemented with fresh media and selected with 1–2 µg/mL of puromycin for 10 days. To generate a single clonal population of NEK1 KO cells, we seeded 1–2 cells per well in a 96-well plate and grew them until confluency, and then transferred them to a bigger dish for expansion. KO efficiency was measured by Western blotting (WB) using anti-NEK1 mouse antibody from Santa Cruz Biotechnology (Dallas, TX, USA, cat# sc-398813).

2.7. Protein Purification

Recombinant His-tagged full-length MK5 and His-tagged NEK1 N-terminal-truncated proteins (NEK1ΔCT) were purified by affinity chromatography. Both MK5 and NEK1ΔCT were transformed into Rosetta2 DE3 strain [23]. Expression of His-MK5 was induced with 1mM Isopropyl β-d-1-thiogalactopyranoside (IPTG) at 37 °C for 3–4 h, and His-NEK1ΔCT expression was induced with 0.5 mM IPTG overnight at 25 °C. Bacteria were pelleted down; dissolved in buffer containing 50 mM sodium phosphate (Na_2HPO_4 + NaH_2PO_4) of pH 8.0, 300 mM NaCl, 20 mM imidazole, and 1mM phenylmethylsulfonyl fluoride (PMSF); and lysed by sonication. Supernatants were incubated with Ni-NTA agarose (Qiagen, cat# 30210), and protein was eluted in buffer containing 50 mM sodium phosphate (Na_2HPO_4 + NaH_2PO_4) of pH 8.0, 300 mM NaCl, and 250 mM imidazole. Eluted proteins were dialyzed overnight at 4 °C using dialysis buffer containing 20 mM sodium phosphate (Na_2HPO_4 + NaH_2PO_4) of pH 7.7, 1 M NaCl, 10 mM β-mercaptoethanol, 0.5 mM ethylenediaminetetraacetic acid (EDTA) of pH 8.0, and 5% glycerol. After the dialysis, protein samples were run in SDS-PAGE gel to check their purity and correct molecular weight.

2.8. ADP Hunter Assay

ADP hunter assays were conducted to determine the catalytic activity of the purified kinases by the fluorescence detection of ATP to ADP conversion using an ADP Hunter Plus Assay kit (Eurofins, DeSoto, TX, USA, cat# 90-0083). Increasing amount of purified recombinant NEK1 or MK5 were incubated with either dephosphorylated α-casein (substrate for NEK1, source: Sigma-Aldrich, St.

Louis, Missouri, USA, cat# C8032) or purified recombinant HSP27 (substrate for MK5, source: Abcam, Cambridge, MA, USA, cat# ab48740). The manufacturer provided kinase buffer, and 50 µM of ATP was added to the reaction, incubating the reaction at 30 °C for 30 min. Afterwards, reagent A and B were added sequentially, incubating the reaction at room temperature for 30 min. Stop solution was added and fluorescence intensity signal was measured at 530/590 nm excitation/emission wavelength. ADP concentration was determined by the standard curve through the serial dilutions of the ADP standards provided with the kit.

2.9. In Vitro Kinase Assay

In vitro kinase (IVK) assays were performed using purified recombinant proteins, kinase buffer, ATP, and/or [γ-^{32}P] ATP. Purified recombinant GST-tagged YAP1 (Novus Biologicals, cat# Centennial, CO, USA, H00010413-P01) was incubated with either purified recombinant His-NEK1ΔCT or purified recombinant His-tagged MK5. Kinase buffer (10X) contains 10 mM Tris-Cl of pH 7.5, 10 mM MgCl$_2$, 10 mM dithiothreitol (DTT), and 10 mM ATP. For radioactive IVK assays, we added 10 µCi of radiolabeled [γ-^{32}P] ATP purchased from Perkin Elmer (cat# BLU002H250UC). The reactions were incubated for 30 min at 30 °C and subsequently were separated by SDS-PAGE, stained with Coomassie Brilliant Blue, and exposed to X-ray film for 72 h. For mass spectrometric (MS) analysis, YAP1 bands were excised after Coomassie staining and sent to the Kentucky MS facility.

2.10. Identification of YAP1 Phosphorylation by Mass Spectrometry

The band corresponding to YAP1 was excised and subjected to dithiothreitol reduction, iodoacetamide alkylation, and in-gel chymotrypsin digestion. Peptides were extracted, concentrated, and subjected to LC–MS/MS analysis at the University of Kentucky Proteomics Core Facility, as previously reported [32]. Briefly, LC–MS/MS analysis was performed using an LTQ-Orbitrap mass spectrometer (Thermo Fisher Scientific, Waltham, MA) coupled with an Eksigent Nanoflex cHiPLC system (Eksigent, Dublin, CA, USA) through a nano-electrospray ionization source. The peptide samples were separated with a reversed-phase cHiPLC column (75 µm × 15 cm) at a flow rate of 300 nL/min. Mobile phase A was water with 0.1% (*v/v*) formic acid, while B was acetonitrile with 0.1% (*v/v*) formic acid. The data-dependent acquisition method consisted of an Orbitrap MS scan (250–1800 m/z) with 60,000 resolution for parent ions, followed by MS/MS for fragmentation of the 10 most intense multiple charged ions. The LC–MS/MS data were submitted to a local Mascot server for MS/MS protein identification via Proteome Discoverer (version 1.3, Thermo Fisher Scientific, Waltham, MA, USA). Typical parameters used in the Mascot MS/MS ion search were chymotrypsin digestion with a maximum of two miscleavages; 10 ppm precursor ion and 0.8 Da fragment ion mass tolerances; and dynamic modifications, including cysteine carbamidomethylation, methionine oxidation, and serine/threonine/tyrosine phosphorylation. The identified phosphorylation sites were illustrated with relevant b and/or y ions labeled.

2.11. Western Blotting

Cells were collected and lysed by sonication in 1X RIPA lysis buffer. Protein concentration was determined using a Pierce BCA protein assay kit (Thermo Scientific, cat# 23225, Waltham, MA, USA). Samples from the lysate or co-IP or IVK assays were separated by SDS-PAGE gels and transferred to polyvinylidene fluoride (PVDF) membrane. The membrane was blocked in 5% non-fat dry milk for 1 h at room temperature and incubated with primary antibodies overnight at 4 °C. Afterwards, HRP-conjugated secondary antibodies were used to incubate the blots for 1 h at room temperature, and finally the specific proteins were detected by chemiluminescence using ECL substrates (Thermo Scientific, Waltham, MA, USA, cat# 32106) or by colorimetry using Opti-4CN substrate kit (Biorad, cat# 1708235, Waltham, MA, USA). The membrane was visualized by Biorad chemidoc imaging system (Biorad, Hercules, CA, USA, cat# 12003154). Densitometric quantifications of each blot in arbitrary units relative to the loading control are shown in Figure S5.

2.12. Real-time Quantitative PCR (RT-qPCR)

Total RNA was isolated using a RNeasy RNA isolation minikit (Qiagen, cat# 74104, Germantown, MD, USA) according to the manufacturer's instructions. Complementary DNA (cDNA) was synthesized using 1µg of RNA/reaction using ProtoScript First Strand RNA synthesis reverse transcriptase and oligo (dT) primers (New England Biolab, cat# E6300L, Ipswich, MA, USA). qPCR was conducted using iQ SYBR green supermix (Biorad, cat# 1708880, Des Plaines, IL, USA) and Bio-Rad CFX96 Fast Real-Time PCR Systems. Gene expression changes were determined by $\Delta\Delta Ct$ relative quantification method. GAPDH mRNA was used as an internal control. All values are presented as mean ± standard error mean (SEM).

2.13. Bioinformatics Analysis

mRNA expression analyses of TCGA patient datasets were conducted using the UALCAN online platform [33]. Oncoprints of the NEK1 and YAP1 protein level of at least more than 0.5-fold increase was generated using Cbioportal [34] from The Cancer Genome Atlas (TCGA-firehose legacy) datasets. Proteomic level of NEK1 and YAP1 based on the immunohistochemistry (IHC) analysis in different cancers were determined using the Human Protein Atlas [35] database. Representative IHC images of high-grade prostate adenocarcinoma (PRAD) and metastatic head and neck squamous cell (HNSC) carcinoma were also obtained from the Human Protein Atlas database. Volcano plot of gene enrichment correlated with NEK1 upregulation of TCGA (firehose legacy) head and neck cancer study was generated using the cBIOPORTAL web tool.

3. Results

3.1. NEK1 Regulated the Stability of YAP

We have previously reported that androgen deprivation in LNCaP cells results in a strong increase in expression of TLK1B. This increase is mTOR-dependent and suppressible with rapamycin [24]. Similar results were obtained with TRAMP-C2 cells [24], and more recently in a AR+/PDX adenocarcinoma model (NSG-TM00298 [25]). This is apparently a critical survival mechanism of AS-PCa cells that implement a DDR in order to arrest in G1 upon androgen deprivation-like treatment with bicalutamide (BIC) [36]. We have recently attributed the probable mechanisms causing this DDR activation to the role played by the AR as a replication licensing factor [37] in combination with the increased expression of TLK1B, and resulting activation of the NEK1>ATR>Chk1 axis [24], which is a key target of TLK1 [23]. Additional work from our lab suggested that this may be a conserved nexus in other cellular models, in the TRAMP mice, and probably in many patients, since the specific activating phosphorylation of NEK1 by TLK1 correlates with the Gleason score [25]. While the significance of the cell cycle arrest upon unfavorable growth conditions (androgen deprivation therapy, ADT) seems clear in order to avoid mitotic catastrophe, it is still unclear how AS-PCa cells eventually adapt to ADT and reprogram to become AI (CRPC progression). Interestingly, we have previously noticed that when LNCaP cells were stably transfected with a wt-NEK1 expression vector, they rapidly (less than 1 week) became tolerant to BIC and resumed growth to form AI colonies [24]. However, this did not happen when we expressed the hypoactive T141A-NEK1 variant [23] that cannot be phosphorylated/activated by TLK1, while these cells also remained AS when injected as xenografts [24]. The rapid resumption of growth of LNCaP-NEK1 cells in the presence of anti-androgen (BIC) could not be readily explained by the implementation of the pro-survival DDR checkpoint, suggesting that NEK1 also promotes the AI conversion. On the basis of a review of the literature (see the Introduction), we suspected that NEK1 may affect the Hippo pathway, and thus we carried out a Western blotting (WB) analysis of YAP expression in LNCaP cells overexpressing wt-NEK1 or NEK1-T141A variant. The cells were also treated or not treated with BIC and thioridazine (THD), which is a rather specific inhibitor of TLKs [38]. In Figure 1A (quantitation in Figure S5), we show that overexpression of the NEK1-T141A variant results in reduced levels of YAP (lane 1 vs. 5), along with evidence of an elevated cleaved product (Cl-YAP). Decreased YAP levels and evidence of Cl-YAP were also seen in parental LNCaP cells treated with THD (+/− BIC, lane 3 and 4 vs. 1). In contrast, LNCaP cells that overexpress wt-NEK1 showed elevated expression of YAP and no evidence of Cl-YAP (lanes 9–12), where a possible mechanism is that the phosphorylation of YAP by elevated wt-NEK1 mediates a process of stabilization to counteract its degradation when TLK activity (upstream of NEK1) is suppressed with THD (lane 11 vs. 3). Furthermore, the expression of typical YAP/TEAD-dependent transcripts such as CTGF, CDH2 (N-cadherin), Twist1, and TP53AIP1 were decreased in LNCaP cells treated with THD, while in contrast, the expression of CDH1 (E-cadherin) that drives MET was slightly increased (Figure 1D).

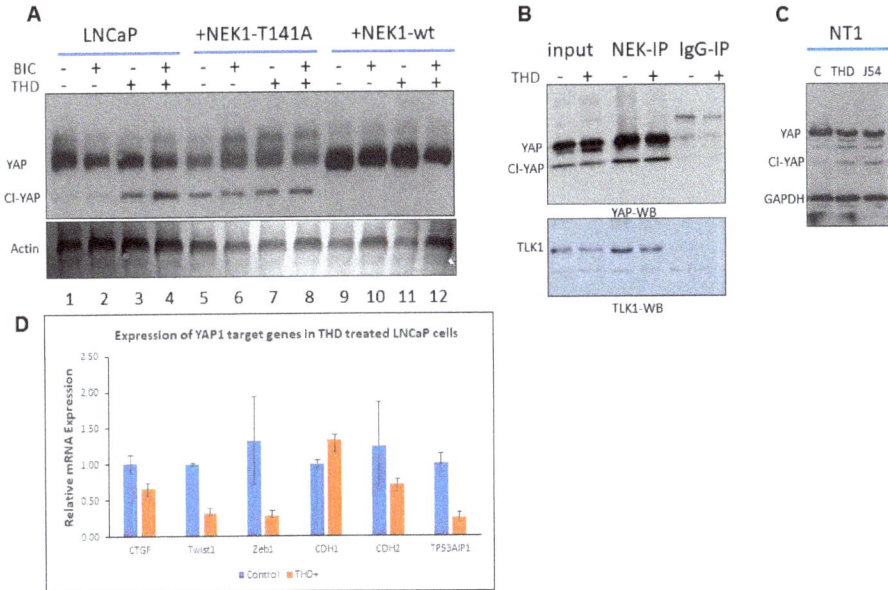

Figure 1. (**A**) The expression of yes-associated protein (YAP) was regulated by never in mitosis gene A (NIMA)-related kinases (NEK) activity and its upstream kinase tousled-like kinase (TLK). Overexpression of wt-NEK1 resulted in elevated YAP expression and conversely in its degradation in LNCaP cells overexpressing the dominant negative mutant NEK1-T141A. Thioridazine (THD) led to degradation of YAP in parental LNCaP cells, even after treatment with bicalutamide (BIC), which led to overexpression of TLK1B. (**B**) YAP interacted with NEK1 and was enriched upon co-immunoprecipitation. TLK1 inhibition with 10 μM THD did not affect NEK1 interaction with YAP, and thus the state of NEK1 kinase activity did not affect YAP binding. (**C**) The expression of YAP was decreased in NT1 cells treated with two different inhibitors of TLK (THD and J54), with a corresponding increase in CL-YAP products. (**D**) Expression of several typical YAP target genes in LNCaP cells treated with THD.

We also show that NEK1 interacted with YAP, as it was enriched by co-IP, and their association was not altered by THD (Figure 1B, top panel; quantitation in Figure S5), indicating that the NEK1 kinase activity was independent of its ability to interact with YAP. As we previously reported [23], the same co-IP also brought down TLK1, and THD did not affect their interaction (Figure 1B, bottom panel; quantitation in Figure S5). There is a possibility that in cells, NEK1, TLK1, and YAP are in a complex, or that NEK1 interacts independently with TLK1 and YAP. In either case, TLK1 was not found to interact directly with YAP [23].

To confirm the effect of inhibition of the TLK1>NEK1 axis on the expression of YAP in a different PCa cell line, we treated Neo-TAg1 (NT1) with two different inhibitors of TLK1: THD or J54. This resulted in a reduction of YAP level and appearance of a set of cleavage products (Figure 1C; quantitation in Figure S5).

3.2. NEK1 KO in NeoTag1 Cells Resulted in Reduced YAP Levels and Expression of Several of Its Target Genes

Consistent with our initial observations that NEK1 activity is critical for YAP stabilization, we found that YAP expression was concomitantly reduced in CRISPR-mediated KO of NEK1 in the PCa line NT1 (Figure 2A; quantitation in Figure S5). Likewise, the expression of several YAP target genes (e.g., CTGF, Zeb1, Twist1) that drive Epithelial to Mesenchymal Transition (EMT) and invasiveness of these cells was suppressed in all the positive NEK1 KO clones (Figure 2B). Conversely, inhibition of TLK1 with THD, which we showed leads to reduced NEK1 activity [23], can inhibit cell migration via suppression of EMT-related genes such as Claudin1, E-cadherin, N-cadherin, Twist1, Snail3, Slug, FOXC2, MMP3, and MMP9 in Hepato Cellular Carcinoma (HCC) cells [39]. We now suggest this observation derives from reduction of YAP expression concomitant with loss of NEK1 (activity) due to inhibition of TLK. In fact, we showed in Figure 2C (quantitation in Figure S5) that YAP expression was reduced in LNCaP cells treated with THD, while conversely, pYAP(S127), which is a phospho-degron leading to its proteasomal degradation, was elevated.

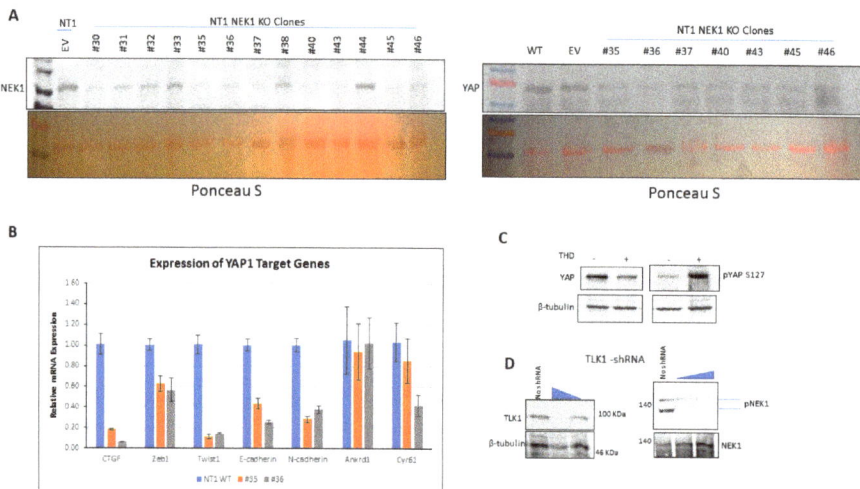

Figure 2. (**A**) CRISPR/Cas9-mediated loss of NEK1 resulted in reduced levels of YAP protein, possibly due to instabilization (EV = empty vector). (**B**) Expression of several typical YAP target genes is reduced in NEK1 KO clones. GAPDH mRNA was used as an internal control. (**C**) Treatment of LNCaP cells with THD, a specific inhibitor of TLKs, resulted in reduced YAP protein level and conversely in its S127 hyperphosphorylation. (**D**) Reduction of TLK1 expression via (short hairpin) shRNA transfection led to loss of pNEK1-T141.

In order to confirm with a genetic approach that the inhibition of TLK1 results in suppression of the pathway that leads to activation of NEK1 and subsequent stabilization of YAP, we knocked down TLK1 with shRNA in HeLa cells. Effective knockdown of TLK1 was achieved in a dose-dependent manner with the shRNA (Figure 2D; quantitation in Figure S5), and importantly, activated NEK1 levels, i.e., pNEK1(T141) were similarly suppressed. This suggests that at least in these cells, TLK1 is the principal kinase responsible for the phosphorylation and activation of NEK1—note that the T141 residue resides in the kinase domain of the protein adjacent to the activation loop [40] that we have previously shown to be important for NEK1 kinase activity [23].

3.3. NEK1 Phosphorylated YAP In Vitro on Several Residues

In order to determine if NEK1 could phosphorylate YAP in vitro, we first purified a recombinant His-tagged NEK1-NT fragment spanning nearly half of the entire protein (total NEK1 protein = 1258 AA, Singh et al. (2017) [ref 23]) following standard protocol and determined its catalytic activity using dephosphorylated α-casein by ADP Hunter assay (Figure 3A,B, see the Section 2). ADP hunter assay revealed that our lab-purified truncated NEK1 is catalytically active, as the incubation of increasing amounts of NEK1 resulted in corresponding ATP to ADP conversion (Figure 3B). Afterwards, we carried out a preliminary in vitro kinase (IVK) reaction by incubating purified recombinant His-tagged NEK1 with purified recombinant GST-YAP (Novus Biologicals) and [γ-^{32}P] ATP. For comparison, we also carried out the IVK reaction using recombinant MK5, which was recently reported to be a novel YAP1 kinase [41]. The purity of all recombinant proteins is shown in the Coomassie Blue-stained SDS/PAGE, and the autoradiography of the gel is shown above it (Figure 3C; quantitation in Figure S5). Notably, NEK1 was capable of strongly phosphorylating YAP, even when small amounts were used (see stained gel). In contrast, MK5 (even in high amount) was a very weak kinase for YAP, if at all, although it was clearly highly active since it was capable of auto-phosphorylation (see autoradiogram) and when tested with ADP Hunter reagent.

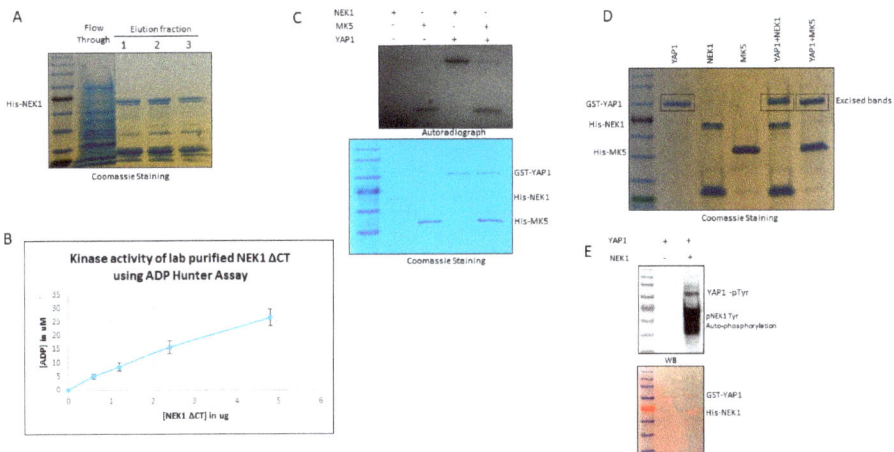

Figure 3. (**A**) Expression and purification of His-NEK1 kinase domain (NEK1ΔCT). (**B**) NEK1ΔCT was catalytically active and ATP/ADP conversion (kinase activity) was linear with the enzyme amount. (**C**) In vitro phosphorylation reactions of YAP using His-NEK1 and MK5 kinases in presence of [γ-^{32}P] ATP. (**D**) In vitro phosphorylation of YAP using His-NEK1 and MK5 kinases for preparative isolation for MS determination of phosphopeptides. (**E**) His-NEK1 also phosphorylated YAP on Tyr, as demonstrated by immunoreactivity with pY antibody.

The IVK reactions were repeated with greater amounts of proteins for preparative isolation for MS analysis for assignment of the phosphorylated residues (Figure 3D). The bands corresponding to YAP incubated with NEK1, MK5, or mock were excised. Determination of the phosphorylated peptides and assignment of the phospho-amino acids were carried out at the University of Kentucky Proteomics facility. The YAP bands were digested with chymotrypsin and analyzed with an LTQ-Orbitrap mass spectrometer. MS datasets were searched with MASCOT against a custom database containing only human YAP1 and NEK1. A synopsis of the results is that (1) when searched against YAP1 and NEK1, only YAP was detected in these samples (well separated on the gel), with 43–49% peptide coverage and protein scores of 2573-3321; (2) potential phosphorylation sites S163/S164 were detected in all three samples (including the YAP1 no kinase sample), which can be explained as a basal phosphorylated residue of recombinant YAP isolated from wheat germ; and (3) six unique phosphorylation sites were detected in the YAP_NEK1 sample: T83, T361, S366, S388, S406, Y407, or T493 (Figure 4 and Figures S1–S4; Table S1). However, no unique phosphorylation site was detected in the YAP_MK5 sample, which we now suggest is not an authentic YAP kinase. Interestingly, in the paper that purported MK5 as an important YAP kinase, the authors did not report whether they attempted to verify that MK5 can phosphorylate YAP in vitro, nor did they identify the phosphorylation target in vivo [41]. In Figure 4, we present an example of data identifying Y407 and T493, which we currently assume are the most interesting.

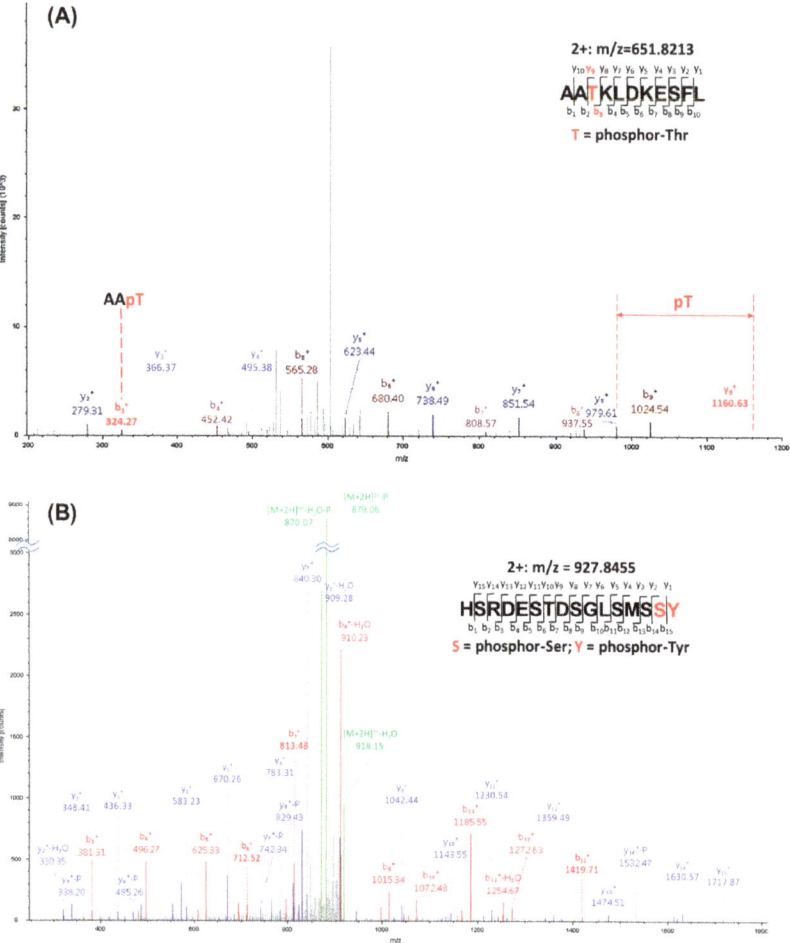

Figure 4. MS/MS spectra demonstrating the phosphorylation sites at T493 (**A**) and S406/Y407 (**B**) as examples of LC–MS/MS determinations.

All of the phosphorylated residues listed in Table S1 have been reported in MS studies in cells, according to the report of Phosphosite Plus, except for S406 (putative) and T493, which, as such, are the first report of phosphorylation of these residues specifically by NEK1. The phosphorylation of Y407 (putative) should not be surprising, since NEK1 is a dual specificity kinase that was originally identified as a tyrosine kinase [42]. Note that although the MS/MS spectrum could not distinguish the exact phosphorylation site at S406 or Y407, a phospho-Tyr Western blot (Figure 3E; quantitation in Figure S5) supported the conclusion that Y407 (the only identified pTyr in the MS analysis) was phosphorylated. It is also noteworthy that the NEK1 protein was also phosphorylated on Tyr (Figure 3E), as we previously reported that it is in fact auto-phosphorylated on Y315 [23], confirming the specificity of the antiserum.

3.4. Bioinformatic Studies Suggest NEK1 Mediated Stabilization of YAP1 in Different Cancers

We analyzed mRNA expression of both NEK1 and YAP1 in prostate adenocarcinoma (PRAD) and head and neck squamous cell (HNSC) carcinoma patients from TCGA datasets using the UALCAN online platform. In PRAD, no significant alteration in mRNA expression of NEK1 was observed (Figure 5A), while YAP1 mRNA level was consistently downregulated with respect to the tumor Gleason score (Figure 5B). However, reverse phase protein array (RPPA)-based protein profiling of NEK1 and YAP1 in PRAD patients from TCGA datasets revealed upregulation of YAP1 level (Figure 5D), but no change in NEK1 protein level (Figure 5C). In addition, proteomic analysis based on immunohistochemistry (IHC) data from the Human Protein Atlas web server revealed a higher protein level of NEK1 and YAP1 in high-grade PRAD patients (Figure 5G,H). Representative IHC analysis revealed intense staining of both NEK1 and YAP1 in high-grade PRAD compared to normal prostate tissue (Figure 5I). This supports our hypothesis of NEK1 implication in YAP1 protein stabilization/accumulation in advanced PCa, despite YAP1 transcript downregulation.

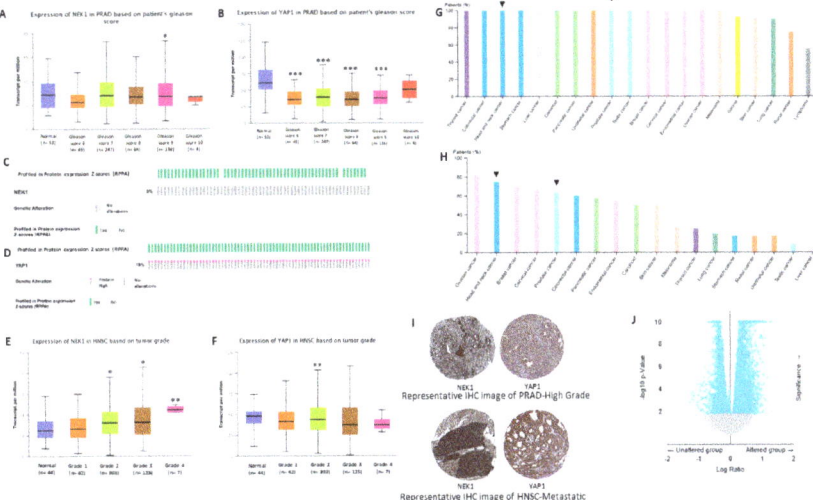

Figure 5. Gene expression of (**A**) NEK1 and (**B**) YAP1 of prostate adenocarcinoma (PRAD) patients on the basis of the Gleason score extracted from The Cancer Genome Atlas (TCGA) datasets using the UALCAN web tool. OncoPrint representation of the protein level alteration of (**C**) NEK1 and (**D**) YAP1 of PRAD patients by reverse phase protein array (RPPA) extracted from TCGA (firehose legacy) datasets using cBIOPORTAL online platform. Gene expression of (**E**) NEK1 and (**F**) YAP1 in head and neck squamous cell (HNSC) patients on the basis of the tumor grade extracted from TCGA datasets using the UALCAN web tool. Percentage of patients of different types of cancer with higher level of (**G**) NEK1 and (**H**) YAP1 on the basis of immunohistochemistry (IHC) staining generated using the Human Protein Atlas database. Staining intensity correlated with the color code. Deeper color represents high staining intensity. (**I**) Representative IHC images of NEK1 and YAP1 of high-grade PRAD (top panel) and metastatic HNSC samples (bottom panel). (**J**) Volcano plot of gene enrichment analysis based on NEK1 overexpression in HNSC patients extracted from TCGA (firehose legacy) datasets using cBIOPORTAL online platform. * represents $p < 0.05$, ** represents $p < 0.005$, and *** represents $p < 0.0005$. All comparisons were with the normal tissue.

Similarly, in head and neck squamous cell carcinoma (Figure 5F), glioblastoma, and other cancers (data not shown), there was no significant upregulation of YAP1 mRNA expression; nonetheless, YAP1 protein level was elevated in high-grade metastatic tumors (Figure 5). Moreover, gene set enrichment analysis significantly correlated NEK1 expression with several YAP1 target genes such as Zeb1, BirC2, BirC6, Ankrd11, and ARID1B (Figure 5J; Table 1). Overall, these data suggest NEK1 increases YAP1 level by reducing YAP1 protein turnover rate in different cancers.

Table 1. Some of the YAP target genes significantly upregulated with NEK1 upregulation in head and neck squamous cell (HNSC) carcinoma (TCGA, firehose legacy) analyzed using cBIOPORTAL.

Gene Name	Mean Log2 mRNA Expression ± SD in NEK1-Overexpressed Group	p-Value	q-Value
Zeb1	8.57 ± 1.00	3.68×10^{-7}	5.153×10^{-6}
Zeb2	8.80 ± 1.05	7.237×10^{-6}	6.617×10^{-5}
Ankrd36B	4.33 ± 0.93	1.410×10^{-4}	8.367×10^{-4}
Ankrd11	11.55 ± 0.49	1.159×10^{-3}	4.984×10^{-3}
BirC2	10.46 ± 0.96	0.0187	0.0498
BirC6	11.13 ± 0.49	3.91×10^{-12}	2.80×10^{-10}
HoxB3	6.44 ± 2.11	0.0169	0.0458
ARID1B	10.84 ± 0.46	4.14×10^{-10}	1.57×10^{-8}
WSB2	11.05 ± 0.45	2.016×10^{-4}	1.136×10^{-3}
CAT	10.01 ± 0.68	3.621×10^{-4}	1.872×10^{-3}
ABCB1	5.11 ± 1.45	0.0111	0.0327
PTX3	5.33 ± 2.12	1.994×10^{-4}	1.126×10^{-3}

4. Discussion

During studies aimed at elucidating the process of ADT adaptation of AS PCa cell (initially in LNCaP), which proceeds through a process of activating the DDR and increased activity of the kinases TLK1B and NEK1 [11,24,25], we made the observation that overexpression of wt-NEK1, but not the hypoactive NEK1-T141A variant that cannot be activated by TLK, resulted in a rapid adaptation to bicalutamide and formation of AI colonies. From a review of the literature on the process of AI conversion of LNCaP and other studies of CRPC progression, we suspected the involvement of Hippo pathway deregulation and, in particular, YAP-driven gene expression (for a recent review, see [43]). Moreover, Yim et al. reported that NEK1 can phosphorylate TAZ and regulates its turnover rate [18]. Since YAP1 and TAZ are two highly homologous proteins that possess several conserved phospho-residues, we set out to investigate the protein level of YAP in LNCaP overexpressing wt-NEK1 and the T141A mutant in conjunction with a TLK inhibitor (THD) to suppress the activating phosphorylation of NEK1. Interestingly, we observed an increased degradation of YAP in cells overexpressing NEK1-T141A mutant or parental LNCaP treated with THD, in contrast to elevated level of YAP (and no degradation) in cells that overexpress wt-NEK1 (Figure 1). Furthermore, treatment of LNCaP cells with THD resulted in downregulated expression of several YAP-dependent transcripts (Figure 1D). As an indication that this is in fact a general phenomenon in PCa, increased degradation of YAP1 after inhibition of the TLK1>NEK1 axis with THD or J54 was independently verified in mouse NT1 cells (Figure 1C). In addition, genetic depletion of NEK1 resulted in YAP1 loss and YAP1 target gene downregulation in NT1 cells (Figure 2). It should be noted that YAP is a generally unstable protein whose turnover rate is strongly regulated by multiple stabilizing [44] or de-stabilizing phosphorylation events controlled by multiple kinases (see [19,20,26] for some reviews). Large tumor suppressor 1 and 2 (LATS1/2), the core kinases of the Hippo signaling pathway, can phosphorylate YAP1 on Ser127 residue, which creates a binding site for 14-3-3 proteins. The 14-3-3 binding of YAP leads to the cytoplasmic sequestration of YAP [45,46]. Sequential phosphorylation by LATS1/2 on YAP Ser397 primes it for further phosphorylation by Casein Kinase CK1δ/ε on Ser400 and Ser403, which creates a phosphodegron motif for (Skp Cullin F box) β-TrCP/SCF E3 ubiquitin ligase-mediated proteasomal degradation [47]. Recent findings also identify factors such as NR4A1 (nuclear receptor superfamily) that regulate the 14-3-3 interaction with YAP1 and promote its ubiquitination and degradation [48]. Several other kinases independent of the Hippo pathway can regulate the stability of YAP1 protein. For instance, nuclear Dbf2-related kinase (NDR1/2) can also phosphorylate YAP on Ser127 residue and can promote its cytoplasmic retention, thereby negatively regulating YAP stability [49]. Evidence suggests that the protein kinase B/AKT can also phosphorylate YAP on Ser127 residue, leading to binding of 14-3-3 and cytoplasmic retention [45]. In contrast, several members of the Src family of kinases such as Src, Yes, and c-Abl can positively regulate YAP stability. c-Abl/Src/Yes are known to phosphorylate YAP on Tyr357 residue, which results in the nuclear translocation and, hence, stabilization of YAP [44,50,51]. Moreover, Ras-associated factor isoform 1C (RASSF1C) is known to promote tyrosine phosphorylation of YAP1 (Tyr357) through activated Src (pTyr416) and cause nuclear localization of YAP1 [52]. Similarly, mitogen-activated protein kinases such as c-Jun-N-terminal kinases (JNK1/2) are also reported to be YAP kinases that phosphorylate YAP on Ser317 and Thr362, promoting YAP nuclear translocation and stabilization [53]. Thus, post-translational modifications such as phosphorylation determine YAP turnover rate and activity.

Therefore, we propose the phosphorylation of Y407 as one potential mechanism of YAP stabilization and increased transcriptional output, although the other 5-phosphorylation sites could be equally important (Figure 4 and Figures S1–S4; Table S1). There are examples in YAP and TAZ where phosphorylation of some residues impairs ubiquitination and subsequent proteasomal degradation, as in one example, phosphorylation of S128 by NLK competed for the destabilizing LATS1-dependent S127 phosphorylation [54]. However, we currently favor a pY407-related mechanism based on the equivalent pY316 of TAZ, where it was shown that the phosphorylation of that residue, reportedly by c-Abl, was necessary to mediate its interaction with the transcription factor NFAT5 [55]. This was implicated in an inhibitory pathway of NFAT5—a major osmoregulatory transcription factor—during hyperosmotic stress. Similarly, JNK1/2-mediated phosphorylation of YAP1 on Ser317 and Thr362 promotes YAP's ability to bind and stabilize both pro-apoptotic p73 and pro-proliferative ΔNp63α in different cell types [53,56]. We think that, likewise, pY407 promotes the interaction of YAP with some of its transcriptional partners, and hence promotes its nuclear translocation, function, and stabilization, away from cytoplasmic degradation. Importantly, while the phosphorylation of Y407 was identified in proteomic studies [57], to our knowledge, the kinase responsible for it has not been reported.

Resistance to androgen deprivation therapy (ADT) promotes androgen-independent growth and proliferation of PCa cells, which requires efficient DNA damage response (DDR) and repair mechanisms, activation of compensatory signaling pathways, transcription factors, and co-factors to drive castration resistance. Findings from our lab and others suggest that ADT activates the TLK1-NEK1 signaling pathway that promotes PCa progression by activating the DDR [11,24]. Hyper-activation of NEK1 may also lengthen G2/M checkpoints, which provides the cells sufficient time to repair their damaged DNA after ADT or radiation therapy [7,58]. However, DDR alone may not be able to induce androgen-insensitive growth of PCa cells. Thus, we hypothesize that TLK1-NEK1 may be implicated in some other signaling pathway, leading to AI growth. YAP1 is a major oncoprotein that drives many different types of malignancies, including PCa [59], head and neck cancer [59], gastric cancer [60], colon cancer [60], thyroid cancer [61], lung cancer [62], ovarian cancer [63], and liver cancer [64]. NEK1-mediated phosphorylation of YAP1 (most probably on Tyr407 and/or Thr493) may induce a conformational change that counteracts the sequential phosphorylation by LATS1/2 and CK1δ/ε and subsequently protects YAP from proteasomal degradation. Moreover, Tyr407 lies on the transcriptional activation domain of YAP1, which may increase its interaction affinity to its assigned transcriptional factors [65]. Ectopic YAP expression was reported to drive LNCaP cells from androgen-sensitive to androgen-insensitive states [19]. Reducing the turnover rate will increase cellular accumulation of YAP, which can enable its oncogenic properties to drive castration resistance by several mechanisms. Previous studies reported that YAP can mediate PI (3)K-mTOR signaling and activate AKT [66–68]. Activation of mTOR will lead to enhanced translation of TLK1B that can, in turn, increase YAP1 phosphorylation through TLK1-NEK1 nexus. This suggests a positive feed-forward mechanism for YAP accumulation. Elevated YAP can also activate ERK that will promote cell proliferation in absence of AR signaling. Kuser-Abali et al. reported that AR and YAP can interact, and this interaction contributes to the switch from androgen-dependent to castration-resistant phenotype [27]. Overexpression of YAP can also regulate the expression of AR target genes, including PSA, NKX3.1, PGC-1, and KLK2, which suggests that YAP may control AR activity. YAP Tyr407 phosphorylation could increase the binding affinity of AR and AR ligand-insensitive variant AR-V7, thus contributing to androgen refractory growth of PCa cells. Therapy-induced YAP overexpression may also induce EMT activation by upregulating EMT-specific genes. Increasing the stemness of PCa cells can be another mechanism by which stabilized YAP can promote castration-resistant growth of PCa cells, which will further contribute to chemo-resistance of cancer cells [69]. Our bioinformatics analyses also suggested a link between NEK1 and YAP1 in different cancers (Figure 5). YAP1 protein level is abundant in high-grade PCa tumors, despite the progressive downregulation of YAP1 mRNA expression. Other groups also reported that YAP protein is positively correlated with the Gleason score, consistent with the findings of our bioinformatics analysis [70]. We propose that the signaling of TLK1>NEK1-mediated YAP phosphorylation and stabilization contributes not only to PCa progression, but also many other cancers. Importantly, we found a correlation between increased phosphorylated NEK1(T141) in relation to the Gleason score [25] and YAP1 protein expression, whereas the mRNA for YAP1 actually decreased (Figure 5), consistent with our model of post-transcriptional protein stabilization.

5. Conclusions

YAP's transcriptional activity and degradation is mainly regulated by phosphorylation through several kinases dependent and independent of the Hippo pathway. Using small molecule inhibitors against YAP cannot completely abolish YAP transcriptional activity and is not very effective in treating YAP-driven cancers. Inhibitors such as verteporfin that can disrupt the YAP–TEAD interaction, but still cannot result in complete inhibition, as YAP can bind with other transcription factors such as TEF, SMADs, or TBX5. The majority of YAP kinases negatively regulate YAP by promoting its nuclear egress or degradation; however, NEK1 is found to stabilize YAP protein by phosphorylating it on several residues. Thus, targeting NEK1 or the TLK1–NEK1 axis can bring about therapeutic benefits in the clinical management of YAP-driven malignancies.

Supplementary Materials: The following are available online at http://www.mdpi.com/2072-6694/12/12/3666/s1: Figure S1: MS/MS spectrum of the phosphor-peptide N_{70}AVMNPKTANVPQTVPMRL$_{88}$ to determine pT83, Figure S2. MS/MS spectrum of the phosphor-peptide R_{161}QSSFEIPDDVPLPAGW$_{177}$ to determine pS163/pS164, Figure S3. MS/MS spectrum of the phosphor-peptide A_{347}LRSQLPTLEQDGGTQNPVSSPGmSQEL$_{374}$ to determine pT361/pS366, Figure S4. MS/MS spectrum of the phosphor-peptide R_{375}TMTTNSSDPFLNSGTY$_{391}$ to determine pS388, Figure S5. Densitometry of the original uncropped blots and gel images with their respective numbers from the main figures, Table S1. Assigned phosphorylated sites.

Author Contributions: Conception and design: M.I.K., V.S., I.G., A.D.B. Development of methodology: M.I.K., V.S., I.G., J.C., H.Z., A.D.B. Acquisition of data: M.I.K., V.S., I.G., J.C., H.Z., A.D.B. Analysis and interpretation of data (e.g., statistical analysis, biostatistics, computational analysis): M.I.K., J.C., H.Z., A.D.B. Writing, review, and/or revision of the manuscript: M.I.K., I.G., J.C., H.Z., A.D.B. Administrative, technical, or material support: M.I.K., I.G., J.C., H.Z., A.D.B. Study supervision: A.D.B., H.Z. All authors have read and agreed to the published version of the manuscript.

Funding: This work was supported primarily by DoD-PCRP grant W81XWH-17-1-0417 to A.D.B. LC–MS/MS equipment was acquired using a National Center for Research Resources High-End Instrumentation grant (1S10RR029127 to H.Z.).

Acknowledgments: We thank the Research Core Facility Genomics Core at LSU Health Shreveport for the help with the qPCR analysis. We acknowledge the University of Kentucky Markey Cancer Center's Redox Metabolism Shared Resource Facility partially supported by a National Cancer Institute Center Core support grant (P30 CA177558).

Conflicts of Interest: No potential conflicts of interest are disclosed.

References

1. Osmani, S.A.; Pu, R.T.; Morris, N.R. Mitotic induction and maintenance by overexpression of a G2-specific gene that encodes a potential protein kinase. *Cell* **1988**, *53*, 237–244. [CrossRef]
2. Lu, K.P.; Hunter, T. Evidence for a NIMA-like mitotic pathway in vertebrate cells. *Cell* **1995**, *81*, 413–424. [CrossRef]
3. Meirelles, G.V.; Perez, A.M.; de Souza, E.E.; Basei, F.L.; Papa, P.F.; Melo Hanchuk, T.D.; Cardoso, V.B.; Kobarg, J. "Stop Ne(c)king around": How interactomics contributes to functionally characterize Nek family kinases. *World J. Biol. Chem.* **2014**, *5*, 141–160. [PubMed]
4. Moniz, L.; Dutt, P.; Haider, N.; Stambolic, V. Nek family of kinases in cell cycle, checkpoint control and cancer. *Cell Div.* **2011**, *6*, 18. [CrossRef] [PubMed]
5. Chen, Y.; Chen, C.F.; Riley, D.J.; Chen, P.L. Nek1 kinase functions in DNA damage response and checkpoint control through a pathway independent of ATM and ATR. *Cell Cycle* **2011**, *10*, 655–663. [CrossRef] [PubMed]
6. Liu, S.; Ho, C.K.; Ouyang, J.; Zou, L. Nek1 kinase associates with ATR-ATRIP and primes ATR for efficient DNA damage signaling. *Proc. Natl. Acad. Sci. USA* **2013**, *110*, 2175–2180. [CrossRef]
7. Chen, Y.; Chen, P.L.; Chen, C.F.; Jiang, X.; Riley, D.J. Never-in-mitosis related kinase 1 functions in DNA damage response and checkpoint control. *Cell Cycle* **2008**, *7*, 3194–3201. [CrossRef]
8. Pelegrini, A.L.; Moura, D.J.; Brenner, B.L.; Ledur, P.F.; Maques, G.P.; Henriques, J.A.; Saffi, J.; Lenz, G. Nek1 silencing slows down DNA repair and blocks DNA damage-induced cell cycle arrest. *Mutagenesis* **2010**, *25*, 447–454. [CrossRef]
9. Chen, Y.; Chen, C.F.; Chiang, H.C.; Pena, M.; Polci, R.; Wei, R.L.; Edwards, R.A.; Hansel, D.E.; Chen, P.L.; Riley, D.J. Mutation of NIMA-related kinase 1 (NEK1) leads to chromosome instability. *Mol. Cancer* **2011**, *10*, 5. [CrossRef]
10. Chen, Y.; Gaczynska, M.; Osmulski, P.; Polci, R.; Riley, D.J. Phosphorylation by Nek1 regulates opening and closing of voltage dependent anion channel 1. *Biochem. Biophys. Res. Commun.* **2010**, *394*, 798–803. [CrossRef]
11. Singh, V.; Khalil, M.I.; De Benedetti, A. The TLK1/Nek1 axis contributes to mitochondrial integrity and apoptosis prevention via phosphorylation of VDAC1. *Cell Cycle* **2020**, *9*, 1–13. [CrossRef] [PubMed]
12. Chen, Y.; Chen, C.F.; Polci, R.; Wei, R.; Riley, D.J.; Chen, P.L. Increased Nek1 expression in renal cell carcinoma cells is associated with decreased sensitivity to DNA-damaging treatment. *Oncotarget* **2014**, *5*, 4283–4294. [CrossRef] [PubMed]
13. Higelin, J.; Catanese, A.; Semelink-Sedlacek, L.L.; Oezteurk, S.; Lutz, A.K.; Bausinger, J.; Barbi, G.; Speit, G.; Andersen, P.M.; Ludolph, A.C.; et al. NEK1 loss-of-function mutation induces DNA damage accumulation in ALS patient-derived motoneurons. *Stem Cell Res.* **2018**, *30*, 150–162. [CrossRef] [PubMed]
14. Naruse, H.; Ishiura, H.; Mitsui, J.; Takahashi, Y.; Matsukawa, T.; Yoshimura, J.; Doi, K.; Morishita, S.; Goto, J.; Toda, T.; et al. Loss-of-function variants in NEK1 are associated with an increased risk of sporadic ALS in the Japanese population. *J. Hum. Genet.* **2020**, *12*, 020–00830. [CrossRef]
15. Mahjoub, M.R.; Trapp, M.L.; Quarmby, L.M. NIMA-related kinases defective in murine models of polycystic kidney diseases localize to primary cilia and centrosomes. *J. Am. Soc. Nephrol.* **2005**, *16*, 3485–3489. [CrossRef]
16. Shalom, O.; Shalva, N.; Altschuler, Y.; Motro, B. The mammalian Nek1 kinase is involved in primary cilium formation. *FEBS Lett.* **2008**, *582*, 1465–1470. [CrossRef]
17. Surpili, M.J.; Delben, T.M.; Kobarg, J. Identification of proteins that interact with the central coiled-coil region of the human protein kinase NEK1. *Biochemistry* **2003**, *42*, 15369–15376. [CrossRef]
18. Yim, H.; Sung, C.K.; You, J.; Tian, Y.; Benjamin, T. Nek1 and TAZ interact to maintain normal levels of polycystin 2. *J. Am. Soc. Nephrol. JASN* **2011**, *22*, 832–837. [CrossRef]
19. Zhang, L.; Yang, S.; Chen, X.; Stauffer, S.; Yu, F.; Lele, S.M.; Fu, K.; Datta, K.; Palermo, N.; Chen, Y.; et al. The hippo pathway effector YAP regulates motility, invasion, and castration-resistant growth of prostate cancer cells. *Mol. Cell. Biol.* **2015**, *35*, 1350–1362. [CrossRef]
20. Zhao, B.; Li, L.; Lei, Q.; Guan, K.L. The Hippo-YAP pathway in organ size control and tumorigenesis: An updated version. *Genes Dev.* **2010**, *24*, 862–874. [CrossRef]
21. Chang, L.; Azzolin, L.; Di Biagio, D.; Zanconato, F.; Battilana, G.; Lucon Xiccato, R.; Aragona, M.; Giulitti, S.; Panciera, T.; Gandin, A.; et al. The SWI/SNF complex is a mechanoregulated inhibitor of YAP and TAZ. *Nature* **2018**, *563*, 265–269. [CrossRef] [PubMed]

22. Cheng, S.; Prieto-Dominguez, N.; Yang, S.; Connelly, Z.M.; StPierre, S.; Rushing, B.; Watkins, A.; Shi, L.; Lakey, M.; Baiamonte, L.B.; et al. The expression of YAP1 is increased in high-grade prostatic adenocarcinoma but is reduced in neuroendocrine prostate cancer. *Prostate Cancer Prostatic Dis.* **2020**, *23*, 661–669. [CrossRef] [PubMed]
23. Singh, V.; Connelly, Z.M.; Shen, X.; De Benedetti, A. Identification of the proteome complement of humanTLK1 reveals it binds and phosphorylates NEK1 regulating its activity. *Cell Cycle* **2017**, *16*, 915–926. [CrossRef] [PubMed]
24. Singh, V.; Jaiswal, P.; Ghosh, I.; Koul, H.K.; Yu, X.; De Benedetti, A. Targeting the TLK1/NEK1 DDR axis with Thioridazine suppresses outgrowth of Androgen Independent Prostate tumors. *Int. J. Cancer* **2019**, *145*, 1055–1067. [CrossRef] [PubMed]
25. Singh, V.; Jaiswal, P.K.; Ghosh, I.; Koul, H.K.; Yu, X.; De Benedetti, A. The TLK1-Nek1 axis promotes prostate cancer progression. *Cancer Lett.* **2019**, *453*, 131–141. [CrossRef] [PubMed]
26. Yu, F.X.; Zhao, B.; Guan, K.L. Hippo Pathway in Organ Size Control, Tissue Homeostasis, and Cancer. *Cell* **2015**, *163*, 811–828. [CrossRef]
27. Kuser-Abali, G.; Alptekin, A.; Lewis, M.; Garraway, I.P.; Cinar, B. YAP1 and AR interactions contribute to the switch from androgen-dependent to castration-resistant growth in prostate cancer. *Nat. Commun.* **2015**, *6*, 8126. [CrossRef]
28. Noh, M.-G.; Kim, S.S.; Hwang, E.C.; Kwon, D.D.; Choi, C. Yes-Associated Protein Expression Is Correlated to the Differentiation of Prostate Adenocarcinoma. *J. Pathol. Transl. Med.* **2017**, *51*, 365–373. [CrossRef]
29. Nguyen, L.T.; Tretiakova, M.S.; Silvis, M.R.; Lucas, J.; Klezovitch, O.; Coleman, I.; Bolouri, H.; Kutyavin, V.I.; Morrissey, C.; True, L.D.; et al. ERG Activates the YAP1 Transcriptional Program and Induces the Development of Age-Related Prostate Tumors. *Cancer Cell* **2015**, *27*, 797–808. [CrossRef]
30. Wang, Y.; Kasper, S.; Yuan, J.; Jin, R.J.; Zhang, J.; Ishii, K.; Wills, M.L.; Hayward, S.W.; Matusik, R.J. Androgen-dependent prostate epithelial cell selection by targeting ARR(2)PBneo to the LPB-Tag model of prostate cancer. *Lab. Investig.* **2006**, *86*, 1074–1088. [CrossRef]
31. Singh, V.; Bhoir, S.; Chikhale, R.; Hussain, J.; Dwyer, D.; Bryce, R.; Kirubakaran, S.; De Benedetti, A. Generation of Phenothiazine with Potent Anti-TLK1 Activity for Prostate Cancer Therapy. *iScience* **2020**, *23*. [CrossRef] [PubMed]
32. Kamelgarn, M.; Chen, J.; Kuang, L.; Arenas, A.; Zhai, J.; Zhu, H.; Gal, J. Proteomic analysis of FUS interacting proteins provides insights into FUS function and its role in ALS. *Biochim. Biophys. Acta* **2016**, *1862*, 2004–2014. [CrossRef] [PubMed]
33. UALCAN. Available online: http://ualcan.path.uab.edu/ (accessed on 16 October 2020).
34. cBIOPORTAL. Available online: https://www.cbioportal.org/ (accessed on 16 October 2020).
35. The Human Protein Atlas. Available online: https://www.proteinatlas.org/ (accessed on 16 October 2020).
36. Lu, S.; Tan, Z.; Wortman, M.; Dong, Z. Preferential induction of G1 arrest in androgen-responsive human prostate cancer cells by androgen receptor signaling antagonists DL3 and antiandrogen bicalutamide. *Cancer Lett.* **2010**, *298*, 250–257. [CrossRef]
37. Litvinov, I.V.; Vander Griend, D.J.; Antony, L.; Dalrymple, S.; De Marzo, A.M.; Drake, C.G.; Isaacs, J.T. Androgen receptor as a licensing factor for DNA replication in androgen-sensitive prostate cancer cells. *Proc. Natl. Acad. Sci. USA* **2006**, *103*, 15085–15090. [CrossRef] [PubMed]
38. Ronald, S.; Awate, S.; Rath, A.; Carroll, J.; Galiano, F.; Dwyer, D.; Kleiner-Hancock, H.; Mathis, J.M.; Vigod, S.; De Benedetti, A. Phenothiazine Inhibitors of TLKs Affect Double-Strand Break Repair and DNA Damage Response Recovery and Potentiate Tumor Killing with Radiomimetic Therapy. *Genes Cancer* **2013**, *4*, 39–53. [CrossRef] [PubMed]
39. Lu, M.; Li, J.; Luo, Z.; Zhang, S.; Xue, S.; Wang, K.; Shi, Y.; Zhang, C.; Chen, H.; Li, Z. Roles of dopamine receptors and their antagonist thioridazine in hepatoma metastasis. *Onco Targets Ther.* **2015**, *8*, 1543–1552. [CrossRef] [PubMed]
40. Melo-Hanchuk, T.D.; Slepicka, P.F.; Meirelles, G.V.; Basei, F.L.; Lovato, D.V.; Granato, D.C.; Pauletti, B.A.; Domingues, R.R.; Leme, A.F.P.; Pelegrini, A.L.; et al. NEK1 kinase domain structure and its dynamic protein interactome after exposure to Cisplatin. *Sci. Rep.* **2017**, *7*, 5445. [CrossRef]
41. Seo, J.; Kim, M.H.; Hong, H.; Cho, H.; Park, S.; Kim, S.K.; Kim, J. MK5 Regulates YAP Stability and Is a Molecular Target in YAP-Driven Cancers. *Cancer Res.* **2019**, *79*, 6139–6152. [CrossRef]

42. Letwin, K.; Mizzen, L.; Motro, B.; Ben-David, Y.; Bernstein, A.; Pawson, T. A mammalian dual specificity protein kinase, Nek1, is related to the NIMA cell cycle regulator and highly expressed in meiotic germ cells. *EMBO J.* **1992**, *11*, 3521–3531. [CrossRef]
43. Salem, O.; Hansen, C.G. The Hippo Pathway in Prostate Cancer. *Cells* **2019**, *8*, 370. [CrossRef]
44. Levy, D.; Adamovich, Y.; Reuven, N.; Shaul, Y. Yap1 phosphorylation by c-Abl is a critical step in selective activation of proapoptotic genes in response to DNA damage. *Mol. Cell* **2008**, *29*, 350–361. [CrossRef] [PubMed]
45. Basu, S.; Totty, N.F.; Irwin, M.S.; Sudol, M.; Downward, J. Akt phosphorylates the Yes-associated protein, YAP, to induce interaction with 14-3-3 and attenuation of p73-mediated apoptosis. *Mol. Cell* **2003**, *11*, 11–23. [CrossRef]
46. Piccolo, S.; Dupont, S.; Cordenonsi, M. The biology of YAP/TAZ: Hippo signaling and beyond. *Physiol. Rev.* **2014**, *94*, 1287–1312. [CrossRef] [PubMed]
47. Zhao, B.; Li, L.; Tumaneng, K.; Wang, C.Y.; Guan, K.L. A coordinated phosphorylation by Lats and CK1 regulates YAP stability through SCF(beta-TRCP). *Genes Dev.* **2010**, *24*, 72–85. [CrossRef] [PubMed]
48. He, L.; Yuan, L.; Yu, W.; Sun, Y.; Jiang, D.; Wang, X.; Feng, X.; Wang, Z.; Xu, J.; Yang, R.; et al. A Regulation Loop between YAP and NR4A1 Balances Cell Proliferation and Apoptosis. *Cell Rep.* **2020**, *33*, 108284. [CrossRef]
49. Zhang, L.; Tang, F.; Terracciano, L.; Hynx, D.; Kohler, R.; Bichet, S.; Hess, D.; Cron, P.; Hemmings, B.A.; Hergovich, A.; et al. NDR functions as a physiological YAP1 kinase in the intestinal epithelium. *Curr. Biol.* **2015**, *25*, 296–305. [CrossRef]
50. Li, B.; He, J.; Lv, H.; Liu, Y.; Lv, X.; Zhang, C.; Zhu, Y.; Ai, D. C-Abl regulates YAPY357 phosphorylation to activate endothelial atherogenic responses to disturbed flow. *J. Clin. Investig.* **2019**, *129*, 1167–1179. [CrossRef]
51. Sugihara, T.; Werneburg, N.W.; Hernandez, M.C.; Yang, L.; Kabashima, A.; Hirsova, P.; Yohanathan, L.; Sosa, C.; Truty, M.J.; Vasmatzis, G.; et al. YAP Tyrosine Phosphorylation and Nuclear Localization in Cholangiocarcinoma Cells Are Regulated by LCK and Independent of LATS Activity. *Mol. Cancer Res.* **2018**, *16*, 1556–1567. [CrossRef]
52. Vlahov, N.; Scrace, S.; Soto Manuel, S.; Grawenda Anna, M.; Bradley, L.; Pankova, D.; Papaspyropoulos, A.; Yee Karen, S.; Buffa, F.; Goding Colin, R.; et al. Alternate RASSF1 Transcripts Control SRC Activity, E-Cadherin Contacts, and YAP-Mediated Invasion. *Curr. Biol.* **2015**, *25*, 3019–3034. [CrossRef]
53. Tomlinson, V.; Gudmundsdottir, K.; Luong, P.; Leung, K.Y.; Knebel, A.; Basu, S. JNK phosphorylates Yes-associated protein (YAP) to regulate apoptosis. *Cell Death Dis.* **2010**, *1*, e29. [CrossRef]
54. Moon, S.; Kim, W.; Kim, S.; Kim, Y.; Song, Y.; Bilousov, O.; Kim, J.; Lee, T.; Cha, B.; Kim, M.; et al. Phosphorylation by NLK inhibits YAP-14-3-3-interactions and induces its nuclear localization. *EMBO Rep.* **2017**, *18*, 61–71. [CrossRef] [PubMed]
55. Jang, E.J.; Jeong, H.; Han, K.H.; Kwon, H.M.; Hong, J.H.; Hwang, E.S. TAZ suppresses NFAT5 activity through tyrosine phosphorylation. *Mol. Cell. Biol.* **2012**, *32*, 4925–4932. [CrossRef] [PubMed]
56. Danovi, S.A.; Rossi, M.; Gudmundsdottir, K.; Yuan, M.; Melino, G.; Basu, S. Yes-associated protein (YAP) is a critical mediator of c-Jun-dependent apoptosis. *Cell Death Differ.* **2008**, *15*, 217–219. [CrossRef] [PubMed]
57. Iliuk, A.B.; Martin, V.A.; Alicie, B.M.; Geahlen, R.L.; Tao, W.A. In-depth analyses of kinase-dependent tyrosine phosphoproteomes based on metal ion-functionalized soluble nanopolymers. *Mol. Cell Proteom.* **2010**, *9*, 2162–2172. [CrossRef]
58. Freund, I.; Hehlgans, S.; Martin, D.; Ensminger, M.; Fokas, E.; Rödel, C.; Löbrich, M.; Rödel, F. Fractionation-Dependent Radiosensitization by Molecular Targeting of Nek1. *Cells* **2020**, *9*, 1235. [CrossRef]
59. Jiang, N.; Hjorth-Jensen, K.; Hekmat, O.; Iglesias-Gato, D.; Kruse, T.; Wang, C.; Wei, W.; Ke, B.; Yan, B.; Niu, Y.; et al. In vivo quantitative phosphoproteomic profiling identifies novel regulators of castration-resistant prostate cancer growth. *Oncogene* **2015**, *34*, 2764–2776. [CrossRef]
60. Kang, W.; Tong, J.H.; Chan, A.W.; Lee, T.L.; Lung, R.W.; Leung, P.P.; So, K.K.; Wu, K.; Fan, D.; Yu, J.; et al. Yes-associated protein 1 exhibits oncogenic property in gastric cancer and its nuclear accumulation associates with poor prognosis. *Clin. Cancer Res.* **2011**, *17*, 2130–2139. [CrossRef]
61. Lee, S.E.; Lee, J.U.; Lee, M.H.; Ryu, M.J.; Kim, S.J.; Kim, Y.K.; Choi, M.J.; Kim, K.S.; Kim, J.M.; Kim, J.W.; et al. RAF kinase inhibitor-independent constitutive activation of Yes-associated protein 1 promotes tumor progression in thyroid cancer. *Oncogenesis* **2013**, *2*, e55. [CrossRef]

62. Xu, C.M.; Liu, W.W.; Liu, C.J.; Wen, C.; Lu, H.F.; Wan, F.S. Mst1 overexpression inhibited the growth of human non-small cell lung cancer in vitro and in vivo. *Cancer Gene Ther.* **2013**, *20*, 453–460. [CrossRef]
63. Steinhardt, A.A.; Gayyed, M.F.; Klein, A.P.; Dong, J.; Maitra, A.; Pan, D.; Montgomery, E.A.; Anders, R.A. Expression of Yes-associated protein in common solid tumors. *Hum. Pathol.* **2008**, *39*, 1582–1589. [CrossRef]
64. Zhou, D.; Conrad, C.; Xia, F.; Park, J.S.; Payer, B.; Yin, Y.; Lauwers, G.Y.; Thasler, W.; Lee, J.T.; Avruch, J.; et al. Mst1 and Mst2 maintain hepatocyte quiescence and suppress hepatocellular carcinoma development through inactivation of the Yap1 oncogene. *Cancer Cell* **2009**, *16*, 425–438. [CrossRef] [PubMed]
65. Yu, Y.; Su, X.; Qin, Q.; Hou, Y.; Zhang, X.; Zhang, H.; Jia, M.; Chen, Y. Yes-associated protein and transcriptional coactivator with PDZ-binding motif as new targets in cardiovascular diseases. *Pharmacol. Res.* **2020**, *159*, 105009. [CrossRef] [PubMed]
66. Tumaneng, K.; Schlegelmilch, K.; Russell, R.C.; Yimlamai, D.; Basnet, H.; Mahadevan, N.; Fitamant, J.; Bardeesy, N.; Camargo, F.D.; Guan, K.L. YAP mediates crosstalk between the Hippo and PI(3)K–TOR pathways by suppressing PTEN via miR-29. *Nat. Cell Biol.* **2012**, *14*, 1322–1329. [CrossRef] [PubMed]
67. Xin, M.; Kim, Y.; Sutherland, L.B.; Qi, X.; McAnally, J.; Schwartz, R.J.; Richardson, J.A.; Bassel-Duby, R.; Olson, E.N. Regulation of insulin-like growth factor signaling by Yap governs cardiomyocyte proliferation and embryonic heart size. *Sci. Signal.* **2011**, *4*, ra70. [CrossRef] [PubMed]
68. Xu, M.Z.; Chan, S.W.; Liu, A.M.; Wong, K.F.; Fan, S.T.; Chen, J.; Poon, R.T.; Zender, L.; Lowe, S.W.; Hong, W.; et al. AXL receptor kinase is a mediator of YAP-dependent oncogenic functions in hepatocellular carcinoma. *Oncogene* **2011**, *30*, 1229–1240. [CrossRef]
69. Yan, B.; Jiang, Z.; Cheng, L.; Chen, K.; Zhou, C.; Sun, L.; Qian, W.; Li, J.; Cao, J.; Xu, Q.; et al. Paracrine HGF/c-MET enhances the stem cell-like potential and glycolysis of pancreatic cancer cells via activation of YAP/HIF-1α. *Exp. Cell Res.* **2018**, *371*, 63–71. [CrossRef]
70. Sheng, X.; Li, W.B.; Wang, D.L.; Chen, K.H.; Cao, J.J.; Luo, Z.; He, J.; Li, M.C.; Liu, W.J.; Yu, C. YAP is closely correlated with castration-resistant prostate cancer, and downregulation of YAP reduces proliferation and induces apoptosis of PC-3 cells. *Mol. Med. Rep.* **2015**, *12*, 4867–4876. [CrossRef]

Publisher's Note: MDPI stays neutral with regard to jurisdictional claims in published maps and institutional affiliations.

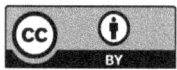

© 2020 by the authors. Licensee MDPI, Basel, Switzerland. This article is an open access article distributed under the terms and conditions of the Creative Commons Attribution (CC BY) license (http://creativecommons.org/licenses/by/4.0/).

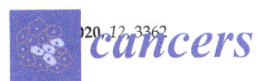

Article

Two Secreted Proteoglycans, Activators of Urothelial Cell–Cell Adhesion, Negatively Contribute to Bladder Cancer Initiation and Progression

Vasiliki Papadaki [1,2,†], Ken Asada [3,4,†], Julie K. Watson [5,6,7,†], Toshiya Tamura [1,8], Alex Leung [1], Jack Hopkins [1], Margaret Dellett [1,9], Noriaki Sasai [1,10], Hongorzul Davaapil [1,11], Serena Nik-Zainal [12,13], Rebecca Longbottom [1,14], Makoto Nakakido [1,15], Ryo Torii [16], Abhi Veerakumarasivam [5,17], Syuzo Kaneko [3], Mandeep S. Sagoo [1,18,19,20], Gillian Murphy [5,6], Akihisa Mitani [21], Kohei Tsumoto [15], John D. Kelly [5,22], Ryuji Hamamoto [3,4,5,15,*] and Shin-ichi Ohnuma [1,5,*]

1. UCL Institute of Ophthalmology, University College London, 11-43 Bath Street, London EC1V 9EL, UK; vpapadaki@fleming.gr (V.P.); toshiya.tamura@axcelead.com (T.T.); alex.leung.18@ucl.ac.uk (A.L.); jack.hopkins.18@ucl.ac.uk (J.H.); m.dellett@ulster.ac.uk (M.D.); noriakisasai@bs.naist.jp (N.S.); hd410@cam.ac.uk (H.D.); e.longbottom@nsh.net (R.L.); nakakido@protein.t.u-tokyo.ac.jp (M.N.); m.sagoo@ucl.ac.uk (M.S.S.)
2. Institute of Fundamental Biological Research, Biomedical Sciences Research Center "Alexander Fleming", 16672 Vari, Greece
3. Division of Molecular Modification and Cancer Biology, National Cancer Center Research Institute, 5-1-1 Tsukiji, Chuo-ku, Tokyo 104-0045, Japan; ken.asada@riken.jp (K.A.); sykaneko@ncc.go.jp (S.K.)
4. Cancer Translational Research Team, RIKEN Center for Advanced Intelligence Project, 1-4-1 Nihonbashi, Chuo-ku, Tokyo 103-0027, Japan
5. The Hutchison/MRC Research Centre, Department of Oncology, University of Cambridge, Hills Road, Cambridge CB2 2XZ, UK; julie.watson@stemcell.com (J.K.W.); abhiv@sunway.edu.my (A.V.); gm290@cam.ac.uk (G.M.); j.d.kelly@ucl.ac.uk (J.D.K.)
6. Cancer Research UK Cambridge Institute, University of Cambridge, Cambridge CB2 0RE, UK
7. Stem Cell Technologies, Building 7100, Cambridge Research Park, Beach Drive, Waterbeach, Cambridge CB25 9TL, UK
8. Integrated Biology, Research Division Axcelead Drug Discovery Partners, Inc. 26-1, Muraoka-Higashi 2-chome, Fujisawa, Kanagawa 251-0012, Japan
9. C-TRIC, Altnagelvin Hospital Campus, NI Centre for Stratified Medicine, Glenshane Road, Derry/Londonderry BT47 6SB, UK
10. Developmental Biomedical Science, Graduate School of Biological Sciences, Nara Institute of Science and Technology, 8916-5, Takayama-cho, Ikoma 630-0192, Japan
11. Cambridge Biomedical Campus, Jeffrey Cheah Biomedical Centre, Puddicombe Way, Wellcome—MRC Cambridge Stem Cell Institute, Cambridge CB2 0AW, UK
12. MRC Cancer Unit University of Cambridge Hutchison/MRC Research Centre, Box 197, Cambridge Biomedical Campus, Cambridge CB2 0XZ, UK; snz@mrc-cu.cam.ac.uk
13. Academic Laboratory of Medical Genetics, Box 238, Lv 6 Addenbrooke's Treatment Centre, Addenbrooke's Hospital, Cambridge CB2 0QQ, UK
14. Critical Care, University College London Hospital, 3rd floor, 235 Euston Road, London NW1 2PG, UK
15. Institute of Medical Science, The University of Tokyo, 4-6-1 Shirokanedai, Minato-ku, Tokyo 108-8639, Japan; tsumoto@bioeng.t.u-tokyo.ac.jp
16. Department of Mechanical Engineering, University College London, Torrington Place, London WC1E 7JE, UK; r.torii@ucl.ac.uk
17. Department of Biological Sciences, School of Science and Technology, Sunway University, Bandar Sunway, Selangor Darul Ehsan 47500, Malaysia
18. Retinoblastoma Service, Royal London Hospital, Whitechapel Road, London E1 1BB, UK
19. Ocular Oncology Service, Moorfields Eye Hospital, City Road, London EC1V 2PD, UK
20. National Institute for Health Research Biomedical Research Centre at Moorfields Eye Hospital NHS Foundation Trust and UCL Institute of Ophthalmology, City Road, London EC1V 2PD, UK

21 Department of Respiratory Medicine, The University of Tokyo Hospital, 7-3-1 Hongo, Bunkyo-ku, Tokyo 113-8655, Japan; mitania-tky@umin.ac.jp
22 Division of Surgery and Interventional Science, University College London, 74 Huntley Street, London WC1E 6AU, UK
* Correspondence: rhamamot@ncc.go.jp (R.H.); s.ohnuma@ucl.ac.uk (S.-i.O.); Tel.: +44-20-7608-4062 (S.-i.O.)
† These authors contributed equally to this work.

Received: 23 September 2020; Accepted: 3 November 2020; Published: 13 November 2020

Simple Summary: Epithelial–mesenchymal transition (EMT) is associated with cancer progression. Here, we found that two secreted proteins of osteomodulin (OMD) and proline/arginine-rich end leucine repeat protein (PRELP) were selectively expressed in bladder umbrella epithelial cells, and they were suppressed in bladder cancer. We revealed that $OMD^{-/-}$ or $PRELP^{-/-}$ knockout mice caused a breakdown of the umbrella cell layer through weakening cell–cell integrity and the activation of partial EMT, which resulted in the formation of early bladder cancer-like structures, while OMD or PRELP application to bladder cancer cells inhibited cancer progression through reversing EMT, which was mediated by the inhibition of TGF-β and EGF. Our result indicates that OMD and PRELP function as tumor-suppressing proteins through inhibiting EMT. OMD and PRELP may be potential therapeutic targets in bladder cancer.

Abstract: Osteomodulin (OMD) and proline/arginine-rich end leucine repeat protein (PRELP) are secreted extracellular matrix proteins belonging to the small leucine-rich proteoglycans family. We found that OMD and PRELP were specifically expressed in umbrella cells in bladder epithelia, and their expression levels were dramatically downregulated in all bladder cancers from very early stages and various epithelial cancers. Our in vitro studies including gene expression profiling using bladder cancer cell lines revealed that OMD or PRELP application suppressed the cancer progression by inhibiting TGF-β and EGF pathways, which reversed epithelial–mesenchymal transition (EMT), activated cell–cell adhesion, and inhibited various oncogenic pathways. Furthermore, the overexpression of OMD in bladder cancer cells strongly inhibited the anchorage-independent growth and tumorigenicity in mouse xenograft studies. On the other hand, we found that in the bladder epithelia, the knockout mice of OMD and/or PRELP gene caused partial EMT and a loss of tight junctions of the umbrella cells and resulted in formation of a bladder carcinoma in situ-like structure by spontaneous breakdowns of the umbrella cell layer. Furthermore, the ontological analysis of the expression profiling of an OMD knockout mouse bladder demonstrated very high similarity with those obtained from human bladder cancers. Our data indicate that OMD and PRELP are endogenous inhibitors of cancer initiation and progression by controlling EMT. OMD and/or PRELP may have potential for the treatment of bladder cancer.

Keywords: OMD; PRELP; tumor suppression gene; bladder cancer initiation; tight junction; partial EMT

1. Introduction

Small leucine-rich proteoglycans (SLRPs) are a family of 17 secreted extracellular matrix (ECM) proteoglycans [1]. SLRP members function not only as modifiers of ECM organization but also as regulators of ligand-induced signaling pathways [1–4]. For example, Tsukushi regulates the Notch, Wnt, FGF, BMP4, and Nodal pathways through interactions with extracellular components in a context-dependent manner [5–8]. The expression of SLRPs is often altered in tumors. Biglycan, lumican, and fibromodulin are overexpressed in various types of cancer, whilst decorin is overexpressed in some types of cancer and suppressed in others [9]. High expression levels of lumican are associated with a poorer survival in colorectal tumors, and they are also presented with increased metastasis in lung cancers [10]. Conversely, the overexpression of lumican in melanoma cells inhibited tumor formation in an animal model [11], whereas low expression levels of lumican and decorin are associated with a poorer patient survival in breast tumors and spindle cell carcinomas, respectively [12]. Thirty percent of decorin knockout mice develop intestinal tumors [13], and decorin/p53 double knockout mice demonstrate an enhanced susceptibility to thymic lymphoma [14]. Decorin suppressed squamous cell carcinoma in vitro by binding to EGFR to regulate downstream signaling pathways, while it also inhibited tumor formation and metastasis in a xenograft model [1,15,16]. However, no mutations or deletions of these genes have been reported so far in human cancers. Thus, their relevance to human carcinogenesis remains unclear.

With the development of epithelial malignancies, major changes occur in the organization of ECM, which normally provides the microenvironment for the maintenance of epithelial cell integrity. Many oncogenes cannot initiate a tumor if the extracellular microenvironment is normally maintained [17]. Moreover, in some cases, breakdown of the extracellular microenvironment by itself can trigger tumorigenesis [18]. These studies further demonstrate the importance of ECM proteins in cancer development.

Bladder cancer is one of the most common cancers worldwide, with 549,400 new cases and 200,000 deaths annually [19]. Our study shows that the two SLRPs or secreted ECM, osteomodulin (OMD) and proline/arginine-rich end leucine repeat protein (PRELP) are expressed in bladder and critical regulators of bladder cancer initiation and progression via altering cell–cell adhesion, probably through the regulation of epithelial–mesenchymal transition (EMT). Our findings can explain the mechanism of cancer initiation and can contribute to new therapeutic applications.

2. Results

2.1. OMD and PRELP Expression and the Association with the Early Stages of Bladder Cancer

We analyzed the expression levels of SLRP members in various epithelial cancers including bladder cancer using two independent microarray-based expression-profiling databases drawn from a worldwide population: Oncomine (Figure 1a,b; Figure S1) and Gene Logic Inc (Figure S2). Interestingly, the expression levels of *OMD* and *PRELP* are strongly suppressed in the majority of epithelial cancer types.

Next, we performed a detailed expression analysis of 126 bladder cancer samples and 31 normal control samples (Figure 1c–f; Table S1). The expression of both *OMD* and *PRELP* in tumors was drastically lower compared to normal tissues (Figure 1d,f) and declined progressively with cancer stage (Figure 1c,e; Table S1). No associations were found with gender or recurrence status, nor with age or tumor size (Table S1). *OMD* and *PRELP* were also downregulated in bladder cancer cell lines compared to normal bladder tissue (Figure S3a,b). Moderate *OMD* expression was seen only in the non-invasive bladder cell lines RT4 and LHT1376.

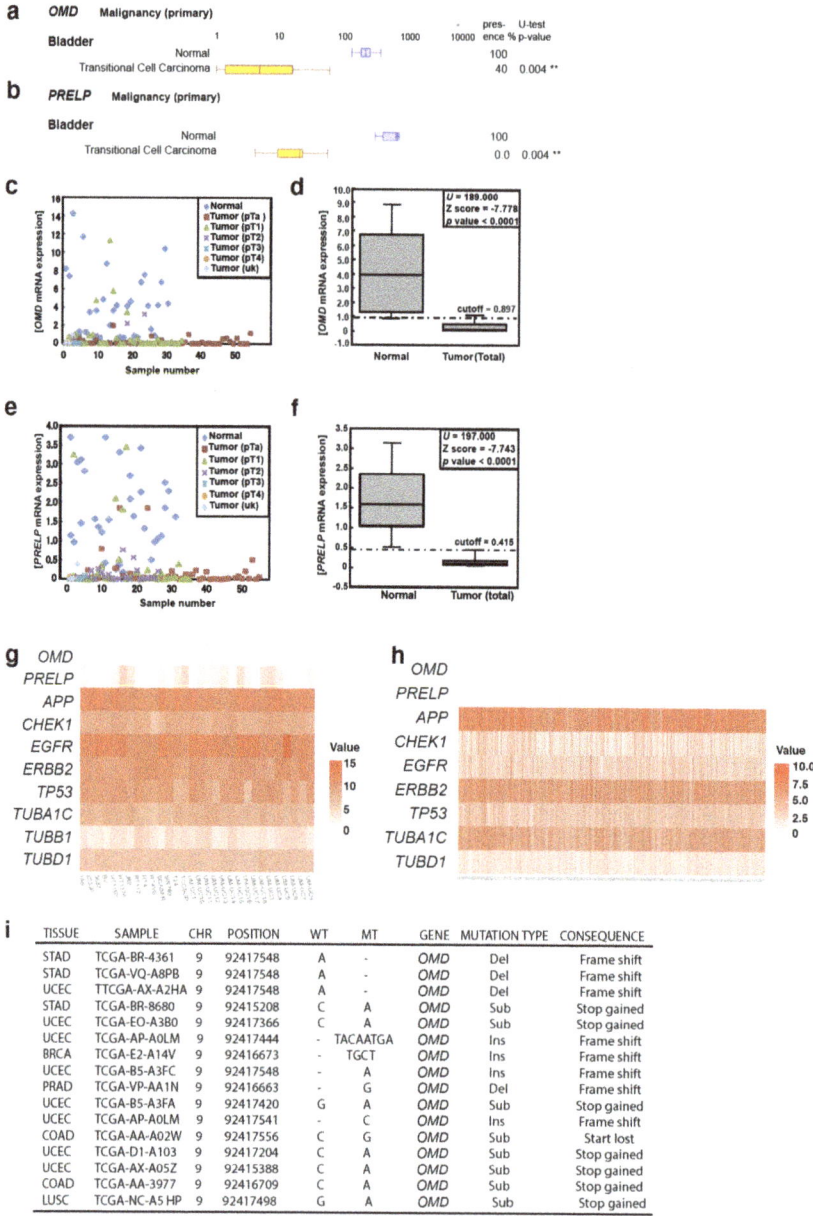

Figure 1. Expression of osteomodulin (OMD) and proline/arginine-rich end leucine repeat protein (PRELP) in cancer (**a**,**b**). Microarray analysis of *OMD* (**a**) and *PRELP* (**b**) expression in human bladder cancer samples and normal bladder tissues. (**c**) Quantitative analysis of *OMD* expression in bladder cancer at different stages by qPCR. (**d**) Box–whisker plot (median 50% boxed) of (**c**). Cutoff value (dash line) was determined as described in Materials and Methods. (**e**) Quantitative analysis of *PRELP* expression in bladder cancer at different stages by qPCR. (**f**) Box–whisker plot of (**e**). (**g**) Expression analysis of *OMD* and *PRELP* in bladder cell lines. Published expression profiling data of MIBC cell lines (GSE97768) are re-examined to elucidate the relative expression of *OMD* and *PRELP* in comparison

with known overexpressing genes in bladder cancer; *APP*, *CHEK1*, *EGFR*, *ERBB2*, and *TP53* and with housekeeping genes of *TUBA1C*, *TUBB*, and *TUBD1*. (**h**) Expression analysis of *OMD* and *PRELP* in bladder tissues samples from patients. Published expression profiling data of non- Non-muscle-invasive bladder cancer (NMIBC)(E-MTAB-4321) are re-examined to elucidate the relative expression of *OMD* and *PRELP* in comparison with *APP*, *CHEK1*, *EGFR*, *ERBB2*, and *TP53* and with housekeeping genes of *TUBA1C* and *TUBD1*. Details of both (**g**,**h**) analyses are in Materials and Methods. (**i**) Somatic mutations in human cancer samples that are predicted to generate a loss of function of *OMD*. Detail of cancers is described in Materials and Methods in the section of OMD and PRELP Expression Analysis in muscle-invasive bladder cancer (MIBC) cell lines and NMIBC Patient Samples. ** indicates $p < 0.01$.

To assess the potential role of OMD and PRELP as diagnostic markers, we set cutoff values to distinguish tumor samples from normal tissues through calculation of the interquartile range. The expression levels of *OMD* and *PRELP* in almost all normal bladder tissues were above the cutoff value (specificity: 83.9% (*OMD*) and 90.3% (*PRELP*)), while expression in the vast majority of tumor tissues was below the cutoff (sensitivity: 88.9% (*OMD*) and 90.5% (*PRELP*), Table S2). Expression levels of *OMD* and *PRELP* in the Ta (early) stage of almost all tumor tissues were below the cutoff value (sensitivity: 88.9% (OMD) and 88.9% (PRELP), Table S2). When we combined the data for *OMD* and *PRELP*, the expression of both genes below the cutoff value was found only in tumor samples and in none of the normal tissues (specificity 100%). These results show that the expression levels of *OMD* and *PRELP* genes are powerful markers for the prediction of the presence of urothelial carcinomas. The suppression of *OMD* and *PRELP* was also observed when we analyzed previously published expression profiling data for muscle-invasive bladder cancer (MIBC) and non-muscle-invasive bladder cancer (NMIBC) (Figure 1g,h) [20,21]. An examination of mutation analysis using The Cancer Genome Atlas (TCGA) (Figure 1i) found a total of 3,142,246 somatic substitutions/indels were interrogated from 33,096 primary human cancers, and the somatic mutations predicted to generate a loss-of-function effect in OMD are summarized in Figure 1i. However, relatively few mutations were observed (95 for OMD and 158 for PRELP) (unpublished data).

2.2. Cell–Cell Adhesion and Cancer Signaling Regulated by OMD and PRELP

To further assess the role of OMD and PRELP in cancer, we overexpressed or underexpressed the two proteins in cultured cells and performed gene expression analysis using microarrays (Affimetrix GeneChip® System). The T-Rex-293T system was used to express the genes at a near-physiological level without causing adverse effects due to their insertion site. To ablate gene expression, 5637 bladder cancer cells, expressing *OMD* and *PRELP* at a low level, were transfected with siRNA constructs for *OMD* or *PRELP*. After validating the altered expression of *OMD* and *PRELP* by RT-PCR, gene expression profiling was performed.

Figure 2a,b show the numbers of genes that are negatively and positively transcriptionally regulated by OMD and/or PRELP, respectively. The genes affected by OMD and PRELP include many oncogenes and tumor-suppressor genes such as *NF-kB*, *Ras*, and *c-Fos*. For example, 107 genes were activated by both OMD and PRELP overexpression, while 139 genes were suppressed by the double-depletion (Figure 2b). These observations indicate that OMD and PRELP have a functional redundancy while they also regulate various distinct target genes.

Next, to elucidate the affected signaling pathways, biological events, and mechanisms, the gene expression profiling data were analyzed with a data mining program (Ingenuity Pathway Analysis, IPA, Qiagen, (https://digitalinsights.qiagen.com/products-overview/discovery-insights-portfolio/analysis-and-visualization/qiagen-ipa/?cmpid=QDI_GA_IPA&gclid=CjwKCAiAtK79BRAIEiwA4OskBpDKfEsg5CJdSERKm3IEd_0gZRXNEGfgu7XJjKoC9hVggrFtzQnvxBoCY_wQAvD_BwE). Using the Functional Analysis mode, "molecular mechanism of cancer" was identified as one of the most significantly affected biological functions and/or diseases in all four conditions of OMD overexpression, OMD depletion, PRELP overexpression, and PRELP depletion (Figure 2c; Figure S3c–f). In total, 304 and 388 genes related to the "cancer" category are significantly affected by the altered expression of

OMD and PRELP, including members of the p53 pathway, the NF-kB pathway, the Ras pathway, the RB1 pathway, the Jun/Fos pathway, and the Myc pathway (Figure 2d).

Our analysis also revealed that both OMD and PRELP strongly influence cell–cell adhesion mediated by tight junctions (Figure 2e). Tight junctions are a type of cell–cell junction that binds the apical sides of epithelial cells. The breakdown of tight junctions has been proposed as a critical step in cancer initiation [22,23]. Tight junction components such as Zonula occlugens-1 (ZO-1) and Nectin were transcriptionally activated by OMD or PRELP overexpression, while they were suppressed in OMD or PRELP depletion, suggesting that OMD and PRELP have the ability to positively regulate tight junctions (Figure 2e).

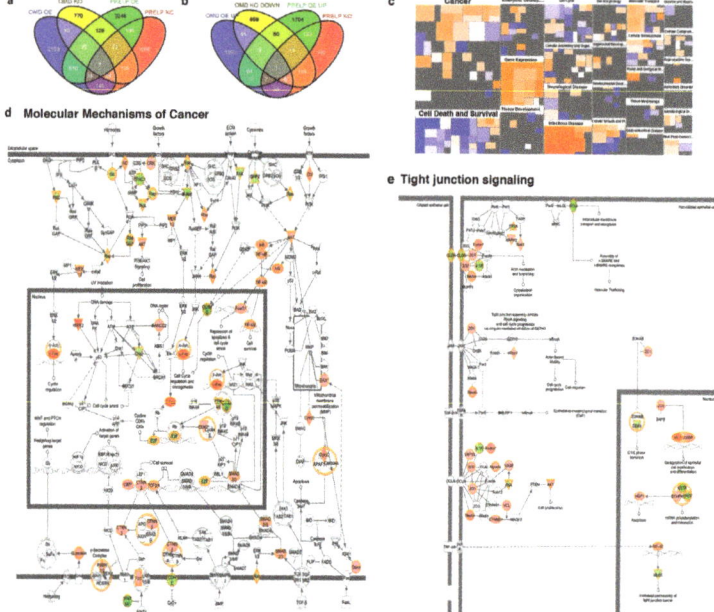

Figure 2. Gene expression profiling in OMD/PRELP overexpressing or deleted cells. Gene expression profiling was performed under seven conditions; OMD overexpression in T-Rex-293T cells, PRELP overexpression in T-Rex-293T cells, control T-Rex-293T cells, OMD depletion in the 5637 bladder cancer cells, PRELP depletion in the 5637 cells, two controls of the 5637 cells. Details are in Materials and Methods. Then, genes with statistical significant changes of mRNA levels have been identified. Data were analyzed, and the following figures were made through the use of Ingenuity Pathway Analysis (IPA) (QIAGEN Inc., https://www.qiagenbioinformatics.com/products/ingenuitypathway-analysis). (**a**) Gene numbers significantly inhibited by OMD overexpression or PRELP overexpression but activated by OMD depletion or PRELP depletion. (**b**) Gene numbers activated by OMD overexpression or PRELP overexpression but suppressed by OMD depletion or PRELP depletion. (**c**) Heat map of signaling pathways significantly affected by OMD overexpression. This heat map was created using IPA software. Similar heat maps were observed in other three conditions of OMD depletion, PRELP overexpression, and PRELP depletion. (**d,e**) Schematic drawing of the most strongly influenced biological events regulated by OMD overexpression. "Molecular Mechanism of Cancer" (**d**) and "Tight junction signaling" (**e**) category. Both images of (**d,e**) were created by Ingenuity Pathway Analysis according to their rule. This pathway is one of the most strongly influenced ones by any of four conditions (OMD overexpression, OMD depletion, PRELP overexpression, PRELP depletion).

2.3. OMD or PRELP Overexpression in EJ28 Bladder Cancer Cells

To investigate the roles of OMD and PRELP at the molecular level, we constructed stable cell lines that overexpressed OMD, OMD-myc, PRELP, and PRELP-myc using the EJ28 bladder cancer cell line, as their endogenous expression is strongly suppressed.

Under standard cell culture using non-coated culture dish with non-confluent conditions, control EJ28 cells had a flattened fibroblast-like shape. In contrast, many OMD overexpressing cells had a markedly different round shape with many pin-like extensions (Figure 3a). PRELP overexpression also resulted in a change of cell morphology to round cells similar to OMD overexpressors together with elongated cells with protruding stress fiber-like filamentous extensions (Figure 3a). To evaluate relevant changes in the cytoskeletal structure, we stained for actin and tubulin. We found that there are many pin-like actin structures on the surface of the round OMD-expressing cells, similar to the phenotype induced by cdc42 activation [24]. On the other hand, PRELP overexpression resulted in both round cells with pin-like structures and elongated cells with long clear actin fibers (Figure 3b). These abnormal morphological changes were also observed with tubulin staining (Figure 3c).

We next analyzed the effect of OMD/PRELP overexpression on cell proliferation and survival. First, expression levels of *OMD* and *PRELP* in EJ28 cells were analyzed by qRT-PCR (S4a and b) and by Western blotting using the myc antibody for myc-tag protein expression (S8n and S8p). OMD and OMD-myc cells exhibited reduced proliferation, both in standard proliferation and BrdU incorporation assays (Figure S4c,d), while cell cycle analysis by flow cytometry revealed an enhanced G1 phase transition (Figure S4e). Finally, OMD and OMD-myc cells presented a small but significant increase in apoptosis, as assayed by annexin staining (Figure S4f). The overexpression of OMD, OMD-myc, and PRELP resulted in a slight but significant suppression of cell growth with modulation of the cell cycle phase distribution. In addition, OMD and PRELP overexpression slightly increased apoptosis, although the majority of cells remained non-apoptotic. Overall, we conclude that the overexpression of OMD and PRELP proteins results in a subtle but significant suppression of cell growth with the modulation of cell cycle phase distribution.

Anchorage-independent growth is a well-established property of transformed cancer cells. Therefore, we examined the effect of OMD or PRELP overexpression on anchorage-independent growth (Figure 3d,e). OMD or PRELP-myc overexpression completely abolished colony formation. These results indicate that OMD and PRELP suppression might be important for the transition from normal epithelial cells to mesenchymal-like cancer cells. Additionally, we tested the cell growth in a 3D environment using Matrigel to investigate growth under partial anchorage conditions. Control EJ28 cells grew well and showed a "spread-like" morphology (Figure 3f), as observed in standard cell culture dishes. However, OMD or PRELP overexpressing cells tended to make cell aggregates, suggesting that OMD and PRELP may influence cell migration. To address this, we performed the Boyden chamber assay with Matrigel-coated transwells. The assay clearly demonstrated that the overexpression of OMD or PRELP strongly suppressed cell migration and invasion (Figure 3g,h). The effect of OMD and PRELP overexpression on cell migration was also tested in standard 2D conditions with the scratch wound assay, where a small inhibition of the wound recovery was observed (Figure S4g). Collectively, these results suggest that the two proteins affect colony formation, migration, and invasion capabilities of cancer cells in a substrate-dependent manner.

As OMD and PRELP are secreted proteins, to confirm that the observed effects are mediated by the extracellular forms, we performed a co-culture assay, in which EJ28 cells (Cell A) overexpressing OMD or PRELP were cultured in the chamber above tester EJ28 cells (Cell B) (Figure 3i). OMD and PRELP significantly suppressed the growth of the lower layer of EJ28 tester cells (Figure 3j), as we expected.

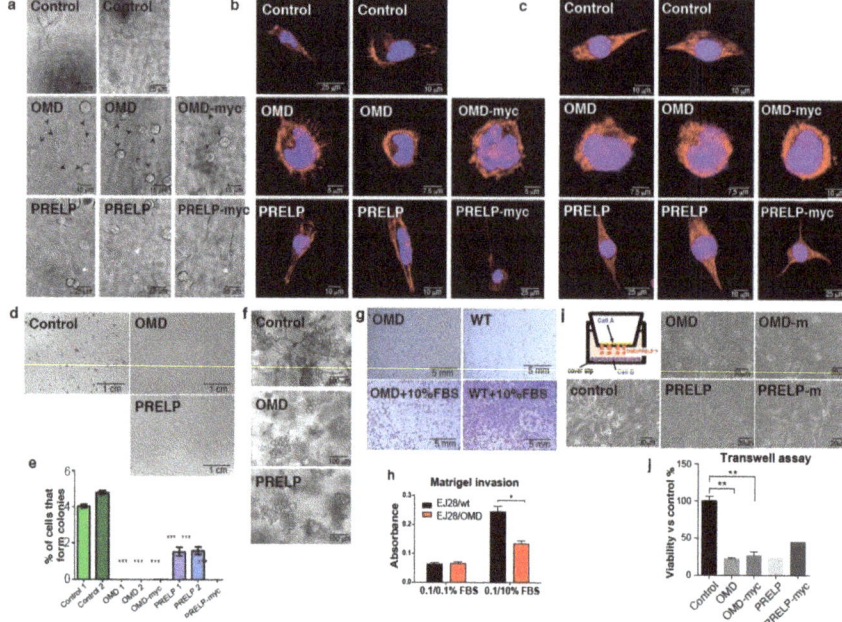

Figure 3. Effect of OMD or PRELP overexpression in bladder cancer cell lines. (**a**) Cell morphology of EJ28 bladder cancer cells transfected with OMD, OMD-myc, PRELP, or PRELP-myc constructs, observed by differential interference contrast (DIC) microscope. Round cells are indicated as arrowheads. (**b**) Phalloidin staining of the transfected EJ28 cells. Phalloidin (red) and DAPI (blue). Pin-like structures of OMD overexpressing cells are phalloidin-positive. PRELP overexpression results in clear long actin fiber formation. (**c**) Anti-tubulin antibody staining. Tubulin (red) and 4′,6-diamidlino-2-phenylindole (DAPI) (blue). (**d,e**) Anchorage-independent growth using the soft agar. Photos of control, OMD, and PRELP overexpressing colonies formed in the top agar layer (**d**). Quantification of the cell percentage that formed colonies (**e**). (**f**) Cell growth in the Matrigel. (**g,h**) Cell migration and invasion assay using the Boyden chamber. Photos of cells that invaded to the bottom side of membrane after the addition of fetal bovine serum (FBS) as a chemoattractant (**g**). Quantification of cell migration/invasion in (**g,h**). (**i,j**) Transwell co-culture assay to evaluate the effect of secreted OMD/PRELP on non-contacting cells. Schematic drawing of the assay system and photos of EJ28 cells cultured at the button chambers (**i**). Quantification of viable cell density in the bottom well by trypan blue staining (**j**). *, **, *** indicate $p < 0.01$, $p < 0.005$, $p < 0.001$, respectively.

2.4. The Relation between OMD or PRELP and Tight Junction Formation

We examined the status of tight junctions of EJ28 cells using antibodies against occludin (Figure 4a–i), ZO-1 (Figure 4j–l), and cingulin (Figure 4m–o). In confluent monolayers of the control EJ28 cells, we observed partial staining at cell–cell interfaces, covering around 40% of the total cell–cell surface for occludin, (40% of total cell–cell surface), ZO-1 (46%), and cingulin (30%) (Figure 4p–r). This appearance of partial junction staining is found in cancer cell lines (personal communication, Karl Matter). Interestingly, the overexpression of OMD resulted in enhanced and continuous junctional staining of all three markers, covering almost the whole cell periphery (Figure 4b,h,k,n). PRELP overexpression had a similar effect, where tight junction formation was also markedly increased compared to the control cells. This enhanced junctional staining was accompanied by a reduction of the cytoplasmic staining of the corresponding markers. To further confirm the formation of tight junctions, the control EJ28 cells and OMD overexpressing cells were examined by electron microscopy.

A large number of tight junctions were observed in OMD overexpressing cells (Figure 4s–u). However, we failed to detect any tight junctions in the control EJ28 cells (Figure 4v,w).

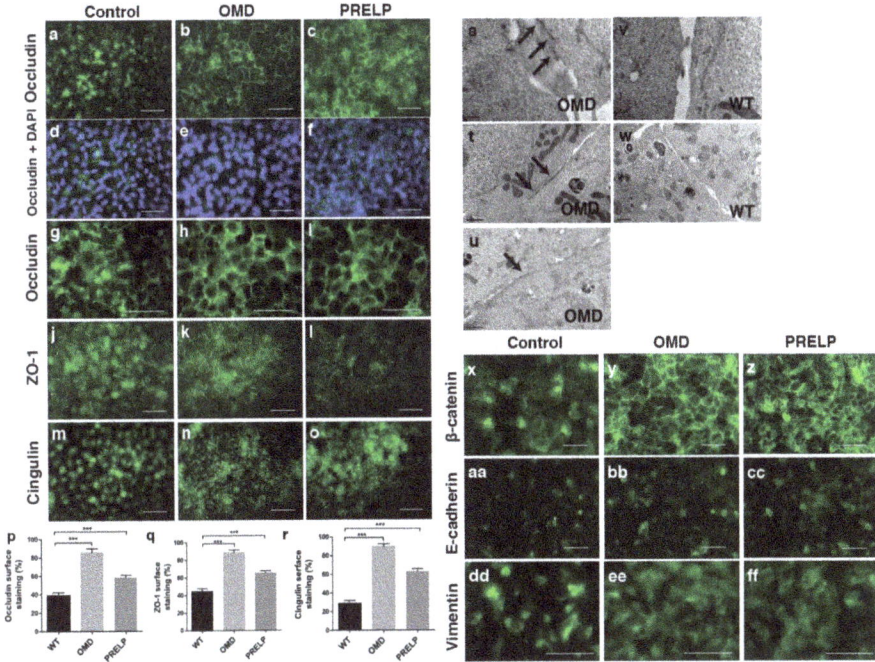

Figure 4. Effect of OMD or PRELP overexpression on tight junction in EJ28 cells. (**a–i**) Occludin antibody staining of OMD or PRELP expressing EJ28 cells; low magnification (**a–c**), overlaid with DAPI (**d–f**), enlarged (**g–i**). (**j–l**) ZO-1 staining. (**m–o**) Cingulin staining. Scale bar represents 100 μm (**a–o**). (**p**) Quantification of occluding staining. (**q**) Quantification of ZO-1 staining. (**r**) Quantification of cingulin staining. (**s–w**) Electron microscope (EM) analysis of cell-cell junction. OMD expressing EJ28 cells (**s–u**) and wild type (WT) EJ28 cells (**v,w**). Tight junctions are indicated by arrows. Scale bar represents 1 μm (**t,u,w**) and 0.5 μm (**s,v**). OMD overexpression strongly activates tight junction formation. (**x–ff**) Antibody staining of confluent monolayer; β-catenin (**x–z**), E-cadherin (**aa–cc**), and vimentin (**dd–ff**). Scale bar represents 100 μm (**x–ff**). *** indicates $p < 0.001$.

Subsequently, to determine the effect on adherens junctions, we examined the expression of β-catenin, E-cadherin, and vimentin. Figure 4x shows that in the control group, many cells have a weak β-catenin localization in the nuclei. On the other hand, in OMD or PRELP overexpressing cells, β-catenin was almost exclusively localized at the plasma membrane, and the strength of the staining was much higher than the control (Figure 4x–z). E-cadherin staining was slightly enhanced (Figure 4aa–cc), indicating that OMD and PRELP activate adherens junctions. To test how OMD and PRELP regulated cell–cell adhesion, we examined the expression of vimentin, an EMT marker. The major characteristics of epithelial cells are cell polarity, strong cell–cell integrity, and anchorage-dependent growth. Cancer initiation in epithelia is always associated with EMT [25,26]. After conversion to mesenchymal cells, these cells can grow in an anchorage-independent manner, as observed in almost all cancer cells. Figure 4dd–ff shows that vimentin was more localized around or in the nucleus, while OMD or PRELP-expressing cells showed a diffuse expression of vimentin in the cytosol. This suggests that OMD and PRELP may regulate cell–cell adhesion through EMT.

2.5. Signal Pathways Regulated by OMD and PRELP

The gene expression profiling experiment revealed that OMD and PRELP were involved in the regulation of various components of several ligand-induced signaling pathways, including the IGF-1, Wnt, EGF, and TGF-β pathways. We aimed to determine the molecular mechanisms of OMD/PRELP activity using EJ28 stable cell lines that overexpress the two proteins. In the expression profiling data (Figure 2d), the Akt level was significantly affected by both OMD and PRELP. We found that OMD and PRELP overexpression downregulated the phosphorylation of Akt (Figure 5a), and OMD overexpression downregulated the phosphorylation of ERK1/2 (Figure 5b). Akt phosphorylation is known to be regulated by the EGF and IGF pathways [27,28]. Figure 5a and b show that upon EGF treatment (10 ng/mL), Akt phosphorylation was decreased in the OMD overexpressing cells compared to the control. EGF induced the phosphorylation of tyrosine-1068 of the EGFR, and this phosphorylation was suppressed by OMD expression (Figure 5b). ERK1/2 phosphorylation was elevated by exogenous EGF, and this phosphorylation was also suppressed by OMD (Figure 5b). Co-immunoprecipitation assays revealed that OMD was bound to the EGFR (Figure 5c). Total EGFR protein was reduced in OMD transfected cells (Figure 5d). Inhibition of the EGF pathway is known to lead β-catenin localization to the cell membrane [29], which we observed in OMD/PRELP activation (Figure 4x).

IGF activated Akt through the phosphorylation of the IGF-1R; however, OMD overexpression did not inhibit the IGF-mediated phosphorylation of Akt (Figure 5e) in our assays. In addition, we did not detect any direct interaction of OMD with the IGF receptor (Figure 5f). All the SLRP family members previously studied directly interact with TGF-β family members and regulate transcription of their targets via the phosphorylation of Smad2 [2]. Indeed, OMD and PRELP directly bound to TGF-β protein (Figure 5g) and resulted in Smad2 phosphorylation suppression, particularly in OMD (Figure 5h). The effect of OMD and PRELP on EGFR, β-catenin, and Smad2 were quantitated and the results are shown in Figure S5.

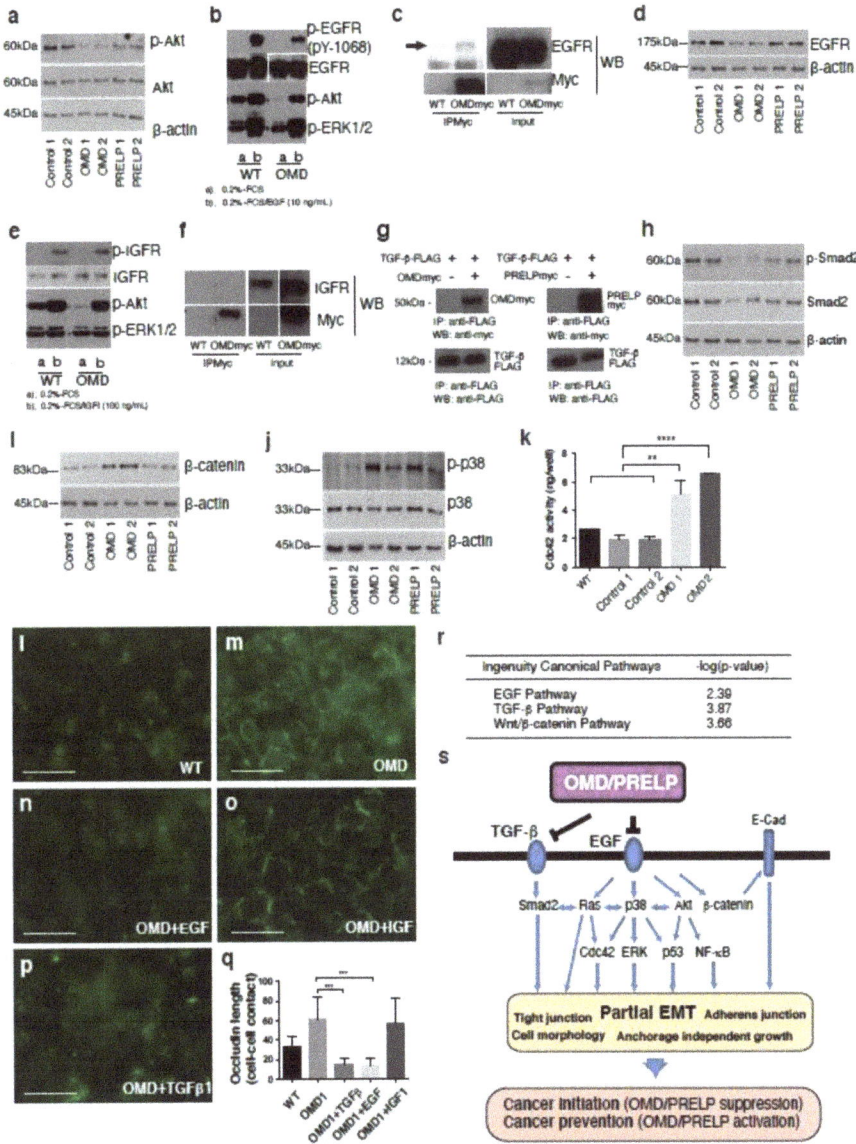

Figure 5. Mechanism of OMD or PRELP-mediated regulation of tight junction. Various effects of OMD and PRELP were examined in vitro using OMD or PRELP stably overexpressing EJ28 bladder cancer cell lines. OMD1 and OMD2 indicate different stable clones. (**a**) Effect of OMD or PRELP overexpression on Akt phosphorylation. (**b**) Effects of OMD overexpression and EGF application on EGF receptor, Akt, and ERK phosphorylation. (**c**) Interaction between OMD and EGF receptor. (**d**) Effect of OMD or PRELP on the total amount of EGF receptor. (**e**) Effects of OMD overexpression and IGF-1 application on phosphorylation of the IGF receptor, Akt, and ERK. (**f**) Interaction between the OMD and IGF receptors. (**g**) Binding of OMD or PRELP with TGF-β. (**h**) Effect of OMD or PRELP on Smad2 phosphorylation. (**i**) Effect of OMD and PRELP on the total levels of β-catenin protein expression. (**j**) Effect of OMD or PRELP on phosphorylation of p38. All original Western blotting data

are shown in Figure S8. (**k**) Effect of OMD on cdc42 activity. (**l–p**) Effect of EGF, IGF-1, and TGF-β 1 application on tight junction formation of confluent OMD overexpressing EJ28 cell monolayers. Occludin staining of normal EJ28 cells (**l**) and OMD expressing EJ28 cells (**m**). Effect of 10 ng/mL EGF (**n**), 100 ng/mL IGF-1 (**o**), or 10 ng/mL TGF-β 1 (**p**) on occludin staining of EJ28 cells overexpressing OMD. Scale bar represents 100 μm. (**q**) Quantification of occludin-positive cell–cell junctions. (**r**) TGF-β, EGF, and Wnt pathways are affected in OMD$^{-/-}$ mouse bladder. Ontological analysis of the expression profiling data obtained in Figure 8. (**s**) Schematic model of OMD/PRELP function. The uncropped Western Blot figure in Supplementary Figure S8. **, **** indicate $p < 0.01$, $p < 0.0001$, respectively.

We found that OMD overexpression significantly increased the total amount of β-catenin (Figure 5i). However, we could not detect a change of Wnt-mediated transcription activity by the TOPFLASH assay (unpublished data). Taken together with our finding that OMD causes the translocation of β-catenin to the plasma membrane (Figure 4x–z), this suggests that the increased β-catenin mainly contributes to its adherens junction-related function.

The downstream segments of ligand-induced signaling pathways are remarkably interconnected with each other in context-dependent manners. Thus, we examined two common downstream components of the EGF and TGF-β pathways, p38 and cdc42, as the OMD or PRELP mediated in vitro phenotypes reported in this paper are similar to those caused by p38 or cdc42 modulation [30–32]. Moreover, our expression profiling analysis indicated the importance of the cdc42 and p38 pathways in this context (Figure 2d). We found that OMD and PRELP overexpression increased the phosphorylation of p38 (Figure 5j), and OMD activated cdc42 (Figure 5k).

Finally, we examined the contribution of OMD-mediated inhibition of pathways to the regulation of tight junctions. TGF-β, IGF, and EGF pathways are well known as major pathways to regulate EMT and mesenchymal–epithelial transition (MET). OMD overexpressing EJ28 cells were treated with either EGF (10 ng/mL), TGF-β (10 ng/mL), or IGF-1 (100 ng/mL) protein, and their effects on tight junction formation were assessed. Cellular response was confirmed by analysis of phosphorylation of ERK1/2, AKT, and Smad2. Figure 5l–q shows that EGF and TGF-β strongly inhibited OMD-induced tight junction formation, while IGF-1 had no effect, suggesting that the OMD-mediated regulation of both EGF and TGF-β pathways is important for the regulation of tight junctions. In addition, OMD overexpression induced the translocation of β-catenin to the plasma membrane (Figure 4x), which was accompanied by an increase in the total expression levels of β-catenin (Figure 5i). Such effects were previously reported as phenotypes caused by EGF pathway inhibition [29]. Later, we will show another gene expression profiling using bladder tissues isolated from OMD$^{-/-}$ or PRELP$^{-/-}$ mice (Figure 8). The ontological analysis shows that indeed, OMD/PRELP regulate EGF and TGF-β pathways (Figure 5r)

Our results demonstrate that the OMD-mediated simultaneous regulation of TGF-β and EGF pathways is important for the maintenance of cell–cell adhesion (Figure 5s).

2.6. Tumor Progression in a Mouse Xenograft Model

In order to examine the in vivo effects of OMD overexpression in cancer development, we performed mouse xenograft experiments using stably transformed EJ28 cells. When EJ28 cells were grafted in nude mice, the control EJ28 cancer cells grew well, while OMD-expressing EJ28 cells did not grow at all (Figure 6a). These observations are in accordance with the decreased anchorage-independent growth we observed in vitro (Figure 3d–e). Haemotoxylin and Eosin (H&E) staining of tumor sections showed that the density of nuclei was reduced and the nuclear–cytoplasmic ratio was increased in OMD-overexpressing samples (Figure 6b–e). Moreover, occludin staining revealed that OMD-expressing EJ28 cells have a more organized structure and stronger tight junctions (Figure 6f–h). Next, we analyzed the ultrastructure of the xenografted cells by electron microscopy. This analysis showed that adjacent cells of the control samples intercellular spaces between neighboring cells are always visible, and almost no tight junctions can be observed (Figure 6i,j), while the OMD-expressing xenografts are in close contact and form multiple tight junctions (Figure 6k,l). These results confirmed that OMD/PRELP overexpression enhances cell–cell adhesion and suppresses cancer development in vivo.

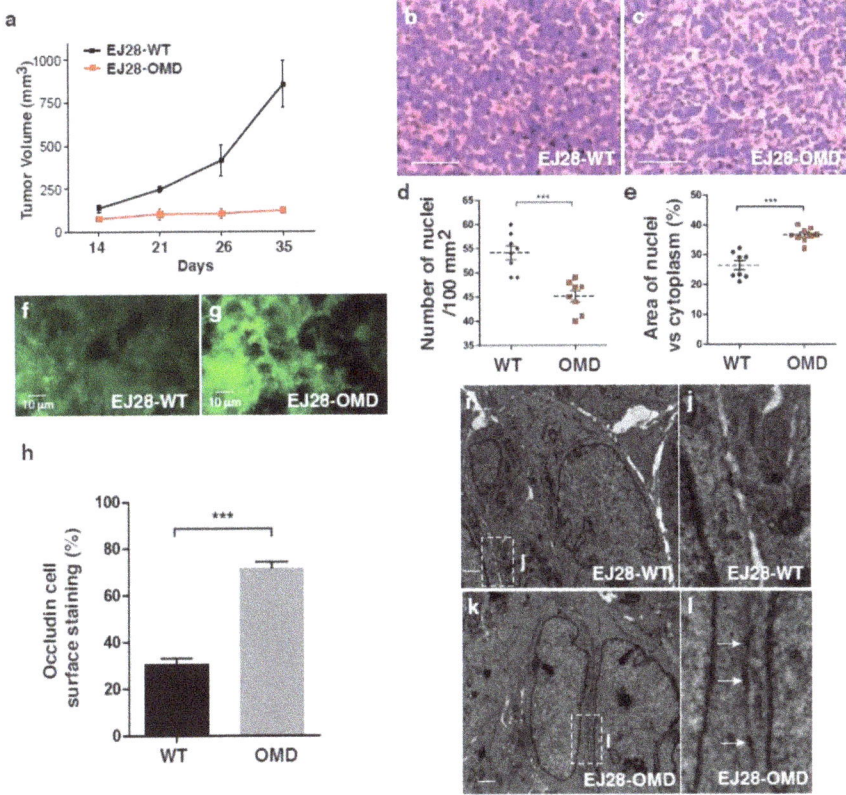

Figure 6. Mouse xenograft model overexpression of OMD. (**a**) Xenograft of EJ28 cells stably expressing OMD. Tumor volume progression graph. EJ28-*WT* ($n = 5$) and EJ28-OMD ($n = 5$). (**b–e**) Histology of xenografted tissues; H&E staining of control EJ28 cells (**b**) and EJ28 cells overexpressing OMD (**c**), comparison of the number of nuclei in 100 µm^2 of sections (**d**), comparison of the ratio of nucleus vs cytosol. (**e**) Scale bar represents 100 µm (**b**,**c**). (**f**,**g**) Occludin staining of control EJ28 tumor (**f**) and OMD overexpressing EJ28 tumor (**g**). (**h**) Quantification of occludin staining. The stained percentage of cell surfaces was measured. (**i**) EM of control EJ28 cells. (**j**) Enlarged from (**i**). (**k**) EM of OMD-overexpressing EJ28 tumor cells. Scale bar represents 1 µm (**i**,**k**). (**l**) Enlarged from (**k**). Tight junctions are shown with arrows. *** indicates $p < 0.001$.

2.7. $OMD^{-/-}$ or $PRELP^{-/-}$ Mice and Tight Junctions between Umbrella Cells

Next, we established constitutive $OMD^{-/-}$, $PRELP^{-/-}$, and $OMD^{-/-}/PRELP^{-/-}$ double knockout mice (Figure S6a–d). The knockouts were designed to target exons 2 and 3, resulting in the complete removal of protein coding sequences while knocking in the β-galactosidase gene under the *OMD* and *PRELP* promoters, respectively. The mice were viable and fertile, and no severe developmental defects were observed. *OMD* and *PRELP* expression in mice were analyzed by qRT-PCR (Figure S6e,f).

OMD and *PRELP* were expressed in all organs tested in various levels (Figure S6g,h for mouse, Figure S6i,j for human). To characterize the expression in the bladder, we assayed β-galactosidase activity in heterozygous $OMD^{+/-(LacZ)}$ and $PRELP^{+/-(LacZ)}$ mice. We observed β-gal-positive cells only in the epithelial layer (Figure S6k,l). A similar pattern was found by the in situ hybridization with the *OMD* or *PRELP* gene probe (Figure S6m,n). The bladder epithelium contains three cell types: basal cells, intermediate cells, and superficial umbrella cells [33]. To identify which cell types express OMD or PRELP, bladder sections were co-stained with β-gal and uroplakin-III (umbrella), CK18 (umbrella), CK5 (basal), or laminin (basement membrane of epithelium) antibody. In $OMD^{+/-}$ mice, β-gal positive cells were always co-localized with a subpopulation of the uroplakin-III and CK18 positive cells, but not with CK5 or laminin (Figure S6o–r). We also stained with Ki67 (proliferative) markers (Figure S6s), but there was no overlap staining. PRELP showed an expression pattern similar to that of OMD (Figure S6t–x). These results indicate that at any one time, the active transcription of *OMD* and *PRELP* is occurring in a subpopulation of umbrella cells.

Umbrella cells are connected to each other strongly by tight and adherens junctions [33]. We examined the effect of OMD or PRELP deficiency on umbrella cell junctions. Electron microscopy images indicated that the apical–lateral interfaces between *WT* bladder umbrella cells were tightly sealed by dense tight junctions (Figure 7a,b). However, strong tight junctions were markedly reduced in $OMD^{-/-}$, $PRELP^{-/-}$, or the double knockout mice (Figure 7c–e). The reduction at the lateral surface was confirmed by immunostaining with the tight junction marker ZO-1. In the *WT*, ZO-1 staining was located at the lateral cell surface (Figure 7f). In $OMD^{-/-}$ or $PRELP^{-/-}$ bladder tissues, the ZO-1 signal at the lateral cell surface was significantly reduced (Figure 7g–j). Adherens junctions are localized in the lateral cell–cell surface between umbrella cells, below the tight junction level. In *WT* mice, the adherens junctions were visible in the basolateral surface of umbrella cells, as marked by E-cadherin staining (Figure 7k), while in $OMD^{-/-}$, $PRELP^{-/-}$, and the double knockout mice, E-cadherin was localized in the whole cell surface (Figure 7l–n). This demonstrates that the disruption of tight junctions enables E-cadherin to migrate to the apical side of the cell membrane. These observations indicate that OMD or PRELP depletion results in the induction of a partial EMT state, which is characterized by the loss of tight junctions but not adherens junctions (Figure 7o).

One of the major functions of tight junctions in the bladder is to form the blood–urine barrier to block the leakage of fluids into the bladder [34]. In accordance with this function, deletion of the *PRELP* gene resulted in the formation of clots containing fibrin/fibrinogen in the bladder lumen (Figure 7p,q) and the leakage of proteins into the urine (Figure 7r).

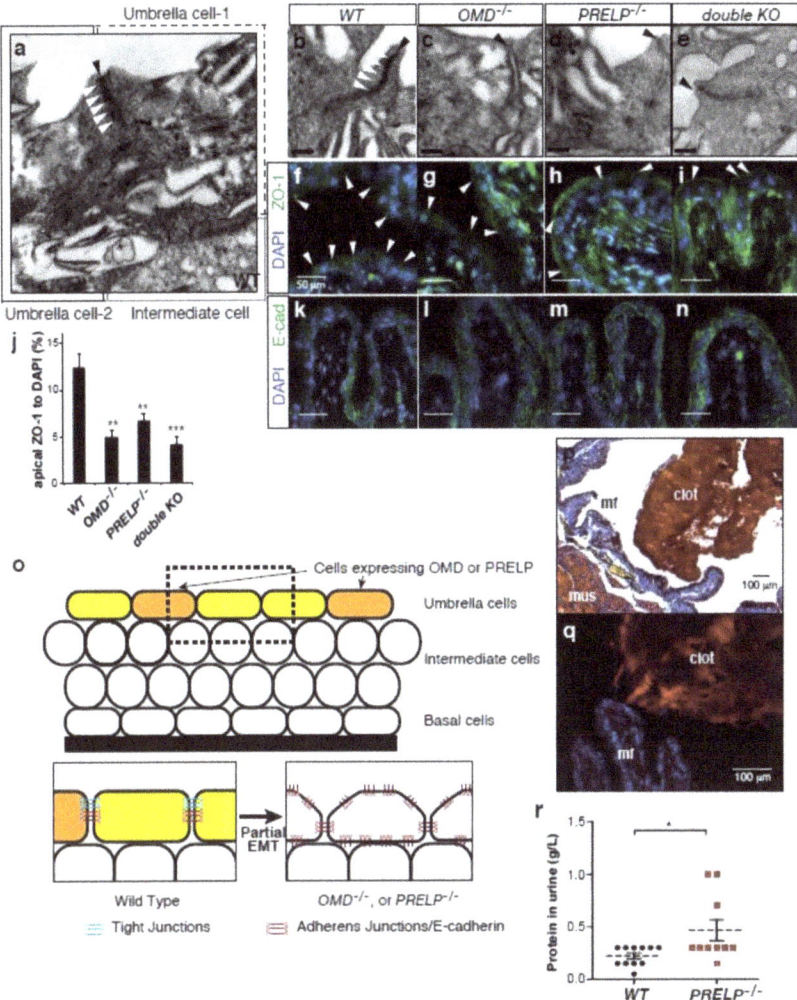

Figure 7. *OMD* or *PRELP* knockout resulted in a loss of tight junctions between bladder umbrella cells. (**a–e**) EM analysis of *WT* (**a,b**), $OMD^{-/-}$ (**c**), $PRELP^{-/-}$ (**d**), and their double (**e**) knockout bladders at 3 months old. A wide view of *WT* bladder epithelia, which includes two umbrella cells and an intermediate cell. The apical side of the cell–cell surface of umbrella cells (black arrowhead) are strongly sealed by dense tight junctions (white arrowheads) (**a**). Apical side of umbrella cell–cell interfaces. Black arrowheads; cell–cell interfaces. White arrowheads; tight junctions (**b–e**). Scale bar represents 200 nm. (**f–j**) Analysis of ZO-1 staining of a 3-month-old bladder. ZO-1 staining between umbrella cells is indicated by white arrowheads (**f**). Quantification of ZO-1 staining (**j**). (**k–n**) E-cadherin staining of a 3-month-old bladder. (**o**) Model of cell–cell adhesion in bladder epithelial cells. (**p**) Phosphotungstic acid hematoxylin (PATH) staining of 3-month-old $PRELP^{-/-}$ bladder. PATH staining stains fibrin and erythrocytes. (**q**) Fibrin antibody staining of 3-month-old $PRELP^{-/-}$ bladder. (**r**) Analysis of urinary fibrin. Urine samples were collected from *WT* and $PRELP^{-/-}$ mice at the morning and were tested using Multistix (SIEMENS). *, **, *** indicate $p < 0.05$, $p < 0.01$, $p < 0.001$, respectively.

2.8. Expression Profiling of $OMD^{-/-}$, $PRELP^{-/-}$ Bladder Epithelia

To consolidate our hypothesis that OMD and PRELP contribute to the maintenance of cell–cell adhesion and the inhibition of EMT, we performed gene expression profiling by RNA-seq using isolated bladder epithelia from WT mice (n = 3), $OMD^{-/-}$ (n = 5), and $PRELP^{-/-}$ (n = 3). Similarly to our previous gene expression analysis data (Figure 2), 148 genes were commonly affected both in $OMD^{-/-}$ and in $PRELP^{-/-}$ (Figure 8a), indicating their partial functional redundancy.

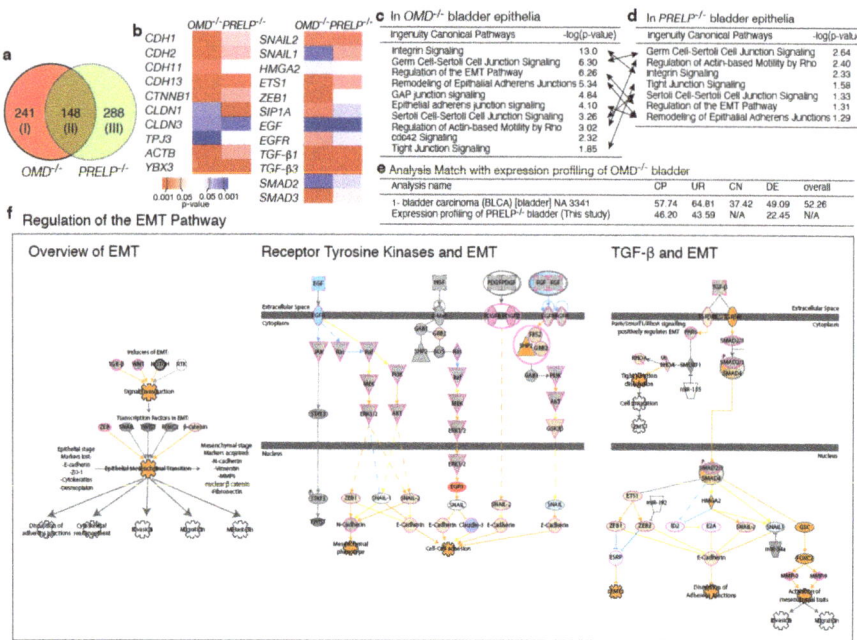

Figure 8. Expression profiling of $OMD^{-/-}$, $PRELP^{-/-}$ mouse bladder epithelia. Expression profiling was performed using $OMD^{-/-}$, $PRELP^{-/-}$ mouse bladder epithelia. Data were analyzed, and the following figures were made through the use of IPA (QIAGEN Inc., https://www.qiagenbioinformatics.com/products/ingenuitypathway-analysis). (**a**) Significantly affected gene numbers, including both up and downregulated. (**b**) Expression of genes related to cell–cell adhesion and EMT. (**c,d**) Significantly affected cell adhesion-related pathways in $OMD^{-/-}$ (**c**) and $PRELP^{-/-}$ (**d**). The same pathways are connected by arrows. (**e**) Similarity of expression profiling data. Using Analysis Match software (Ingenuity Pathway Analysis, IPA, Qiagen), we examined the similarity of expression profiling data of $OMD^{-/-}$ retina with the already deposited publicly available expression profiling dataset and those of $PRELP^{-/-}$ retina. $OMD^{-/-}$ retina data showed high similarity with $PRELP^{-/-}$ retina. The public database search revealed that bladder cancer-related datasets showed high similarity in all categories. CP; canonical pathways, UR; upstream regulators, CN; causal networks, DE; downstream effectors. (**f**) Schematic drawing of "Regulation of the EMT pathway" in $OMD^{-/-}$ vs. WT. Drawing was slightly modified from the original of "Regulation of the EMT Pathway". This image was created by Ingenuity Pathway Analysis according to their rule.

These genes include components of cell–cell adhesion and EMT (Figure 8b). Ontological analysis using the IPA showed that EMT-related events such as "Regulation of the Epithelial–Mesenchymal Transition Pathway" ($OMD^{-/-}$, z = 6.26, $PRELP^{-/-}$, z = 1.31) (Figure 8c–e) were significantly affected in both $OMD^{-/-}$ and $PRELP^{-/-}$ bladder epithelia. Additionally, cell–cell adhesion-related pathways, which is a consequence of EMT, such as "Tight Junction Signaling", and "Germ Cell–Sertoli Cell Junction Signaling", were significantly affected both in $OMD^{-/-}$ and $PRELP^{-/-}$, confirming their involvement in the maintenance of the epithelial junctional barrier.

The ontological analysis also revealed that many cancer-related pathways are more strongly affected (Figure S7a,b), even to a higher extend compared to the gene expression profiling performed in cell lines (Figure 2). Many oncogenes and tumor-suppressor genes are strongly affected (Figure S7c). Figure S6d shows the schematic diagram of "Molecular Mechanisms of Cancer" pathway, affected in $OMD^{-/-}$ ($z = 15.2$), indicating that a majority of cancer-related regulators such as NF-kB, p53, myc, Ras, c-Jun/c-Fos, TGF-β R1/2, and RB are significantly affected. Since the host mouse strain C57BL/6J is not known to hold tumorigenic mutations in the above proteins, these data confirm that in parallel with their ability to regulate EMT and cell–cell integrity, OMD and PRELP have the ability to influence cancer-related activities. Furthermore, in order to know how deeply the OMD suppression in bladder cancer contributes to the properties of bladder cancer, we searched already deposited publicly available expression profiling datasets that showed similarities with that of $OMD^{-/-}$ retina. This analysis revealed that many cancer-related public datasets showed strong similarity with our $OMD^{-/-}$ dataset. In particular, as shown in Figure 8e, both bladder transitional cell carcinoma and bladder carcinoma showed the strong similarity [35,36]. This result demonstrates the significant contribution of OMD suppression in human bladder cancer initiation and/or progression. In addition, we examined the similarity between the $OMD^{-/-}$ and $PRELP^{-/-}$ expression profiling datasets using the Analysis Match software. Figure 8e shows the high similarity between $OMD^{-/-}$ and $PRELP^{-/-}$, supporting the results in Figure 8a–d.

2.9. Breakdown of the Umbrella Cell Layer in $OMD^{-/-}$ and $PRELP^{-/-}$ Mice

We made 10 μm paraffin section series from whole bladder specimens of *WT*, $OMD^{-/-}$, $PRELP^{-/-}$, and double knockout mice and examined the fine structure of the urothelium. In the *WT* mice, bladder umbrella cells form a clear single epithelial layer at the apical side of the urothelium and function as a barrier to the toxic bladder fluid (Figure 9a–c). In contrast, all of the bladder tissue samples from $OMD^{-/-}$, $PRELP^{-/-}$, and the double knockout mice showed points of breakdown/dysplasia of the urothelium (Figure 9d–l). We here termed these histological structures as "epithelial bursts". Furthermore, histological observation and bladder marker staining showed that the spread cells of the epithelial bursts originated from umbrella cells expressing uroplakin-III (Figure 9m,n), while their number was significantly increased in $OMD^{-/-}$ or $PRELP^{-/-}$ mice (Figure 9o). Of note, no obvious abnormalities were seen in the basal and intermediate cell layers (Figure 9p). To investigate whether the epithelial bursts are associated with aberrant cell proliferation, we performed immunohistochemical analysis using the Ki67 proliferation marker. There are few Ki67-positive cells in the *WT* bladder urothelium, and their number is only slightly increased in the $OMD^{-/-}$ and the double knockout samples, suggesting that the epithelial bursts do not result from increased proliferation (Figure 9q).

In humans, carcinoma in situ (CIS) appears histologically as a flat dysplasia of umbrella cells and is recognized as an early sign of malignant bladder cancer. However, an epithelial burst-type dysplasia, as seen in the $OMD^{-/-}$ and $PRELP^{-/-}$ mouse bladders, has not been recognized. The luminal mouse bladder is consistently covered by convex mucosal folds, while the human bladder surface is relatively flat or slightly concave. During our histological analysis, we observed a simple flat dysplasia of umbrella cells in the concave areas of mouse bladder as in human CIS (Figure 9r–t), suggesting that the structural difference of dysplasia might result from the different urothelium structure: convex vs. concave. To address this, we developed a mathematical simulation to visualize the direction of epithelial layer breakdown through the calculation of the forces created on convex and concave structures (Figure 9u). The model demonstrated that in a convex structure, the basal side of the epithelial layer was sealed, and the epithelial cells tended to escape to the apical side, similar to an epithelial burst. On the other hand, in a concave structure, the apical side was sealed, and the dysplasia cells tended to move under the epithelial layer. Supporting our analysis, Messal et al. has recently reported that a mechanical tension model for tissue curvature can instruct the direction of cancer morphogenesis [37]. These model-based analyses suggest that OMD and/or PRELP deletion can result in a defect in maintenance of the umbrella cell layer, as observed in human bladder CIS.

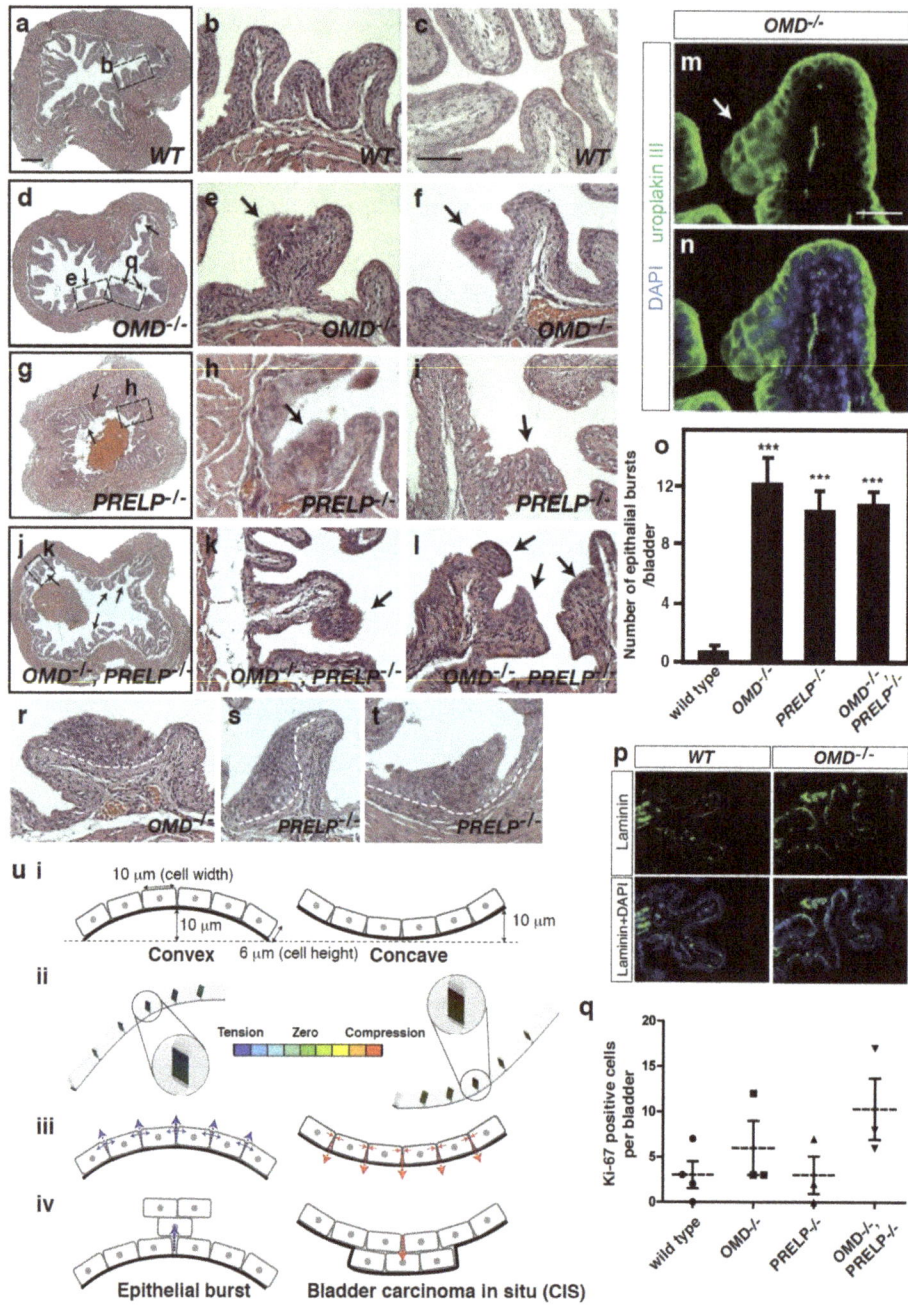

Figure 9. $OMD^{-/-}$, $PRELP^{-/-}$, and their double knockout mice spontaneously initiate bladder papillary cancer. (**a–l**) 3-month-old bladder of WT (**a–c**), $OMD^{-/-}$ (**d–f**), $PRELP^{-/-}$ (**g–i**), and their double knockout (**j–l**). A low magnification and two high magnification images are shown in order. Epithelial bursts are indicated as arrows. Some enlarged areas are indicated as boxes in low-magnification images. Scale bar represents 500 μm (**a,d,g,j**) and 100 μm (**b,c,e,f,h,i,k,l**). (**m–o**) Uroplakin III antibody staining

of an epithelial burst of $OMD^{-/-}$. Uroplakin staining (m), overlaid view of uroplakin III and DAPI (n). Scale bar represents 50 µm (m,n). Quantification of epithelial burst number per bladder; WT ($n = 7$), $OMD^{-/-}$ ($n = 7$), $PRELP^{-/-}$ ($n = 6$), $OMD^{-/-}$, $PRELP^{-/-}$ ($n = 3$) (o). In quantification, we examined six to seven 10 µm slices from each bladder. Each slice was separated around 200 µm in the bladder, and these slices covered the whole bladder except their edges. (p) Laminin antibody staining of WT and $OMD^{-/-}$ bladders. (q) Ki-67 staining positive cells in bladder. (r–t) Carcinoma in situ (CIS)-like structures in $OMD^{-/-}$ (r) and $PRELP^{-/-}$ (s,t). (u) Computational models for the mouse and human epithelial dysplasia. Conditions of models (u-i). Calculated forces between cells (u-ii). Direction of dysplasia (u-iii). Epithelial burst-like dysplasia and carcinoma in situ-like dysplasia (u-iv). *** indicates $p < 0.001$.

2.10. Some $PRELP^{-/-}$ Mice Spontaneously Initiate Bladder Papillary Cancer

On analysis of bladders from $OMD^{-/-}$, $PRELP^{-/-}$, and the double knockout mice, we found that $OMD^{-/-}$, $PRELP^{-/-}$, and double KO bladders showed a slightly increased number of mucosal folds with multiple branches (Figure 10a,b). Interestingly, in one-third of the $PRELP^{-/-}$ and double knockout mice but not in $OMD^{-/-}$ mice, the bladder developed abnormal urothelia with hyperplasia, resulting in a pattern of papillary growth on a normal muscularis (Figure 10c,e in WT, d, f–o in PRELP). This phenotype seen in some $PRELP^{-/-}$ bladders is similar to some types of human bladder papillary cancer (https://www.proteinatlas.org/learn/dictionary/pathology/urothelial+cancer).

We observed various stages of papillary cancer progression such as mucosal folds with multiple branches (Figure 10g), partially fused mucosal folds (Figure 10h), and completely fused mucosal folds (Figure 10i,j). The process of clot formation was also observed, including small aggregates of proteinaceous material secreted from umbrella cells (Figure 10i), larger aggregates in which clumps of cells were embedded (Figure 10k,l), and large acellular clots covered with a single layer of cells (Figure 10m). We observed early signs of cancer invasions into the underlying muscularis (Figure 10n,o).

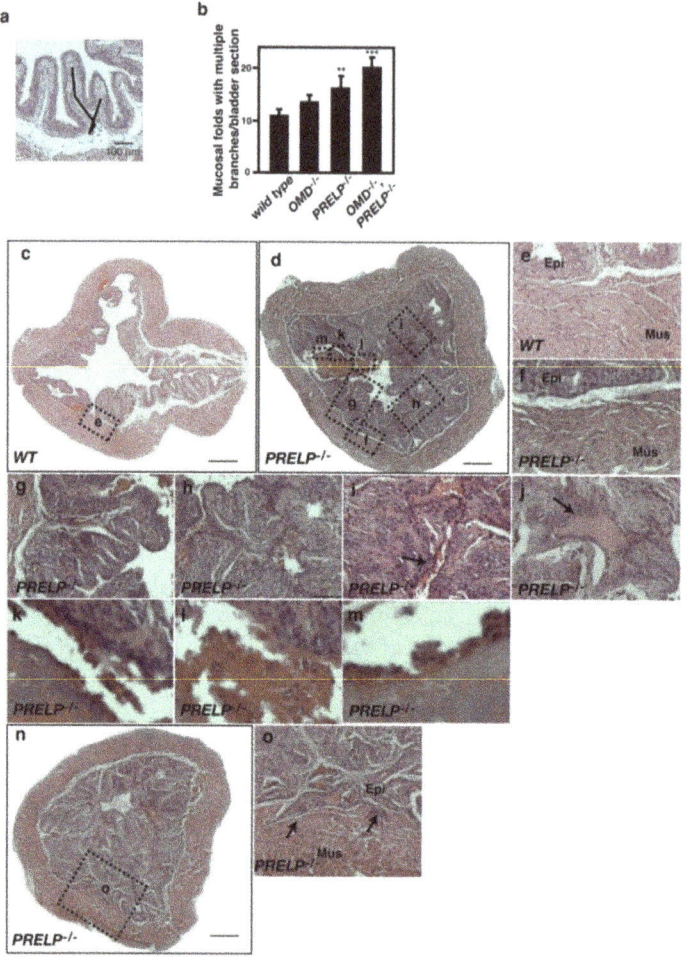

Figure 10. *PRELP* knockout mice spontaneously initiate early stages of bladder cancer. (**a**) H&E-stained section showing a branched mucosal fold. (**b**) Number of mucosal folds with multiple branches. In each bladder, we have examined two sections in the medial region of bladder. (**c**) H&E-stained section of a WT mouse bladder at 3 months of age. (**d**) Bladder papillary cancer in $PRELP^{-/-}$ at 3 months. Scale bar represents 500 µm (**c,d**). The bladder lumen is almost completely filled by mucosal folds with multiple branches and fused mucosal folds. Clots formation is observed. Enlarged regions in the following panels are indicated by the dotted boxes. (**e**) WT bladder muscularis (Mus) and epithelial tissue (Epi). (**f**) $PRELP^{-/-}$ bladder muscularis. (**g**) Mucosal fold with multiple branches. (**h**) Partially fused mucosal folds with multiple branches. (**i**) Fused mucosal folds. The arrow points secretion of materials to lumen. (**j**) Fused mucosal folds. Deposited material is enriched in fused folds (arrow). (**k**) Separation of epithelial cells with sticky material. (**l**) Aggregation of separated cells with clot materials. (**m**) The clot is covered by a layer of cells. (**n**) T1 stage bladder cancer in $PRELP^{-/-}$ at 3 months. (**o**) Epithelial papillary cancer integration into muscularis (arrows). ** and *** indicate $p < 0.005$, and $p < 0.001$, respectively.

3. Discussion

3.1. ECM Proteins and Cancer Initiation

OMD and PRELP are secreted ECM proteins, belonging to the Class II SLRP subfamily [38–40]. SLRP family members were originally identified as abundant proteins within the ECM of cartilage, connecting tissues and differentiating osteoblasts [41–43]. ECM proteins of the tumor microenvironment play important roles in many aspects of cancer initiation and progression [44]. One member of the SLRP family, decorin expression, decreases on the malignant transformation of tumor cells. Thirty percent (30%) of decorin knockout mice developed spontaneous intestinal tumors [13]. On the other hand, in an inflammation murine model, decorin is upregulated in endothelial cells and facilitates the downregulation of tight junctions [45]. This suggests that inflammation may affect OMD and PRELP function.

Here, we have demonstrated that OMD and PRELP function to maintain epithelial cell–cell integrity in urothelial cells through the inhibition of partial EMT. At epithelial cancer initiation, EMT is required, while MET is observed at cancer metastasis. Recent comprehensive expression profiling analyses in bladder and other epithelial cancers have revealed a novel concept of partial EMT [46–49]. The typical partial EMT state is the loss of tight junctions without affecting adherens junctions [48]. This is particularly important for understanding cancer initiation. In bladder cancer, a loss of E-cadherin expression is used as a marker of advanced bladder cancer, suggesting that the partial EMT state might be associated with early-stage bladder cancer. The tight junctions between umbrella cells in $OMD^{-/-}$ and $PRELP^{-/-}$ mice disappeared, while adherens junctions were maintained, indicating a typical partial EMT state. The loss of tight junctions resulted in disruption of the apical–basal polarity of umbrella cells, which is demonstrated by uniform E-cadherin staining around umbrella cells. Moreover, the partial EMT state we observed is susceptible for breakdown of the umbrella-cell layer, which might be related to cancer initiation. Collectively, our findings might be the first demonstration of partial EMT state and associated bladder cancer initiation in mice.

3.2. OMD and PRELP and NMIBC Initiation

$OMD^{-/-}$ or $PRELP^{-/-}$ mice showed many breakdown sites in the umbrella-cell layer, and one-third of $PRELP^{-/-}$ developed large-scale papillary cancer without muscle invasion. A large region of chromosome 9q, including the *OMD* gene, is deleted in half of NMIBC cases [50]. The deletion is associated with the initiation of NMIBC [51]. *PTCH* and *TSC1* were proposed to be the critical tumor-suppressor genes in 9q deletions [52,53], but this hypothesis is controversial [54]. Rather, with the present study, we propose *OMD* as a novel 9q-residing tumor-suppressor gene involved in cancer bladder initiation.

NMIBC is clinically classified as Ta, T1, or CIS. CIS is proposed to originate from umbrella cells because the cells in CIS are positive to umbrella cell markers such as CK20 [55]. Recent comprehensive expression profiling analysis classified NMIBC into three classes. Among these, Class 2 has the expression of CIS type markers, and Class 2 is defined based on the expression of EMT marker genes [20]. $OMD^{-/-}$ or $PRELP^{-/-}$ showed two types of breakdown of the umbrella layer: epithelial bursts and CIS-like structures. Our mathematical model indicates that the difference between the two breakdowns reflects the structural differences of the epithelia. We propose that umbrella-layer breakdown mediated by the loss of OMD and PRELP may initiate CIS. Some bladder cancers are thought to originate from the umbrella cells [51], because selective overexpression of a mutant H-Ras in umbrella cells resulted in low-grade papillary tumors [56–58].

Additionally, $PRELP^{-/-}$ mice tended to form protein clots, including fibrin, in the bladder. The fibrin/fibrinogen degradation products in human urine samples have been used as a bladder cancer marker [59]. The leakage of fibrin is regulated by the blood–urine barrier in bladder epithelial cells. This suggests that damage to the blood urine barrier is associated with bladder cancer initiation and that PRELP may have the ability to regulate the blood–urine barrier. Interestingly, we have found that in $OMD^{-/-}$ and $PRELP^{-/-}$ mice, umbrella cells are connected to each other by adherens junctions. It is known that the loss of E-cadherin is a marker of conversion from benign to malignant bladder cancer. Thus, double knockout of *OMD/PRELP* and E-cadherin may reveal the process of malignant cancer initiation.

3.3. EMT/MET Regulated by OMD and PRELP

During malignant transformation, cancer cells have acquired mesenchymal-like characteristics such as anoikis resistance and invade adjacent tissues. Our results showed that OMD or PRELP overexpression in bladder cancer cells resulted in an increase of epithelial-like properties such as tight junction induction and adherens junction activation as well as a change of EMT markers. A cardinal feature of cancer is the ability for anchorage-independent growth, which changes the properties of cell–cell and cell–matrix adhesion conferred at EMT.

Umbrella cells secrete signaling proteins such as EGF and TGF-β [60]. The concept that OMD or PRELP mediated the inhibitory activity of TGF-β and EGF pathways could be important for the regulation of EMT/MET, because the TGF-β/Smad2 pathway is the biggest common target of all SLRP family members [2] and is a well-known regulator of EMT/MET [46]. In addition, EGF is known as a major regulator of EMT/MET [46] and is one of the most established targets of cancer treatment [61]. Previously, we reported that the simultaneous regulation of Xnr2, FGF, and BMP pathways by Tsukushi, another SLRP member, had an increased synergistic effect compared to the single regulation of each pathway alone [6].

OMD and PRELP are selectively expressed in the ciliary body of the retina and in ependymal cells in the brain (paper in preparation) that are characterized by strong tight junctions forming the blood–CSF barrier. The expression of many components of tight junctions is associated with tumorigenesis [62]. However, so far, there is no report showing that the knockout of any tight junction component by itself can spontaneously lead to tumor formation, although, hyperplasia of the gastric epithelium has been observed in an occludin knockout model [63]. This suggests that the loss of tight junctions alone is not sufficient to initiate bladder cancer. TGF-β and EGF pathways are involved in the regulation of many cancer-associated signaling pathways, suggesting that in addition to the loss of tight junctions in an $OMD^{-/-}$ or $PRELP^{-/-}$ bladder, further regulation of TGF-β and EGF downstream signaling components might be required for cancer initiation. Of note, one limitation of our study is that although the TGF-β-flag protein bound with OMDmyc and PRELPmyc proteins directly, the binding affinities of secreted TGF-β to the OMD and PRELP is unknown; therefore, further studies are required.

3.4. The Similarity and Difference between OMD and PRELP

Both OMD and PRELP were downregulated, especially in bladder cancer. Our results indicated that although OMD and PRELP share considerable amount of signal pathways, there are some differences in the observed phenotypes: branching, proliferation, bladder cancer progression, and protein expression. Functional difference between OMD and PRELP may be associated with certain cancer phenotypes. This indicates that they would play a redundant and non-redundant function in bladder cancer.

3.5. Diagnostic and Therapeutic Potential of OMD and PRELP in Bladder Cancer

OMD and *PRELP* are expressed in normal human epithelia. However, in many epithelial cancers, they are strongly downregulated. Particularly, their expression in the bladder is drastically reduced even in very early stages of cancer. This potentially means that it is possible to classify a patient's clinical state based solely on their OMD and PRELP expression status from early-stage cancers. So far, several diagnostic markers of bladder cancer have been used in clinics such as BTA-Stat (sensitivity 50–70%, specificity 67–78%) and fibrin degradation products (FDP) (sensitivity 52–68.4%, specificity 79.6–91%) [64]. With our findings, we show that the assessment of *OMD* and *PRELP* expression status can be used as a novel, more sensitive, criterion in assessing the initiation and progression of bladder cancer. We also observed a similar evaluation in renal cell carcinoma and retinoblastoma (paper in preparation), proposing their diagnostic potential in various epithelial cancers, possibly through using new technology such as quench bodies to detect loss-of-function regions [65]. This study demonstrates that the functions of OMD and PRELP are partially redundant in the regulation of both cell–cell integrity and cancer initiation/progression, and they are potentially important, especially for bladder cell therapeutics.

4. Materials and Methods

Materials and Methods are described in the Supplementary Materials and Methods. The accession number for the raw and processed data of microarray and RNA-seq data from *OMD* and *PRELP* knockdown experiments reported in this paper is GEO: GSE63955 and GSE144295. Other data supporting our findings can be found either in this article or in the supplementary materials. Please contact the corresponding author for all "unpublished data" and "paper in preparation" requests.

The research protocol was reviewed and approved by the Ethical Committee of Addenbrooke's Hospital, Cambridgeshire Local Research Ethics Committee (No. 03/018).

5. Conclusions

In this study, we demonstrated that two SLRP proteins, OMD and PRELP, are novel activators of the cell–cell integrity by inhibiting EMT through the simultaneous inhibition of TGF-β and EGF signaling. The downregulation of OMD and PRELP expression was observed in all of the cancers we analyzed, including bladder cancer. We showed that in association with a change of EMT states, OMD or PRELP suppression in mice resulted in an initiation of bladder cancer, while the activation of OMD or PRELP inhibited bladder cancer progression in vitro and in vivo. We propose that OMD and PRELP-mediated regulation of EMT is important for the initiation of human bladder cancer.

Supplementary Materials: The following are available online at http://www.mdpi.com/2072-6694/12/11/3362/s1, Figure S1: Microarray analysis of *OMD* and *PRELP* expression in various cancers and normal tissues; Figure S2: Expression analysis of OMD and PRELP in various human cancers using Gene Logic Inc. Figure S3: *OMD* and *PRELP* expression analysis in various cancer cells and ontological analysis of expression profiling data; Figure S4: Effect of OMD or PRELP on cell properties under standard cell culture conditions; Figure S5: Quantification of OMD and PRELP effects; Figure S6: PRELP is expressed in subpopulation of bladder umbrella epithelial cells; Figure S7: The ontological analysis in $OMD^{-/-}$ and $PRELP^{-/-}$ bladder epithelia; Figure S8: Original Western Blotting images used in Figure 5.; Table S1: Statistical analysis of *OMD* and *PRELP* expression levels in clinical bladder tissues; Table S2: Relationship between *OMD* and *PRELP* expression levels and carcinogenesis; Table S3: Primer sequences for quantitative RT-PCR.

Author Contributions: V.P., R.H., K.A., T.T., J.K.W., A.L., J.H., M.D., N.S., H.D., S.N.-Z., R.L., M.N., R.T., A.V. and S.-i.O. participated in project conception, performed the experiments, and analyzed the data. V.P., R.H., K.A., T.T., J.K.W., and S.-i.O. wrote the original draft. V.P., R.H., K.A., T.T., J.K.W., A.L., J.H., M.D., N.S., H.D., S.N.-Z., R.L., M.N., R.T., A.V., S.K., M.S.S., G.M., A.M., K.T., J.D.K., and S.-i.O. discussed the data, reviewed and edited the manuscript. R.H., G.M., K.T., J.D.K., and S.-i.O. supervised the experiments. All authors have read and agreed to the published version of the manuscript.

Funding: This work is partially supported by Santen SensyT PhD studentships to A.L., Cancer Research UK (C1528/A2690), The Great Britain Sasakawa Foundation (B85), St Peter's Trust for Kidney Bladder & Prostate Research (NA), Fight for Sight (F94), and Childhood Eye Cancer Trust (24CEC12) to S.O.

Acknowledgments: We thank Bruce Ponder and David E. Neal for their initial contributions to this project and all members of the Ohnuma lab, particularly Stephen Bolsover, Ryohei Sekido, and Kevin Broad for critical reading of the manuscript. We also thank Tatsuhiko Tsunoda for assistance in cancer genome data analysis, to Karl Matter, Maria Balda, Vassiliki Saloura for helpful discussion and reagents, and to Stewart McArthur for the network analysis. We thank Alex Freeman for uropathological analysis.

Conflicts of Interest: The authors declare no conflict of interest.

References

1. Schaefer, L.; Iozzo, R.V. Biological Functions of the Small Leucine-rich Proteoglycans: From Genetics to Signal Transduction. *J. Biol. Chem.* **2008**, *283*, 21305–21309. [CrossRef] [PubMed]
2. Dellett, M.; Hu, W.; Papadaki, V.; Ohnuma, S.-I. Small leucine rich proteoglycan family regulates multiple signalling pathways in neural development and maintenance. *Dev. Growth Differ.* **2012**, *54*, 327–340. [CrossRef] [PubMed]
3. Vogel, K.G.; Paulsson, M.; Heinegård, D.; Uldbjerg, N.; Danielsen, C.C.; De O Sampaio, L.; Bayliss, M.T.; Hardingham, T.E.; Muir, H.; Kuwaba, K.; et al. Specific inhibition of type I and type II collagen fibrillogenesis by the small proteoglycan of tendon. *Biochem. J.* **1984**, *223*, 587–597. [CrossRef] [PubMed]
4. Hocking, A.M.; Shinomura, T.; McQuillan, D.J. Leucine-rich repeat glycoproteins of the extracellular matrix. *Matrix Biol.* **1998**, *17*, 1–19. [CrossRef]
5. Kuriyama, S.; Lupo, G.; Ohta, K.; Ohnuma, S.-I.; Harris-Warrick, R.; Tanaka, H. Tsukushi controls ectodermal patterning and neural crest specification in Xenopus by direct regulation of BMP4 and X-delta-1 activity. *Development* **2006**, *133*, 75–88. [CrossRef]
6. Morris, S.A.; Almeida, A.D.; Tanaka, H.; Ohta, K.; Ohnuma, S.-I. Tsukushi Modulates Xnr2, FGF and BMP Signaling: Regulation of Xenopus Germ Layer Formation. *PLoS ONE* **2007**, *2*, e1004. [CrossRef]
7. Ohta, K.; Kuriyama, S.; Okafuji, T.; Gejima, R.; Ohnuma, S.-I.; Tanaka, H. Tsukushi cooperates with VG1 to induce primitive streak and Hensen's node formation in the chick embryo. *Development* **2006**, *133*, 3777–3786. [CrossRef]
8. Ohta, K.; Lupo, G.; Kuriyama, S.; Keynes, R.; Holt, C.E.; Harris, W.A.; Tanaka, H.; Ohnuma, S.-I. Tsukushi Functions as an Organizer Inducer by Inhibition of BMP Activity in Cooperation with Chordin. *Dev. Cell* **2004**, *7*, 347–358. [CrossRef]
9. Appunni, S.; Anand, V.; Khandelwal, M.; Gupta, N.; Rubens, M.; Sharma, A. Small Leucine Rich Proteoglycans (decorin, biglycan and lumican) in cancer. *Clin. Chim. Acta* **2019**, *491*, 1–7. [CrossRef]
10. Matsuda, Y.; Yamamoto, T.; Kudo, M.; Kawahara, K.; Kawamoto, M.; Nakajima, Y.; Koizumi, K.; Nakazawa, N.; Ishiwata, T.; Naito, Z. Expression and roles of lumican in lung adenocarcinoma and squamous cell carcinoma. *Int. J. Oncol.* **2008**, *33*, 1177–1185.
11. Vuillermoz, B.; Khoruzhenko, A.; D'Onofrio, M.-F.; Ramont, L.; Venteo, L.; Perreau, C.; Antonicelli, F.; Maquart, F.-X.; Wegrowski, Y. The small leucine-rich proteoglycan lumican inhibits melanoma progression. *Exp. Cell Res.* **2004**, *296*, 294–306. [CrossRef] [PubMed]
12. Troup, S.; Njue, C.; Kliewer, E.V.; Parisien, M.; Roskelley, C.; Chakravarti, S.; Roughley, P.J.; Murphy, L.C.; Watson, P.H. Reduced expression of the small leucine-rich proteoglycans, lumican, and decorin is associated with poor outcome in node-negative invasive breast cancer. *Clin. Cancer Res.* **2003**, *9*, 207–214. [PubMed]
13. Bi, X.; Tong, C.; Dockendorff, A.; Bancroft, L.; Gallagher, L.; Guzman, G.; Iozzo, R.V.; Augenlicht, L.H.; Yang, W. Genetic deficiency of decorin causes intestinal tumor formation through disruption of intestinal cell maturation. *Carcinogenesis* **2008**, *29*, 1435–1440. [CrossRef] [PubMed]
14. Iozzo, R.V.; Chakrani, F.; Perrotti, D.; McQuillan, D.J.; Skorski, T.; Calabretta, B.; Eichstetter, I. Cooperative action of germ-line mutations in decorin and p53 accelerates lymphoma tumorigenesis. *Proc. Natl. Acad. Sci. USA* **1999**, *96*, 3092–3097. [CrossRef]
15. Araki, K.; Wakabayashi, H.; Shintani, K.; Morikawa, J.; Matsumine, A.; Kusuzaki, K.; Sudo, A.; Uchida, A. Decorin Suppresses Bone Metastasis in a Breast Cancer Cell Line. *Oncology* **2009**, *77*, 92–99. [CrossRef]
16. Satonaka, H.; Wakabayashi, H.; Iino, T.; Uchida, A.; Araki, K.; Wakabayashi, T.; Matsubara, T.; Matsumine, A.; Kusuzaki, K.; Morikawa, J.; et al. Decorin suppresses lung metastases of murine osteosarcoma. *Oncol. Rep.* **2008**, *19*, 1533–1539. [CrossRef]
17. Nelson, C.M.; Bissell, M.J. Of Extracellular Matrix, Scaffolds, and Signaling: Tissue Architecture Regulates Development, Homeostasis, and Cancer. *Annu. Rev. Cell Dev. Biol.* **2006**, *22*, 287–309. [CrossRef]
18. Sternlicht, M.D.; Lochter, A.; Sympson, C.J.; Huey, B.; Rougier, J.-P.; Gray, J.W.; Pinkel, D.; Bissell, M.J.; Werb, Z. The Stromal Proteinase MMP3/Stromelysin-1 Promotes Mammary Carcinogenesis. *Cell* **1999**, *98*, 137–146. [CrossRef]
19. Bray, F.; Me, J.F.; Soerjomataram, I.; Siegel, R.L.; Torre, L.A.; Jemal, A. Global cancer statistics 2018: GLOBOCAN estimates of incidence and mortality worldwide for 36 cancers in 185 countries. *CA A Cancer J. Clin.* **2018**, *68*, 394–424. [CrossRef]

20. Hedegaard, J.; Lamy, P.; Nordentoft, I.; Algaba, F.; Høyer, S.; Ulhøi, B.P.; Vang, S.; Reinert, T.; Hermann, G.G.; Mogensen, K.; et al. Comprehensive Transcriptional Analysis of Early-Stage Urothelial Carcinoma. *Cancer Cell* **2016**, *30*, 27–42. [CrossRef]
21. Robertson, A.G.; Kim, J.; Al-Ahmadie, H.; Bellmunt, J.; Guo, G.; Cherniack, A.D.; Hinoue, T.; Laird, P.W.; Hoadley, K.A.; Akbani, R.; et al. Comprehensive Molecular Characterization of Muscle-Invasive Bladder Cancer. *Cell* **2017**, *171*, 540–556.e25. [CrossRef] [PubMed]
22. Tsukita, S.; Yamazaki, Y.; Katsuno, T.; Tamura, A. Tight junction-based epithelial microenvironment and cell proliferation. *Oncogene* **2008**, *27*, 6930–6938. [CrossRef] [PubMed]
23. Tracey, A.M. Tight junctions in cancer metastasis. *Front. Biosci.* **2011**, *16*, 898. [CrossRef]
24. Nobes, C.D.; Hall, A. Rho, rac and cdc42 GTPases: Regulators of actin structures, cell adhesion and motility. *Biochem. Soc. Trans.* **1995**, *23*, 456–459. [CrossRef]
25. Ye, X.; Weinberg, R.A. Epithelial–Mesenchymal Plasticity: A Central Regulator of Cancer Progression. *Trends Cell Biol.* **2015**, *25*, 675–686. [CrossRef]
26. De Craene, B.; Berx, G. Regulatory networks defining EMT during cancer initiation and progression. *Nat. Rev. Cancer* **2013**, *13*, 97–110. [CrossRef]
27. Pollak, M. The insulin and insulin-like growth factor receptor family in neoplasia: An update. *Nat. Rev. Cancer* **2012**, *12*, 159–169. [CrossRef]
28. Takeuchi, K.; Ito, F. EGF receptor in relation to tumor development: Molecular basis of responsiveness of cancer cells to EGFR-targeting tyrosine kinase inhibitors. *FEBS J.* **2009**, *277*, 316–326. [CrossRef]
29. Lee, C.-H.; Hung, H.-W.; Hung, P.-H.; Shieh, Y.-S. Epidermal growth factor receptor regulates β-catenin location, stability, and transcriptional activity in oral cancer. *Mol. Cancer* **2010**, *9*, 64. [CrossRef]
30. Nobes, C.D.; Hall, A. Rho, Rac, and Cdc42 GTPases regulate the assembly of multimolecular focal complexes associated with actin stress fibers, lamellipodia, and filopodia. *Cell* **1995**, *81*, 53–62. [CrossRef]
31. Shiizaki, S.; Naguro, I.; Ichijo, H. Activation mechanisms of ASK1 in response to various stresses and its significance in intracellular signaling. *Adv. Biol. Regul.* **2013**, *53*, 135–144. [CrossRef] [PubMed]
32. Cerione, R. Cdc42: New roads to travel. *Trends Cell Biol.* **2004**, *14*, 127–132. [CrossRef] [PubMed]
33. Khandelwal, P.; Abraham, S.N.; Apodaca, G. Cell biology and physiology of the uroepithelium. *Am. J. Physiol. Physiol.* **2009**, *297*, F1477–F1501. [CrossRef] [PubMed]
34. Kreft, M.E.; Hudoklin, S.; Jezernik, K.; Romih, R. Formation and maintenance of blood–urine barrier in urothelium. *Protoplasma* **2010**, *246*, 3–14. [CrossRef]
35. Riester, M.; Taylor, J.M.; Feifer, A.; Koppie, T.; Rosenberg, J.E.; Downey, R.J.; Bochner, B.H.; Michor, F. Combination of a Novel Gene Expression Signature with a Clinical Nomogram Improves the Prediction of Survival in High-Risk Bladder Cancer. *Clin. Cancer Res.* **2012**, *18*, 1323–1333. [CrossRef]
36. Sjödahl, G.; Lauss, M.; Lövgren, K.; Chebil, G.; Gudjonsson, S.; Veerla, S.; Patschan, O.H.; Aine, M.; Fernö, M.; Ringnér, M.; et al. A Molecular Taxonomy for Urothelial Carcinoma. *Clin. Cancer Res.* **2012**, *18*, 3377–3386. [CrossRef]
37. Messal, H.A.; Alt, S.; Ferreira, R.M.M.; Gribben, C.; Wang, V.M.-Y.; Cotoi, C.G.; Salbreux, G.; Behrens, A. Tissue curvature and apicobasal mechanical tension imbalance instruct cancer morphogenesis. *Nat. Cell Biol.* **2019**, *566*, 126–130. [CrossRef]
38. Wendel, M.; Sommarin, Y.; Heinegård, D. Bone Matrix Proteins: Isolation and Characterization of a Novel Cell-binding Keratan Sulfate Proteoglycan (Osteoadherin) from Bovine Bone. *J. Cell Biol.* **1998**, *141*, 839–847. [CrossRef]
39. Sommarin, Y.; Wendel, M.; Shen, Z.; Hellman, U.; Heinegård, D. Osteoadherin, a Cell-binding Keratan Sulfate Proteoglycan in Bone, Belongs to the Family of Leucine-rich Repeat Proteins of the Extracellular Matrix. *J. Biol. Chem.* **1998**, *273*, 16723–16729. [CrossRef]
40. Bengtsson, E.; Aspberg, A.; Heinegård, D.; Sommarin, Y.; Spillmann, D. The Amino-terminal Part of PRELP Binds to Heparin and Heparan Sulfate. *J. Biol. Chem.* **2000**, *275*, 40695–40702. [CrossRef]
41. Heinegård, D.; Larsson, T.; Sommarin, Y.; Franzén, A.; Paulsson, M.; Hedbom, E. Two novel matrix proteins isolated from articular cartilage show wide distributions among connective tissues. *J. Biol. Chem.* **1986**, *261*, 13866–13872. [PubMed]
42. Rehn, A.P.; Chalk, A.M.; Wendel, M. Differential regulation of osteoadherin (OSAD) by TGF-β1 and BMP-2. *Biochem. Biophys. Res. Commun.* **2006**, *349*, 1057–1064. [CrossRef] [PubMed]

43. Stanford, C.M.; Jacobson, P.A.; Eanes, E.D.; Lembke, L.A.; Midura, R.J. Rapidly Forming Apatitic Mineral in an Osteoblastic Cell Line (UMR 10601 BSP). *J. Biol. Chem.* **1995**, *270*, 9420–9428. [CrossRef] [PubMed]
44. Wong, G.S.; Rustgi, A.K. Matricellular proteins: Priming the tumour microenvironment for cancer development and metastasis. *Br. J. Cancer* **2013**, *108*, 755–761. [CrossRef] [PubMed]
45. Hoettels, B.A.; Wertz, T.S.; Birk, D.E.; Oxford, J.T.; Beard, R.S., Jr. The Extracellular Matrix Proteoglycan Decorin is Upregulated by Endothelial Cells During Inflammation and Contributes to Blood-Brain Barrier Dysfunction. *FASEB J.* **2017**, *31*, 682.4. [CrossRef]
46. Lamouille, S.; Xu, J.; Derynck, R. Molecular mechanisms of epithelial–mesenchymal transition. *Nat. Rev. Mol. Cell Biol.* **2014**, *15*, 178–196. [CrossRef]
47. Aiello, N.M.; Maddipati, R.; Norgard, R.J.; Balli, D.; Li, J.; Yuan, S.; Yamazoe, T.; Black, T.; Sahmoud, A.; Furth, E.E.; et al. EMT Subtype Influences Epithelial Plasticity and Mode of Cell Migration. *Dev. Cell* **2018**, *45*, 681–695.e4. [CrossRef]
48. Nieto, M.A.; Huang, R.Y.-J.; Jackson, R.A.; Thiery, J.P. EMT: 2016. *Cell* **2016**, *166*, 21–45. [CrossRef]
49. Puram, S.V.; Tirosh, I.; Parikh, A.S.; Patel, A.P.; Yizhak, K.; Gillespie, S.; Rodman, C.; Luo, C.L.; Mroz, E.A.; Emerick, K.S.; et al. Single-Cell Transcriptomic Analysis of Primary and Metastatic Tumor Ecosystems in Head and Neck Cancer. *Cell* **2017**, *171*, 1611–1624.e24. [CrossRef]
50. Hurst, C.D.; Alder, O.; Platt, F.M.; Droop, A.; Stead, L.F.; Burns, J.E.; Burghel, G.J.; Jain, S.; Klimczak, L.J.; Lindsay, H.; et al. Genomic Subtypes of Non-invasive Bladder Cancer with Distinct Metabolic Profile and Female Gender Bias in KDM6A Mutation Frequency. *Cancer Cell* **2017**, *32*, 701–715.e7. [CrossRef]
51. Castillo-Martin, M.; Domingo-Domenech, J.; Karni-Schmidt, O.; Matos, T.; Cordon-Cardo, C. Molecular pathways of urothelial development and bladder tumorigenesis. *Urol. Oncol. Semin. Orig. Investig.* **2010**, *28*, 401–408. [CrossRef] [PubMed]
52. Hamed, S.; LaRue, H.; Hovington, H.; Girard, J.; Jeannotte, L.; Latulippe, E.; Fradet, Y. Accelerated induction of bladder cancer in patched heterozygous mutant mice. *Cancer Res.* **2004**, *64*, 1938–1942. [CrossRef] [PubMed]
53. Knowles, M.A.; Habuchi, T.; Kennedy, W.; Heavens, D. Mutation spectrum of the 9q34 tuberous sclerosis gene TSC1 in transitional cell carcinoma of the bladder. *Cancer Res.* **2003**, *63*, 7652–7656. [PubMed]
54. Thievessen, I.; Wolter, M.; Prior, A.; Seifert, H.-H.; Schulz, W.A. Hedgehog signaling in normal urothelial cells and in urothelial carcinoma cell lines. *J. Cell. Physiol.* **2005**, *203*, 372–377. [CrossRef] [PubMed]
55. Harnden, P.; Eardley, I.; Joyce, A.; Southgate, J. Cytokeratin 20 as an objective marker of urothelial dysplasia. *BJU Int.* **1996**, *78*, 870–875. [CrossRef] [PubMed]
56. Mo, L.; Zheng, X.; Huang, H.-Y.; Shapiro, E.; Lepor, H.; Cordon-Cardo, C.; Sun, T.-T.; Wu, X.-R. Hyperactivation of Ha-ras oncogene, but not Ink4a/Arf deficiency, triggers bladder tumorigenesis. *J. Clin. Investig.* **2007**, *117*, 314–325. [CrossRef]
57. Cheng, J.; Huang, H.; Zhang, Z.-T.; Shapiro, E.; Pellicer, A.; Sun, T.-T.; Wu, X.-R. Overexpression of epidermal growth factor receptor in urothelium elicits urothelial hyperplasia and promotes bladder tumor growth. *Cancer Res.* **2002**, *62*, 4157–4163. [PubMed]
58. Zhang, Z.T.; Pak, J.; Shapiro, E.; Sun, T.T.; Wu, X.R. Urothelium-specific expression of an oncogene in transgenic mice induced the formation of carcinoma in situ and invasive transitional cell carcinoma. *Cancer Res.* **1999**, *59*, 3512–3517. [PubMed]
59. Jeong, S.; Park, Y.; Cho, Y.; Kim, Y.R.; Kim, H.-S. Diagnostic values of urine CYFRA21-1, NMP22, UBC, and FDP for the detection of bladder cancer. *Clin. Chim. Acta* **2012**, *414*, 93–100. [CrossRef]
60. Balestreire, E.M.; Apodaca, G. Apical Epidermal Growth Factor Receptor Signaling: Regulation of Stretch-dependent Exocytosis in Bladder Umbrella Cells. *Mol. Biol. Cell* **2007**, *18*, 1312–1323. [CrossRef]
61. Seshacharyulu, P.; Ponnusamy, M.P.; Haridas, D.; Jain, M.; Ganti, A.K.; Batra, S.K. Targeting the EGFR signaling pathway in cancer therapy. *Expert Opin. Ther. Targets* **2012**, *16*, 15–31. [CrossRef] [PubMed]
62. Runkle, E.A.; Mu, D. Tight junction proteins: From barrier to tumorigenesis. *Cancer Lett.* **2013**, *337*, 41–48. [CrossRef] [PubMed]
63. Saitou, M.; Furuse, M.; Sasaki, H.; Schulzke, J.-D.; Fromm, M.; Takano, H.; Noda, T.; Tsukita, S. Complex Phenotype of Mice Lacking Occludin, a Component of Tight Junction Strands. *Mol. Biol. Cell* **2000**, *11*, 4131–4142. [CrossRef] [PubMed]
64. Parker, J.; Spiess, P.E. Current and Emerging Bladder Cancer Urinary Biomarkers. *Sci. World J.* **2011**, *11*, 1103–1112. [CrossRef]

65. Abe, R.; Ohashi, H.; Iijima, I.; Ihara, M.; Takagi, H.; Hohsaka, T.; Ueda, H. "Quenchbodies": Quench-Based Antibody Probes That Show Antigen-Dependent Fluorescence. *J. Am. Chem. Soc.* **2011**, *133*, 17386–17394. [CrossRef]

Publisher's Note: MDPI stays neutral with regard to jurisdictional claims in published maps and institutional affiliations.

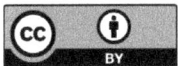

© 2020 by the authors. Licensee MDPI, Basel, Switzerland. This article is an open access article distributed under the terms and conditions of the Creative Commons Attribution (CC BY) license (http://creativecommons.org/licenses/by/4.0/).

MDPI
St. Alban-Anlage 66
4052 Basel
Switzerland
Tel. +41 61 683 77 34
Fax +41 61 302 89 18
www.mdpi.com

Cancers Editorial Office
E-mail: cancers@mdpi.com
www.mdpi.com/journal/cancers

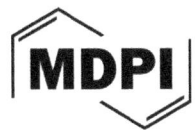

www.ingramcontent.com/pod-product-compliance
Lightning Source LLC
LaVergne TN
LVHW070141100526
838202LV00015B/1868